INTRAPERITONEAL CANCER THERAPY
PRINCIPLES AND PRACTICE

EDITED BY

WIM P. CEELEN
Ghent University, Ghent, Belgium

EDWARD A. LEVINE
Wake Forest University, Winston-Salem, North Carolina, USA

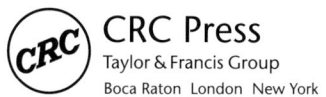

CRC Press
Taylor & Francis Group
Boca Raton London New York

CRC Press is an imprint of the
Taylor & Francis Group, an **informa** business

CRC Press
Taylor & Francis Group
6000 Broken Sound Parkway NW, Suite 300
Boca Raton, FL 33487-2742

© 2016 by Taylor & Francis Group, LLC
CRC Press is an imprint of Taylor & Francis Group, an Informa business

No claim to original U.S. Government works

Printed and bound in India by Replika Press Pvt. Ltd.

Printed on acid-free paper
Version Date: 20150917

International Standard Book Number-13: 978-1-4822-6118-9 (Pack - Book and Ebook)

Dedication

In honor of our brave patients and with thanks to our wives

Joan and Michèle

Contents

Preface

Despite the advances made in the surgical and medical treatment of metastatic cancer, the management of peritoneal carcinomatosis remains a substantial clinical and research challenge. Traditionally, patients with peritoneal metastases were approached with therapeutic nihilism and relegated to palliative therapy or hospice care. Over the past three decades, cytoreductive surgery combined with intraperitoneal drug delivery has been established as an additional therapeutic option in selected patients with peritoneal metastatic disease. In parallel with the increasing adoption of this clinical strategy, significant research efforts have been directed toward the elucidation of the pharmacology and physiology of intraperitoneal drug treatment.

This book is one of the first to combine the latest clinical developments in the treatment of patients with peritoneal surface disease and the scientific principles that underlie the concept of intraperitoneal cancer therapy. It covers basic concepts such as anatomy, physiology, pharmacology, mathematical models of drug transport, as well as practical clinical applications, highlighted with results from clinical trials and promising novel preclinical developments.

With this book, the editors aim to provide a useful and state-of-the-art reference for surgical and medical oncologists interested in the treatment of carcinomatosis. In addition, they hope it will further establish and promote basic and translational research interest in the field of intraperitoneal drug delivery, which has the potential to improve the outcome for this dreaded condition. Further, we hope to justify a better approach to our patients with peritoneal dissemination of malignant disease.

Wim P. Ceelen, MD
Edward A. Levine, MD

Contributors

H. Richard Alexander, Jr.
Division of Surgical Oncology
Department of Surgery
and
Marlene and Stewart Greenebaum Cancer Center
University of Maryland Medical Center
Baltimore, Maryland

Deborah Armstrong
The Sidney Kimmel Comprehensive Cancer Center
Johns Hopkins University
Baltimore, Maryland

Jessie L.-S. Au
Optimum Therapeutics, LLC
San Diego, California

and

College of Pharmacy
The Ohio State University
Columbus, Ohio

and

Medical University of South Carolina
Charleston, South Carolina

and

Taipei Medical University
Taipei, Taiwan, Republic of China

Itzhak Avital
U.S. Army Medical Corps
Uniformed Services University of the Health Sciences
Bethesda, Maryland

David L. Bartlett
Division of Surgical Oncology
University of Pittsburgh Cancer Institute
Pittsburgh, Pennsylvania

Joel M. Baumgartner
Department of Surgery
Division of Surgical Oncology
Moores Cancer Center
University of California, San Diego
San Diego, California

Marc Bracke
Laboratory for Experimental Cancer Research
Ghent University
Ghent, Belgium

Wim P. Ceelen
Academic Department of Surgery
Ghent University
and
Department of Gastrointestinal Surgery
Ghent University
Ghent, Belgium

Haroon A. Choudry
Division of Surgical Oncology
University of Pittsburgh Cancer Institute
Pittsburgh, Pennsylvania

Pieter Colin
Laboratory of Medical Biochemistry and Clinical
Analysis
Ghent University
and
Department of Surgery
Ghent University Hospital
Ghent, Belgium

and

Department of Anesthesiology
University Medical Center Groningen
Groningen, the Netherlands

George R. Dakwar
Laboratory for General Biochemistry and Physical
Pharmacy
Ghent University
Ghent, Belgium

Baratti Dario
Department of Surgery
National Cancer Institute
Milan, Italy

Erienne M.V. de Cuba
Department of Pathology
VU University Medical Center
Amsterdam, the Netherlands

Pieter Demetter
Department of Pathology
Erasme University Hospital
Brussels Free University
Brussels, Belgium

Stefaan S.C. De Smedt
Laboratory for General Biochemistry and Physical
Pharmacy
Ghent University
Ghent, Belgium

Elly De Vlieghere
Laboratory of Experimental Cancer Research
Ghent University
Ghent, Belgium

Olivier De Wever
Laboratory of Experimental Cancer Research
Ghent University
Ghent, Belgium

Katharina G.M.A. D'Herde
Department of Basic Medical Sciences
Ghent University
Ghent, Belgium

Sean P. Dineen
Department of Surgical Oncology
MD Anderson Cancer Center
University of Texas
Houston, Texas

Cathy Eng
Department of Gastrointestinal Medical
Oncology
MD Anderson Cancer Center
The University of Texas
Houston, Texas

Jesus Esquivel
Department of Surgical Oncology
Cancer Treatment Centers of America
Philadelphia, Pennsylvania

Michael F. Flessner
National Institute of Diabetes and Digestive and Kidney
Diseases
National Institutes of Health
Bethesda, Maryland

Keith F. Fournier
Department of Surgical Oncology
MD Anderson Cancer Center
University of Texas
Houston, Texas

Valerie Francescutti
Department of Surgical Oncology
Roswell Park Cancer Institute
Buffalo, New York

Lauren Gillory
Department of General Surgery
Wake Forest University
Winston-Salem, North Carolina

Félix Gremonprez
Department of Surgery
Ghent University Hospital
Ghent, Belgium

Markus M. Heiss
Department of Abdominal, Vascular and Transplant
Surgery
Cologne Merheim Medical Center
Witten/Herdecke University
Cologne, Germany

Sarah E. Herrick
Faculty of Medical and Human Sciences
Institute of Inflammation and Repair
and
Manchester Academic Health Science Centre
University of Manchester
Manchester, United Kingdom

John M. Kane III
Department of Surgical Oncology
Roswell Park Cancer Institute
Buffalo, New York

Kaitlyn J. Kelly
Department of Surgery
Division of Surgical Oncology
Moores Cancer Center
University of California, San Diego
San Diego, California

Manuel J. Koppe
Department of Surgery
Netherlands Cancer Institute
Amsterdam, the Netherlands

Riom Kwakman
Department of Surgery
VU University Medical Center
Amsterdam, the Netherlands

Lisa M. Landrum
Section of Gynecology Oncology
University of Oklahoma Health Sciences Center
Oklahoma City, Oklahoma

Edward A. Levine
Department of General Surgery
Wake Forest University
Winston-Salem, North Carolina

Bettina Lieske
Division of Colorectal Surgery
Department of Surgery
University Surgical Cluster
National University Hospital
Singapore, Singapore

Andrew M. Lowy
Department of Surgery
Division of Surgical Oncology
Moores Cancer Center
University of California, San Diego
San Diego, California

Ze Lu
Optimum Therapeutics, LLC
San Diego, California

Paul Mansfield
Department of Surgical Oncology
MD Anderson Cancer Center
Houston, Texas

Deraco Marcello
Department of Surgery
National Cancer Institute
Milan, Italy

Brendan Moran
Pseudomyxoma Peritonei Centre
North Hampshire Hospital
Hampshire, United Kingdom

Steven E. Mutsaers
Institute for Respiratory Health
and
Centre for Respiratory Health
and
Centre for Cell Therapy and Regenerative Medicine
School of Medicine and Pharmacology
University of Western Australia
Crawley, Australia

and

Harry Perkins Institute of Medical Research
Nedlands, Australia

Chukwuemeka Obiora
Department of General Surgery
Wake Forest University
Winston-Salem, North Carolina

Colette Pameijer
Division of Surgical Oncology
Department of Surgery
Penn State College of Medicine
Hershey, Pennsylvania

Katie Planche
Department of Radiology
Royal Free Hospital
London, United Kingdom

Cecilia M. Prêle
Institute for Respiratory Health
and
Centre for Respiratory Health
and
Centre for Cell Therapy and Regenerative Medicine
School of Medicine and Pharmacology
University of Western Australia
Crawley, Australia

and

Harry Perkins Institute of Medical Research
Nedlands, Australia

Mladjan Protić
Faculty of Medicine
Department of Surgery
University of Novi Sad
Novi Sad, Serbia

and

Clinic of Surgical Oncology
Oncology Institute of Vojvodina
Sremska Kamenica, Serbia

Katrien Remaut
Laboratory of General Biochemistry and Physical Pharmacy
Ghent University
Ghent, Belgium

Marc A. Reymond
Division of Surgical Oncology
Marien Hospital Herne
Ruhr-University Bochum
Bochum, Germany

Richard E. Royal
Department of Surgical Oncology
MD Anderson Cancer Center
Houston, Texas

Kusamura Shigeki
Department of Surgery
National Cancer Institute
Milan, Italy

Abdulrahman Sinno
Department of Gynecology and Obstetrics
Johns Hopkins University School of Medicine
Baltimore, Maryland

Joseph J. Skitzki
Department of Surgical Oncology
Roswell Park Cancer Institute
Buffalo, New York

Nina R. Sluiter
Department of Surgery
VU University Medical Center
Amsterdam, the Netherlands

W. Solass
Institute of Pathology
Medical School Hanover
Hanover, Germany

Joanna Stachowska-Pietka
Nalecz Institute of Biocybernetics and Biomedical
Engineering
Polish Academy of Sciences
Warsaw, Poland

John H. Stewart, IV
Department of General Surgery
Wake Forest University
Winston-Salem, North Carolina

Alexander Stojadinovic
Uniformed Services University of the Health Sciences
Bethesda, Maryland

Michael A. Ströhlein
Department of Abdominal, Vascular and Transplant Surgery
Cologne Merheim Medical Center
Witten/Herdecke University
Cologne, Germany

Paul H. Sugarbaker
Washington Cancer Institute
Center for Gastrointestinal Malignancies
MedStar Washington Hospital Center
Washington, DC

Bo Sun
Department of Industrial and Physical Pharmacy
Purdue University
West Lafayette, Indiana

Melissa Taggart
Department of Pathology
MD Anderson Cancer Center
Houston Texas

C. Tempfer
Department of Gynecology and Obstetrics
Marien Hospital Herne
Ruhr-University Bochum
Bochum, Germany

Elisabeth (Lisette) A. te Velde
Department of Surgery
VU University Medical Center
Amsterdam, the Netherlands

Kiran Turaga
Division of Surgical Oncology
Medical College of Wisconsin
Milwaukee, Wisconsin

Keli M. Turner
Department of Surgery
School of Medicine
University of Maryland
Baltimore, Maryland

Kurt Van der Speeten
Department of Surgical Oncology
Ziekenhuis Oost-Limburg
Genk, Belgium

and

Department of Life Sciences
BIOMED Research Institute
Oncology Research Cluster
Universiteit Hasselt
Hasselt, Belgium

Laurine Verset
Department of Pathology
Erasme University Hospital
Brussels Free University
Brussels, Belgium

Konstantinos I. Votanopoulos
Department of General Surgery
Wake Forest University
Winston-Salem, North Carolina

Joan L. Walker
Section of Gynecology Oncology
University of Oklahoma Health Sciences Center
Oklahoma City, Oklahoma

Jacek Waniewski
Nalecz Institute of Biocybernetics and Biomedical
Engineering
Polish Academy of Sciences
Warsaw, Poland

M. Guillaume Wientjes
Optimum Therapeutics, LLC
San Diego, California

Yoon Yeo
Department of Industrial and Physical Pharmacy
and
Weldon School of Biomedical Engineering
Purdue University
West Lafayette, Indiana

Jennifer L. Zadlo
MD Anderson Cancer Center
The University of Texas
Houston, Texas

PART 1

Peritoneum:
Embryology, anatomy, and physiology

Embryology and anatomy of the peritoneal cavity

JESUS ESQUIVEL

INTRODUCTION

The peritoneum is the largest and most complexly arranged serous membrane in the body. It is a closed sac in males, but in females it is not closed since the free extremities of the Fallopian tubes open directly into the peritoneal cavity and communicate with the extraperitoneal pelvis exteriorly through the uterus and vagina. An accurate examination and knowledge of its intricate anatomy is imperative to the understanding of the pathological processes that affect it.

The abdominal cavity is divided into the peritoneal and extraperitoneal compartments, separated by the posterior parietal peritoneum. It extends from the diaphragm to the pelvic floor. The visceral peritoneum covers the intraperitoneal and part of the pelvic organs. The parietal and visceral layers of the peritoneum are in contact; the potential space between them is called the peritoneal cavity and is a part of the embryologic abdominal cavity or primitive coelomic duct. Both types of peritoneum consist of a single layer of simple low-cuboidal epithelium called a mesothelium. A capillary film of serous fluid (approximately 50–100 mL) separates the parietal and visceral layers of peritoneum from one another and lubricates the peritoneal surfaces. The spreading of different diseases is dependent not only on the force of gravity and negative pressure but also on the numerous peritoneal recesses and folds [1]. A total of 11 large ligaments and mesenteries comprise the complex structures within the abdominal cavity, the peritoneal recesses and folds, or compartments. An appreciation of the embryologic development of the peritoneal cavity is crucial to understanding the anatomy and determining the cause and extent of peritoneal dissemination in gynecological and gastrointestinal cancers [2]. This chapter reviews the embryology and anatomy of the peritoneal cavity.

EMBRYOLOGY

Until the end of the second gestational week, the embryo disk, known as the blastodisc, consists of two germ layers, the endoderm and ectoderm, separated from each other by a basal membrane. Both germ layers participate in forming the third layer, the mesoderm, which develops between the two. During the course of the third week, the mesoderm starts separating endoderm from ectoderm. They stay in contact only in the areas of the buccopharyngeal and cloacal membranes.

The blastodisc folds along a sagittal plane (craniocaudal) and a horizontal (lateral) plane. The lateral and craniocaudal folding of the embryo leads to the development of an endodermal tube. Initially, this tube consists only of a crania and a caudal part. The pressure difference between the amniotic and chorionic cavities is the main catalyst for the lateral folding motion. The amniotic fluid increases in volume, which stimulates surface growth of the amnion and directs this growth into an anterior, lateral expansion toward the chorionic cavity (extraembryonic coelom).

The lateral folding movement occurs simultaneously with the formation of somites, also known as primitive segments. Paraxial mesoderm becomes organized and is segmented into somites, while the lateral plate mesoderm splits into somatopleuric and splanchnopleuric mesoderm.

Somatopleuric mesoderm later forms the parietal serous lining of the body cavities (parietal peritoneum), while splanchnopleuric mesoderm forms the serous membrane ensheathing visceral organs (visceral peritoneum) [3]. They do not participate in segmentation. Later, the mesoderm of the somites migrates to the somatopleuric layer, leading to a secondary segmentation, which then precipitates the innervation of the parietal peritoneum.

Initially, the digestive tube arising through all these processes is embedded in mesenchymal tissue and runs sagittally. The double-layered mesentery, which later develops from the mesenchyme, connects the visceral and parietal mesoderm layers. Lateral folding of the mesoderm leads to the formation of a cavity, the intraembryonic coelom. The intraembryonic coelom begins as one continuous cavity, that is, the peritoneal, pericardial, and pleural cavities are connected to each other via pleuroperitoneal canals. Once the diaphragm develops, it splits off the peritoneal cavity.

The primitive gut forms within the peritoneal cavity and is suspended by a plane composed of two peritoneal reflections called the primitive mesenteries, which cover the extension of the subperitoneal space from the abdominal walls. The position of the gut within the primitive mesentery plane divides the primitive mesentery into ventral and dorsal portions, which undergo specialization throughout fetal life and create a right and left cavity. Vascular and lymphatic vessels and nerves that supply the abdominal viscera are enfolded within the plane of the primitive mesentery. The liver grows ventral from the gut within the ventral plane. The ventral mesentery anterior to the liver attaches to the anterior abdominal wall, forming the falciform ligament, and the ventral mesentery between the liver and stomach forms the gastrohepatic and hepatoduodenal ligaments. The spleen and pancreas and a major portion of the gut grow within the dorsal plane. Once visceral descent is completed, the gut and other intraperitoneal organs grow further and change their positions in the abdominal cavity. The stomach moves toward the left, while the duodenum rotates to the right and then attaches to the posterior parietal peritoneum. The attachment of the descending duodenum to the posterior parietal peritoneum via Treitz's fascia is the most secure attachment in the peritoneum. The duodenum grows and moves to the left, where the duodenojejunal junction attaches via the suspensory muscle of the duodenum (muscle of Treitz) to the diaphragm. This constitutes the top pole of the midgut rotation. At the distal end of the sagittal tube (hindgut), the bottom pole arises from a fixation of a structure, which later develops into the descending colon. This structure attaches to the posterior parietal peritoneum while rotating and ascending laterally and to the left. The visceral peritoneum, the left mesentery, and the posterior parietal peritoneum fuse to form the left Toldt's line. The top and bottom poles become the fixed points for the subsequent rotational growth of the midgut. The sigmoid colon also grows between two fixed points, that is, the original medial mesenteric root and the secondarily attached Toldt's line of the descending colon. The rotations, descents, and resorption of the mesenteric plane take place throughout fetal life. Regardless of the complexity of adult mesenteries, they are derived from a single plane and remain interconnected [2].

ANATOMY OF THE PERITONEAL CAVITY

The peritoneum is the largest serous membrane in the body. The peritoneal cavity is a potential space between the parietal peritoneum, which lines the abdominal wall, and the visceral peritoneum, which envelopes the abdominal organs [4]. The free surface of the membrane is smooth, covered by a layer of flattened epithelium, and lubricated by a small quantity of serous fluid. Hence, the viscera can glide freely against the wall of the cavity or upon one another with the least possible amount of friction. The attached surface is rough, being connected to the viscera and inner surface of the abdominal wall by means of areolar tissue, termed the subserous areolar tissue. The parietal portion is loosely connected with the fascial lining of the abdomen and pelvis but is more closely adherent to the under surface of the diaphragm and also in the middle of the abdomen.

The space between the parietal and visceral peritoneums is named the peritoneal cavity. Under normal conditions, this cavity is a virtual one since the parietal and visceral layers are in contact. The peritoneal cavity is a complex structure consisting of ligaments, the greater and lesser omentum, as well as the mesenteries and several peritoneal folds. A mesentery is a double layer of peritoneum and attaches the vasculature and nerves to the intraperitoneal organs. A ligament is made up of two layers of visceral peritoneum and supports one organ or structure within the peritoneal cavity. It can contain lymph nodes, vasculature, and ducts and is usually named after the two structures or organs that it interconnects. The peritoneal cavity is subdivided by a constriction, termed the foramen of Winslow, into two sacs, a greater and a lesser. The greater sac is opened when the abdominal wall is incised; the lesser sac is situated behind the stomach and adjoining structures and may be regarded as a diverticulum from the greater sac [5].

An omentum is also a duplication of the visceral peritoneum and contains fatty tissue with lymph nodes and blood vessels. If the stomach is drawn downward, a fold of peritoneum will be seen stretching from its lesser curvature to the transverse fissure of the liver. This is the gastrohepatic, or small (lesser), omentum and consists of two layers; these, on being traced downward, split to envelop the stomach, covering, respectively, its anterosuperior and posteroinferior surfaces. At the greater curvature of the stomach, they again come into contact and are continued downward in front of the transverse colon, forming the anterior two layers of the greater or gastrocolic omentum. Reaching the free edge of this fold, they are reflected upward as its two posterior layers, and thus the greater omentum actually consists of four layers of peritoneum. Followed upward the two posterior layers separate to enclose the transverse colon, above which they once more come into contact and pass backward to the abdominal wall as the transverse mesocolon. Reaching the abdominal wall at the upper border of the transverse part of the duodenum, the two layers of the transverse mesocolon become separated from each other and take different directions. The upper or anterior layer, known as the ascending layer of the transverse mesocolon, ascends in front of the pancreas. The lower or posterior layer is carried downward, as the anterior layer of the mesentery, by the superior mesenteric vessels to the small intestine around which it may be followed and subsequently traced upward as the posterior layer of the mesentery to the abdominal wall. From the posterior abdominal wall, it sweeps downward over the aorta into the pelvis, where it invests the first portion of the rectum and attaches it to the front of the sacrum by a fold termed the mesorectum or pelvic mesocolon. Leaving first the sides and then the front of the rectum, it is reflected on to the back of the bladder and, after covering the posterior and upper aspects of the bladder, is carried by the urachus and obliterated hypogastric arteries on to the posterior surface of the anterior abdominal wall. Between the rectum and bladder, it forms a pouch, the rectovesical pouch, the bottom of which is about on a level with the middle of the seminal vesicles. In females the peritoneum is reflected from the rectum on to the upper part of the posterior vaginal wall, forming the rectovaginal pouch or pouch of Douglas, which is bounded on each side by a crescentic fold, the fold of Douglas. It is then carried over the posterior aspect and fundus of the uterus on to its anterior surface, which it covers as far as the junction of the body and cervix uteri, forming a second, but shallower depression, the uterovesical pouch. It is also reflected from the sides of the uterus to the lateral walls of the pelvis as two expanded folds, the broad ligaments of the uterus; in the free margin of each can be felt a thickened cord-like structure, the Fallopian tube [6].

On following the parietal peritoneum upward on the back of the anterior abdominal wall, it is seen to be reflected around a fibrous band, the ligamentum teres or obliterated umbilical vein, which reaches from the umbilicus to the undersurface of the liver. Here, the membrane forms a somewhat triangular fold, the falciform or suspensory ligament of the liver, which attaches the upper and anterior surfaces of the liver to the diaphragm and abdominal wall. With the exception of the line of attachment of this ligament, the peritoneum covers the under surface of the anterior part of the diaphragm and is reflected from it on to the upper surface of the right lobe of the liver as the superior layer of the coronary ligament and on to the upper surface of the left lobe as the superior layer of the left lateral ligament of the liver. Covering the upper and anterior surface of the liver, it is reflected round its sharp margins on to its under surface, where if present the following relations apply: (1) It covers the lower aspect of the quadrate lobe and the under and lateral aspects of the gallbladder and at the transverse fissure is continuous with the anterior layer of the lesser omentum. (2) It invests the under surface and posterior border of the left lobe and is reflected from its upper surface on to the diaphragm as the superior layer of the left

lateral ligament of the liver. (3) It covers the under aspect of the right lobe of the liver, from the back part of which it is reflected on to the upper extremity of the right kidney, forming, in this situation, the inferior layer of the coronary ligament; from the kidney it is carried to the duodenum and the hepatic flexure of the colon.

Between the two layers of the coronary ligament, there is a large triangular surface of the liver devoid of peritoneal covering; this is known as the bare area of the liver and it is attached to the diaphragm by areolar tissue. If the two layers of the coronary ligament be traced toward the right margin of the liver, they gradually approach each other and ultimately fuse to form a small triangular fold that connects the right lobe to the diaphragm, which is termed the right lateral ligament of the liver [6,7]. The apex of the triangular bare area corresponds with the point of meeting of the two layers of the coronary ligament, its base with the fossa for the inferior vena cava.

The posterior layer of the lesser omentum is reflected on to the caudate and Spigelian lobes of the liver and is continued from the upper extremity of the latter lobe to the diaphragm, forming the upper limit of the lesser sac of the peritoneum. Between the two layers of the lesser omentum, the hepatic artery and portal vein ascend to the liver, while the bile duct descends from the liver. When followed to the right, the lesser omentum is seen to form a distinct free border, and if a finger is introduced behind this free border, it passes into the lesser sac of the peritoneum through a constricted ring termed the foramen of Winslow. This foramen forms the communication between the greater and lesser sacs of the peritoneum and can be entered toward the left along the neck of the gallbladder. It is bounded, anteriorly, by the free border of the lesser omentum; posteriorly, by the parietal layer of peritoneum covering the inferior vena cava; superiorly, by the caudate lobe of the liver; and inferiorly, by the first part of the duodenum and by the peritoneum, which covers the hepatic artery as the latter passes forward beneath the foramen of Winslow, before ascending between the two layers of the lesser omentum.

The lesser sac of the peritoneum is merely a diverticulum of the greater sac. Anteriorly, the lesser sac is bounded, from above downward, by the Spigelian lobe of the liver, the lesser omentum, the stomach, and the anterior two layers of the greater omentum; posteriorly, it is limited from below upward by the two posterior layers of the greater omentum, the transverse colon, and the ascending layer of the transverse mesocolon, which covers the upper surface of the pancreas, the capsule of the left adrenal gland, and the upper pole of the left kidney. To the right of the esophageal opening of the diaphragm, it is formed by that portion of the diaphragm that supports the Spigelian lobe of the liver. Laterally, the lesser sac extends from the foramen of Winslow to the spleen, where it is limited by the posterior layer of the gastrosplenic ligament. The extent of the lesser sac and its relations to the surrounding structures can be easily identified by opening the lesser omentum and inserting the hand through the opening.

PERITONEAL SPACES

Knowledge of the peritoneal spaces and the routes of communication between them is extremely important in order to understand the patterns of dissemination of peritoneal metastases. The peritoneal cavity is divided into two main compartments by the transverse colon and its mesentery that connects the colon to the posterior abdominal wall: (1) the supramesocolic compartment (Table 1.1) and (2) the inframesocolic compartment (Table 1.2) [8].

Supramesocolic compartment

The supramesocolic compartment can be divided into right and left peritoneal spaces, which in turn are arbitrarily divided into several subspaces; these spaces are normally in communication but often become separated by adhesions [9]. The right supramesocolic space has three subspaces:

1. The right subphrenic space, which extends over the diaphragmatic surface of the right lobe of the liver to the right coronary ligament posteroinferiorly and the falciform ligament medially, which separates it from the left subphrenic space.

2. The right subhepatic space, which can be further divided into anterior and posterior compartments. The anterior compartment is limited inferiorly by the transverse colon and its mesentery. The posterior compartment, also known as the hepatorenal fossa or Morrison's pouch, extends posteriorly to the parietal peritoneum overlying the right kidney. Superiorly, the subhepatic space is bounded by the inferior surface of the right lobe of the liver. Both the right subphrenic and right subhepatic spaces communicate freely with the right paracolic gutter.

3. The lesser sac extends behind the stomach, anterior to the pancreas, communicating with the rest of the peritoneal cavity through a narrow inlet, the epiploic foramen or foramen of Winslow. A prominent oblique fold of peritoneum is raised on the posterior wall of the lesser sac by the left gastric artery, dividing it into two major recesses. The smaller superior recess completely encloses the caudate lobe of the liver. It extends superiorly deep into the fissure for the ligamentum venosum and lies adjacent to the right crus of the diaphragm. The larger recess lies between the stomach and the visceral surface of the spleen. It is bounded inferiorly by the transverse colon and its mesentery but can extend for a variable distance between the leaves of the greater omentum.

Table 1.1 Supramesocolic compartment

Ligament	Relation to organs	Landmarks
Gastrohepatic	Lesser curvature of the stomach to the liver	Left gastric vessels
Hepatoduodenal	From the duodenum to the hepatic hilum	Portal vein, proper hepatic artery, extrahepatic bile duct
Gastrocolic	Greater curvature of the stomach to transverse colon	Perigastric branches of left and right gastroepiploic vessels
Gastrosplenic	Continues to the left of gastrocolic ligament, from greater curvature of the stomach to splenic helium	Short gastric vessels and left gastroepiploic vessels
Splenorenal	Between spleen and pancreatic tail	Distal splenic artery or proximal splenic vein

Source: Adapted from *Oncologic Imaging: A Multidisciplinary Approach*, 1st edn., Le, O., Part VIII: Metastatic disease, peritoneal cavity and gastrointestinal tract, pp. 633–652, Copyright 2012, with permission from Elsevier.

Table 1.2 Inframesocolic compartment

Ligament	Relation to organs	Landmarks
Root of mesentery	Horizontal portion of the duodenum to the right iliac fossa	SMA, SMV, and ileocolic artery vein
Ileal mesentery	From the root of the mesentery to the ileum	Ileal artery and veins
Ascending mesocolon	From the root of the mesentery to the ascending colon	Right colic vessels, cecal vessels
Jejunal mesentery	From the root of the mesentery to the jejunum	Jejunal artery and vein
Descending mesocolon	Base of the transverse mesocolon along the tail of the pancreas to the descending colon	Left colic artery and vein
Sigmoid mesocolon	Root of the sigmoid colon	Sigmoid arteries, superior hemorrhoidal artery and vein

Source: Adapted from *Oncologic Imaging: A Multidisciplinary Approach*, 1st edn., Le, O., Part VIII: Metastatic disease, peritoneal cavity and gastrointestinal tract, pp. 633–652, Copyright 2012, with permission from Elsevier.

The left supramesocolic space has four arbitrary communicating spaces:

1. The left anterior perihepatic space bounded medially by the falciform ligament, posteriorly by the liver surface, and anteriorly by the diaphragm.
2. The left posterior perihepatic space, also called the gastrohepatic recess, follows the inferior surface of the lateral segment of the left hepatic lobe [10].
3. The left anterior subphrenic space lies between the anterior wall of the stomach and the left hemidiaphragm, communicating inferiorly with the left anterior perihepatic space.
4. The posterior subphrenic (perisplenic) space covers the superior and inferolateral surfaces of the spleen.

The phrenicocolic ligament, extending from the splenic flexure of the colon to the diaphragm, partially separates the perisplenic space from the rest of the peritoneal cavity. It forms a partial barrier to the spread of fluid and/or tumor deposits from the left paracolic gutter into the left subphrenic space, explaining why left subphrenic collections and tumor deposits are less common than those on the right subphrenic space.

Inframesocolic compartment

The inframesocolic compartment is divided into two unequal spaces by the root of the small bowel mesentery, as it runs from the duodenojejunal flexure in the left upper quadrant to the ileocecal valve in the right lower quadrant of the abdomen:

1. The smaller right infracolic space is bounded inferiorly by the small bowel mesentery, extending from the duodenojejunal flexure to the ileocecal valve.
2. The larger left infracolic space is in free communication with the pelvis, except where it is bounded by the sigmoid mesocolon.

The paracolic gutters are the peritoneal recesses on the posterior abdominal wall lateral to the ascending and descending colon. The right paracolic gutter is larger than its counterpart on the left and is continuous superiorly with the right subhepatic and subphrenic spaces. Both paracolic gutters are in continuity with the pelvic peritoneal space.

Inferiorly the peritoneum is reflected over the fundus of the bladder, the anterior and posterior surfaces of the uterus in females, and on the superior part of the rectum. The urinary bladder subdivides the pelvis into right and left paravesical spaces. In men, there is only one potential space for fluid and/or tumor collections posterior to the bladder, the rectovesical pouch. In women, there are two potential spaces posterior to the bladder, the uterovesical pouch, and posterior to the uterus, the rectouterine pouch, better known as the pouch of Douglas [9].

TELA SUBSEROSA (SUBSEROSA)

The liver is encased by a capsule made of connective tissue, the so-called Glisson capsule. It is a protuberance of the peritoneum outside the bare area in the region of the diaphragm. It runs to the liver as a septum. The part of the Glisson capsule that covers the intrahepatic portal vein apparatus is called the Glisson envelope. The Glisson capsule is directly connected to the subserosa by the gastrohepatic and hepatoduodenal ligaments.

The subserosa is one layer of connective tissue beneath the serosa, which is partially adherent and partially loosely connected to the serosa. The anatomic continuity of the subserosa enables the spread of diseases, not only between the intraperitoneal structures but also between intra- and extraperitoneal spaces. A clinical example would be Cullen's sign, which is the result of a subserosal spread of inflammation. This phenomenon also occurs during acute severe pancreatitis and is characterized by the spreading of exudates to the ventral abdominal wall by the inflamed hepatoduodenal ligament and along the falciform ligament. Free air, inflammation, tumors, or other proliferative diseases can also spread along the subserosa. Clinically significant as well is the so-called Sister Mary Joseph nodule in the umbilicus due to peritoneal spread from gastric or ovarian cancers.

CONCLUSION

The spread of malignant diseases within the peritoneal cavity is determined by numerous recesses and folds in addition to the force of gravity, the subdiaphragmatic pressure, and the phagocytic activity of the lesser and greater omentums. To understand the complex anatomical structures and a variety of folds and recesses of the peritoneum, an appreciation of the embryologic development of the peritoneal cavity is crucial.

This solid knowledge, combined with modern imaging modalities, facilitates the illustration of the anatomic reflections and compartments of the peritoneum, especially when intraperitoneal fluid is present. Consequently, the morphology, the localization, and the spreading pattern of peritoneal diseases are thus more easily and distinctly characterized, assisting clinicians with establishing a diagnosis and formulating a therapeutic plan for their patients.

REFERENCES

1. Meyers MA. Intraperitoneal spread of infections. In: Meyers MA, ed., *Dynamic Radiology of the Abdomen: Normal and Pathologic Anatomy*, 4th edn., Berlin, Germany: Springer, 1994. pp. 55–113.
2. Helsmoortel J, Hirth T, Wuhrl P. Peritoneal and intraperitoneal viscera. In: *Visceral Osteopathy: The Peritoneal Organs*, Seattle, WA: Eastland Press, 2010. pp. 11–15.

3. Moore K. *Developing Human: Clinically Oriented Embryology,* Philadelphia, PA: Saunders, 1982. pp. 227–229.
4. Temel T, Sandrasegaran K, Patel A, Hollar M, Tejada J, Tann M, Akisik F, Lappas J. Peritoneal and retroperitoneal anatomy and its relevance for cross-sectional imaging. *RadioGraphics.* 2012;32:437–451.
5. Ba-Ssalamah A, Fakhrai N, Baroud S, Shirkhoda A. Mesentery, omentum, peritoneum: Embryology, normal anatomy and anatomic variants. *Abdominal Imaging.* 2013;101:1563–1575.
6. Henry Gray F.R.S. *The Complete Gray's Anatomy,* 16th edn., East Moseley, U.K.: Merchant Book Company, 2003. pp. 1058–1061.
7. Mirilas P, Skandalakis JE. Benign anatomical mistakes: Right and left coronary ligaments. *The American Surgeon.* 2002;68:832–835.
8. Le O, Part VIII: Metastatic disease, peritoneal cavity and gastrointestinal tract. In: Paul, Silverman MD, ed. *Oncologic Imaging: A Multidisciplinary Approach,* 1st edn., Philadelphia, PA: Elsevier, 2012. pp. 633–652.
9. Healy JC, Reznek RH. The peritoneum, mesenteries and omenta: Normal anatomy and pathological processes. *European Radiology.* 1998;8:886–900.
10. Kim S, Kim TU, Lee JW. The perihepatic space: Comprehensive anatomy and CT features of pathologic conditions. *RadioGraphics.* 2007;27(1):129–143.

2

Structure and function of the mesothelial cell

STEVEN E. MUTSAERS, CECILIA M. PRÊLE, AND SARAH E. HERRICK

INTRODUCTION

Mesothelial cells form a monolayer of cobblestone-like cells that line the peritoneal, pleural, and pericardial cavities and most internal organs. They are embryologically derived from the mesoderm but express many epithelial cell characteristics including junctional complexes, apical/basal polarity, cytokeratins, and surface microvilli. Under normal conditions, mesothelial cells form a monolayer, termed the mesothelium, and play important roles in maintaining normal serosal membrane integrity and function. These cells are essential in embryological development as they can undergo mesothelial to mesenchymal transition (MMT) and differentiate into cells of different mesenchymal phenotypes. Mesothelial cells control fibrin deposition and breakdown and secrete mediators that initiate serosal inflammation and tissue repair, as well as regulate the immune response by presenting antigen to T cells. The mesothelium provides a nonadhesive protective surface to allow the movement of organs within the serosal cavities and provides a semipermeable membrane regulating transport of fluid and cells across the serosa. This layer also provides a barrier to the dissemination of peritoneal metastases, but equally, tumor cells may cause mesothelial cells to transition into cells that support tumor growth and dissemination. This chapter will describe the morphology and structure of the mesothelium and discuss some of the many roles mesothelial cells play under normal and pathological conditions.

MORPHOLOGY

Mesothelial cells form a sheet of epithelial-like cells that cover the coelomic cavities (peritoneal, pleural, and pericardial) to form the mesothelium. The mesothelium was first described in 1827 by Bichart but it was not until 1890 that Minot coined the term mesothelium, following a detailed study of its embryological origin showing that this layer was the "epithelial lining of mammalian mesodermic cavities" [1].

Mesothelial cells are generally morphologically similar, regardless of their anatomical site and species (Figure 2.1a). In general, they exhibit an elongated, flattened, and squamous morphology, approximately 25 μm in diameter, with a central oval nucleus and characteristic apical microvilli and occasional cilia [2]. The microvilli vary in length and density between adjacent cells and different organs that may reflect functional adaptation [2,3]. The role of the microvilli is to increase the surface area of the cells to enhance absorption and secretion and prevent frictional injury to the mesothelial cells. They are also likely to be involved in a variety of other cellular functions such as regulation of energy metabolism, gating of ion flux, generation and modulation of membrane potential, Ca^{2+} signaling, and mechanoreception [4].

In some regions, mesothelial cells display a cuboidal phenotype such as the septal folds of the mediastinal pleura, parenchymal organs (liver, spleen), the "milky spots" of the omentum, and the peritoneal side of the diaphragm overlying the lymphatic lacunae (Figure 2.1b) [2]. Mesothelial cells can also become cuboidal when activated following injury or stimulation by exposure to pathogenic antigens or materials such as asbestos. These cells have a larger nucleus with prominent nucleoli and an abundance of intracellular organelles including mitochondria, rough endoplasmic reticulum, Golgi bodies, and vesicles [5].

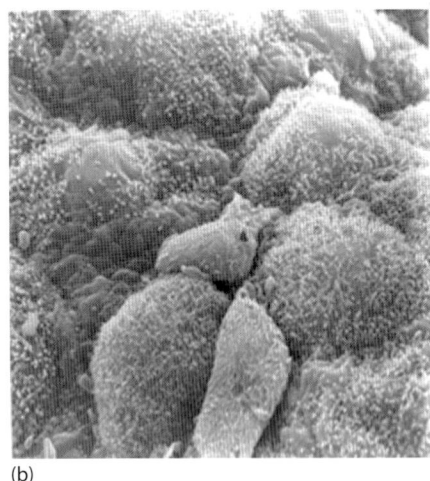

(a)   (b)

Figure 2.1 Scanning electron micrographs showing different mesothelial cell phenotypes. **(a)** Squamous-like visceral mesothelium with a carpet of microvilli on the surface of the cells. Cell borders are not easily discernible. Bar 7.5 μm. **(b)** Cuboidal omental mesothelial cells with clearly discernible cell borders. Bar 15 μm.

Mesothelial cells are embryologically derived from the mesoderm and display classic mesenchymal features including cytoskeletal proteins vimentin and desmin and, upon stimulation, alpha smooth muscle actin (α-SMA). However, they also express many other epithelial characteristics including junctional complexes; tight junctions, adherens junctions, gap junctions, and desmosomes; E-, N-, and P-cadherins; apical/basal polarity; cytokeratins (6, 8, 18, and 19), a developed system of vesicles and vacuoles, and the ability to secrete a basement membrane [5].

Mesothelial cells rest on a thin basement membrane supported by connective tissue stroma containing blood vessels, lymphatics, resident macrophages, lymphocytes, and fibroblast-like cells [6]. Mesothelial cells also line stomata, openings at the junction of two or more mesothelial cells, which provides direct access to the underlying submesothelial lymphatics, permitting clearance of fluid, cells, and other particles from the coelomic cavities [7]. Furthermore, mesothelium is bathed in a small volume of fluid that increases with disease severity. In the pleural space, this fluid has been reported to be 0.26 ± 0.1 mL/kg in humans and contains approximately 1.7×10^3 cells/mL, comprising approximately 75% macrophages, 23% lymphocytes, less than 3% polymorphonuclear cells, and 1%–2% free-floating mesothelial cells [8]. Although the volume is likely to be higher in the peritoneum, cell proportions are thought to be similar although this needs to be confirmed. It has also been suggested that a proportion of free-floating cells are stem-like cells although this needs further investigation [9].

EPITHELIAL TO MESENCHYMAL TRANSITION AND MESOTHELIAL TO MESENCHYMAL TRANSITION

Epithelial to mesenchymal transition (EMT) is a basic biological process that is involved in embryogenesis, tissue repair, and numerous pathologies, including organ fibrosis,

malignant transformation, and cancer progression. The processes that occur during pathological EMT are thought to be comparable to physiological EMT as they are controlled by similar signaling pathway regulators and effector molecules. When exposed to certain growth factors and/or injurious agents, epithelial cells undergo a complex morphological transition and acquire a mesenchymal phenotype. This complex process is primarily controlled by three main families of transcription factors: snail family zinc finger (SNAI1, SNAI2), basic helix-loop-helix (TWIST1), and zinc finger E-box-binding homeobox (ZEB1, ZEB2) [10]. Epithelial cells initially lose cell–cell junctions, attachment to basement membrane, and apical–basal cell polarity. Of importance, loss of cell surface junctional protein E-cadherin is a prerequisite for EMT. With subsequent migration and invasion through the basement membrane and a change in cytoskeletal components, a full change to a mesenchymal phenotype occurs. Expression of a multitude of mesenchymal markers, including α-SMA, EDA-fibronectin, vimentin, and fibroblast-specific protein-1, is proposed to be an indicator that EMT has occurred [11]. The profibrotic mediator, transforming growth factor-β1 (TGF-β_1), represents a major inducer of EMT, whereas bone morphogenic protein 7 has been identified as a repressor in certain tissues [12]. MicroRNAs (miRs) have recently emerged as important regulators of EMT as they are able to target multiple signaling pathways [13].

Mesothelial cells are unique in that they function as an epithelium but express both epithelial and mesenchymal markers and have an inherent ability to undergo EMT, a process that has recently been termed MMT [14]. Mesothelium-specific genetic lineage tracing systems used in mice have clearly demonstrated that during development mesothelial cells contribute to smooth muscle in the nascent vasculature of the gut, heart, liver, and lungs through MMT [15–19]. Wilms tumor 1 (WT1), a zinc finger transcription factor, expressed by mesothelium, has been found to regulate its functional properties during development. For example, during lung development, WT1-expressing mesothelial cells migrate into lung parenchyma and undergo a transition to form subpopulations of bronchial smooth muscle cells, vascular smooth muscle cells, and fibroblasts [17,20]. This transition requires the direct action of sonic hedgehog signaling [20]. Recent interest has focused on whether this phenomenon can occur in the adult with evidence to support such an event coming from a number of different groups [21–23]. In particular, Lachaud et al. [24] isolated murine uterine-derived mesothelial cells and stimulated them to undergo MMT and become functional vascular smooth muscle-like cells expressing smoothelin-B, typical of contractile cells. In addition, we have demonstrated that human and rat adult mesothelial cells undergo MMT and can be induced to differentiate into osteoblasts and adipocytes in culture [25].

In patients, MMT is proposed to be the predominant mechanism underlying the development of peritoneal sclerosis following long-term peritoneal dialysis [26]. The hyperosmotic, hyperglycemic, and acidic nature of dialysis fluid causes chronic injury and inflammation of the peritoneum, resulting in denuding of mesothelial cells and fibrosis. Such events may be accelerated by recurrent or severe cases of peritonitis. Yanez-Mo et al. [27] initially demonstrated that the extent of MMT in mesothelial cells, isolated from dialysis effluent of patients undergoing peritoneal dialysis, corresponded to the length of time on dialysis. Furthermore, biopsies from these patients showed evidence of mesothelial markers in fibroblast-like cells in the subepithelial layer, suggesting a transition of surface cells.

Numerous groups have shown upregulation of mesenchymal markers and downregulation of junctional protein components by human mesothelial cells, following exposure to various injurious agents *in vitro*. TGF-β_1 in particular is a recognized potent inducer of MMT. In human mesothelial cell cultures isolated from the pleura, omentum, or mesenteric tissue, TGF-β_1 induced MMT with downregulation of junctional components (E-cadherin, ZO-1) and upregulation of mesenchymal markers (α-SMA) and deposition of extracellular matrix (ECM) [22,28,29]. Furthermore, a number of studies have shown an upregulation of transcription factors in mesothelial cells associated with MMT (SNAI1/SNAI2, ZEB1/ZEB2, TWIST1) following exposure to TGF-β_1 as well as other cytokines including hepatocyte growth factor (HGF), platelet-derived growth factor (PDGF)-BB, and interleukin (IL)-1β [30–33].

MMT is proposed to play a role in the establishment of endometriosis where retrograde menstrual tissue embeds on the peritoneal surface and forms an active lesion. The early pathogenesis of endometriosis remains to be elucidated with regard to the initial interaction between menstrual tissue and mesothelial cells; however, Demir et al. showed in a series of studies that menstrual effluent induced MMT *in vitro* [34,35]. Furthermore, they suggested that soluble factors including tumor necrosis factor (TNF)-α, α-enolase, and hemoglobin present in menstrual effluent were major inducers of this process [34,35].

Lipopolysaccharide (LPS), a derivative of bacterial cell wall, has also been found to induce MMT and is proposed to be a possible mechanism whereby peritonitis is linked to peritoneal fibrosis [36]. *In vivo*, a number of studies have reported the importance of mesothelial cells in the development of fibrosis following injury. We have shown, using a rat peritoneal scrape injury model, that DiI-labeled rat mesothelial cells injected into the peritoneal cavity are incorporated into the mesothelial layer, eventually appearing in the subserosa [37]. Furthermore, adenovirus-mediated overexpression of TGF-β_1 in the lung and peritoneum induced fibrosis in mice that was associated with MMT and reduced epithelial cell (E-cadherin) and increased myofibroblast (collagen type 1, α-SMA, matrix metalloproteinase [MMP]-2 and MMP-9) marker expression [38,39]. Li et al. [14], using conditional cell lineage murine studies, also demonstrated that hepatic stellate cells and myofibroblasts are derived from mesothelial cells expressing WT1 that had undergone MMT during liver fibrogenesis. In a study using similar techniques, WT1-positive pleural mesothelial cells migrated into the lung parenchyma leading to idiopathic lung fibrosis following TGF-β_1 treatment in mice [40].

In terms of a role in cancer progression, primary effusion lymphoma cells induced human MMT with the upregulation of EMT-associated transcriptional repressors (SNAI1, Slug, ZEB1, Sip1), whereas mesothelial cells were shown to modulate lymphoma cell turnover by increasing resistance to apoptosis and proliferation [41]. Moreover, the protective role of mesothelial cells on lymphoma cells was retained even after transition to a mesenchymal phenotype but could be inhibited by interferon (IFN)-α2b treatment.

ROLE OF MESOTHELIAL CELLS

Mesothelial cells are metabolically active cells that play important roles in maintaining serosal homeostasis. This review will focus on the role of the mesothelial cell in inflammation and immune regulation and tumor cell dissemination. Other roles for the mesothelium are discussed in reviews by Mutsaers and colleagues [2,42].

Inflammation and immune regulation

Mesothelial cells act as a barrier to invading organisms, injurious agents, and tumor cells and are one of the first cell types to initiate defense mechanisms. They have a well-developed surface glycocalyx and are in contact with serosal fluid containing immunoglobulins, complement, lysozyme, and other proteins that aid in killing microorganisms and prevent them from adhering to the mesothelial surface [43]. Mesothelial cells have multiple pattern recognition receptors that recognize carbohydrates and LPSs on the surface of microbial pathogens and, in response, release inflammatory mediators to initiate inflammation and activate immunomodulatory pathways.

Toll-like receptors (TLRs), nucleotide-binding oligomerization domain–like receptors, RIG-I-like receptors, and

C-type lectin-like receptors bind to microorganisms such as bacteria, fungi, and viruses [44,45]. Mesothelial cells constitutively express *TLR1–6* mRNA. TLR2 recognizes numerous microbial molecules such as Gram-positive bacteria and is upregulated in response to proinflammatory cytokines including IFN-γ, TNF-α, and IL-1β [46–48]. TLR4 responds to Gram-negative bacteria through recognition of LPS [49] and is upregulated by Angiotensin II [50]. Human mesothelial cells also express TLR3 and other viral receptors RIG-1 and MDA5, which recognize viral double-stranded RNA and are also upregulated following stimulation with IFN-γ, TNF-α, and IL-1β [51]. TLR3 induces upregulation of MMP-9 and tissue inhibitor of MMP (TIMP)-1 [52] as well as IFN-inducible protein 10 (IP-10) in mesothelial cells. IP-10 is also upregulated by IFN-α, IFN-β, and IFN-γ [53]. Upregulation of early response genes by bacterial infection of mesothelial cells may contribute to mesothelial cell apoptosis.

Protease-activated receptor (PAR)-2 is also a transmembrane receptor expressed on mesothelial cells that can induce inflammation [54,55]. PAR-2 is activated by tryptase, trypsin, and coagulation factor Xa. Activation of PAR-2 stimulates the release of cytokines and chemokines including TNF-α, IL-8, macrophage inflammatory protein-2 [55], growth-related oncogene-α (GRO-α), monocyte chemoattractant protein-1, RANTES [56,57], eotaxin [58], IP-10, and stromal cell-derived factor-1 (SDF-1) [59] and induces neutrophil recruitment [55]. SDF-1 stimulates the growth of B lymphocyte precursors (B1a) and this is potentiated by the action of IL-10 that is produced by B1a lymphocytes [54]. These two mediators secreted by mesothelial cells therefore may account for the selective accumulation of B1 lymphocytes in body cavities.

LEUKOCYTE MIGRATION

An effective inflammatory response requires rapid recruitment of leukocytes from the bloodstream to the site of injury through the generation of a chemotactic gradient across the mesothelium. Chemokines secreted by mesothelial cells can interact with their high-affinity seven transmembrane G protein–coupled receptors to induce intracellular signaling, as well as bind glycosaminoglycans located on the cell surface and in basement membranes [60], which prevents chemokines from undergoing proteolysis and induces oligomerization to establish a more activated form of the chemokines [61].

Migration of leukocytes to the site of serosal injury also requires interaction with integrins and adhesion molecules on the surface of mesothelial cells, including vascular and intercellular adhesion molecules (VCAM-1 and ICAM-1), cadherins, and several types of selectins and α- and β-integrins [56,62,63]. Leukocytes express β$_2$-integrins, lymphocyte function-associated antigen-1 (LFA-1) (CD11a/CD18), and Mac-1 (CD11b/CD18), which are counter receptors for ICAM-1. Interaction between LFA-1/Mac-1 and ICAM-1 leads to the transmigration of leukocytes across the mesothelial cell monolayer. Prestimulation

of pleural mesothelial cells with antibodies directed against ICAM-1 or VCAM-1 significantly inhibits adhesion, activation, and effector regulatory T-cell expansion induced by pleural mesothelial cells [64]. ICAM-1 and VCAM-1 are only expressed on the microvilli of mesothelial cells [65], suggesting that leukocytes may crawl along the microvilli.

The expression of different adhesion molecules on mesothelial cells is also likely to regulate specific cell movement. For example, α6β1- and α4β1-integrins selectively mediate adhesion and migration of Th1 and Th2 T-cell subsets across human mesothelial cell monolayers [66], respectively. We have also shown that clearance of macrophages from the peritoneum is controlled through integrin-mediated regulation of macrophage–mesothelial cell interactions involving very late antigen (VLA)-4 and VLA-5 [67]. This suggests that differential integrin expression and selective cell recruitment may have significant effects on immune regulation and resolution of inflammation.

Mesothelial cells express class II major histocompatibility complex molecules and therefore can also modulate the immune response through antigen presentation. Mesothelial cells have been shown to present *Candida albicans* bodies and tetanus toxoid to peripheral blood mononuclear cells and T cells [68]. IFN-γ also stimulates mesothelial cells to induce CD4+ T-cell proliferation in the presence of antigen and secrete the T-cell growth factor and activator IL-15 [69] following CD40 activation [70]. CD40 ligation with IFN-γ also induces RANTES production by mesothelial cells, which increases mononuclear cell infiltration during peritonitis [71,72]. It has also been shown in tuberculous pleurisy that antigen presentation by mesothelial cells stimulates CD4+ T-cell proliferation and both Th22- and Th9-cell differentiation [73,74].

Mesothelial cells also secrete a wide range of cytokines, growth factors, and ECM molecules that participate in the inflammatory and tissue repair process and are likely to play significant roles in immune regulation. For example, mesothelial cells produce IL-6, heat shock proteins 72/73, granulocyte colony-stimulating factor, granulocyte-macrophage colony-stimulating factor, and IL-1, which are upregulated in response to mediators such as LPS, IL-1β, TNF-α, and epidermal growth factor (EGF) [56,75,76]. IL-6 is often induced together with proinflammatory cytokines IL-1 and TNF-α, and circulating IL-6 plays an important role in the induction of acute-phase reactions [77]. In addition, mesothelial cells produce reactive nitrogen and oxygen species in response to cytokines, bacterial products, and asbestos [78] as well as antioxidants [79,80]. They can also regulate the inflammatory response by releasing anti-inflammatory prostaglandins and prostacyclin both constitutively and following induction by inflammatory mediators [81].

Mesothelial cells release growth factors that initiate autocrine- and paracrine-induced cell proliferation, differentiation, and migration of mesothelial and other resident cells. TGF-β, PDGF, fibroblast growth factor, HGF, keratinocyte growth factor, and members of the EGF family (EGF, heparin-binding EGF, and vascular EGF [VEGF]) are some of the factors likely to regulate these processes [42,82]. Mesothelial cells also synthesize ECM molecules that are important for cell function and tissue repair including collagen types I, III, and IV, elastin, fibronectin, and laminin [83,84]. They can be further stimulated when exposed to peritoneal effluents from patients with acute peritonitis [85] or various cytokines and growth factors such as IL-1β, TNF-α, EGF, PDGF, and TGF-β [84]. Overexpression of TGF-β_1 in serosal tissues leads to fibrosis and adhesion formation [39,86]. Mesothelial cells are likely to regulate ECM turnover by secreting proteases and antiproteases such as MMPs and TIMPs, respectively, and factors such as decorin and biglycan, which inhibit TGF-β activity [87,88].

Tumor dissemination

Intraperitoneal dissemination is the primary metastatic route of ovarian cancers and a common progression for gastrointestinal malignancies [89]. Tumor cells spread through the peritoneal cavity by two main approaches. The first is by transversal growth, where tumor cells exfoliate from the primary tumor into the peritoneal cavity preoperatively [90]. The second is intraperitoneal spread, where surgical trauma can cause the release of tumor cells from the primary tumor or through resection of blood and lymph vessels. Once detached, the cells spread rapidly through the peritoneum, transported by serosal fluid. Detachment is the first of four basic steps for dissemination of peritoneal tumors: (1) detachment of cancer cells from the primary tumor, (2) attachment to distant peritoneum, (3) invasion into subperitoneal space, and (4) proliferation and vascular neogenesis [91]. The mesothelial cell is likely to play significant roles in trying to prevent tumor cell attachment, invasion, and growth, but inflammatory cytokines released by tumor and immune cells compromise the protective, antiadhesive mesothelial cell monolayer and expose the underlying ECM, through which the cancer cells can attach. Here, we will discuss some of the possible mechanisms both in the prevention and induction of tumor dissemination (Figure 2.2).

CELL ADHESION

A number of sites within the peritoneal cavity show increased tumor cell implantation. One common site is the greater omentum, in particular within areas of milky spots, as they do not have a continuous mesothelial layer [92]. This is particularly important as cancer cells preferentially attach to exposed ECM. Interestingly, it has also been proposed that milky spot macrophages can be stimulated by gastric cancer cells to induce mesothelial cell apoptosis that would further promote tumor cell attachment [93]. Similarly, after surgery, traumatized mesothelial surfaces are privileged sites for tumor cell adhesion due to the exposure of the submesothelial connective tissue [94]. Furthermore, inflammatory cytokines including TNF-α and IL-1β, released following surgery or secreted by tumor cells, cause the protective mesothelial cells to retract,

exposing underlying ECM [95,96]. Clearly, mesothelial cells play a protective role against tumor cell adhesion by maintaining an intact barrier. When tumor spheroids of a human ovarian cancer cell line were inoculated onto submesothelial matrix, there was rapid attachment of the spheroids followed by rapid dissemination and growth of tumor cells. However, when cells were seeded onto an intact mesothelium, the attachment time increased and led to an almost complete inhibition of tumor cell dissemination [97]. Interestingly, this inhibition appears to be lost *in vivo* as biopsies taken from tumors attached to peritoneal organs showed that mesothelial cells were not present under tumor masses. Iwanicki et al. showed that ovarian cancer spheroids utilize integrin- and talin-dependent activation of myosin and traction force to promote mesothelial cell displacement from underneath a tumor cell spheroid [98]. Davidowitz et al. [99] subsequently showed that ovarian tumor cells that were able to promote mesothelial cell clearance overexpressed the EMT-transcription factors SNAI1, TWIST1, and ZEB1, and knockdown of these genes attenuated clearance.

Although normally protective, mesothelial cells can also be directly involved in carcinomatosis through direct mesothelial-tumor cell adhesion, implantation, invasion, and subsequent growth. Tumor cells can attach to mesothelium due to upregulation of adhesion molecules on mesothelial cells in response to inflammatory mediators released following surgery or by the tumors themselves [100]. Cancer cells bind to mesothelial cell surface receptors ICAM-1 and/or VCAM-1, which are upregulated on the cell surface by inflammatory mediators including IL-1β, TNF-α, IL-6, and IFN-γ [101–106]. It has also been suggested that mesothelial adhesive properties are dependent on cell senescence [107]. Increased oxidative stress leads to an increase in ICAM-1 and fibronectin expression in senescent mesothelial cells, and incubation of these cells in the presence of a strong antioxidant significantly reduced the senescence-associated increase in cancer cell binding [102,108]. ICAM-1 binds to tumors expressing CD43 and this binding can be blocked *in vitro* using antibodies against ICAM-1 or CD43 [106,109]. Heparin treatment can also downregulate ICAM-1 expression on mesothelial cells *in vitro* [106,109] and prevent tumor growth in rats [101]. In addition, blocking VCAM-1 expression on mesothelial cells significantly decreased transmigration of ovarian cancer cells through mesothelial monolayers *in vitro* and decreased tumor burden and increased survival in a mouse model of ovarian cancer metastases [103], suggesting that blocking ICAM-1 and VCAM-1 expression may have therapeutic antimetastatic potential. Other adhesion molecules are also important in inducing tumor cell adhesion and migration on peritoneal surfaces. MUC16/CA-125, which is a transmembrane mucin present on ovarian tumor cells, can bind to mesothelin expressed on mesothelial cells and promote attachment [110]. Membrane type 1 (MT1)-MMP, also called MMP-14, a transmembrane collagenase highly expressed in ovarian cancer cells, induces MUC16/CA-125 ectodomain shedding, reducing adhesion

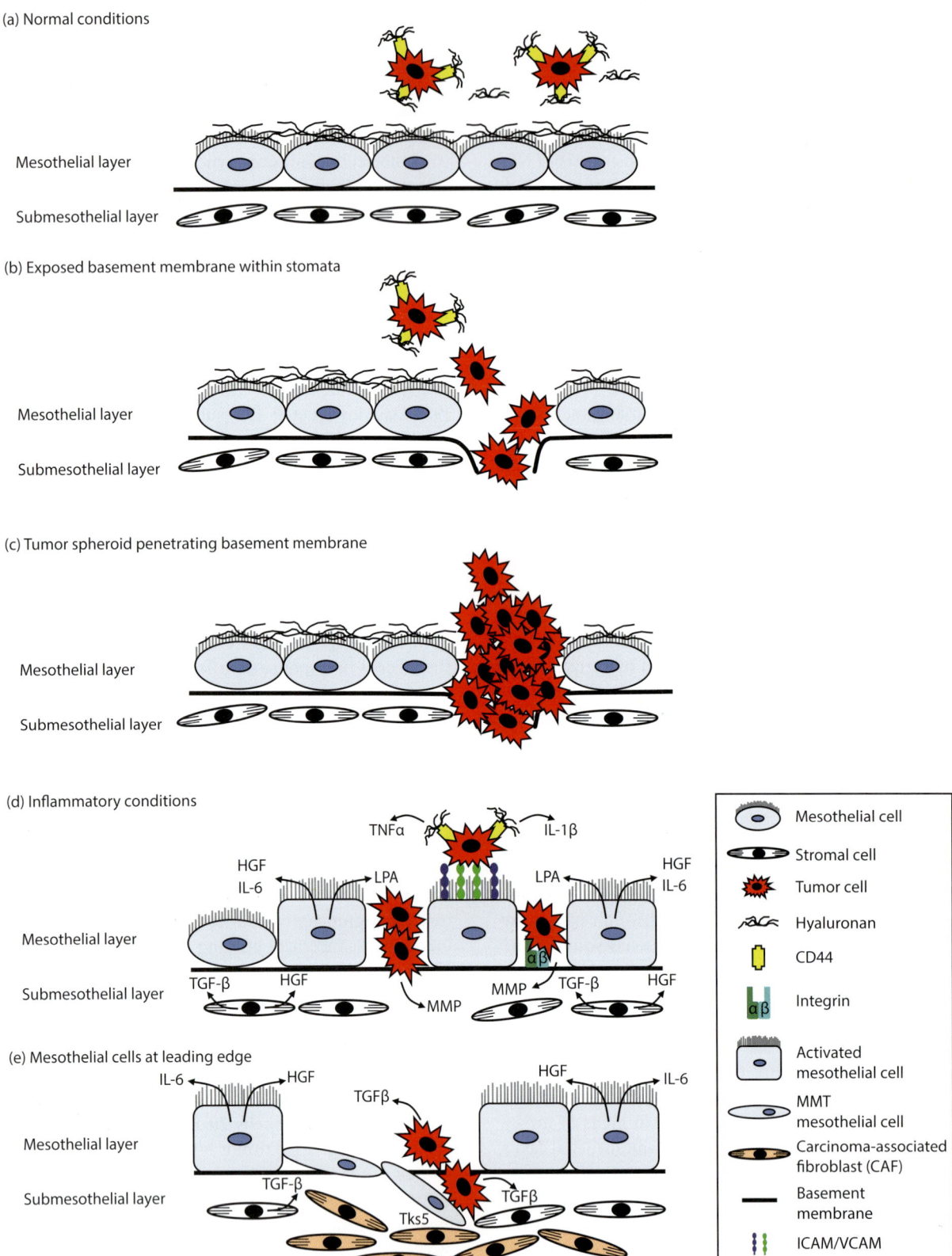

(a) Normal conditions

Mesothelial layer

Submesothelial layer

(b) Exposed basement membrane within stomata

Mesothelial layer

Submesothelial layer

(c) Tumor spheroid penetrating basement membrane

Mesothelial layer

Submesothelial layer

(d) Inflammatory conditions

TNFα   IL-1β
HGF   LPA   LPA   HGF
IL-6   IL-6
Mesothelial layer
TGF-β   HGF   MMP   TGF-β   HGF
Submesothelial layer   MMP
αβ

(e) Mesothelial cells at leading edge

IL-6   HGF   HGF   IL-6
TGFβ
Mesothelial layer
TGF-β   TGFβ
Submesothelial layer   Tks5

Legend:
- Mesothelial cell
- Stromal cell
- Tumor cell
- Hyaluronan
- CD44
- αβ Integrin
- Activated mesothelial cell
- MMT mesothelial cell
- Carcinoma-associated fibroblast (CAF)
- Basement membrane
- ICAM/VCAM

Figure 2.2 Mechanisms leading to peritoneal dissemination of tumors. **(a)** Under normal conditions, free hyaluronan in the serosal fluid binds to CD44 on tumor cells reducing tumor binding to hyaluronan on the surface of mesothelial cells. **(b)** Tumor cells selectively attach to stomata and milky spots. **(c)** Cancer spheroids promote mesothelial cell displacement. **(d)** During inflammation, mediators produced by activated mesothelial cells, submesothelial fibroblasts, and tumor cells induce rounding up of mesothelial cells and exposure of the ECM. **(e)** Tumor cells secrete MMT-promoting factors that induce mesenchymal conversion of mesothelial cells into CAFs that promote tumor cell invasion and growth.

to cultured mesothelial cells and peritoneal explants, but may then expose integrins for high-affinity cell binding to peritoneal tissues [111]. P-cadherin facilitates the assembly of floating epithelial ovarian cancer cells into spheroids and promotes attachment to mesothelial cells *in vitro*. In mice, inhibition of P-cadherin decreased the aggregation and survival of floating tumor cells in ascites and reduced the number of tumor implants on peritoneal surfaces [112]. Loss of E-cadherin in epithelial tumor cells also triggers peritoneal dissemination. TWIST regulates EMT and is one of the E-cadherin repressors. Suppression of TWIST in epithelial ovarian carcinoma cells promotes a more epithelial phenotype and inhibits the adhesion of these cells to mesothelial monolayers [113].

The hyaluronan receptor CD44, which is expressed by many cancer cell types including ovarian and colorectal cancer, enables these cells to bind to the hyaluronan-rich apical surface of mesothelial cells [114–116]. A wide variety of malignancies of epithelial and mesenchymal origin express high levels of CD44 [117], although the degree of adhesion does not necessarily relate to the amount of CD44 expressed [118,119]. This may be due to differences in CD44 glycosylation [119] or variant forms of CD44 [117]. Blocking interaction between CD44 and hyaluronan using various approaches reduced tumor cell adhesion and inhibited cell migration [114–116,119–121].

Although mesothelial cells either directly or indirectly appear to promote tumor dissemination and growth, intact hyaluronan can also inhibit the adhesion of tumor cells to mesothelium [115]. Ovarian carcinoma cell lines with high levels of surface hyaluronan were less adherent to mesothelial cells than ovarian carcinoma lines with low hyaluronan levels [122]. Furthermore, conditioned medium from a confluent mesothelial cell culture containing high amounts of hyaluronan prevented tumor cell adhesion [123]. Free hyaluronan binds to CD44 molecules on the tumor cells, preventing their binding to the mesothelial hyaluronan pericellular coat. Therefore, under normal physiological conditions, secretion of hyaluronan by mesothelial cells into the serosal fluid may protect the serosa from tumor implantation.

It is clear that integrins play a major role in peritoneal tumor dissemination. For example, the β1-integrin is common to many integrin molecules and can bind a variety of ECM proteins.

Blocking β1-integrin, which is upregulated by IL-1β [124], inhibits tumor cell attachment and migration on ECM substrates and to confluent mesothelial cell monolayers in culture [114,116,125]. In addition, migration of ovarian carcinoma cell lines toward fibronectin, type I and IV collagen, and laminin was blocked by antibodies against α5β1, α2β1, and α6β1, respectively [115,126–129]. Similarly, adhesion of gastric carcinoma cells to mesothelial cells was blocked by antibodies against β1, α2, and α3 subunits, indicating that α2β1 and possibly to an even greater extent α3β1-integrins play a role in gastric carcinoma cell adhesion to peritoneum [130]. This is supported by the observation that expression of

these two integrins also correlates with increased metastatic potential [131]. The α3β1-integrin also binds strongly with laminin-5, a major component of submesothelial basement membranes, to enhance production of MMP-9 by gastric carcinoma cells and facilitate their invasion via degradation of the matrix [132].

TGF-β has been shown to induce mesothelial cell apoptosis [133] and promote cancer cell attachment [134] and proliferation and the activation of MMP-2 and MMP-9 [135]. This appears to be induced through downregulation of the miR-200 family by TGF-β, as restoration of the expression of miR-200 family members in mesothelial cells suppressed cancer cell attachment and proliferation. Importantly, delivery of the miR-200s to mesothelial cells in mice inhibited ovarian cancer cell implantation and dissemination [135]. SDF-1α also promotes attachment between ovarian carcinoma cells and mesothelial cells or ECM components, and this appears linked to the expression of CXC chemokine receptor type 4 [136].

CELL INVASION

Mesothelial cells are also likely to play a role in cancer cell invasion. Mesothelial cells produce lysophosphatidic acid (LPA), which is a biologically active lipid able to stimulate adhesion, migration, and invasion of ovarian cancer cells [137,138]. LPA produced by cultured mesothelial cells induced ovarian cancer cell migration, cell adhesion to collagen type I, and cell invasion across a mesothelial monolayer, involving LPA_1 and LPA_2 receptors. LPA has also been shown to stimulate the proliferation and motility of mesothelioma cells through LPA_1 and LPA_2 receptors [139]. Furthermore, LPA stimulates VEGF production by mesothelial cells that may play a significant role in tumor angiogenesis [140]. Various studies have examined ways to block LPA-induced tumor cell proliferation, chemotaxis, and invasion. Ovarian cancer cells treated with secreted protein acidic and rich in cysteine inhibited LPA-induced mesothelial–ovarian cancer cell crosstalk through the regulation of both LPA-induced IL-6 production and function [141]. The knockdown of cofilin/ADF, LIM kinase-1 (LIMK1), or Slingshot (SSH)1/SSH2 expression by small interfering RNAs significantly decreased the LPA-induced transcellular migration of rat hepatoma cells and their motility in 2D culture. The knockdown of LIMK1 also suppressed fibronectin-mediated cell attachment and focal adhesion formation [142].

For tumor cells to invade the stroma, they require various proteases such as MMPs. MMP-1, MMP-2, and MMP-7 have been implicated in the progression of gastric and ovarian cancer [91,143,144]. MMP-2 is known to break down collagen type IV, laminin, and fibronectin (all components of basement membrane), while MMP-1 acts on collagen types I and III. *In vitro* studies have shown that mesothelial cells spontaneously express MMP-1 and MMP-2 when in contact with tumor cells, which leads to enhanced tumor invasion [91]. Mesothelin enhances ovarian cancer invasion by MMP-7 expression through the MAPK/ERK and JNK signal transduction pathways [143]. MMP-7, also known as matrilysin, degrades a range of ECM proteins including collagen type IV, laminin-1, fibronectin, proteoglycan, type 1 gelatin, and insoluble elastin. MT1-MMP, which cleaves gelatin, fibronectin, and laminin, is also important for transmigration of cancer cells through stroma and basement membrane and has also been shown to promote the formation and dissemination of multicellular aggregates or spheroids, which may be important for ovarian carcinoma metastasis [145,146]. Burleson et al. [125] were able to inhibit tumor invasion by addition of broad-scale MMP inhibitors, highlighting the importance of proteases in tumor dissemination. However, clinical trials using broad-range MMP inhibitors have yielded disappointing outcomes, possibly due to inhibitor concentrations at too low levels to accomplish the inhibition of critical MMPs [147].

The protease inhibitor, plasminogen activator inhibitor-1 (PAI-1), has also been implicated in peritoneal tumor cell invasion and metastasis [148]. Mesothelial cells upregulate PAI-1 in response to growth factors such as TGF-β_1 secreted directly by tumor cells, which facilitate tumor cell adhesion, invasion, and dissemination [148].

A recent study by Satoyoshi et al. [149], using human tissue and a mouse model of scirrhous gastric cancer, suggests that peritoneal mesothelial cells in peritoneal carcinomatosis undergo MMT and acquire invasive properties and then guide the invasion of cancer cells. They showed that Tks5, an adaptor protein required for podosome and invadopodia formation by certain cells and a substrate for Src family kinases, was upregulated in mesothelial cells exposed to cancer cells. If Tks5 was blocked, invasion did not occur. Likewise, if Tks5 expression was reinstated, invasion progressed. This is an important finding as it shows that mesothelial cells can be "hijacked" by cancer cells to support their invasion and growth.

TUMOR GROWTH

For tumors to grow, they need an appropriate environment with support stroma and vasculature. Interestingly, it has been demonstrated that peritoneal fibrosis provides a favorable environment for the dissemination of gastric cancer [134]. Carcinoma-associated fibroblasts (CAFs) are prominent within the tumor stroma and participate in most stages of tumor progression [150]. CAFs have many characteristics consistent with myofibroblasts and produce a wide array of growth factors and ECM components, thereby contributing to the growth and vascularization of solid tumors [151]. The origin of these CAFs is unclear and they may originate from different cell types between different cancers and within different areas of individual tumors [152]. The most likely source of peritoneal CAFs is from resident peritoneal fibroblasts that respond to a variety of stimuli and differentiate into myofibroblasts. However, it has also been proposed that these cells may be derived from bone marrow progenitor cells, endothelial cells, epithelial cells, and most recently peritoneal mesothelial cells [153].

There is now strong evidence that mesothelial cells are a source of CAFs and promote tumor cell growth. Sandoval et al. [153] showed that CAFs located within or nearby peritoneal carcinoma implants expressed mesothelial cell markers and that in vitro, carcinoma cells secreted MMT-promoting factors and that the mesenchymal conversion of mesothelial cells favored cell–cell interaction with tumor cells.

TGF-β_1 secreted by scirrhous gastric cancer cells also induced mesothelial cells to differentiate into myofibroblasts and increase adhesion and invasion of scirrhous gastric cancer cells [154,155]. Blocking TGF-β_1 in a mouse model partially attenuated early-stage gastric cancer peritoneal dissemination [156]. In vitro studies showed that mesothelial cells became more invasive and increased proliferation of human gastric cancer–derived MKN45 cells following direct cell–cell contact [157], and when MKN45 cells were cocultured with human peritoneal mesothelial cells, they also acquired anchorage-independent cell growth and decreased expression of E-cadherin. When tumors derived from injection of MKN45 cells were grown in mice, the largest tumors were from MKN45 cells that had been cocultured with mesothelial cells. Furthermore, these tumors contained mesothelial cell-derived fibrous tissue. Similarly, ovarian cancer cells secrete TGF-β_1, which induces MMT. These differentiated mesothelial cells upregulated production of fibronectin, which, when blocked in vitro and in murine models, decreased adhesion, invasion, proliferation, and metastasis of ovarian cancer cells [158].

Mesothelial cells also produce various growth factors that are increased within the peritoneal fluid following surgery and may enhance local and distant tumor growth [159–161]. One example is HGF, a potent mitogen and motogen on a range of cell types including ovarian, gastric, pancreatic, and colorectal cancers [162]. Furthermore, the HGF receptor c-Met is overexpressed in several peritoneal cancers including gastric and ovarian cancers [163,164]. As well as directly stimulating tumor cell responses, HGF also induces mesothelial cell retraction, exposing underlying ECM [82,165]. Blocking c-Met on an ovarian cancer cell line inhibited adhesion of the cancer cells to different ECM components as well as cultured mesothelial cells and mouse peritoneum in vivo. This was paralleled by a significant reduction in α5β1-integrin and a reduction of urokinase and MMP-2 and MMP-9 activities [166], also implicated in tumor cell adhesion and dissemination. IL-1β and TNF-α also stimulate similar responses in mesothelial cells [104], but they may act through HGF as both IL-1β and TNF-α upregulate HGF and c-Met expression in cells [167,168]. Interestingly, Fujiwara and colleagues [169] suppressed gastric cancer dissemination and increased survival time in mice following intraperitoneal injection of an adenovirus vector encoding the NK4 gene, a competitive antagonist for HGF. Many studies have examined the role of HGF/c-Met in various cancers and several types of inhibitors are currently in clinical trial [170].

IL-6 is a pleiotropic cytokine produced by mesothelial cells, fibroblasts, macrophages, and tumor cells with anti- and proinflammatory and proangiogenic roles [171]. Its expression correlates with a poor prognosis in ovarian carcinoma [172] and it has been associated with chemoresistance [173]. The IL-6 receptor is overexpressed in ovarian cancer cells compared to normal ovarian cells [174], and the cytokine promotes tumor cell proliferation and metastasis of ovarian cancer cell lines and prevents their apoptosis [175].

Interestingly, senescent mesothelial cells have also been shown to secrete proangiogenic mediators VEGF, CXCL1/GRO-α, CXCL8/IL-8, and CCL2/MCP-1, which may also contribute to accelerated intraperitoneal cancer progression, particularly in the elderly [176].

CONCLUSION

The mesothelial cell is an important cell in the maintenance of normal serosal integrity in health and disease. However, cancer cells can "hijack" mesothelial cells and induce them to promote tumor cell attachment, invasion, and growth on and across the peritoneal and other serosal surfaces. A better understanding of the mechanisms tumor cells use to influence mesothelial cell morphology and function will enable the development of better therapeutic approaches to help stop peritoneal carcinomatosis and improve patient survival.

ACKNOWLEDGMENTS

We wish to express our gratitude to Dr. Hassan Sulaiman who provided the scanning electron micrograph of the omental mesothelium.

REFERENCES

1. Minot CS. The mesoderm and the coelom of vertebrates. *The American Naturalist*. 1890;24:877–898.
2. Mutsaers SE. Mesothelial cells: Their structure, function and role in serosal repair. *Respirology*. September 2002;7(3):171–191.
3. Mutsaers SE, Whitaker D, Papadimitriou JM. Changes in the concentration of microvilli on the free surface of healing mesothelium are associated with alterations in surface membrane charge. *The Journal of Pathology*. November 1996;180(3):333–339.
4. Lange K. Fundamental role of microvilli in the main functions of differentiated cells: Outline of an universal regulating and signaling system at the cell periphery. *Journal of Cellular Physiology*. April 2011;226(4):896–927.
5. Mutsaers SE, Whitaker D, Papadimitriou JM. Stimulation of mesothelial cell proliferation by exudate macrophages enhances serosal wound healing in a murine model. *The American Journal of Pathology*. February 2002;160(2):681–692.
6. Albertine KH, Wiener-Kronish JP, Roos PJ, Staub NC. Structure, blood supply, and lymphatic vessels of the sheep's visceral pleura. *American Journal of Anatomy*. 1982;165(3):277–294.
7. Nakatani T, Ohtani O, Tanaka S. Lymphatic stomata in the murine diaphragmatic peritoneum: The timing of their appearance and a map of their distribution. *The Anatomical Record*. 1996;244(4):529–539.
8. Noppen M, De Waele M, Li R, Gucht KV, D'Haese J, Gerlo E et al. Volume and cellular content of normal pleural fluid in humans examined by pleural lavage. *American Journal of Respiratory and Critical Care Medicine*. September 2000;162(3 Pt. 1):1023–1026.
9. Herrick SE, Mutsaers SE. The potential of mesothelial cells in tissue engineering and regenerative medicine applications. *The International Journal of Artificial Organs*. June 2007;30(6):527–540.
10. Thiery JP, Acloque H, Huang RY, Nieto MA. Epithelial-mesenchymal transitions in development and disease. *Cell*. November 25, 2009;139(5):871–890.
11. Zeisberg M, Neilson EG. Biomarkers for epithelial-mesenchymal transitions. *The Journal of Clinical Investigation*. June 2009;119(6):1429–1437.
12. Zeisberg M, Kalluri R. The role of epithelial-to-mesenchymal transition in renal fibrosis. *Journal of Molecular Medicine*. March 2004;82(3):175–181.
13. Lamouille S, Subramanyam D, Blelloch R, Derynck R. Regulation of epithelial-mesenchymal and mesenchymal-epithelial transitions by microRNAs. *Current Opinion in Cell Biology*. April 2013;25(2):200–207.
14. Li Y, Wang J, Asahina K. Mesothelial cells give rise to hepatic stellate cells and myofibroblasts via mesothelial-mesenchymal transition in liver injury. *Proceedings of the National Academy of Sciences of the United States of America*. February 5, 2013;110(6):2324–2329.
15. Asahina K, Zhou B, Pu WT, Tsukamoto H. Septum transversum-derived mesothelium gives rise to hepatic stellate cells and perivascular mesenchymal cells in developing mouse liver. *Hepatology*. March 2011;53(3):983–995.
16. Cai CL, Martin JC, Sun Y, Cui L, Wang L, Ouyang K et al. A myocardial lineage derives from Tbx18 epicardial cells. *Nature*. July 3, 2008;454(7200):104–108.
17. Que J, Wilm B, Hasegawa H, Wang F, Bader D, Hogan BL. Mesothelium contributes to vascular smooth muscle and mesenchyme during lung development. *Proceedings of the National Academy of Sciences of the United States of America*. October 28, 2008;105(43):16626–16630.
18. Wilm B, Ipenberg A, Hastie ND, Burch JB, Bader DM. The serosal mesothelium is a major source of smooth muscle cells of the gut vasculature. *Development (Cambridge, England)*. December 2005;132(23):5317–5328.

19. Zhou B, Ma Q, Rajagopal S, Wu SM, Domian I, Rivera-Feliciano J et al. Epicardial progenitors contribute to the cardiomyocyte lineage in the developing heart. *Nature*. July 3, 2008;454(7200): 109–113.

20. Dixit R, Ai X, Fine A. Derivation of lung mesenchymal lineages from the fetal mesothelium requires hedgehog signaling for mesothelial cell entry. *Development (Cambridge, England)*. November 2013;140(21):4398–4406.

21. Kawaguchi M, Bader DM, Wilm B. Serosal mesothelium retains vasculogenic potential. *Developmental Dynamics: An Official Publication of the American Association of Anatomists*. November 2007;236(11):2973–2979.

22. van Tuyn J, Atsma DE, Winter EM, van der Velde-van Dijke I, Pijnappels DA, Bax NA et al. Epicardial cells of human adults can undergo an epithelial-to-mesenchymal transition and obtain characteristics of smooth muscle cells in vitro. *Stem Cells*. February 2007;25(2):271–278.

23. Wada AM, Smith TK, Osler ME, Reese DE, Bader DM. Epicardial/mesothelial cell line retains vasculogenic potential of embryonic epicardium. *Circulation Research*. March 21, 2003;92(5):525–531.

24. Lachaud CC, Pezzolla D, Dominguez-Rodriguez A, Smani T, Soria B, Hmadcha A. Functional vascular smooth muscle-like cells derived from adult mouse uterine mesothelial cells. *PLOS ONE*. 2013;8(2):e55181.

25. Lansley SM, Searles RG, Hoi A, Thomas C, Moneta H, Herrick SE et al. Mesothelial cell differentiation into osteoblast- and adipocyte-like cells. *Journal of Cellular and Molecular Medicine*. October 2011;15(10):2095–2105.

26. Aroeira LS, Aguilera A, Sanchez-Tomero JA, Bajo MA, del Peso G, Jimenez-Heffernan JA et al. Epithelial to mesenchymal transition and peritoneal membrane failure in peritoneal dialysis patients: Pathologic significance and potential therapeutic interventions. *Journal of the American Society of Nephrology*. July 2007;18(7):2004–2013.

27. Yanez-Mo M, Lara-Pezzi E, Selgas R, Ramirez-Huesca M, Dominguez-Jimenez C, Jimenez-Heffernan JA et al. Peritoneal dialysis and epithelial-to-mesenchymal transition of mesothelial cells. *The New England Journal of Medicine*. January 30, 2003;348(5):403–413.

28. Nasreen N, Mohammed KA, Mubarak KK, Baz MA, Akindipe OA, Fernandez-Bussy S et al. Pleural mesothelial cell transformation into myofibroblasts and haptotactic migration in response to TGF-beta1 in vitro. *American Journal of Physiology Lung Cellular and Molecular Physiology*. July 2009;297(1):L115–L124.

29. Yang AH, Chen JY, Lin JK. Myofibroblastic conversion of mesothelial cells. *Kidney International*. April 2003;63(4):1530–1539.

30. Liu Q, Mao H, Nie J, Chen W, Yang Q, Dong X et al. Transforming growth factor {beta}1 induces epithelial-mesenchymal transition by activating the JNK-Smad3 pathway in rat peritoneal mesothelial cells. *Peritoneal Dialysis International: Journal of the International Society for Peritoneal Dialysis*. June 2008;28(Suppl. 3):S88–S95.

31. Patel P, West-Mays J, Kolb M, Rodrigues JC, Hoff CM, Margetts PJ. Platelet derived growth factor B and epithelial mesenchymal transition of peritoneal mesothelial cells. *Matrix Biology: Journal of the International Society for Matrix Biology*. March 2010;29(2):97–106.

32. Strippoli R, Benedicto I, Perez Lozano ML, Cerezo A, Lopez-Cabrera M, del Pozo MA. Epithelial-to-mesenchymal transition of peritoneal mesothelial cells is regulated by an ERK/NF-kappaB/Snail1 pathway. *Disease Models & Mechanisms*. November to December 2008;1(4–5):264–274.

33. Zhou Q, Yang M, Lan H, Yu X. miR-30a negatively regulates TGF-beta1-induced epithelial-mesenchymal transition and peritoneal fibrosis by targeting Snai1. *The American Journal of Pathology*. September 2013;183(3):808–819.

34. Demir AY, Groothuis PG, Dunselman GA, Schurgers L, Evers JL, de Goeij AF. Molecular characterization of soluble factors from human menstrual effluent that induce epithelial to mesenchymal transitions in mesothelial cells. *Cell and Tissue Research*. November 2005;322(2):299–311.

35. Demir AY, Groothuis PG, Nap AW, Punyadeera C, de Goeij AF, Evers JL et al. Menstrual effluent induces epithelial-mesenchymal transitions in mesothelial cells. *Human Reproduction*. January 2004;19(1):21–29.

36. Liu J, Zeng L, Zhao Y, Zhu B, Ren W, Wu C. Selenium suppresses lipopolysaccharide-induced fibrosis in peritoneal mesothelial cells through inhibition of epithelial-to-mesenchymal transition. *Biological Trace Element Research*. November 2014;161(2):202–209.

37. Foley-Comer AJ, Herrick SE, Al-Mishlab T, Prele CM, Laurent GJ, Mutsaers SE. Evidence for incorporation of free-floating mesothelial cells as a mechanism of serosal healing. *Journal of Cell Science*. April 1, 2002;115(Pt. 7):1383–1389.

38. Decologne N, Kolb M, Margetts PJ, Menetrier F, Artur Y, Garrido C et al. TGF-beta1 induces progressive pleural scarring and subpleural fibrosis. *Journal of Immunology*. November 1, 2007;179(9):6043–6051.

39. Margetts PJ, Bonniaud P, Liu L, Hoff CM, Holmes CJ, West-Mays JA et al. Transient overexpression of TGF-{beta}1 induces epithelial mesenchymal

transition in the rodent peritoneum. *Journal of the American Society of Nephrology.* February 2005;16(2):425–436.

40. Karki S, Surolia R, Hock TD, Guroji P, Zolak JS, Duggal R et al. Wilms' tumor 1 (Wt1) regulates pleural mesothelial cell plasticity and transition into myofibroblasts in idiopathic pulmonary fibrosis. *FASEB Journal: Official Publication of the Federation of American Societies for Experimental Biology.* March 2014;28(3):1122–1131.

41. Lignitto L, Mattiolo A, Negri E, Persano L, Gianesello L, Chieco-Bianchi L et al. Crosstalk between the mesothelium and lymphomatous cells: Insight into the mechanisms involved in the progression of body cavity lymphomas. *Cancer Medicine.* February 2014;3(1):1–13.

42. Mutsaers SE, Wilkosz S. Structure and function of mesothelial cells. *Cancer Treatment and Research.* 2007;134:1–19.

43. Jantz MA, Antony VB. Pathophysiology of the pleura. *Respiration; International Review of Thoracic Diseases.* 2008;75(2):121–133.

44. Plato A, Hardison SE, Brown GD. Pattern recognition receptors in antifungal immunity. *Seminars in Immunopathology.* November 25, 2014.

45. Tosi MF. Innate immune responses to infection. *The Journal of Allergy and Clinical Immunology.* August 2005;116(2):241–249; quiz 50.

46. Colmont CS, Raby AC, Dioszeghy V, Lebouder E, Foster TL, Jones SA et al. Human peritoneal mesothelial cells respond to bacterial ligands through a specific subset of Toll-like receptors. *Nephrology, Dialysis, Transplantation: Official Publication of the European Dialysis and Transplant Association—European Renal Association.* December 2011;26(12):4079–4090.

47. Hussain T, Nasreen N, Lai Y, Bellew BF, Antony VB, Mohammed KA. Innate immune responses in murine pleural mesothelial cells: Toll-like receptor-2 dependent induction of beta-defensin-2 by staphylococcal peptidoglycan. *American Journal of Physiology Lung Cellular and Molecular Physiology.* September 2008;295(3):L461–L470.

48. Kim TH, Lee KB, Kang MJ, Park JH. Critical role of Toll-like receptor 2 in *Bacteroides fragilis*-mediated immune responses in murine peritoneal mesothelial cells. *Microbiology and Immunology.* November 2012;56(11):782–788.

49. Kato S, Yuzawa Y, Tsuboi N, Maruyama S, Morita Y, Matsuguchi T et al. Endotoxin-induced chemokine expression in murine peritoneal mesothelial cells: The role of toll-like receptor 4. *Journal of the American Society of Nephrology.* May 2004;15(5):1289–1299.

50. Wu J, Yang X, Zhang YF, Zhou SF, Zhang R, Dong XQ et al. Angiotensin II upregulates Toll-like receptor 4 and enhances lipopolysaccharide-induced CD40 expression in rat peritoneal mesothelial cells. *Inflammation Research: Official Journal of the European Histamine Research Society* [et al.]. August 2009;58(8):473–482.

51. Wornle M, Sauter M, Kastenmuller K, Ribeiro A, Roeder M, Schmid H et al. Novel role of toll-like receptor 3, RIG-I and MDA5 in poly (I:C) RNA-induced mesothelial inflammation. *Molecular and Cellular Biochemistry.* February 2009;322(1–2):193–206.

52. Merkle M, Ribeiro A, Sauter M, Ladurner R, Mussack T, Sitter T et al. Effect of activation of viral receptors on the gelatinases MMP-2 and MMP-9 in human mesothelial cells. *Matrix Biology: Journal of the International Society for Matrix Biology.* April 2010;29(3):202–208.

53. Merkle M, Sauter M, Ribeiro A, Mussack T, Ladurner R, Sitter T et al. Synthetic double-stranded RNA stimulates the expression of interferon-inducible protein 10 in human mesothelial cells. *Clinical and Vaccine Immunology.* January 2011;18(1):176–179.

54. Balabanian K, Foussat A, Bouchet-Delbos L, Couderc J, Krzysiek R, Amara A et al. Interleukin-10 modulates the sensitivity of peritoneal B lymphocytes to chemokines with opposite effects on stromal cell-derived factor-1 and B-lymphocyte chemoattractant. *Blood.* January 15, 2002;99(2):427–436.

55. Lee YC, Knight DA, Lane KB, Cheng DS, Koay MA, Teixeira LR et al. Activation of proteinase-activated receptor-2 in mesothelial cells induces pleural inflammation. *American Journal of Physiology Lung Cellular and Molecular Physiology.* April 2005;288(4):L734–L740.

56. Jonjic N, Peri G, Bernasconi S, Sciacca FL, Colotta F, Pelicci P et al. Expression of adhesion molecules and chemotactic cytokines in cultured human mesothelial cells. *The Journal of Experimental Medicine.* October 1, 1992;176(4):1165–1174.

57. Visser CE, Tekstra J, Brouwer-Steenbergen JJ, Tuk CW, Boorsma DM, Sampat-Sardjoepersad SC et al. Chemokines produced by mesothelial cells: huGRO-alpha, IP-10, MCP-1 and RANTES. *Clinical and Experimental Immunology.* May 1998;112(2):270–275.

58. Katayama H, Yokoyama A, Kohno N, Sakai K, Hiwada K, Yamada H et al. Production of eosinophilic chemokines by normal pleural mesothelial cells. *American Journal of Respiratory Cell and Molecular Biology.* April 2002;26(4):398–403.

59. Foussat A, Balabanian K, Amara A, Bouchet-Delbos L, Durand-Gasselin I, Baleux F et al. Production of stromal cell-derived factor 1 by mesothelial cells and effects of this chemokine on peritoneal B lymphocytes. *European Journal of Immunology.* February 2001;31(2):350–359.

60. Johnson Z, Power CA, Weiss C, Rintelen F, Ji H, Ruckle T et al. Chemokine inhibition—Why, when, where, which and how? *Biochemical Society Transactions.* April 2004;32(Pt. 2):366–377.

61. Parish CR. The role of heparan sulphate in inflammation. *Nature Reviews Immunology.* September 2006;6(9):633–643.

62. Ross JA, Ansell I, Hjelle JT, Anderson JD, Miller-Hjelle MA, Dobbie JW. Phenotypic mapping of human mesothelial cells. *Advances in Peritoneal Dialysis Conference on Peritoneal Dialysis.* 1998;14:25–30.

63. Simsir A, Fetsch P, Mehta D, Zakowski M, Abati A. E-cadherin, N-cadherin, and calretinin in pleural effusions: The good, the bad, the worthless. *Diagnostic Cytopathology.* March 1999;20(3):125–130.

64. Yuan ML, Tong ZH, Jin XG, Zhang JC, Wang XJ, Ma WL et al. Regulation of CD4(+) T cells by pleural mesothelial cells via adhesion molecule-dependent mechanisms in tuberculous pleurisy. *PLOS ONE.* 2013;8(9):e74624.

65. Liang Y, Sasaki K. Expression of adhesion molecules relevant to leukocyte migration on the microvilli of liver peritoneal mesothelial cells. *The Anatomical Record.* January 1, 2000;258(1):39–46.

66. Wang HH, Lee TY, Lin CY. Integrins mediate adherence and migration of T lymphocytes on human peritoneal mesothelial cells. *Kidney International.* September 2008;74(6):808–816.

67. Bellingan GJ, Xu P, Cooksley H, Cauldwell H, Shock A, Bottoms S et al. Adhesion molecule-dependent mechanisms regulate the rate of macrophage clearance during the resolution of peritoneal inflammation. *The Journal of Experimental Medicine.* December 2, 2002;196(11):1515–1521.

68. Valle MT, Degl'Innocenti ML, Bertelli R, Facchetti P, Perfumo F, Fenoglio D et al. Antigen-presenting function of human peritoneum mesothelial cells. *Clinical and Experimental Immunology.* July 1995;101(1):172–176.

69. Hausmann MJ, Rogachev B, Weiler M, Chaimovitz C, Douvdevani A. Accessory role of human peritoneal mesothelial cells in antigen presentation and T-cell growth. *Kidney International.* February 2000;57(2):476–486.

70. Yang X, Ye R, Kong Q, Yang Q, Dong X, Yu X. CD40 is expressed on rat peritoneal mesothelial cells and upregulates ICAM-1 production. *Nephrology, Dialysis, Transplantation: Official Publication of the European Dialysis and Transplant Association—European Renal Association.* June 2004;19(6):1378–1384.

71. Basok A, Shnaider A, Man L, Chaimovitz C, Douvdevani A. CD40 is expressed on human peritoneal mesothelial cells and upregulates the production of interleukin-15 and RANTES. *Journal of the American Society of Nephrology.* April 2001;12(4):695–702.

72. Mazar J, Agur T, Rogachev B, Ziv NY, Zlotnik M, Chaimovitz C et al. CD40 ligand (CD154) takes part in regulation of the transition to mononuclear cell dominance during peritonitis. *Kidney International.* April 2005;67(4):1340–1349.

73. Ye ZJ, Yuan ML, Zhou Q, Du RH, Yang WB, Xiong XZ et al. Differentiation and recruitment of Th9 cells stimulated by pleural mesothelial cells in human Mycobacterium tuberculosis infection. *PLOS ONE.* 2012;7(2):e31710.

74. Ye ZJ, Zhou Q, Yuan ML, Du RH, Yang WB, Xiong XZ et al. Differentiation and recruitment of IL-22-producing helper T cells stimulated by pleural mesothelial cells in tuberculous pleurisy. *American Journal of Respiratory and Critical Care Medicine.* March 15, 2012;185(6):660–669.

75. Lanfrancone L, Boraschi D, Ghiara P, Falini B, Grignani F, Peri G et al. Human peritoneal mesothelial cells produce many cytokines (granulocyte colony-stimulating factor [CSF], granulocyte-monocyte-CSF, macrophage-CSF, interleukin-1 [IL-1], and IL-6) and are activated and stimulated to grow by IL-1. *Blood.* 1992;80(11):2835–2842.

76. Topley N, Jorres A, Luttmann W, Petersen MM, Lang MJ, Thierauch KH et al. Human peritoneal mesothelial cells synthesize interleukin-6: Induction by IL-1 beta and TNF alpha. *Kidney International.* 1993;43(1):226–233.

77. Ataie-Kachoie P, Pourgholami MH, Richardson DR, Morris DL. Gene of the month: Interleukin 6 (IL-6). *Journal of Clinical Pathology.* November 2014;67(11):932–937.

78. Choe N, Tanaka S, Kagan E. Asbestos fibers and interleukin-1 upregulate the formation of reactive nitrogen species in rat pleural mesothelial cells. *American Journal of Respiratory Cell and Molecular Biology.* August 1998;19(2):226–236.

79. Janssen YM, Marsh JP, Absher MP, Gabrielson E, Borm PJ, Driscoll K et al. Oxidant stress responses in human pleural mesothelial cells exposed to asbestos. *American Journal of Respiratory and Critical Care Medicine.* March 1994;149(3 Pt. 1):795–802.

80. Kinnula VL, Everitt JI, Mangum JB, Chang LY, Crapo JD. Antioxidant defense mechanisms in cultured pleural mesothelial cells. *American Journal of Respiratory Cell and Molecular Biology.* July 1992;7(1):95–103.

81. Hott JW, Godbey SW, Antony VB. Mesothelial cell modulation of pleural repair: Thrombin stimulated mesothelial cells release prostaglandin E2. *Prostaglandins, Leukotrienes, and Essential Fatty Acids.* November 1994;51(5):329–335.

82. Warn R, Harvey P, Warn A, Foley-Comer A, Heldin P, Versnel M et al. HGF/SF induces mesothelial cell migration and proliferation by autocrine and paracrine pathways. *Experimental Cell Research*. July 15, 2001;267(2):258–266.

83. Rennard SI, Jaurand MC, Bignon J, Kawanami O, Ferrans VJ, Davidson J et al. Role of pleural mesothelial cells in the production of the submesothelial connective tissue matrix of lung. *The American Review of Respiratory Disease*. 1984;130(2):267–274.

84. Saed GM, Zhang W, Chegini N, Holmdahl L, Diamond MP. Alteration of type I and III collagen expression in human peritoneal mesothelial cells in response to hypoxia and transforming growth factor-beta1. *Wound Repair and Regeneration: Official Publication of the Wound Healing Society [and] the European Tissue Repair Society*. 1999;7(6):504–510.

85. Perfumo F, Altieri P, Degl'Innocenti ML, Ghiggeri GM, Caridi G, Trivelli A et al. Effects of peritoneal effluents on mesothelial cells in culture: Cell proliferation and extracellular matrix regulation. *Nephrology, Dialysis, Transplantation: Official Publication of the European Dialysis and Transplant Association—European Renal Association*. 1996;11(9):1803–1809.

86. Margetts PJ, Kolb M, Galt T, Hoff CM, Shockley TR, Gauldie J. Gene transfer of transforming growth factor-beta1 to the rat peritoneum: Effects on membrane function. *Journal of the American Society of Nephrology*. October 2001;12(10):2029–2039.

87. Ma C, Tarnuzzer RW, Chegini N. Expression of matrix metalloproteinases and tissue inhibitor of matrix metalloproteinases in mesothelial cells and their regulation by transforming growth factor-beta1. *Wound Repair and Regeneration: Official Publication of the Wound Healing Society [and] the European Tissue Repair Society*. November to December 1999;7(6):477–485.

88. Yung S, Thomas GJ, Stylianou E, Williams JD, Coles GA, Davies M. Source of peritoneal proteoglycans. Human peritoneal mesothelial cells synthesize and secrete mainly small dermatan sulfate proteoglycans. *The American Journal of Pathology*. 1995;146(2):520–529.

89. Sodek KL, Murphy KJ, Brown TJ, Ringuette MJ. Cell-cell and cell-matrix dynamics in intraperitoneal cancer metastasis. *Cancer Metastasis Reviews*. June 2012;31(1–2):397–414.

90. Terzi C, Arslan NC, Canda AE. Peritoneal carcinomatosis of gastrointestinal tumors: Where are we now? *World Journal of Gastroenterology*. October 21, 2014;20(39):14371–14380.

91. Yonemura Y, Endou Y, Fujita H, Fushida S, Bandou E, Taniguchi K et al. Role of MMP-7 in the formation of peritoneal dissemination in gastric cancer. *Gastric Cancer: Official Journal of the International Gastric Cancer Association and the Japanese Gastric Cancer Association*. September 29, 2000;3(2):63–70.

92. Tsujimoto H, Hagiwara A, Shimotsuma M, Sakakura C, Osaki K, Sasaki S et al. Role of milky spots as selective implantation sites for malignant cells in peritoneal dissemination in mice. *Journal of Cancer Research and Clinical Oncology*. 1996;122(10):590–595.

93. Liu XY, Miao ZF, Zhao TT, Wang ZN, Xu YY, Gao J et al. Milky spot macrophages remodeled by gastric cancer cells promote peritoneal mesothelial cell injury. *Biochemical and Biophysical Research Communications*. September 27, 2013;439(3):378–383.

94. Cunliffe WJ, Sugarbaker PH. Gastrointestinal malignancy: Rationale for adjuvant therapy using early postoperative intraperitoneal chemotherapy. *The British Journal of Surgery*. 1989;76(10):1082–1090.

95. Mochizuki Y, Nakanishi H, Kodera Y, Ito S, Yamamura Y, Kato T et al. TNF-alpha promotes progression of peritoneal metastasis as demonstrated using a green fluorescence protein (GFP)-tagged human gastric cancer cell line. *Clinical & Experimental Metastasis*. 2004;21(1):39–47.

96. Stadlmann S, Raffeiner R, Amberger A, Margreiter R, Zeimet AG, Abendstein B et al. Disruption of the integrity of human peritoneal mesothelium by interleukin-1beta and tumor necrosis factor-alpha. *Virchows Archiv: An International Journal of Pathology*. November 2003;443(5):678–685.

97. Stadlmann S, Feichtinger H, Mikuz G, Marth C, Zeimet AG, Herold M et al. Interactions of human peritoneal mesothelial cells with serous ovarian cancer cell spheroids—Evidence for a mechanical and paracrine barrier function of the peritoneal mesothelium. *International Journal of Gynecological Cancer: Official Journal of the International Gynecological Cancer Society*. February 2014;24(2):192–200.

98. Iwanicki MP, Davidowitz RA, Ng MR, Besser A, Muranen T, Merritt M et al. Ovarian cancer spheroids use myosin-generated force to clear the mesothelium. *Cancer Discovery*. July 2011;1(2):144–157.

99. Davidowitz RA, Selfors LM, Iwanicki MP, Elias KM, Karst A, Piao H et al. Mesenchymal gene program-expressing ovarian cancer spheroids exhibit enhanced mesothelial clearance. *The Journal of Clinical Investigation*. June 2, 2014;124(6):2611–2625.

100. van der Wal BC, Hofland LJ, Marquet RL, van Koetsveld PM, van Rossen ME, van Eijck CH. Paracrine interactions between mesothelial and colon-carcinoma cells in a rat model. *International Journal of Cancer (Journal International du Cancer)*. 1997;73(6):885–890.

101. Alkhamesi NA, Ziprin P, Pfistermuller K, Peck DH, Darzi AW. ICAM-1 mediated peritoneal carcinomatosis, a target for therapeutic intervention. *Clinical & Experimental Metastasis*. 2005;22(6):449–459.

102. Ksiazek K, Mikula-Pietrasik J, Catar R, Dworacki G, Winckiewicz M, Frydrychowicz M et al. Oxidative stress-dependent increase in ICAM-1 expression promotes adhesion of colorectal and pancreatic cancers to the senescent peritoneal mesothelium. *International Journal of Cancer (Journal International du Cancer)*. July 15, 2010;127(2):293–303.

103. Slack-Davis JK, Atkins KA, Harrer C, Hershey ED, Conaway M. Vascular cell adhesion molecule-1 is a regulator of ovarian cancer peritoneal metastasis. *Cancer Research*. February 15, 2009;69(4):1469–1476.

104. van Grevenstein WM, Hofland LJ, Jeekel J, van Eijck CH. The expression of adhesion molecules and the influence of inflammatory cytokines on the adhesion of human pancreatic carcinoma cells to mesothelial monolayers. *Pancreas*. May 2006;32(4):396–402.

105. van Rossen ME, Hofland LJ, van den Tol MP, van Koetsveld PM, Jeekel J, Marquet RL et al. Effect of inflammatory cytokines and growth factors on tumour cell adhesion to the peritoneum. *The Journal of Pathology*. 2001;193(4):530–537.

106. Ziprin P, Ridgway PF, Pfistermuller KL, Peck DH, Darzi AW. ICAM-1 mediated tumor-mesothelial cell adhesion is modulated by IL-6 and TNF-alpha: A potential mechanism by which surgical trauma increases peritoneal metastases. *Cell Communication & Adhesion*. May to June 2003;10(3):141–154.

107. Ranieri D, Raffa S, Parente A, Rossi Del Monte S, Ziparo V, Torrisi MR. High adhesion of tumor cells to mesothelial monolayers derived from peritoneal wash of disseminated gastrointestinal cancers. *PLOS ONE*. 2013;8(2):e57659.

108. Ksiazek K, Mikula-Pietrasik J, Korybalska K, Dworacki G, Jorres A, Witowski J. Senescent peritoneal mesothelial cells promote ovarian cancer cell adhesion: The role of oxidative stress-induced fibronectin. *The American Journal of Pathology*. April 2009;174(4):1230–1240.

109. Ziprin P, Alkhamesi NA, Ridgway PF, Peck DH, Darzi AW. Tumour-expressed CD43 (sialophorin) mediates tumour-mesothelial cell adhesion. *Biological Chemistry*. August 2004;385(8):755–761.

110. Rump A, Morikawa Y, Tanaka M, Minami S, Umesaki N, Takeuchi M et al. Binding of ovarian cancer antigen CA125/MUC16 to mesothelin mediates cell adhesion. *The Journal of Biological Chemistry*. March 5, 2004;279(10):9190–9198.

111. Bruney L, Conley KC, Moss NM, Liu Y, Stack MS. Membrane-type I matrix metalloproteinase-dependent ectodomain shedding of mucin16/ CA-125 on ovarian cancer cells modulates adhesion and invasion of peritoneal mesothelium. *Biological Chemistry*. October 1, 2014;395(10):1221–1231.

112. Usui A, Ko SY, Barengo N, Naora H. P-cadherin promotes ovarian cancer dissemination through tumor cell aggregation and tumor-peritoneum interactions. *Molecular Cancer Research*. April 2014;12(4):504–513.

113. Terauchi M, Kajiyama H, Yamashita M, Kato M, Tsukamoto H, Umezu T et al. Possible involvement of TWIST in enhanced peritoneal metastasis of epithelial ovarian carcinoma. *Clinical & Experimental Metastasis*. 2007;24(5):329–339.

114. Burleson KM, Casey RC, Skubitz KM, Pambuccian SE, Oegema TR, Jr., Skubitz AP. Ovarian carcinoma ascites spheroids adhere to extracellular matrix components and mesothelial cell monolayers. *Gynecologic Oncology*. April 2004;93(1):170–181.

115. Casey RC, Skubitz AP. CD44 and beta1 integrins mediate ovarian carcinoma cell migration toward extracellular matrix proteins. *Clinical & Experimental Metastasis*. 2000;18(1):67–75.

116. Lessan K, Aguiar DJ, Oegema T, Siebenson L, Skubitz AP. CD44 and beta1 integrin mediate ovarian carcinoma cell adhesion to peritoneal mesothelial cells. *The American Journal of Pathology*. May 1999;154(5):1525–1537.

117. Zeng C, Toole BP, Kinney SD, Kuo JW, Stamenkovic I. Inhibition of tumor growth in vivo by hyaluronan oligomers. *International Journal of Cancer (Journal International du Cancer)*. 1998;77(3):396–401.

118. Catterall JB, Gardner MJ, Jones LM, Turner GA. Binding of ovarian cancer cells to immobilized hyaluronic acid. *Glycoconjugate Journal*. 1997;14(5):647–649.

119. Catterall JB, Jones LM, Turner GA. Membrane protein glycosylation and CD44 content in the adhesion of human ovarian cancer cells to hyaluronan. *Clinical & Experimental Metastasis*. 1999;17(7):583–591.

120. Harada N, Mizoi T, Kinouchi M, Hoshi K, Ishii S, Shiiba K et al. Introduction of antisense CD44S CDNA down-regulates expression of overall CD44 isoforms and inhibits tumor growth and metastasis in highly metastatic colon carcinoma cells. *International Journal of Cancer (Journal International du Cancer)*. 2001;91(1):67–75.

121. Li CZ, Liu B, Wen ZQ, Li HY. Inhibition of CD44 expression by small interfering RNA to suppress the growth and metastasis of ovarian cancer cells in vitro and in vivo. *Folia Biologica*. 2008;54(6):180–186.

122. Tamada Y, Takeuchi H, Suzuki N, Aoki D, Irimura T. Cell surface expression of hyaluronan on human ovarian cancer cells inversely correlates with their adhesion to peritoneal mesothelial cells. *Tumour Biology: The Journal of the International Society for Oncodevelopmental Biology and Medicine*. August 2012;33(4):1215–1222.

123. Jones LM, Gardner MJ, Catterall JB, Turner GA. Hyaluronic acid secreted by mesothelial cells: A natural barrier to ovarian cancer cell adhesion. *Clinical & Experimental Metastasis.* 1995;13(5):373–380.

124. Watanabe T, Hashimoto T, Sugino T, Soeda S, Nishiyama H, Morimura Y et al. Production of IL1-beta by ovarian cancer cells induces mesothelial cell beta1-integrin expression facilitating peritoneal dissemination. *Journal of Ovarian Research.* 2012;5(1):7.

125. Burleson KM, Hansen LK, Skubitz AP. Ovarian carcinoma spheroids disaggregate on type I collagen and invade live human mesothelial cell monolayers. *Clinical & Experimental Metastasis.* 2004;21(8):685–697.

126. Ahmed N, Riley C, Rice G, Quinn M. Role of integrin receptors for fibronectin, collagen and laminin in the regulation of ovarian carcinoma functions in response to a matrix microenvironment. *Clinical & Experimental Metastasis.* 2005;22(5):391–402.

127. Fishman DA, Kearns A, Chilukuri K, Bafetti LM, O'Toole EA, Georgacopoulos J et al. Metastatic dissemination of human ovarian epithelial carcinoma is promoted by alpha2beta1-integrin-mediated interaction with type I collagen. *Invasion & Metastasis.* 1998;18(1):15–26.

128. Moser TL, Pizzo SV, Bafetti LM, Fishman DA, Stack MS. Evidence for preferential adhesion of ovarian epithelial carcinoma cells to type I collagen mediated by the alpha2beta1 integrin. *International Journal of Cancer (Journal International du Cancer).* September 4, 1996;67(5):695–701.

129. Oosterling SJ, van der Bij GJ, Bogels M, ten Raa S, Post JA, Meijer GA et al. Anti-beta1 integrin antibody reduces surgery-induced adhesion of colon carcinoma cells to traumatized peritoneal surfaces. *Annals of Surgery.* January 2008;247(1):85–94.

130. Takatsuki H, Komatsu S, Sano R, Takada Y, Tsuji T. Adhesion of gastric carcinoma cells to peritoneum mediated by alpha3beta1 integrin (VLA-3). *Cancer Research.* September 1, 2004;64(17):6065–6070.

131. Kawamura T, Endo Y, Yonemura Y, Nojima N, Fujita H, Fujimura T et al. Significance of integrin alpha2/beta1 in peritoneal dissemination of a human gastric cancer xenograft model. *International Journal of Oncology.* April 2001;18(4):809–815.

132. Saito Y, Sekine W, Sano R, Komatsu S, Mizuno H, Katabami K et al. Potentiation of cell invasion and matrix metalloproteinase production by alpha3beta1 integrin-mediated adhesion of gastric carcinoma cells to laminin-5. *Clinical & Experimental Metastasis.* April 2010;27(4):197–205.

133. Lv ZD, Yang ZC, Wang HB, Li JG, Kong B, Wang XG et al. The cytotoxic effect of TGF-beta1 on mesothelial cells via apoptosis in early peritoneal carcinomatosis. *Oncology Reports.* June 2012;27(6):1753–1758.

134. Lv ZD, Na D, Liu FN, Du ZM, Sun Z, Li Z et al. Induction of gastric cancer cell adhesion through transforming growth factor-beta1-mediated peritoneal fibrosis. *Journal of Experimental & Clinical Cancer Research.* 2010;29:139.

135. Sugiyama K, Kajiyama H, Shibata K, Yuan H, Kikkawa F, Senga T. Expression of the miR200 family of microRNAs in mesothelial cells suppresses the dissemination of ovarian cancer cells. *Molecular Cancer Therapeutics.* August 2014;13(8):2081–2091.

136. Kajiyama H, Shibata K, Terauchi M, Ino K, Nawa A, Kikkawa F. Involvement of SDF-1alpha/CXCR4 axis in the enhanced peritoneal metastasis of epithelial ovarian carcinoma. *International Journal of Cancer (Journal International du Cancer).* January 1, 2008;122(1):91–99.

137. Ren J, Xiao YJ, Singh LS, Zhao X, Zhao Z, Feng L et al. Lysophosphatidic acid is constitutively produced by human peritoneal mesothelial cells and enhances adhesion, migration, and invasion of ovarian cancer cells. *Cancer Research.* March 15, 2006;66(6):3006–3014.

138. Symowicz J, Adley BP, Woo MM, Auersperg N, Hudson LG, Stack MS. Cyclooxygenase-2 functions as a downstream mediator of lysophosphatidic acid to promote aggressive behavior in ovarian carcinoma cells. *Cancer Research.* March 15, 2005;65(6):2234–2242.

139. Yamada T, Yano S, Ogino H, Ikuta K, Kakiuchi S, Hanibuchi M et al. Lysophosphatidic acid stimulates the proliferation and motility of malignant pleural mesothelioma cells through lysophosphatidic acid receptors, LPA1 and LPA2. *Cancer Science.* August 2008;99(8):1603–1610.

140. Sako A, Kitayama J, Shida D, Suzuki R, Sakai T, Ohta H et al. Lysophosphatidic acid (LPA)-induced vascular endothelial growth factor (VEGF) by mesothelial cells and quantification of host-derived VEGF in malignant ascites. *The Journal of Surgical Research.* January 2006;130(1):94–101.

141. Said NA, Najwer I, Socha MJ, Fulton DJ, Mok SC, Motamed K. SPARC inhibits LPA-mediated mesothelial-ovarian cancer cell crosstalk. *Neoplasia.* January 2007;9(1):23–35.

142. Horita Y, Ohashi K, Mukai M, Inoue M, Mizuno K. Suppression of the invasive capacity of rat ascites hepatoma cells by knockdown of Slingshot or LIM kinase. *The Journal of Biological Chemistry.* March 7, 2008;283(10):6013–6021.

143. Chang MC, Chen CA, Chen PJ, Chiang YC, Chen YL, Mao TL et al. Mesothelin enhances invasion of ovarian cancer by inducing MMP-7 through MAPK/ERK and JNK pathways. *The Biochemical Journal.* March 1, 2012;442(2):293–302.

144. Mizutani K, Kofuji K, Shirouzu K. The significance of MMP-1 and MMP-2 in peritoneal disseminated metastasis of gastric cancer. *Surgery Today.* 2000;30(7):614–621.

145. Moss NM, Barbolina MV, Liu Y, Sun L, Munshi HG, Stack MS. Ovarian cancer cell detachment and multicellular aggregate formation are regulated by membrane type 1 matrix metalloproteinase: A potential role in I.p. metastatic dissemination. *Cancer Research*. September 1, 2009;69(17):7121–7129.

146. Nonaka T, Nishibashi K, Itoh Y, Yana I, Seiki M. Competitive disruption of the tumor-promoting function of membrane type 1 matrix metalloproteinase/matrix metalloproteinase-14 in vivo. *Molecular Cancer Therapeutics*. August 2005;4(8):1157–1166.

147. Dorman G, Cseh S, Hajdu I, Barna L, Konya D, Kupai K et al. Matrix metalloproteinase inhibitors: A critical appraisal of design principles and proposed therapeutic utility. *Drugs*. May 28, 2010;70(8):949–964.

148. Hirashima Y, Kobayashi H, Suzuki M, Tanaka Y, Kanayama N, Terao T. Transforming growth factor-beta1 produced by ovarian cancer cell line HRA stimulates attachment and invasion through an up-regulation of plasminogen activator inhibitor type-1 in human peritoneal mesothelial cells. *The Journal of Biological Chemistry*. July 18, 2003;278(29):26793–26802.

149. Satoyoshi R, Aiba N, Yanagihara K, Yashiro M, Tanaka M. Tks5 activation in mesothelial cells creates invasion front of peritoneal carcinomatosis. *Oncogene*. June 11, 2015;34(24):3176–3187.

150. Liotta LA, Kohn EC. The microenvironment of the tumour-host interface. *Nature*. May 17, 2001;411(6835):375–379.

151. Orimo A, Weinberg RA. Stromal fibroblasts in cancer: A novel tumor-promoting cell type. *Cell Cycle*. August 2006;5(15):1597–1601.

152. Cirri P, Chiarugi P. Cancer-associated-fibroblasts and tumour cells: A diabolic liaison driving cancer progression. *Cancer Metastasis Reviews*. June 2012;31(1–2):195–208.

153. Sandoval P, Jimenez-Heffernan JA, Rynne-Vidal A, Perez-Lozano ML, Gilsanz A, Ruiz-Carpio V et al. Carcinoma-associated fibroblasts derive from mesothelial cells via mesothelial-to-mesenchymal transition in peritoneal metastasis. *The Journal of Pathology*. December 2013;231(4):517–531.

154. Lv ZD, Na D, Ma XY, Zhao C, Zhao WJ, Xu HM. Human peritoneal mesothelial cell transformation into myofibroblasts in response to TGF-ss1 in vitro. *International Journal of Molecular Medicine*. February 2011;27(2):187–193.

155. Lv ZD, Wang HB, Dong Q, Kong B, Li JG, Yang ZC et al. Mesothelial cells differentiate into fibroblast-like cells under the scirrhous gastric cancer microenvironment and promote peritoneal carcinomatosis in vitro and in vivo. *Molecular and Cellular Biochemistry*. May 2013;377(1–2):177–185.

156. Miao ZF, Zhao TT, Wang ZN, Miao F, Xu YY, Mao XY et al. Transforming growth factor-beta1 signaling blockade attenuates gastric cancer cell-induced peritoneal mesothelial cell fibrosis and alleviates peritoneal dissemination both in vitro and in vivo. *Tumour Biology: The Journal of the International Society for Oncodevelopmental Biology and Medicine*. April 2014;35(4):3575–3583.

157. Tsukada T, Fushida S, Harada S, Yagi Y, Kinoshita J, Oyama K et al. The role of human peritoneal mesothelial cells in the fibrosis and progression of gastric cancer. *International Journal of Oncology*. August 2012;41(2):476–482.

158. Kenny HA, Chiang CY, White EA, Schryver EM, Habis M, Romero IL et al. Mesothelial cells promote early ovarian cancer metastasis through fibronectin secretion. *The Journal of Clinical Investigation*. October 1, 2014;124(10):4614–4628.

159. Baker EA, El Gaddal S, Aitken DG, Leaper DJ. Growth factor profiles in intraperitoneal drainage fluid following colorectal surgery: Relationship to wound healing and surgery. *Wound Repair and Regeneration: Official Publication of the Wound Healing Society [and] the European Tissue Repair Society*. July to August 2003;11(4):261–267.

160. Hofer SO, Shrayer D, Reichner JS, Hoekstra HJ, Wanebo HJ. Wound-induced tumor progression: A probable role in recurrence after tumor resection. *Archives of Surgery*. April 1998;133(4):383–389.

161. Whitworth MK, Sheen A, Rosa DD, Duff SE, Ryder D, Burumdayal A et al. Impact of laparotomy and liver resection on the peritoneal concentrations of fibroblast growth factor 2, vascular endothelial growth factor and hepatocyte growth factor. *Journal of Cancer Research and Clinical Oncology*. January 2006;132(1):41–44.

162. Jiang W, Hiscox S, Matsumoto K, Nakamura T. Hepatocyte growth factor/scatter factor, its molecular, cellular and clinical implications in cancer. *Critical Reviews in Oncology/Hematology*. February 1999;29(3):209–248.

163. Ayhan A, Ertunc D, Tok EC, Ayhan A. Expression of the c-Met in advanced epithelial ovarian cancer and its prognostic significance. *International Journal of Gynecological Cancer: Official Journal of the International Gynecological Cancer Society*. July to August 2005;15(4):618–623.

164. Kaji M, Yonemura Y, Harada S, Liu X, Terada I, Yamamoto H. Participation of c-met in the progression of human gastric cancers: Anti-c-met oligonucleotides inhibit proliferation or invasiveness of gastric cancer cells. *Cancer Gene Therapy*. November to December 1996;3(6):393–404.

165. Yashiro M, Chung YS, Inoue T, Nishimura S, Matsuoka T, Fujihara T et al. Hepatocyte growth factor (HGF) produced by peritoneal fibroblasts may affect mesothelial cell morphology and promote peritoneal dissemination. *International Journal of Cancer (Journal International du Cancer)*. 1996;67(2):289–293.

166. Sawada K, Radjabi AR, Shinomiya N, Kistner E, Kenny H, Becker AR et al. c-Met overexpression is a prognostic factor in ovarian cancer and an effective target for inhibition of peritoneal dissemination and invasion. *Cancer Research*. February 15, 2007;67(4):1670–1679.

167. Khan KN, Masuzaki H, Fujishita A, Kitajima M, Hiraki K, Sekine I et al. Interleukin-6- and tumour necrosis factor alpha-mediated expression of hepatocyte growth factor by stromal cells and its involvement in the growth of endometriosis. *Human Reproduction*. October 2005;20(10):2715–2723.

168. Weng J, Mohan RR, Li Q, Wilson SE. IL-1 upregulates keratinocyte growth factor and hepatocyte growth factor mRNA and protein production by cultured stromal fibroblast cells: Interleukin-1 beta expression in the cornea. *Cornea*. July 1997;16(4):465–471.

169. Fujiwara H, Kubota T, Amaike H, Inada S, Takashima K, Atsuji K et al. Suppression of peritoneal implantation of gastric cancer cells by adenovirus vector-mediated NK4 expression. *Cancer Gene Therapy*. February 2005;12(2):206–216.

170. Cui JJ. Targeting receptor tyrosine kinase MET in cancer: Small molecule inhibitors and clinical progress. *Journal of Medicinal Chemistry*. June 12, 2014;57(11):4427–4453.

171. Naka T, Nishimoto N, Kishimoto T. The paradigm of IL-6: From basic science to medicine. *Arthritis Research*. 2002;4(Suppl. 3):S233–S242.

172. Garg R, Wollan M, Galic V, Garcia R, Goff BA, Gray HJ et al. Common polymorphism in interleukin 6 influences survival of women with ovarian and peritoneal carcinoma. *Gynecologic Oncology*. December 2006;103(3):793–796.

173. Wang Y, Niu XL, Qu Y, Wu J, Zhu YQ, Sun WJ et al. Autocrine production of interleukin-6 confers cisplatin and paclitaxel resistance in ovarian cancer cells. *Cancer Letters*. September 1, 2010;295(1):110–123.

174. Rath KS, Funk HM, Bowling MC, Richards WE, Drew AF. Expression of soluble interleukin-6 receptor in malignant ovarian tissue. *American Journal of Obstetrics Gynecology*. September 2010;203(3):230 e1–e8.

175. Syed V, Ulinski G, Mok SC, Ho SM. Reproductive hormone-induced, STAT3-mediated interleukin 6 action in normal and malignant human ovarian surface epithelial cells. *Journal of the National Cancer Institute*. April 17, 2002;94(8):617–629.

176. Ksiazek K, Jorres A, Witowski J. Senescence induces a proangiogenic switch in human peritoneal mesothelial cells. *Rejuvenation Research*. June 2008;11(3):681–683.

3

Applied radiological anatomy of the peritoneal cavity

KATIE PLANCHE

INTRODUCTION

The peritoneal cavity is a complex anatomical structure that envelops and supports the intra-abdominal organs. It provides the framework for the developing gastrointestinal (GI) tract as it transforms from a simple open-ended tube into the elaborately arranged multitude of loops and segments, which constitute the adult bowel. It provides pathways for blood vessels, nerves, and lymphatics, which connect the intra- and extraperitoneal spaces, allowing spread of disease processes in both directions.

The peritoneal recesses within this cavity are in anatomic continuity, punctuated by mesenteries, ligaments, and fasciae, which may confine pathology or provide routes for disease spread.

It should be noted that the abdominal subperitoneal space is continuous with the thorax providing access for the bidirectional spread of disease between the chest and abdomen.

Modern cross-sectional imaging techniques can produce exquisitely detailed imaging of the peritoneal cavity, allowing the assessment and diagnosis of many disease processes affecting this region. Previously, abnormalities within the peritoneal cavity could only be assumed by their secondary effects on the intra-abdominal organs, for example, the displacement of bowel loops by mass effect, as seen on barium studies. The new generation of multidetector computed tomography (CT) scanners can produce volumetric images within seconds with high spatial resolution to visualize fine detail within the peritoneal cavity. Magnetic resonance imaging (MRI) provides images with high contrast resolution, and diffusion-weighted (DW) MRI has the ability to provide some functional information. Positron emission tomography (PET) scans can provide functional information, and when these images are fused with CT images in PET-CT, an accurate anatomical location for pathology can be given.

The following topics will be discussed in this chapter: the embryology and anatomy of the peritoneal cavity, different imaging modalities used to image this region, and the imaging appearance of pathology within the peritoneal cavity.

EMBRYOLOGY

The anatomy of the abdomen, and in particular the peritoneal cavity, initially appears confusing, with multiple interconnections and spaces, which may or may not be visible on imaging. Knowledge of the embryological development of this region can help us understand these interconnections.

The ventral and dorsal mesenteries suspend the primitive gut within the developing peritoneal cavity and divide it into right and left. As the organs develop, they acquire a visceral peritoneal covering, protruding into the peritoneal sac while remaining connected to their extraperitoneal origins via neurovascular and lymphatic structures [1] (Figure 3.1).

Cranial to the transverse mesocolon, the ventral mesentery contains the liver bud and the dorsal mesentery the splenic bud. As development continues, these organs migrate anticlockwise taking their attached mesenteries with them. This migration divides the right peritoneal cavity into the perihepatic space and the lesser sac. The lesser sac, although located in the mid-left abdomen is embryologically part of the right peritoneal cavity, connected to it by the narrow aperture of the epiploic foramen (foramen of Winslow) (Figure 3.1).

The liver splits the ventral mesentery into the falciform ligament anteriorly and the gastrohepatic ligament (lesser omentum) posteriorly. The free margin of the falciform ligament contains the left umbilical vein forming the ligamentum teres. The free margin of the gastrohepatic ligament contains the common bile duct, portal vein, and hepatic artery and is known as the hepatoduodenal ligament [1].

The splenic bud arises in the dorsal mesentery and gives rise to the gastrosplenic ligament, connecting the spleen and stomach, and the splenorenal ligament, connecting the spleen and kidney. The dorsal mesentery also gives rise to the small bowel mesentery, the transverse mesocolon, and the sigmoid mesocolon.

Posteriorly, the dorsal mesentery connecting the pancreas to the body wall fuses with the posterior abdominal wall, to form part of the anterior pararenal space, making this a retroperitoneal organ (Figures 3.1 and 3.2).

The primitive gut undergoes a complex series of rotations and elongations before settling in its final position within the peritoneal cavity. The fusion of certain segments of bowel produces the adult configuration of the abdomen, with some intraperitoneal segments of bowel: stomach, proximal duodenum, small bowel, transverse colon, and sigmoid colon. These retain posterior attachments to the body wall via their mesenteries.

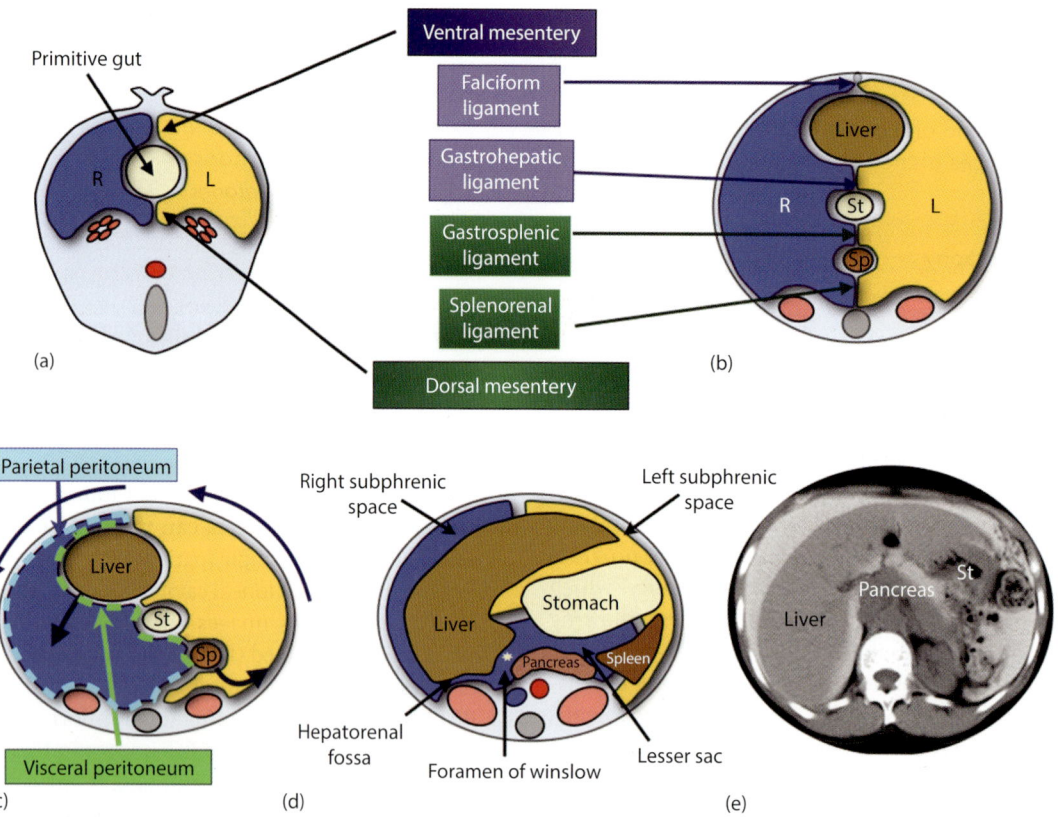

Figure 3.1 Diagrams illustrating the embryological development of the peritoneal spaces: **(a)** 4-week fetus, **(b)** 5-week fetus, **(c)** 10-week fetus, and **(d)** adult. The peritoneal cavity is divided into right and left by the ventral and dorsal mesenteries; the developing viscera invaginate the peritoneum and rotate anticlockwise, taking their mesenteries with them, forming recesses within the peritoneal cavity. **(e)** Axial image from a CT peritoneogram; high-density contrast is seen outlining the peritoneal cavity demonstrating the peritoneal spaces.

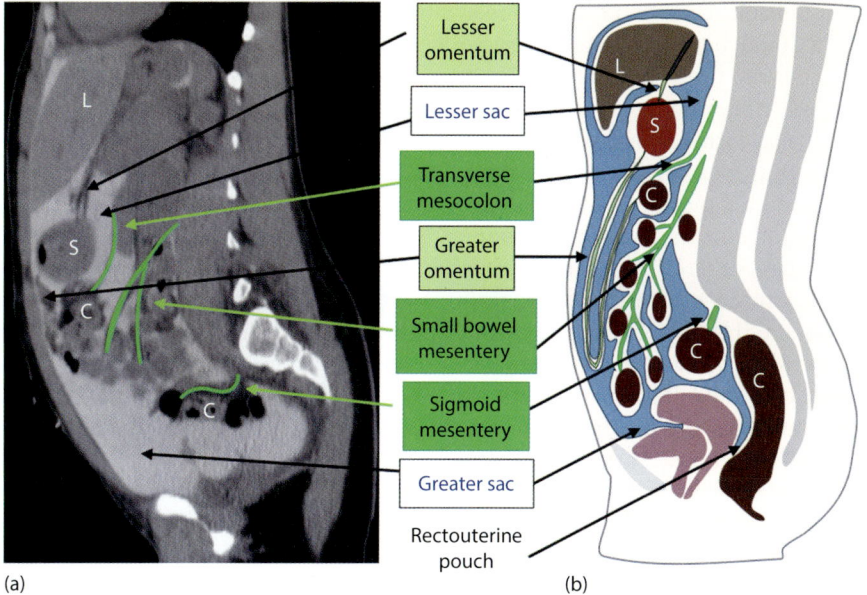

Figure 3.2 **(a)** Sagittal image from a CT peritoneogram with **(b)** diagram illustrating the mesenteries, greater and lesser sac, and omenta. L, liver; S, stomach; C, colon.

The early mesenteries of some segments of bowel fuse with the posterior abdominal wall after they have rotated into position, resulting in extraperitoneal segments: esophagus, majority of the duodenum, ascending colon, descending colon, and rectum.

TERMINOLOGY

The peritoneal cavity is lined by the peritoneum, a large and complex serous membrane, usually less than 1 mm in thickness. It is difficult to see on conventional imaging modalities, but becomes visible when thickened by disease processes such as malignant infiltration or inflammation.

The peritoneum consists of two continuous transparent layers: the parietal and visceral peritoneum. The parietal peritoneum lines the internal surface of the abdominopelvic cavity and has multiple attachments to the abdominal wall. The parietal peritoneum is reflected over the viscera, where it is known as the visceral peritoneum. The peritoneal cavity is a potential space, only becoming apparent on cross-sectional imaging when filled with abnormal fluid or gas [1] (Figure 3.1).

The peritoneal cavity can be divided into two regions: the larger main region being the greater sac and a small diverticulum forming the lesser sac.

Intraperitoneal organs

Strictly speaking, there are no organs within the peritoneal cavity itself, which normally only contains peritoneal fluid. The "intraperitoneal" organs, such as the liver and spleen, invaginate into the peritoneal cavity during embryological development and are completely or almost completely covered by the visceral layer of the peritoneum.

Extra- or retroperitoneal organs, such as the kidneys and pancreas, lie outside the peritoneal cavity, exterior or posterior to the parietal peritoneum. These organs are usually only partially covered anteriorly by peritoneum, with their posterior peritoneal coverings partly resorbed during development [1].

MESENTERIES, LIGAMENTS, AND OMENTA

These terms are used to describe the parts of the peritoneum connecting organs with each other or to the abdominal wall.

A mesentery is a double layer of peritoneum suspending the small or large bowel from the posterior abdominal wall. It acts as a conduit for neurovascular and lymphatic structures between the organ and the subperitoneal space. True mesenteries connect directly to the posterior abdominal wall, whereas specialized mesenteries (the omenta and mesoappendix) are not attached to the posterior abdominal wall (Figure 3.2).

A peritoneal ligament is formed by two layers of peritoneum and supports a structure within the peritoneal cavity. Ligaments are named according to the structures they connect. For example, the gastrosplenic ligament connects the stomach to the spleen; the splenorenal ligament connects the kidney to the spleen (Figure 3.1).

An omentum refers to a double-layered continuation of peritoneal ligaments joining the stomach and proximal duodenum to adjacent structures.

The greater omentum extends from the greater curvature of the stomach and consists of the gastrocolic ligament, the gastrosplenic ligament, and the gastrophrenic ligament. Its descending and ascending layers fuse, forming a four-layered structure in continuity with the lesser sac [2] (Figure 3.2). It drapes over the transverse colon and hangs down a variable length anteriorly as an apron of fat, covering the small bowel allowing free peristalsis. The greater omentum is easily identifiable at surgery but difficult to see on cross-sectional imaging when normal, as it cannot be differentiated from the surrounding mesenteric fat. It can be easily identified when infiltrated with malignant cells, for example, in disseminated ovarian malignancy when it may form an "omental cake."

The lesser omentum extends from the lesser curvature of the stomach to the liver and is made up of the gastro-hepatic and hepatoduodenal ligaments, the hepatoduodenal ligament forming the free edge of the gastrohepatic ligament. These ligaments can be identified on imaging by the structures they contain; the gastrohepatic ligament attaches the lesser curvature of the stomach to the liver and contains the coronary vein and left gastric artery. The hepatoduodenal ligament attaches the duodenum to the liver and contains the portal vein, hepatic artery, common hepatic ducts, and part of the cystic duct [2–4] (Figure 3.2).

ANATOMY OF THE PERITONEAL CAVITY

The peritoneal cavity is divided into interconnecting spaces, the supramesocolic and inframesocolic spaces (divided by the transverse mesocolon) and the pelvic cavity. The small bowel mesentery divides the inframesocolic compartment into two spaces, a larger left compartment, which opens toward the pelvis, and a smaller right compartment [1,5] (Figure 3.3).

The transverse mesocolon suspends the transverse colon from the posterior wall; it lies horizontally across the duodenum and pancreas. The duodenocolic ligament forms the right lateral border where it can be identified by the middle colic vessels. The phrenicocolic ligament forms the left lateral border, between the inferior margin of the spleen and the proximal descending colon.

The small bowel mesentery is a fan-shaped structure that suspends ~600 cm of small bowel from the mesenteric root that extends obliquely over ~15 cm from the region of the duodenojejunal flexure on the left to the region to the right iliac fossa [1] (Figure 3.3).

Supramesocolic compartment

The supramesocolic compartment refers to the intraperitoneal spaces within the upper abdomen above the transverse colon and contains the stomach, liver, and spleen. The falciform ligament divides the supramesocolic compartment into left and right (Figure 3.3).

The right subphrenic space is partially limited postero-inferiorly by the coronary ligament of the liver, which suspends the right lobe of the liver posteriorly, but otherwise communicates freely with the perihepatic and subhepatic spaces, including the hepatorenal fossa (Morison's pouch). The hepatorenal fossa is the most dependent part of the right paravertebral groove in the supine position. It also communicates with the lesser sac via the slit-like epiploic foramen. This is easily closed off from the remainder of the peritoneal cavity by adhesions, so the lesser sac is not a common site for the intraperitoneal spread of infection, and a lesser sac collection is usually the result of local pathology, for example, posterior gastric wall perforation or pancreatitis. The greater and lesser omentum and transverse mesocolon form the lesser sac boundaries and act as pathways for disease spread to and from the anterior pararenal space, mesenteric root, and transverse colon. For example, gastric neoplasms can spread along the greater omentum to involve the superior border of the transverse colon, and vice versa. Similar patterns of spread

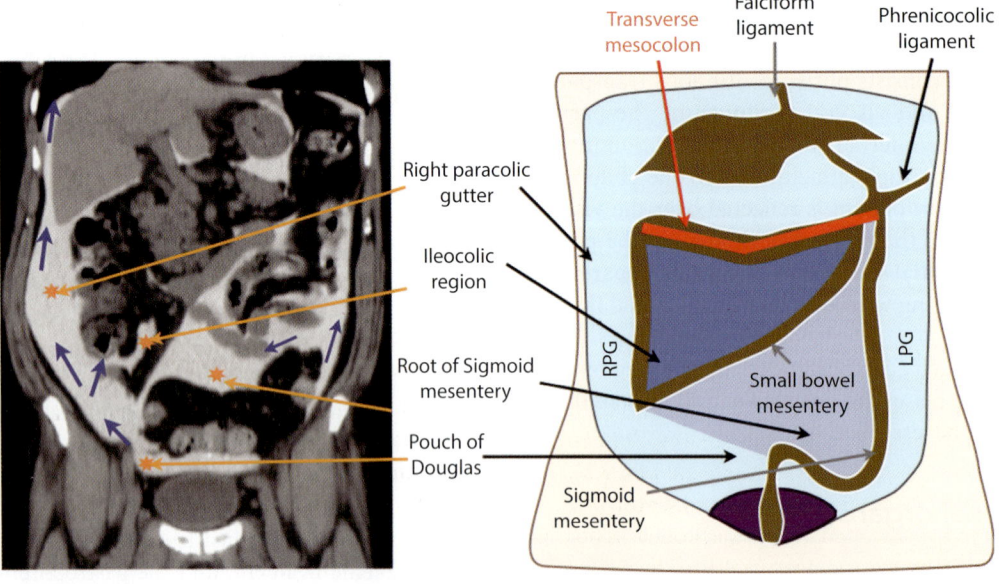

Figure 3.3 Coronal image from a CT peritoneogram with associated diagram showing the direction of flow of peritoneal fluid (blue arrows) and sites of maximum fluid stasis (orange stars). On the diagram, the bowel has been removed to demonstrate the locations of the mesenteries and how these divide the peritoneal spaces. RPG, right paracolic gutter; LPG, left paracolic gutter.

can be seen with pancreatic pathology, which can travel along the transverse mesocolon, with preferential involvement of the inferior border of the transverse colon.

There is no compartmentalization of the left subphrenic space allowing free communication between left subphrenic and perisplenic space. The phrenicocolic ligament, which suspends the splenic flexure of the colon from the diaphragm, separates the left subphrenic space from the left paracolic gutter (Figure 3.3).

Inframesocolic compartment

The inframesocolic compartment lies posterior to the greater omentum, below the transverse mesocolon, medial to the ascending and descending colon and contains the small bowel and ascending and descending colon. It is divided into right and left by the oblique small bowel mesentery, which extends from the duodenojejunal junction, located to the left of midline at the level of the first or second lumbar vertebra to the ileocecal junction in the right iliac fossa (Figure 3.3).

The dorsal mesentery gives rise to the transverse mesocolon, small bowel mesentery, sigmoid mesentery, and mesoappendix. The ventral mesentery regresses below the transverse mesocolon [4,6]. The mesorectum attaches to the posterior pelvis creating the perirectal space. Lateral to the ascending and descending colon are the right and left paracolic gutters. The right paracolic gutter is continuous with the right perihepatic space. On the left, the phrenicocolic ligament prevents direct communication between the left paracolic gutter and the left subphrenic space [7]. This helps to contain pathology, such as a left subphrenic abscess. The phrenicocolic ligament can also act as a conduit for disease, allowing the spread of pancreatic pathologies to the splenic flexure of the transverse colon.

The supramesocolic compartment communicates with the inframesocolic compartments via the right paracolic gutter [1].

Pelvis

The peritoneum reflects over the pelvic organs to form most of the pelvic ligaments and mesenteries, creating the midline rectouterine pouch (pouch of Douglas) in females and the rectovesical pouch in males and the paravesical fossae. The pelvis makes up about one-third of the volume of the peritoneal cavity and is the most dependent part in both the erect and supine position, resulting in fluid stasis in this region, making it a common site for abscesses, fluid collections, and metastatic deposits [1] (Figures 3.2 and 3.3). The pelvis communicates freely with the paracolic gutters.

In females, the broad ligament is a peritoneal reflection forming the mesentery for the ovaries, fallopian tubes, and posterior myometrium. It also drapes over the ureters and round ligament. The peritoneum is discontinuous at the opening of the fallopian tubes in females, allowing spread of disease between intra- and extraperitoneal compartments.

PERITONEAL FLUID CIRCULATION

The peritoneal cavity normally contains only a thin film of fluid, approximately 50–100 mL. This fluid is continually produced, circulated, and resorbed. Direction of flow is determined by diaphragmatic movement and bowel peristalsis. Normally, the pressure in the subdiaphragmatic region is subatmospheric, and during inspiration, pressure decreases further as the outward movement of the rib cage is greater than the descent of the diaphragm. This creates an intra-abdominal pressure gradient encouraging fluid to flow up the paracolic gutters even in a standing position. Limitations to flow are imposed by peritoneal attachments and ligaments. The peritoneal fluid takes the path of least resistance resulting in increased flow up the right paracolic gutter, which is deeper and wider than the left paracolic gutter. The majority of the fluid is resorbed via lymphatics in the subphrenic space [1,5] (Figure 3.3).

Transcoelomic spread of disease is facilitated by this physiological flow of intraperitoneal fluid. Once a primary tumor or malignant lymph node has broken through into the peritoneal cavity, malignant cells will be shed into the peritoneal fluid and are then actively transported around the peritoneal cavity.

Peritoneal fluid is reabsorbed through lymphatic channels in the diaphragm, with 80% of the absorption occurring from the right diaphragm via the submesothelial lymphatic capillaries of the diaphragm, which communicate with a comparable plexus on the pleural surface. This provides another pathway for disease dissemination into the pleural cavity, for example, in metastatic ovarian cancer [1,8].

Areas of preferential stasis

The ligaments of the peritoneal cavity act as watersheds, directing the flow of fluid; the most important are the transverse mesocolon, the small bowel mesentery, the sigmoid mesocolon, and the attachments of the ascending and descending colon.

The areas of preferential fluid stasis within the peritoneal cavity are the most dependent locations and regions where there is slower flow of peritoneal fluid. These are commonly the first sites to be involved in the peritoneal spread of infections and metastases (Figure 3.4). The areas of maximum stasis are the rectovesical/rectouterine pouch, the right lower quadrant at the termination of the small bowel mesentery, the root of the sigmoid mesentery, and the right paracolic gutter (Figure 3.3). Fluid from the right paracolic gutter drains into the right subhepatic space and its inferior extension the hepatorenal fossa (Morison's pouch), the most dependent area of the upper abdomen. The dynamics of peritoneal flow and anatomy of this region explain why intraperitoneal abscesses are twice as commonly seen on the right, with the hepatorenal fossa the most common location [1].

Figure 3.4 **(a)** Sagittal T2 MR and **(b)** sagittal CT image post IV and oral contrast. A 70-year-old female with disseminated intraperitoneal hydatid disease with a large deposit in the rectouterine pouch (of Douglas). The multiple internal septations and loculations are much better demonstrated on the MRI.

INTRAPERITONEAL SPREAD OF DISEASE: RADIOLOGICAL ANALYSIS

The anatomic configuration of the peritoneal cavity and the dynamic flow of intraperitoneal fluid and cells produce pathology with characteristic radiological appearances.

If a patient has a known primary malignancy, such as colorectal cancer, imaging assessment should look for both local disease and distant disease dissemination, with intraperitoneal deposits most likely to be found in the regions of preferential fluid stasis, which must be carefully assessed. The commonest sites for the intraperitoneal seeding of metastases are the pouch of Douglas, root of the small bowel mesentery, sigmoid mesentery, and right paracolic gutter.

If a patient presents with metastatic disease from an unknown primary site, the distribution of peritoneal deposits may point to the primary tumor site. This can be particularly useful in midgut neuroendocrine tumors (NET), which often present with large nodal deposits in the small bowel mesentery and an occult primary site. Careful analysis of the loop of small bowel supplied by that segment of mesentery will often yield an enhancing nodule consistent with the primary tumor (often less than 1 cm in size at the time of diagnosis) particularly if dedicated imaging using CT or MR enterography is used [9].

IMAGING APPEARANCES OF THE PERITONEAL CAVITY

The peritoneal cavity is a potential space and is visible on imaging only when affected by disease processes causing thickening of the peritoneum, or the accumulation of abnormal gas or fluid within the peritoneal cavity.

Imaging is indispensible in the diagnosis, staging, and follow-up of peritoneal disease. Pathological confirmation will almost invariably be required, and imaging can be used both to select an appropriate site for biopsy and to guide this.

The appearance of the peritoneal cavity on different imaging modalities will be outlined in the following text.

Plain film

The plain abdominal radiograph provides extremely limited information on the peritoneal cavity due to the overlapping of relevant structures and has been largely replaced by other imaging modalities. The peritoneum will be visible if calcified, as in encapsulating peritoneal sclerosis. The peritoneal cavity will be visible if there is a large volume of free intraperitoneal gas in the case of a perforated viscus.

Ultrasound

Ultrasound has the advantages of being quick to perform, easily accessible, and relatively cheap, with the benefit of direct patient contact to allow correlation of imaging with patient symptoms. However, it is operator dependent and images may be limited in obese patients [10]. Ultrasound can also be used for the guided drainage of collections or ascites and for the guided biopsy of abnormal regions in order to obtain a tissue diagnosis.

The abdomen is usually scanned with a curvilinear probe of 3.5–5 MHz, which provides sufficient depth penetration (~10–15 cm) for visualization of the intra-abdominal contents. Higher-frequency linear probes (7.5–12 MHz) can be used to provide higher-resolution images, but have more limited depth penetration (3–5 cm), and can be used for superficial structures.

Fluid in the peritoneal cavity can be visualized, and any septation of fluid collections or thickening of the peritoneum is well seen. However, overlying bowel gas may obscure images, and some areas, such as the retroperitoneum, may be difficult to visualize.

In female patients, transvaginal ultrasound can also be performed, as this gives high-resolution images of the pelvis, allowing detailed assessment of the pelvic cavity and pelvic peritoneum for small deposits.

The small bowel mesentery can be visualized on ultrasound in normal patients, as a series of layers stacked on top of each other, each ~1 cm thick; these are more easily visualized in the presence of ascites [11]. Thickening or irregularity of the greater omentum can be demonstrated well with ultrasound, as this is a superficial structure, allowing close assessment with a high-resolution transducer. The thickened omentum may be seen as a "floating cake" within ascitic fluid or may be adherent to underlying small bowel loops.

Ascites occurs following the abnormal accumulation of fluid within the peritoneal cavity. It can be produced by numerous different pathologies; the distribution of fluid and other characteristics seen on ultrasound can help to differentiate between these. Simple ascites is seen as anechoic fluid collecting in the dependent areas of the peritoneal cavity—the rectouterine/rectovesical pouch, the hepatorenal recess, and the paracolic gutters. There are no septations or thickening of the underlying peritoneum.

If ascites is secondary to malignancy or inflammation; other signs such as loculations or septations, displacement of intraperitoneal bowel loops, debris within the fluid, and peritoneal nodularity may be seen.

Pseudomyxoma peritonei produces mucinous ascites, which is seen on ultrasound as echogenic fluid with displacement of small bowel loops, septations, and scalloping of the liver edge [11].

COMPUTED TOMOGRAPHY

Advances in CT technology have transformed image quality in recent years. The advent of multidetector scanners enables the rapid acquisition of volumetric images with high spatial resolution allowing the identification of subcentimeter deposits in the peritoneal cavity. In addition, rapid acquisition time provides high temporal resolution, which minimizes motion artifact from small bowel peristalsis, previously a major problem in imaging of the peritoneal cavity. Multiplanar images are now produced routinely and are useful to analyze lesions on curved surfaces such as the diaphragm and pelvis and to clearly show the relationships of deposits to important vascular structures, which is helpful in surgical planning [12].

The main disadvantage of CT is the exposure to ionizing radiation, although techniques such as iterative reconstruction are reducing dose, making this less of an issue. A further drawback is the need for intravenous iodinated contrast, which may be contraindicated in some patients due to allergy, and restricted in others due to renal impairment.

The normal peritoneum is not routinely seen on CT in its entirety. Some regions of the peritoneum, for instance, the mesorectal fascia and broad ligament, can be identified in normal patients. The location of the peritoneal ligaments can be inferred by the vascular structures they contain. CT is extremely sensitive for the presence of even tiny volumes of free intraperitoneal gas or fluid. Thickening and nodularity of the peritoneum can also be seen in disseminated

malignancies or intraperitoneal infections such as tuberculous peritonitis.

CT is an invaluable tool for the follow-up of patients with metastatic disease, allowing reproducible measurements to be taken to monitor disease progression or response to treatment.

Peritoneal deposits may have a variable appearance on CT. Usually, they will appear as soft tissue nodules, which can coalesce forming plaques over the viscera, which may show postcontrast enhancement or calcification. Deposits may also be of fluid density, for example, in mucinous tumors.

CT techniques

To visualize peritoneal pathology, a scan of the abdomen and pelvis is performed post intravenous contrast. Scans are routinely acquired in the portal venous phase, approximately 60 seconds postcontrast injection; this gives optimum organ and peritoneal enhancement (Figure 3.5).

CT angiography is acquired in the arterial phase (approximately 30 seconds postcontrast) and may be useful if detailed imaging of the arteries is required, for example, to assess patency of encased vessels in patients with extensive mesenteric nodal metastases from metastatic midgut NET.

The CT peritoneogram is a technique used in patients on continuous ambulatory peritoneal dialysis (CAPD) to look for the presence of hernias. Dilute contrast is introduced into the peritoneal cavity via the CAPD catheter and its

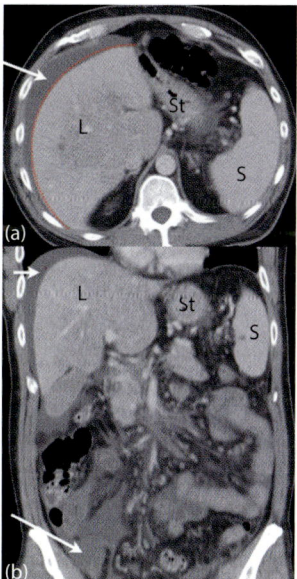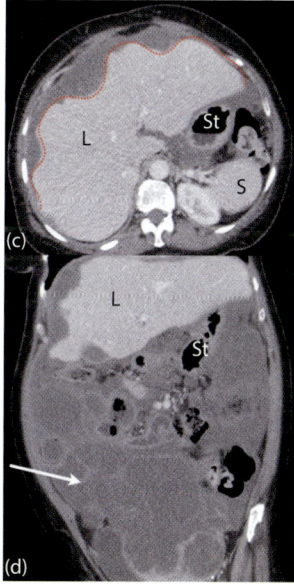

Figure 3.5 **(a)** Axial and **(b)** coronal postcontrast CT images in a 50-year-old man with simple ascites following thrombosis of the superior mesenteric vein. Note the smooth liver edge (red dotted line) and intraperitoneal fluid (arrow). **(c)** Axial and **(d)** coronal images from a postcontrast CT in a patient with pseudomyxoma peritonei; note the scalloping of the liver edge (red dotted line) and extensive loculations (arrow) in the fluid. L = liver, St = stomach, S = spleen.

distribution analyzed. The high-density fluid can be easily identified outlining the peritoneal cavity and showing its recesses and interconnections (Figures 3.1 through 3.3).

MAGNETIC RESONANCE IMAGING

MRI has several advantages over CT. MRI does not involve the use of ionizing radiation but exploits the inherent properties of different tissues to produce different signals after magnetic gradients are applied. This produces images with good soft tissues resolution to allow detailed characterization of masses and fluid collections (Figure 3.4). Contrast enhancement is with gadolinium, which is useful if patients are allergic to iodinated contrast media.

However, MRI of the abdomen and pelvis is a far more time-consuming procedure than CT with scans typically taking 30–45 minutes to acquire. This makes the images more susceptible to motion artifact from small bowel peristalsis, breathing, and patient movement. Additionally, some patients are unable to tolerate MRI due to claustrophobia [13].

Peritoneal deposits enhance slowly postcontrast injection and are best seen on images taken 5–10 minutes postcontrast. Normal peritoneum enhances similarly to liver on MRI, so abnormal enhancement should be suspected if the peritoneum is enhancing more than the liver or if any associated abnormality is seen such as thickening or nodularity [14].

MR diffusion-weighted imaging (DWI) uses the diffusion of water molecules in tissues to produce images and can provide some functional, quantitative information about tissue cellularity to assess tumors and their response to therapy.

DWI does not require any extra equipment and may be added onto standard MRI protocols. An increase in cellularity, for example, in malignancy or inflammation, causes a restriction in the diffusion of water molecules. The more the motion of water molecules is restricted, the more signal is produced. The DW images can be superimposed on anatomic images (in a similar manner to CT-PET) to be viewed as fusion images. Most malignant tumors of the GI tract show increased cellularity, resulting in restricted diffusion, which will be seen as an area of increased signal intensity on DW images. These abnormal areas can then be correlated with the imaging obtained on other MRI sequences. Abnormal areas of diffusion may enable the identification of small lesions, which could be overlooked on standard CT and MR images. This technique can be particularly useful to diagnose small peritoneal deposits, as the signal from normal surrounding organs is suppressed.

Quantitative analysis of DW images can also be performed by calculating the apparent diffusion coefficient (ADC) of different tissues, with a low value produced in areas of restricted diffusion (e.g., malignant deposits). This may be useful in assessing response to treatment, with tumors showing a response to treatment having higher posttreatment ADC values [15,16].

POSITRON EMISSION TOMOGRAPHY–COMPUTED TOMOGRAPHY

PET-CT combines the cross-sectional anatomic information provided by CT with the metabolic information provided by PET. Images are acquired during a single examination and fused to allow accurate localization on the CT images of any region of increased activity seen on the PET images [17]. Standard PET-CT is performed using [18]fluorodeoxyglucose (FDG) and can provide metabolic information about tumor activity. In specific situations, other tracers can be used, for example, in NET; newer agents have been developed for PET to assess somatostatin receptor–positive tumors such as ^{68}Ga-tetraazocyclodecanetetraacetic acid-octreotate (68Ga-DOTATATE), as this is actively taken up by these tumors [9].

PET has the ability to demonstrate abnormal metabolic activity at the molecular level in organs that do not yet demonstrate abnormal morphology, which could be identified on conventional CT or MRI. PET-CT can be useful to differentiate benign from malignant disease, to identify distant spread of disease, and to assess disease response. PET-CT also provides imaging of the entire body so may identify disease at unexpected sites.

The disadvantages of PET-CT include the exposure to ionizing radiation, a whole body PET-CT giving an exposure of ~25 mSv [18] compared to ~10 mSv for a contrast-enhanced CT of the abdomen and pelvis. The PET component of the scan is time consuming, taking ~30 minutes, and also contributes to patient movement artifact. PET-CT is also an expensive resource with limited availability. Certain tumors, for example, mucinous adenocarcinomas, low-grade NET, and certain lymphomas will not show increased activity on PET-CT [19].

The spatial resolution of PET is ~6–10 mm on current scanners [8,17] and it has reduced sensitivity for lesions of less than 1 cm. Normal bowel and urinary uptake can limit the assessment of disease in these regions, so pelvic disease may be difficult to assess.

Images can be interpreted by visual inspection, or using the standardized uptake value (SUV), which can give a quantification of glucose uptake [17]. The SUV is calculated using the formula (tracer activity in tissue /injected radiotracer dose/patient weight). Typically, malignant tumors have an SUV of greater than 2.5–3.0, whereas normal tissues, such as the liver, have SUVs ranging from 0.5 to 2.5 [17]. The SUV can be compared before and after treatment to assess response.

PET-CT can also be used as a problem-solving tool in a patient with discordant clinical and standard CT/MRI findings. For example, in patients with suspected recurrent ovarian cancer, with a rising CA-125 level but negative CT and MR imaging, CT-PET may identify early recurrent disease [8].

On PET-CT, peritoneal deposits appear as nodular soft tissue masses with a variable degree of increased metabolic activity. However, PET-CT is unable to pick up small volume disease (deposits 5–7 mm) or miliary deposits.

Another benefit of PET-CT is that it can accurately identify metastatic disease even in normal-sized lymph nodes on the basis of increased metabolic activity [8].

DISEASE PROCESSES AFFECTING THE PERITONEAL CAVITY

Primary diseases of the peritoneal cavity are uncommon, but this region is a frequent site for secondary spread of disease. Intraperitoneal spread of malignancies and infections, bowel perforations, and trauma are all commonly seen in the peritoneal cavity.

The peritoneal ligaments, mesenteries, and omenta divide the peritoneal cavity into interconnecting spaces and create recesses dictating the location and direction of spread of malignant, inflammatory, and infective processes. These dependent spaces are preferential sites for peritoneal fluid stasis and consequently are common sites for ascites, blood, abscesses, and malignant peritoneal deposits.

Additionally, pathology can spread through the peritoneal cavity via the peritoneal ligaments and mesenteries, which are conduits for lymphatic and vascular structures. These connections allow bidirectional spread of pathology from the peritoneal cavity, via the ligaments and mesenteries to the subperitoneal space and vice versa.

On imaging, the presence of fluid, gas, or soft tissue within the peritoneal cavity indicates underlying pathology and has a wide variety of differential diagnoses. Specific imaging findings can be used to diagnose the cause of these findings.

Fluid

INTRAPERITONEAL FLUID

The finding of fluid within the peritoneal cavity is abnormal, except for the small volume of physiological fluid seen in the pelvis of women of reproductive age. Intraperitoneal fluid is produced due to a combination of factors including lymphatic obstruction, decreased absorption of peritoneal fluid, or increased capillary permeability and fluid production [12]. The causes of fluid accumulation are numerous ranging from low protein states to disseminated malignancies.

Pooling of ascitic fluid occurs maximally within the rectovesical/rectouterine pouch, which is the most dependent part of the peritoneal cavity in the erect or supine position. From here fluid ascends the paracolic gutters, much more so on the right compared to the left, as this is wider and deeper, into the right subhepatic space and its posterior extension the hepatorenal fossa (Morison's pouch) and into the right subphrenic space (Figure 3.3).

The small bowel mesentery forms a series of ruffles as it extends from its narrow base toward the small bowel loops, producing a series of small recesses, and fluid flows down these in a series of rivulets in the axis of the small bowel mesentery from the left upper quadrant to the right lower quadrant, reaching the most inferior point at the level of the ileocecal junction where the largest pool is formed [1]. Fluid is also seen to collect at the superior aspect of the sigmoid mesentery.

When intraperitoneal fluid is identified on imaging, careful assessment needs to be made of the location and composition of the fluid, in addition to any other abnormalities within the peritoneal cavity or elsewhere. These findings can be interpreted with relevant clinical information to provide a likely diagnosis.

SIMPLE FLUID

Simple fluid (ascites) accumulates in conditions such as congestive cardiac failure, low protein states, and chronic liver disease and is seen as low-density fluid in dependent areas of the peritoneal cavity. The first site for fluid collection is usually the rectovesical/rectouterine pouch. Small bowel loops may be seen floating freely in a pool of fluid (Figure 3.5).

COMPLEX FLUID

If ascites is secondary to malignancy or inflammation, loculations/septations, and debris may be seen within the fluid. These features will be best seen on ultrasound or MRI but can be missed on CT due to its inferior soft tissue resolution [13] (Figure 3.4). The fluid tends to form more focal collections, with surrounding enhancing walls seen. There may be displacement of small bowel loops, and the small bowel loops may be matted together by adhesions or peritoneal deposits.

Intraperitoneal abscesses may form secondary to peptic ulcer disease, appendicitis or pancreatitis, or postoperatively, following gastric, biliary, or colonic surgery. Following bacterial contamination of the peritoneal cavity, focal collections are most common at the sites of maximum fluid stasis, especially the pelvis, the hepatorenal recess (Morison's pouch), and right subphrenic space.

Hemorrhage within the peritoneal cavity will alter in appearance with time. Acutely, dense fluid will be seen accumulating at the site of hemorrhage. This can allow the identification of a bleeding site, which may show active extravasation of contrast and blood on CT angiography. The intra- or extraperitoneal location of the hemorrhage will often allow the site of origin to be identified, for example, a splenic laceration will produce intraperitoneal fluid and a renal laceration will produce retroperitoneal fluid. Fluid from bowel injuries may initially bleed between mesenteric folds creating triangular pockets of extraperitoneal fluid, with no fluid/blood seen in the paracolic gutters or pelvis. Conversely, following solid organ injury, blood will initially pool around the injured organ. This will then extend down the paracolic gutters and into the pelvis. Only once these readily accessible spaces are filled, will fluid extend between the mesenteric leaves.

Subacutely, the fluid will produce a layered appearance, as the constituents of blood separate out with more dense fluid seen in dependent areas. This is seen as layers of fluid within the peritoneal cavity, with high-density fluid seen dependently.

Gas

Free gas within the peritoneal cavity is always abnormal. It is often the result of perforation of a viscus, most commonly a gastric/duodenal ulcer or perforated diverticulitis. Other causes include a perforated malignancy of the GI tract and abdominal trauma. Benign causes such as recent instrumentation or pneumatosis intestinalis should also be considered. The site of perforation can usually be ascertained from careful interpretation of CT findings, using knowledge of peritoneal anatomy to interpret the location of free gas (Figure 3.6).

Unlike free fluid, gas will rise to lie against the anterior abdominal wall in the supine patient. The site of perforation and the peritoneal connections it can travel along will determine the location of the gas.

Intraperitoneal segments of the GI tract include the stomach, the proximal duodenum, small bowel, appendix, and transverse and sigmoid colon. Retroperitoneal segments of bowel include the esophagus, part of the duodenum, ascending and descending colon, and rectum. Perforation of the GI tract does not always result in free gas, as surrounding inflammatory change may wall off the abnormal segment, resulting in a fluid/gas collection; this is commonly seen in appendicitis and diverticulitis. CT is the most sensitive imaging technique for the detection of free intraperitoneal air; an accurate diagnosis of the site of perforation can be made on CT in 86% cases [20] (Figure 3.6).

INTRAPERITONEAL GAS

Perforated gastric or duodenal ulcer

Perforation of a peptic ulcer is the most common cause of pneumoperitoneum. Anterior wall ulcers of the stomach and duodenal bulb usually perforate freely into the intraperitoneal space, initially supramesocolic, whereas posterior wall gastric ulcers perforate into the lesser sac. Some ulcers will seal off immediately; the only radiological sign of perforation may be a small locule of gas adjacent to the stomach or in the gastroduodenal ligament. The free gas will pass along the hepatoduodenal ligament into the fissure for ligamentum venosum, adjacent to the portal vein and is seen as discrete locules of gas rather than the branching pattern seen when gas is within the biliary tree (Figure 3.6a).

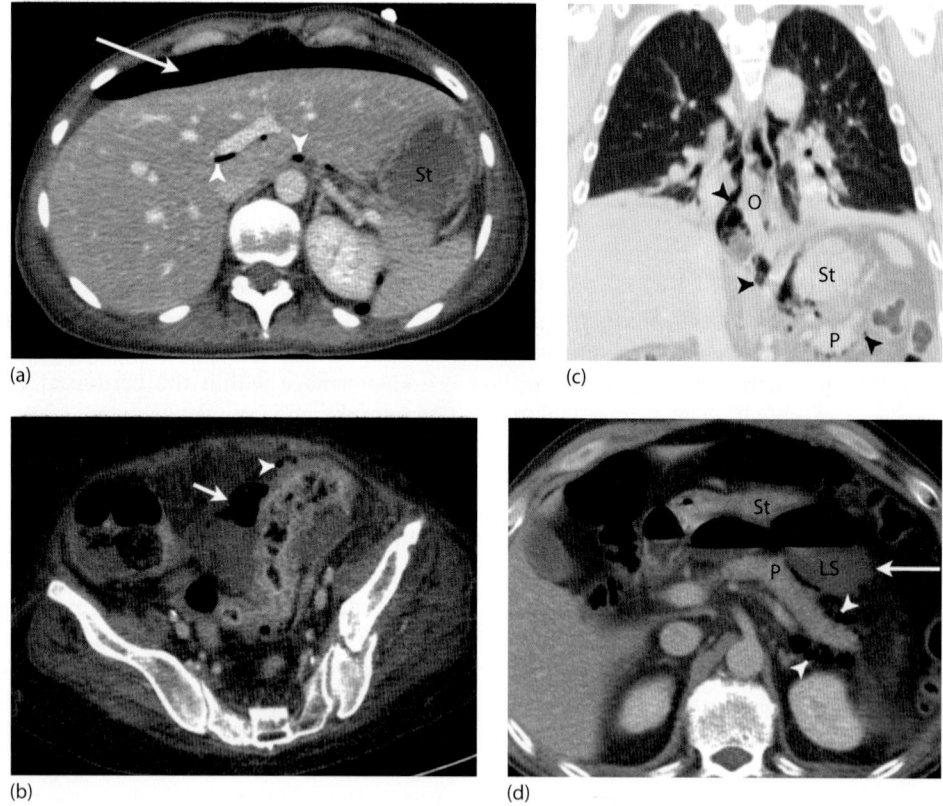

(a)

(c)

(b)

(d)

Figure 3.6 (a) Axial postcontrast CT in a 32-year-old woman with a perforated duodenal ulcer. Note the small locules of free gas (arrowheads) seen in the gastroduodenal ligament and fissure for ligamentum venosum in addition to the large volume of free gas seen anterior to the liver (arrow). (b) Perforated diverticulitis in an 80-year-old woman; free gas can be seen tracking in the sigmoid mesentery (arrowhead), with a gas/fluid collection in the sigmoid mesentery (arrow). (c) Coronal lung windows and (d) axial soft tissue window postcontrast CT in a 55-year-old man with spontaneous esophageal perforation following prolonged vomiting. Note the locules of gas (arrowheads) surrounding the tail of the pancreas (P) and esophagus (E). In addition, there is a gas/fluid collection in the lesser sac (LS) posterior to the stomach (St).

Perforated diverticulitis

When there is perforation of sigmoid diverticulitis, the gas initially tracks into the adjacent sigmoid mesentery before entering the inframesocolic compartment and then the rest of the peritoneal cavity (Figure 3.6b). The differential for a perforated colon includes colorectal cancer. Radiological features suspicious for malignancy include asymmetrical wall thickening (>1.5 cm), shouldering, and large local nodes, but these features are nonspecific and direct visualization will be required in these cases.

Retroperitonal gas

Perforation of a retroperitoneal bowel segment will result in gas in the retroperitoneal spaces.

Esophageal perforation is usually iatrogenic, following endoscopy, but may occasionally rupture spontaneously following severe vomiting (Boerhaave syndrome).

Following esophageal perforation, gas is usually seen on the left just proximal to the esophagogastric junction. From here, free gas can track into the mediastinum, subcutaneously (surgical emphysema), and via the esophageal hiatus, into the retroperitoneum and the peritoneal cavity (Figure 3.6c and d).

Free gas in the anterior pararenal space may be secondary to perforation of the bowel located in this space namely, the duodenum and ascending and descending colon.

In a patient with a pneumothorax, particularly if they are mechanically ventilated, gas may track from the thorax via the subperitoneal space into the retroperitoneal spaces.

Retroperitoneal gas may also be seen associated with infections; peripancreatic collections secondary to pancreatitis may produce gas in the pararenal space or lesser sac. Air in the perirenal space is generally secondary to renal infections, which have spread beyond the capsule.

Soft tissue

Abnormal soft tissue in the peritoneal cavity is usually secondary to transcoelomic spread of malignancy. Other disease processes, such as tuberculous peritonitis and peritoneal lymphomatosis, have similar appearances on imaging, but enlarged nodes, particularly retroperitoneal, are usually more of a feature in these diseases. Pathological confirmation of the diagnosis will generally be required.

INTRAPERITONEAL SPREAD OF METASTASES

Intraperitoneal dissemination of malignancies is not a passive process affecting only the area immediately surrounding the tumor, but, due to the dynamic flow of peritoneal fluid within the peritoneal cavity, an active process transporting free tumor cells shed from the primary around the peritoneal cavity. These cells are removed through lymphatic channels on the diaphragm, mainly located on the right side. Deposits will therefore be frequently seen on the right hemidiaphragm and liver capsule, forming nodules, plaques, or sheetlike masses [1].

The greater omentum contains foci of lymphoid tissue, covered with only loosely connected mesothelial cells,

acting as open lymphatic lacunae, which also absorb peritoneal fluid, bringing any circulating tumor cells into contact with the greater omentum. Omental deposits will initially be seen as discrete nodules, progressing to solid masses forming an "omental cake" appearance (Figure 3.7). Ultrasound may be more sensitive than CT for early changes within the greater omentum.

The pooling of ascitic fluid favors the deposition and growth of malignant cells, which become fixed to the serosal surfaces by fibrinous adhesions [1]. The sites of fluid pooling are therefore common sites for peritoneal deposits (Figure 3.7).

Early peritoneal disease may be seen as subtle diffuse peritoneal thickening and enhancement, enabling the normally inconspicuous peritoneum to be visualized on CT. Peritoneal spread may produce a variety of different patterns on imaging, including thickening, nodularity, and enhancement of the peritoneum and mesenteric fat stranding. Disease in the small bowel mesentery replaces the normal mesenteric fat, making it stiff and losing its normal fold pattern with straightening of the mesenteric vessels producing a pleated or stellate pattern. Small bowel infiltration may lead to small bowel obstruction.

Care must be taken when analyzing lesions surrounding the liver, as deposits on the liver capsule or within the fissures can be misinterpreted as parenchymal liver deposits; these lesions are best assessed using multiplanar reformats on CT or MRI in order to appreciate their relationship to the liver.

PERITONEAL CARCINOMATOSIS

The most common primary sites for peritoneal spread of disease are GI (stomach, colon, appendix, gallbladder, and pancreas) and ovarian (Figure 3.7). Transperitoneal spread of disease may also result in ovarian metastases (Krukenberg tumors) [14].

Patients with ovarian cancer will usually undergo surgery for tumor debulking, but some regions, the diaphragm, splenic hilum, stomach, lesser sac, liver, and mesenteric root are difficult to evaluate at surgery. Imaging is useful to assess these regions preoperatively to determine suitability for neoadjuvant chemotherapy and to follow up response to treatment. It is important to differentiate subcapsular deposits in the liver from parenchymal deposits using multiplanar imaging or reconstructions on CT or MRI to determine suitability for cytoreductive surgery. If implants are seen in the porta hepatis and interlobar fissure, this indicates tumor nonresectability [1].

CT, MRI, and PET have all been used for diagnosis and follow-up, these techniques have different strengths and weaknesses. Usually, a combination of techniques will be required. PET may be useful in patients with negative CT and MRI, but rising tumor markers.

PSEUDOMYXOMA PERITONEI

This is a descriptive term rather than a pathological diagnosis and refers to the presence of large volumes of thick gelatinous material within the peritoneal cavity.

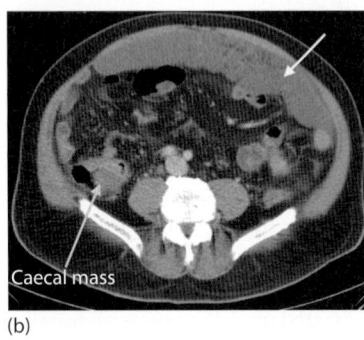
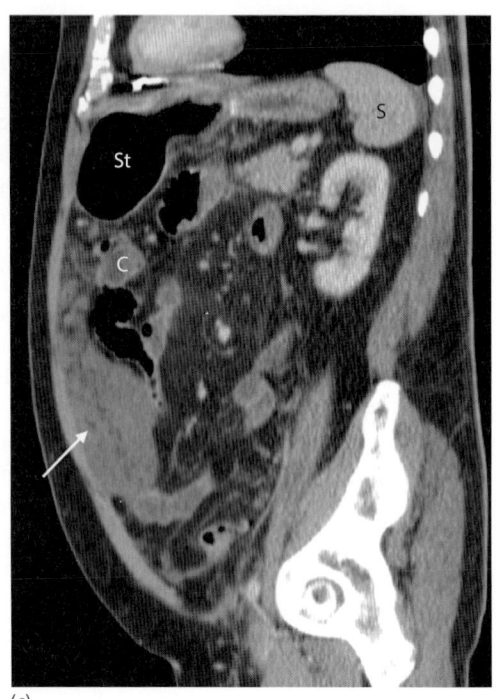

Figure 3.7 (a) and (b) Axial and (c) sagittal images from a postcontrast CT scan in a 74-year-old man with extensive peritoneal disease secondary to colorectal cancer of the cecum. There are peritoneal deposits and stranding seen within the left paracolic gutter (arrowhead) and a large omental cake (arrow).

There are two forms described: Classic pseudomyxoma peritonei is secondary to low-grade mucinous tumors of the appendix, which have ruptured into the peritoneal cavity. It tends to have an indolent course, with its association with ovarian masses likely to be due to secondary ovarian spread [14]. It does not tend to invade visceral organs or pleural spaces or show lymphatic or hematogenous spread.

Mucinous peritoneal carcinomatosis is secondary to mucinous carcinoma of the GI tract or ovary and has a more aggressive course, with a smaller volume of mucin seen. There are commonly associated pathological nodes and pleural extension, with pleural effusions and deposits seen [14].

On ultrasound, pseudomyxoma peritonei is seen as echogenic fluid with internal septations and displacement of bowel loops with scalloping of the liver and spleen. On CT, mucin has low density, often showing some solid elements, with fibrosis of the mesentery, and occasional curvilinear calcification. The mucinous deposits cause extrinsic pressure producing a scalloped effect, seen most easily along the margins of the liver and spleen (Figure 3.5). Close inspection of the appendix should be made, although after rupture, the residual appendix may be small, with no identifiable mass [14].

CONCLUSION

An understanding of peritoneal anatomy is vital for the identification, diagnosis, and follow-up of peritoneal disease.

Ultrasound, CT, MRI, and PET all play a vital role in the assessment of disease processes in the peritoneal cavity.

REFERENCES

1. Meyers MA, Charnsangavej C, Oliphant M. *Meyers' Dynamic Radiology of the Abdomen: Normal and Pathologic Anatomy*, 6th edn., New York: Springer-Verlag, 2011. pp. 9–196.
2. Eunhye Y, Joo HK, Myeong-Jin K, Jeong-Sik Y, Jae-Joon C, Hyung-Sik Y, Ki WK. Greater and lesser omenta: Normal anatomy and pathologic processes. *RadioGraphics*. 2007;27:707–720.
3. Moore KL, Daly AF, Agur, AMR. *Clinically Orientated Anatomy: Abdomen*, 7th edn., Philadelphia, PA: Lippincott Williams & Wilkins, 2013. pp. 181–234.
4. Elsayes KM, Staveteig PT, Narra VR, Leyendecker JR, Lewis, Jr. JS, Brown JJ. MRI of the peritoneum: Spectrum of the abnormalities. *American Journal of Roentgenology*. 2006;186:1368–1379.
5. Patel RR, Planche K. Applied peritoneal anatomy. *Clinical Radiology*. May 2013;68(5):509–520.
6. DeMeo JH, Maj ASF, Austin RF. Anatomic CT demonstration of the peritoneal spaces, ligaments and mesenteries: Normal and pathologic processes. *RadioGraphics*. 1995;15:755–770.
7. Meyers MA, Oliphant M, Berne AS, Feldberg MA. The peritoneal ligaments and mesenteries: Pathways of intraabdominal spread of disease. *Radiology*. 1987;167:593–604.

8. Son H, Khan SM, Rahaman J, Cameron KL, Prasad-Hayes M, Chuang L, Machac J, Heiba S, Kostakoglu, L. Role of FDG PET/CT in staging of recurrent ovarian cancer. *RadioGraphics*. 2011;31:569–583.

9. Woodbridge LR, Murtagh BM, Yu, DFQC, Planche KL. Midgut neuroendocrine tumors: Imaging assessment for surgical resection. *RadioGraphics*. 2014;34:413–426.

10. Hoskins PR, Martin K, Thrush A. *Diagnostic Ultrasound: Physics and Equipment*, 2nd edn., Cambridge, U.K.: Cambridge University Press, 2010.

11. Hanbidge AE, Lynch D, Wilson SR. US of the peritoneum. *RadioGraphics*. 2003;23:663–685.

12. Pannu HK, Bristow RE, Montz FJ, Fishman EK. Multidetector CT of peritoneal carcinomatosis from ovarian cancer. *RadioGraphics*. 2003;23:687–701.

13. Tirkes T, Sandrasegaran K, Patel AA, Hollar MA, Tejada JG, Tann M, Akisik FM, Lappas JC. Peritoneal and retroperitoneal anatomy and its relevance for cross-sectional imaging. *RadioGraphics*. 2012;32:437–451.

14. Levy AD, Shaw JC, Sobin LH. Secondary tumors and tumorlike lesions of the peritoneal cavity: Imaging features with pathologic correlation. *RadioGraphics*. 2009;29:347–373.

15. Sinha R, Rajiah P, Ramachandran I, Sanders S, Murphy PD. Diffusion-weighted MR imaging of the gastrointestinal tract: Technique, indications, and imaging findings. *RadioGraphics*. 2013;33:655–676.

16. Qayyum A. Diffusion-weighted imaging in the abdomen and pelvis: Concepts and applications. *RadioGraphics*. 2009;29:1797–1810.

17. Kapoor V, McCook BM, Torok FS. An introduction to PET-CT imaging. *RadioGraphics*. 2004;24:523–543.

18. Brix G, Lechel U, Glatting G, Ziegler SI, Münzing W, Müller SP, Beyer T. Radiation exposure of patients undergoing whole-body dual-modality 18F-FDG. *Journal of Nuclear Medicine*. 2005;46:608–613.

19. Blake MA, Singh A, Setty BN, Slattery J, Kalra M, Maher MM, Sahani DV, Fischman AJ, Mueller PR. Pearls and pitfalls in interpretation of abdominal and pelvic PET-CT. *RadioGraphics*. 2006;26:1335–1353.

20. Hainaux B, Aneessens E, Bertinotti R, De Maertelaer V, Rubesova E, Capelluto E, Moschopoulos C. Accuracy of MDCT in predicting site of gastrointestinal perforation. *American Journal of Roentgenology*. 2006;187:1179–1183.

4

Peritoneal drug transport

MICHAEL F. FLESSNER

INTRODUCTION

Intraperitoneal (IP) delivery of multiple drugs for the treatment of cancer was developed in the United States by Vincent DeVita and colleagues at the National Cancer Institute in the 1970s and was termed the "belly bath" [1]. Over the last 20 years, IP chemotherapy has increasingly been evaluated for treatment of malignancies localized to the peritoneal cavity [2–17]. Now it is widely used to treat various forms of peritoneal carcinomatosis [18] and is often used intraoperatively, immediately after surgical resection of the primary tumor and any visible peritoneal metastases (>2.5 mm diameter) [19]. IP chemotherapy is now recommended for peritoneal surface metastases of ovarian carcinoma [20], colorectal cancer [21–23], gastric cancer [24,25], and pseudomyxoma peritonei [26,27]. While the overall survival of some patients has been significantly improved [20], the technique, with or without elevated temperature [18], may not be effective in all peritoneal carcinomas [19].

This chapter will outline basic principles of transport across the normal peritoneum and the underlying parenchymal tissue and the challenges of delivery to abnormal carcinomatous tissue. It will include some basic principles of anatomy and physiology, which affect drug transport from the cavity to tissue. These include contact surface area, molecular weight, and solubility of the agent, treatment volume that directly affects IP pressure in the cavity,

and temperature of the therapeutic solution. Comparisons of transport in peritoneal dialysis (non-tumor-bearing tissue) will be made to treatment of metastatic nodules on the peritoneal surface, in order to understand the limitations and the promise of the IP technique. More details of the anatomy, physiology, pharmacokinetics, and specific drugs are discussed in other chapters of this book.

MULTICOMPARTMENTAL CONCEPT FOR IP DRUG DELIVERY

Physiologic characteristics of the peritoneal cavity, which cause it to be advantageous for removal of waste metabolites and poisons from the body, also provide an excellent portal of entry into the body for many drugs. The tissue surrounding the potential space of the cavity is capable of absorbing almost any agent including cell size materials placed in the cavity [28,29]. Figure 4.1 illustrates the complexity of the peritoneal cavity, in terms of pharmacokinetic pathways. Solute and fluid transfer (F_i) as indicated from the peritoneal cavity occurs into the various tissues surrounding the cavity and from there into the body compartment via the circulation. The subperitoneal tissue has been divided into four major compartments: (a) the liver, (b) hollow and other viscera, (c) the abdominal wall and retroperitoneum, and (d) the diaphragm, which is placed in a separate box

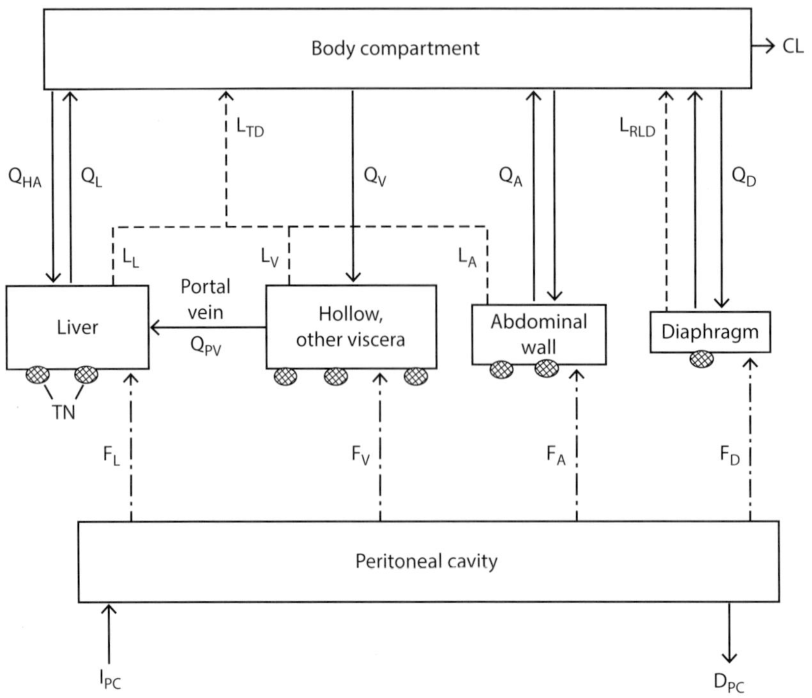

Figure 4.1 Compartmental model concept of intraperitoneal drug delivery in which transport occurs between the cavity and specific tissues surrounding the cavity. The symbols used are as follows: I_i, infusion; CL, clearance; D_i, drainage from the cavity; Q_i, blood flow through organ or vessel; L_i, lymph flow from tissue to body compartment; F_i, rate of convection from the cavity to tissue; and S, rate of solute transfer from the cavity to tissue. The following *subscripts* (L) are used: A, abdominal wall and psoas; BC, body compartment; D, diaphragm; HA, hepatic artery; L, liver, PC, peritoneal cavity; PV, portal vein; RLD, right lymph duct; TD, thoracic duct; TN, tumor nodule invading the peritoneal surface; and V, other viscera including the intestines, stomach, pancreas, and spleen. See text for a full description.

because of its special role in lymphatic drainage of the cavity. Each of these compartments receives blood originating in the body compartment. The blood flows (designated Q_i in the diagram) through capillary exchange vessels distributed throughout the tissue and returns to the body compartment directly or through the hepatic portal system. Lymph flows (designated L_i in the figure) from each tissue space to the body compartment as illustrated in Figure 4.1. Each tissue compartment receives solutes from the peritoneal cavity with a solute mass transfer rate of F_i. In Figure 4.1, the tumor nodules (TNs) overlie the surfaces of the normal tissue. This figure should provide the impression that transfer of drug from the cavity occurs into each tissue system that is connected in turn via the lymphatics or blood flow to the systemic circulation. Although all surfaces are potentially targets for any drug or agent within the peritoneal cavity, *the relative importance of a specific compartment is determined by how much of the surface is in contact with the fluid in the cavity.* This issue is particularly important in the regional administration of antineoplastic agents and will be discussed later.

The peritoneal cavity compartment is assumed to be well mixed; i.e., the concentration is the same throughout the cavity; this is particularly true if the treatment solution is perfused through the cavity via multiple catheters from a reservoir. The cavity has a solute input rate of I_{PC} and a drainage rate of D_{PC}. Note that the cavity does not exchange

directly with the body compartment; transport occurs only with the tissue compartments.

Individual compartments

The *diaphragm* is included as a separate compartment because of the specialized subdiaphragmatic lymphatic system [30–32], which accepts cell sizes up to 25 μm in diameter [28,29] and which accounts for 70%–80% of the total lymph flow from the cavity [33–35]. The diaphragm also experiences relatively large but variable hydrostatic pressure gradients during respiration, because of its position between the thoracic and abdominal cavities. Expiration facilitates direct fluid movement into the diaphragmatic interstitium and into the lacunae of the subdiaphragmatic lymphatic apparatus [30,32]. In later stages of metastatic carcinoma, these lymphatic channels may be obstructed, and ascites typically develop [36].

The *abdominal wall and retroperitoneum* are shown as a separate compartment because their position allows maximum effect of hydrostatic pressure–driven convection that results in significant fluid transfer from the cavity to the body. The abdominal wall itself is of major importance as well because it is likely that much of the macromolecular solute transfer flows through this tissue due to contact with the fluid [37]. In animal experiments, this amounts to 40%–50% of the total fluid movement out of the cavity [34,38,39].

The reason for this fluid movement is due to the hydrostatic pressure gradient across the abdominal wall and retroperitoneum. Since the lymphatics are not well developed in this tissue and therefore do not provide the safety valve that they do in the intestinal tissue [40], this results in the expansion of the interstitial space during therapy that enhances transport of small and large solutes into the muscle space [41,42]. Proteins or other macromolecular drugs such as monoclonal antibodies, which are carried into the muscle tissue as a result of the pressure-driven convection, will transfer to the body compartment slowly [43–45].

The *liver* is separated from the other visceral tissues because of its unique portal circulation coupled with its role in drug metabolism. The liver may be primarily responsible for protein losses into the cavity, but it is likely a minor (~5%) recipient of transfer from the cavity [46].

The "hollow and other viscera" include the spleen, stomach, intestines, and pancreas, which are lumped together in a single tissue compartment. The viscera present the largest portion of the peritoneal surface area, but it is unknown at this time how much of this surface area is in contact with the fluid or the duration of contact time during a therapeutic treatment. As drugs transport into the tissue from the cavity, they will also be taken up by the networks of vessels within each of these tissues and then return to the general circulation. The rate of the drug transfer to the blood is governed by diffusion and convection (solvent drag) within the tissue space, the permeability-surface area-density of the blood exchange vessels, and the rate of blood perfusion. The process of drug uptake from the peritoneal cavity includes the same physiological mechanisms responsible for transport during dialysis except that the direction of transport is reversed.

Table 4.1 lists the human parameters, which are independent of solute size but are necessary to model the system in Figure 4.1. The first two columns concern peritoneal surface area. The first column specifies the percentage of the total peritoneal surface area, while the second tabulates the total surface area in cm². The work of Rubin et al [47] is used because the measurements were more conservative than those of Esperanca and Collins [48], since the mesentery was not included. The areas have been scaled to a 70 kg body weight by the factor (body weight)^0.7 [49]. Despite the fact that these total surface areas have resulted from the dissection of each tissue and surface area measurement by planimetry, *these values may not represent the true area of contact* between the peritoneal fluid and the tissue.

The tissue weights were estimated as follows. The liver weight was taken directly from a table in Ludwig [50]. The "other viscera" weight was computed from the sum of the spleen (0.14 kg) and intestines. The latter were estimated from the product of the total surface area [51], the average thickness of 2.5 mm [52], and the specific gravity of these tissues, which was assumed to equal 1 g/cm³. The thicknesses of the abdominal wall and diaphragm were estimated to be 2 and 0.3 cm [53], respectively, and the tissue weight was calculated in the same fashion as in the case of the hollow viscera.

Tissue perfusion

There have been a number of estimates of the rate of perfusion (q_i) of the abdominal tissues. Measurements in the control animals [47,54] for the parietal wall (0.06 mL/min/g tissue) and diaphragm (0.31) are listed in Table 4.1. Other estimates [55] for the parietal wall tended to be much higher, because of the specific preparation and use of vasodilators in the experiments. The perfusion rates in the "other viscera" and the liver (includes both hepatic artery and portal flow) can be estimated from total organ blood flows [56,57] and divided by the weight of each system. The estimates for the gastrointestinal tract agree with several other measurements made in a variety of tissues from other species [58–60]. The total blood flows for the diaphragm and abdominal wall (Q_i) can be calculated from the product of the organ weight and q_i.

Does blood flow limit transport?

Estimates of the effective blood flow surrounding the peritoneal cavity suggest that transport between the blood and the cavity is not limited by the supply of blood, except in cases of severe hypotension. Physiologists have attempted to estimate the "effective" blood flow by measuring the clearances of various gases from the peritoneal cavity, assuming that these were limited by blood flow only. Gas clearances of hydrogen [61,62] and carbon dioxide [63,64] have been determined in small mammals and found to be equal to 4%–7% of the cardiac output. However, this method of

Table 4.1 Adult human parameters which are independent of solute size (scaled to 70 kg body weight, see text for references)

Tissue	Percentage total surface area	A_i (cm²)	Weight (g)	q_i (ML/min/g)	Q_{tot} (mL/min)	L (mL/min)	F (mL/min)	L/F
Liver	13.2	1056	1800	0.83	1500	0.46	0.07	6.83
Other viscera (intestines, spleen, stomach)	67.9	5432	1700	0.65	1100	0.97	0.33	2.91
Abdominal wall	11	880	1960	0.06	118	0.04	0.67	0.05
Diaphragm	7.9	632	190	0.3	57	0.27	0.27	1.01

determining the effective peritoneal blood flow may actually underestimate the true blood flow. Collins [65], who studied the simultaneous absorption of several inert gases from peritoneal gas pockets in pigs, found almost a threefold range in clearance, which correlated with the gas diffusivity in water. If the transport of these gases was limited by blood flow, the clearance of each gas would have been the same. The results imply that the transport of these gases is not limited by blood flow but by resistance to diffusion in the tissue. Gas clearance data therefore underestimate the true peritoneal blood flow, and the conclusion, based on lumped clearance data, would be that blood flow limitation in the peritoneal cavity is unlikely.

The lumped clearance argument, however, does not rule out specific limitations in a portion of the peritoneal cavity, which may be offset by another set of tissues. To investigate the possibility of blood flow limitation of transport across specific surfaces of the peritoneum, a specialized "chamber" technique was utilized to answer the question of "local" limitations of blood flow on radiolabeled urea (which should diffuse rapidly due to its small molecular weight and which would be more likely to demonstrate blood flow limitations) transport across the liver, stomach, cecum, and abdominal wall [66]. The mass transfer rates of urea were determined under conditions of control blood flow, blood flow reduced by 50%–80%, and no blood flow (postmortem); the blood flow was monitored simultaneously with laser Doppler flowmetry. While all four tissues showed marked decreases in urea transport after cessation of blood flow, only the liver displayed a decrease in the rate of transfer during periods of reduced blood flow. Further studies with the chamber technique tested the effects of blood flow on osmotically induced water flow from the same four tissues; results demonstrated statistically nonsignificant decreases in water flow in the cecum, stomach, and abdominal wall [67]. Analogous to the solute data, the liver demonstrated a significant drop in water transfer with reduced blood flow. Thus, transport of both solute and water across the surface of the liver is limited by blood flow. Zakaria et al. [68] have shown in rats that the liver is responsible for only a very small amount of the actual area of transfer; this implies that a drop in blood flow to the liver would have minimal effects on overall transperitoneal transport. These data support and extend earlier studies of peritoneal dialysis in dogs [69] and rats [70] during conditions of shock and demonstrate relatively small changes in solute transfer. All these support the use of the peritoneal cavity for solute or fluid transfer during periods of low systemic blood pressure that results in low blood perfusion of the organs surrounding the peritoneal cavity.

Lymph flow

Thoracic duct lymph flow has been measured in humans and typically has a flow rate of 1–1.6 mL/h/kg body weight [33,71]. Nonruminant animals have flow rates on the order of 2–3 mL/h/kg body weight [34,72–75]. Morris [72] estimates that the contributions of the liver and gastrointestinal tract amount to 30% and 64%, respectively, of the thoracic duct flow. The remaining 6% of the total flow is from all the skeletal muscle below the diaphragm, including the psoas, the abdominal wall, and the lower limbs. In order to estimate the lymph flow for humans, the mean value for the thoracic duct (1.3 mL/h/kg body weight) was multiplied by the percentages obtained by Morris for each organ system: 30% for the liver and 64% for the other viscera. One-third of the remaining 6% was arbitrarily assumed to be the contribution of the abdominal wall. Total lymph flows were then calculated by multiplying each tissue-specific lymph flow rate by the body weight (70 kg) and converting to mL/min.

Of the lymph that exclusively leaves the peritoneal cavity, 70%–80% occurs through the subdiaphragmatic system [33]. This is a major site for transport of fluids, macromolecules, and cellular materials from the cavity to the blood. Values for flow range from 0.6 to 1.8 mL/h/kg body weight in the anesthetized rat [34] to 0.1 mL/h/kg in anesthetized sheep and 0.50 mL/h/kg in awake sheep [76]. Flow rates in awake, healthy continuous ambulatory peritoneal dialysis patients vary from 0.14 to 0.28 mL/h/kg body weight [71,77]. The rates appear to increase in cirrhosis to 0.43 mL/h/kg [72]. We have chosen the mean rate of 0.23 mL/h/kg and multiplied it by 70 kg to find the diaphragmatic lymph flow rate of 16.1 mL/h.

The next to last column in Table 4.1 lists estimated total flow rates of fluid in mL/min to each tissue compartment from a 2 to 3 L solution in the peritoneal cavity of a 70 kg human. The total flow from the cavity has been estimated from the average of three studies in healthy dialysis patients [60,71,74,77] to be 1.33 mL/min. This flow is driven by the hydrostatic pressure (2–8 mmHg), depending on the position of the body and the measurement reference point [78] in the cavity [30,75,76] and occurs in the face of hyperosmolar solutions, which draw fluid into the cavity [62,70,76]. These studies have shown that protein acts as a marker for fluid movement. The total hourly flow rate has been partitioned to each set of tissues on the basis of the fraction of protein deposition from the cavity of the rat [34] with corrections for the rates of lymph flow from each tissue.

Uncertainty of surface contact area

The area of the peritoneum in contact with the therapeutic solution is typically a fraction of the anatomic area. Research in animals [37,79] and humans [80,81] has clearly demonstrated that during peritoneal dialysis, only about 30% of the total surface area is covered at any one time with the typical volume of 2–3 L. Although, over 24 hours, the entire peritoneum will make contact with an IP solution [82], the duration of contact with specific parts of the peritoneum is unknown. Typical dialysis solutions containing glucose are gradually absorbed from the cavity, and therefore, there is a receding volume and contact surface area after the effective osmolar gradient is lost. An alternative to standard dialysis solutions is one containing 4% of icodextrin (a 20–30 kDa starch), which has been shown to maintain the peritoneal volume at a constant for up to 48 hours [83–85], with a loss of 50% over the next 48 hours. A 7.5% icodextrin solution has been shown to be effective as a drug carrier for 5-fluorouracil (5-FU) [86] for up to 96 hours; this type of solution maintains the volume and the area of contact relatively constant. However, even the icodextrin solutions do not guarantee contact with the target areas for any given length of time. The volume of the solution, the size of the patient, and the patient's position all affect the peritoneal contact area. For example, if the patient is ambulatory, even a large volume (3 L) may pool in the bottom of the peritoneal cavity. Large portions of the peritoneum may not be covered [82], and therefore the residence time of the medication may be a problem for certain regions of the cavity.

The lack of certainty about the surface contact area and the residence time at each tissue surface complicate the implementation of the multicompartmental model of Figure 4.1. There are just no data on which to base a weighting system for fluid contact to a particular tissue. In addition, research in animals has demonstrated that for small molecules (~500 Da), the relative permeabilities of visceral and parietal peritoneal surfaces are nearly the same [87]. For many substances, the model concept of Figure 4.1 requires many defined parameters, and a simpler approach can be employed to calculate transport rates and the pharmacokinetic advantage (see "Simplified Compartmental Model" section).

Approaches to enhance contact area and residence time of IP-administered drugs

Drug delivery to metastatic cancer in the peritoneal cavity requires drug exposure and therefore is vitally dependent on sufficient contact between the therapeutic solution and the targeted TN(s). An approach to improve the contact area is to use a surface-active agent. In experiments with animals, diacetyl-sodium sulfosuccinate (DSS) has been shown to increase the surface contact area and to proportionally increase the rate of mass transfer into the local tissues [37,79,88]. More rapid uptake of the drug would result in a dissipation of the drug concentration from the fluid; this problem could be solved with the use of an automated exchange device such as a peritoneal dialysis machine, programmed to deliver periodic infusions over time of given concentration. Although DSS is used as an oral stool softener (docusate sodium), it unfortunately is quite toxic if administered IP; exposure of fluid containing surfactant to a larger proportion of the peritoneal surface area also accelerated the loss of protein and the dissipation of the drug concentration in the therapeutic solution [79].

In the perioperative setting, drug delivery can be enhanced considerably. Two or more catheters can be placed in the peritoneal cavity: one or more catheters for drug input and the other catheter(s) for removal of solution. Solutions warmed to temperatures greater than body temperature (approximately 41°C) may be infused rapidly into the peritoneal cavity and withdrawn in the second catheter. This technique will set up higher concentrations if solution is fed from a large reservoir that the loss of drug is relatively small.

Heating of the drug causes vasodilation in the surrounding vessels, and there is likely an increase in penetration into both normal tissue and neoplastic tissue [89–93]. Other methods include the surgeon massaging/stirring the treatment solution in situ within the cavity [94]. Either of these techniques may help to solve the problem of residence time. If a greater portion of the peritoneal surface area is covered by the solution and the concentration of the drug is maintained constant, then the area into the curve for the surface contact concentration should be maximized. Randomized controlled trials of these techniques will help in the decision to implement the additional procedures [95].

SIMPLIFIED COMPARTMENTAL MODEL

Simplified model concept

The model concept presented in Figure 4.2 is a simple, two-compartment approach, without regard to the anatomy and physiology of the system. It is the most straightforward concept to estimate transport from the cavity and the resulting pharmacokinetics of the drug delivery. The model consists of two compartments: (1) the systemic blood circulation that circulates through the drug's volume of distribution (V_D) and (2) the peritoneal cavity where the therapeutic drug is in solution. The transfer of drug across the *peritoneal barrier* modeled as a simple transfer of mass is as follows:

$$\text{Rate of mass transfer} = \frac{d(C_P V_P)}{dt} = -\text{MTAC}(C_P - C_B) \quad (4.1)$$

where

MTAC is the overall mass transfer-area coefficient for the drug or solute
C_P is the concentration in the peritoneal cavity
V_P is the volume in the peritoneal cavity
C_B is the concentration in the blood

A mass balance on the body compartment yields

$$\frac{d(C_B V_D)}{dt} = \text{MTAC}(C_P - C_B) - \text{CL}_{BC}(C_B V_D) \quad (4.2)$$

where CL_{BC} is the total body clearance, which is often approximated by the glomerular filtration rate divided by V_D for unbound, water-soluble drugs. Figure 4.3 provides MTACs for water-soluble drugs in normal dialysis patients and in patients undergoing IP chemotherapy [96–98]. These may underestimate or overestimate the mass transfer of particular drugs in tumor-bearing patients, depending on peritoneal contact area and whether vasodilation is present. As can be seen in Figure 4.3, the MTAC for drugs in heated solutions is considerably higher than the nonheated solutions [89,90,93], due to the combination of vasodilation with increased peritoneal blood flow and greater surface contact area with the use of multiple catheters and a continuous flow system. The area is not well defined in these perioperative procedures, but the technique can significantly enhance the

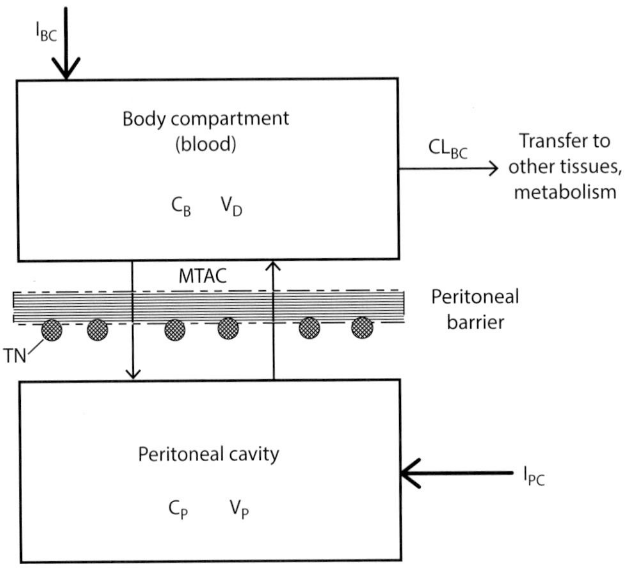

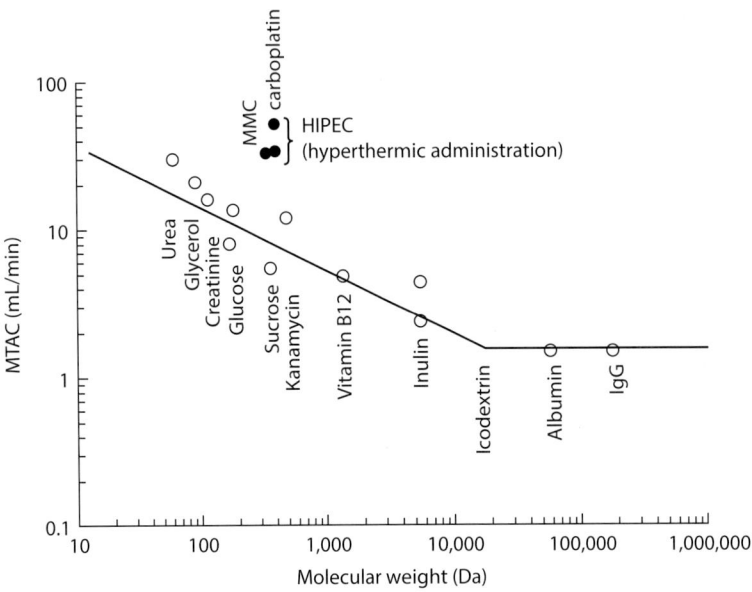

Figure 4.2 Simplified two-compartment model of peritoneal drug transport. MTAC, mass transfer-area coefficient; C_B, concentration in blood; V_D, volume of distribution for drug in body compartment; C_P, concentration in peritoneal cavity; V_P, volume in peritoneal cavity; I_{BC}, drug infusion into the body compartment; I_{PC}, drug infusion into the peritoneal cavity; CL_{BC}, the clearance of drug from the body compartment. See text for more details.

Figure 4.3 Mass transfer-area coefficient from the peritoneal cavity to the body versus molecular weight. See text for more details. (Data replotted from Elias, D. et al., *Ann. Oncol.*, 13, 267, 2002; Steller, M.A. et al., *Cancer Chemother. Pharmacol.*, 43, 106, 1999; Jacquet, P. et al., *Oncology*, 55, 130, 1998; Babb, A.L. et al., *Proc. Eur. Dial. Transplant Assoc.*, 10, 247, 1973; Dedrick, R.L. et al., *Cancer Treat. Rep.*, 62, 1, 1978; Krediet, R.T. et al., *Contrib. Nephrol.*, 89, 161, 1991.)

pharmacokinetic advantage and the efficacy [94,99]. Drugs that are more *lipid soluble* will have an order of magnitude higher rate of clearance from the peritoneal cavity [100–103].

Variation of MTAC with body size

Clearance data (~MTAC) for urea and inulin for the rat, rabbit, dog, and human (200 g to 70 kg) [49] demonstrate an increase as the 0.62–0.74 power of body weight or very close to the 2/3 expected for body-surface-area scaling [49].

Keshaviah et al. [99] demonstrated a linear correlation between the volume at which MTAC was maximum and the body surface area in a study of 10 patients with body surface areas ranging from 1.4 to 2.3 m². Since the characteristic time for absorption from the peritoneal cavity is equal to V_P/MTAC, similar timescales can be achieved in humans and experimental animals if the volume is scaled as the 2/3 power of the body weight. For example, 2 L in the peritoneal cavity of the 70 kg human patient (29 mL/kg) would be equivalent to 40 mL in a 200 g rat (200 mL/kg) because $(200/70{,}000)^{2/3} (2000) = 40$. These scaling criteria permit the design of experiments, which more accurately in small animals reflect treatment that is carried out in humans.

Calculation of the pharmacokinetic advantage

The solution of Equations 4.1 and 4.2 requires the parameters of V_D, CL_{BC}, and the MTAC for each solute and the doses to be given (dose = C × V for each compartment), which are given intravenously (IV) or IP at time = 0. The concentration versus time may then be calculated in each compartment for each route of administration; these concentrations define the pharmacokinetic advantage (R_d).

Alternatively, if a drug is infused at a constant rate into a fixed volume of fluid in the peritoneal cavity until steady state is achieved, then a regional advantage will be observed:

$$R_{ip} = \left(\frac{C_P}{C_B} \right)_{ip} \quad \text{or} \quad R_{ip} = \left(\frac{AUC_P}{AUC_B} \right)_{ip} \qquad (4.3)$$

where

  C_P is the concentration in the peritoneal cavity
  C_B is the concentration in the systemic circulation
  AUC is the area under the concentration versus time curve for an IP-injected drug in the peritoneal cavity (P) or blood (B)
  R_{ip} for cisplatin has been estimated to be 26 [16]

Others have demonstrated regional advantage of 10 for carboplatin to 1000 for paclitaxel [104].

Similarly, if the drug is infused at a constant rate IV with the same fixed IP volume of fluid, then the corresponding concentration ratio may be defined as

$$R_{iv} = \left(\frac{C_P}{C_B} \right)_{iv} \quad \text{or} \quad R_{iv} = \left(\frac{AUC_P}{AUC_B} \right)_{iv} \qquad (4.4)$$

The pharmacokinetic advantage R_d is defined as the ratio

$$R_d = \frac{(C_P/C_B)_{ip}}{(C_P/C_B)_{iv}} \quad \text{or} \quad R_d = \frac{(AUC_P/AUC_B)_{ip}}{(AUC_P/AUC_B)_{iv}} \qquad (4.5)$$

where the subscripts indicate the route of administration (IP, IV). In planning a therapeutic strategy, the physician would like to predict R_d prior to administration of the drug in humans. The pharmacokinetics of a particular drug are based on the transport physiology of the region in which it is administered, as well as pharmacokinetic processes in the rest of the body.

Conceptually, R_d expresses the relative advantage that may be achieved by administration of a drug directly into the peritoneal cavity compared with IV administration. It has been shown [105] that the pharmacokinetic advantage may be expressed as a remarkably simple equation if there is no elimination of the drug from the peritoneal region:

$$R_d = 1 + \frac{CL_{BC}}{MTAC} \qquad (4.6)$$

where CL_{BC} is the total body clearance (cm³/min). The same equation may be used for drug that is not administered by continuous infusion to steady state if the exposure terms are defined as the areas under the peritoneal and plasma concentration curves (AUC_P and AUC_B) following any schedule of administration, if the system is linear in the sense that none of the relevant parameters change with drug concentration or time.

Equation 4.6 indicates a large pharmacokinetic advantage for most hydrophilic drugs administered to the peritoneal cavity. For example, a typical antibiotic would be expected to have a MTAC of the order of 10 mL/min (Figure 4.3). If the drug is cleared from the body by glomerular filtration at the rate of inulin, 125 mL/min [106], then the expected value of R_d is approximately 14.

Many drugs are eliminated by tissues within the peritoneal cavity, particularly the liver. This provides a first-pass effect, which has the effect of increasing the natural pharmacokinetic advantage given by Equation 4.6. The regional advantage expected in the presence of some extraction of the drug by the liver may be obtained from Dedrick [49,96,105]:

$$R_{ip} = \frac{1 + (CL_{BC}/MTAC)}{1 - fE} \qquad (4.7)$$

where f is the fraction of the absorbed drug that enters the liver through the portal system or by direct absorption into its surface, and E is the fraction of that drug that is removed by the liver on a single pass. The quantity $(1 - fE)$ is the fraction of the absorbed drug that reaches the systemic circulation. If this fraction is small, then the natural advantage to regional administration can be considerably enhanced.

We do not have adequate information on the value of f. It is generally thought that small-molecular-weight compounds are absorbed primarily through the portal system [107]; however, there is evidence that some significant fraction of the absorbed drug can bypass the liver [4]. In the Speyer study, concentrations of 5-FU were observed to be higher in a peripheral artery than in the hepatic vein in three of four patients. Calculation of f was not reliable because the analysis of the data depended upon the knowledge on the blood flows in the portal vein and drug metabolism by gastrointestinal tissues, and these were not measured. The fact that about 15%–20% of the peritoneal surface area covers tissues that are not portal to the liver is consistent with these transport observations.

IP-ADMINISTERED DRUG PENETRATION INTO CARCINOMATOUS IMPLANTS

Normal versus neoplastic barriers in the peritoneal cavity

Penetration of 5-FU into tissues surrounding the peritoneal cavity has not been studied experimentally. Collins et al. [108] observed a strong concentration-dependent rate of 5-FU disappearance from the peritoneal cavity of the rat. The peritoneal clearance increased from 0.20 mL/min, consistent with its molecular weight, to 10 times that value as the peritoneal concentration was decreased from 10 mM to 20 µM. This was explained by assuming that the drug is metabolized in tissues adjacent to the peritoneal cavity. A 1D diffusion model with saturable, intratissue metabolism (V_{max} = 36 nmol/min/g, K_M = 5 µM) simulated the peritoneal concentrations reasonably well. The model predicted that the concentration in the tissue would be 10% of its value at the tissue surface at a depth of 0.6 mm following a 12 mM dose; the corresponding 10% level would be reached at only 0.13 mm following a 24 µM dose. Observations that the toxicity profile associated with IP administration is similar to that observed following IV administration [4,109] seem to confirm limited tissue penetration. If the drug had reached the gastrointestinal crypt cells in high concentration, one would expect substantial toxicity there.

Predicting the concentration of the drug at the surface may or may not guarantee penetration of the drug into the tumor to the rapidly dividing tumor cells, which are the real target. The compartmental model concept presented earlier lumps all of the potential barriers to the solute into one entity and does not differentiate between the variety of tissues, which may have different areas of contact and which may experience different transport forces. While Equations 4.1 through 4.5 permit calculation of the pharmacokinetic advantage, the model does not tell us anything about the specific penetration into the tissue. It merely describes the transfer between the two compartments. Illustrated in Figure 4.4 is the distributed model concept [110], in which an idealized tissue space is modeled as a peritoneum overlying a tissue containing parenchymal cells and blood vessels surrounded by an interstitium; mathematical details of this theory are contained in previous publications [110–116] and are beyond the scope of this chapter. Because IP therapy involves drug penetration of normal tissue as well as neoplastic tissue, it is important to differentiate between the properties of both of these. Figure 4.4 displays elements of the normal peritoneum with a carcinomatous nodular implant, which has destroyed the peritoneum and is growing into the tissue. The normal peritoneal barrier is made up of the peritoneum, interstitial matrix, and blood capillary wall. Lymphatic vessels are also located between normal tissue planes within smooth muscle of the intestines or in the diaphragm. The differences between tumor and normal tissue include lack of a mesothelial layer over the tumor, a very altered interstitium, a hyperpermeable microcirculation, and a lack of lymphatics. The following paragraphs will discuss the transport barrier for the normal peritoneum and underlying tissue and the abnormal properties of TNs on the peritoneal surface.

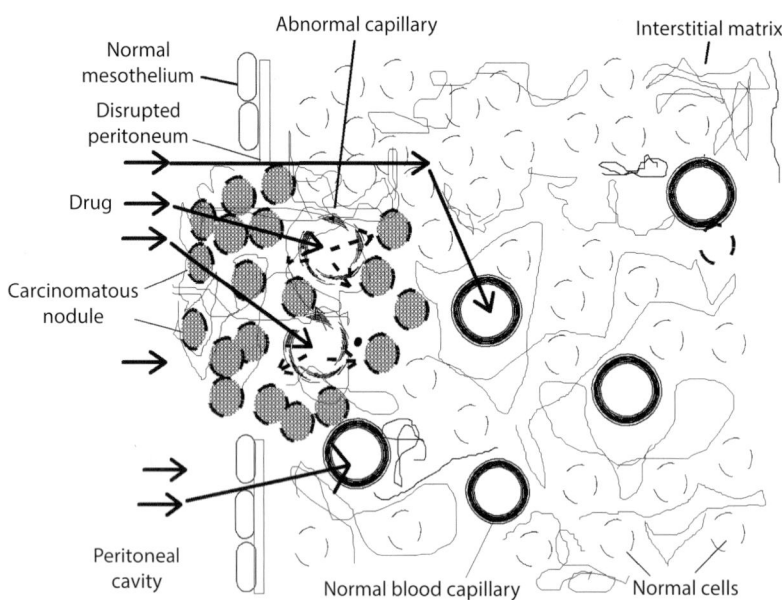

Figure 4.4 Distributed model concept of metastatic cancer and potential barriers to intraperitoneal therapy. Hatched circles represent the tumor metastasis, which have invaded and destroyed the mesothelium in its vicinity. Abnormal capillaries within the carcinomatous nodule (discontinuous circles) are typically more permeable than the normal microcirculation (continuous circles) and set up high interstitial flows and pressures. The tumor microenvironment (interstitium between cells) is often markedly expanded compared to that of normal tissue. See text for details.

Anatomic peritoneum

While the peritoneal barrier is often called the "peritoneal membrane," the actual anatomic peritoneum, made up of a layer of mesothelial cells and several layers of connective tissue [117], is not a significant barrier to molecules up to a molecular weight of 160,000 Da. Studies in rodents and dialysis patients have shown that protein leaves the cavity rates of approximately 10 times the rate at which it appears in blood [118–122]. The only route of transfer of protein in the cavity back to the central circulation is via the lymphatics [33,123,124]. There must be some other pathway for disappearance of this protein. In experiments with rodents, it has been shown that as protein transports across the peritoneum, there is some adsorption (2%–3%) [39] to the glycocalyx of mesothelial cells in which most of the protein deposition is into the subperitoneum. Further experiments demonstrated that removal of the peritoneum does not eliminate the transport properties of the peritoneal barrier [125]. Recent studies in patients undergoing partial or total peritonectomy for treatment of peritoneal carcinomatosis confirm the findings in rodents; the clearance of mitomycin C from the peritoneal cavity was not significantly affected by an extensive peritoneal resection [126]. Although proteins appear to easily pass the mesothelium into the subperitoneum, viral vectors containing gene products are taken up directly into mesothelial cells with little penetration beyond this single cell layer. Adenovirus that contain the reporter gene β-galactosidase have been shown to be quantitatively taken up in mesothelium and not to penetrate into underlying tissues unless there is a break in the mesothelium [127–134].

Penetration into tumor cells replacing peritoneum

The *peritoneum at the site of tumor implantation* will likely be destroyed in most cases of neoplastic cellular infiltration of the peritoneum (see Figure 4.4). The loss of the mesothelium presents problems to the maintenance of the smoothly gliding peritoneal surface of the gut, promotes adhesions, and decreases the function of the immune system. Without the mesothelium, adhesions form between the visceral and parietal surfaces, and the fluid distribution may become markedly abnormal, which may preclude intracavitary therapy [135]. However, viral vectors containing antisense RNA or other gene products as treatment, which might not be capable of passing through the normal mesothelium, have the possibility to penetrate into the tumor from the peritoneal cavity [133]. Other approaches to the optimization of the drug delivery system include the use of drug-eluting beads [136] and the use of microparticles, nanoparticles, liposomes, micelles, implants, and injectable depots [137].

In summary, the normal anatomic peritoneum is not a significant barrier to small solutes or to macromolecules, unless there exists a mechanism of uptake by the mesothelial cells, as in the case of viral vectors. The normal mesothelium may be destroyed by a metastatic tumor, which opens this abnormal tissue to penetration of viral vectors, nanoparticles, and other transport vehicles.

Normal interstitium vs. tumor microenvironment

Normal interstitium (space between the cells) or the so-called microenvironment is made up of collagen fibers linked through adhesion molecules such as β-1 integrins to fibroblasts, parenchymal cells, and other interstitial cells [138,139]. Hyaluronan molecules, which vary from 50,000 Da to 40 million, wrap around the collagen fibers and are likely attached to them at some link point. Large molecules called proteoglycans are attached to the hyaluronan, which also interact with the surrounding cells [140,141]. Hyaluronan molecules are highly negatively charged and imbibe large amounts of water and restrict the passage of negatively charged proteins [142]. Proteins such as immunoglobulins are typically restricted to about 50% of the interstitial space [143,144]. Thus, the interstitial space of normal muscle, which is anywhere from 12% to 20% of the total tissue volume, restricts proteins to 6%–10% of the tissue. The transport of large solutes such as immunoglobulin G (IgG) (150 kD) or adenovirus (900 kD) will be markedly retarded by the microenvironment, as illustrated in Figure 4.5, which compares the concentration profiles of a small solute (mannitol) and a macromolecule (IgG) in normal and neoplastic tissue (replotted from [145–148]).

Alterations in the interstitial pressure can change the relative tissue interstitial water space and the proportion of the tissue available to the solute. It has been shown in animal experiments that the abdominal wall interstitium will double when the IP pressure is increased from 0 to 4 mmHg [41,42]. This will markedly enhance the transport of both small and large solutes through this space, as is illustrated in Figure 4.5 by the MAb profile in normal abdominal wall after 3 hours of a solution dwell at a constant 4 mmHg. The hydraulic conductivity or water permeability of the tissue also increases with increasing IP pressure and washout of hyaluronan from the tissue interstitium [149]. Since the surface contact area is maximized with increasing peritoneal volumes [81,99], attempts to increase the contact area will increase the pressure as well. The IP pressure varies directly with the IP volume [78,150] in normal dialysis patients. The effect of pressure is greatest in the abdominal wall where a nearly linear pressure gradient from the inside of the peritoneal cavity to the outside has been measured in the rat [39]; these profiles may be quite different from those in tumors [147] or in the human abdominal wall. However, patients with adhesions due to extensive surgical resection may have restricted volumes and very different pressure–volume characteristics, with increased pressures at lower volumes than those of dialysis patients. In summary, large volumes in the cavity increase the IP pressure and expand the interstitial space and, in turn, augment the space within the tissue to which both small and large solutes distribute.

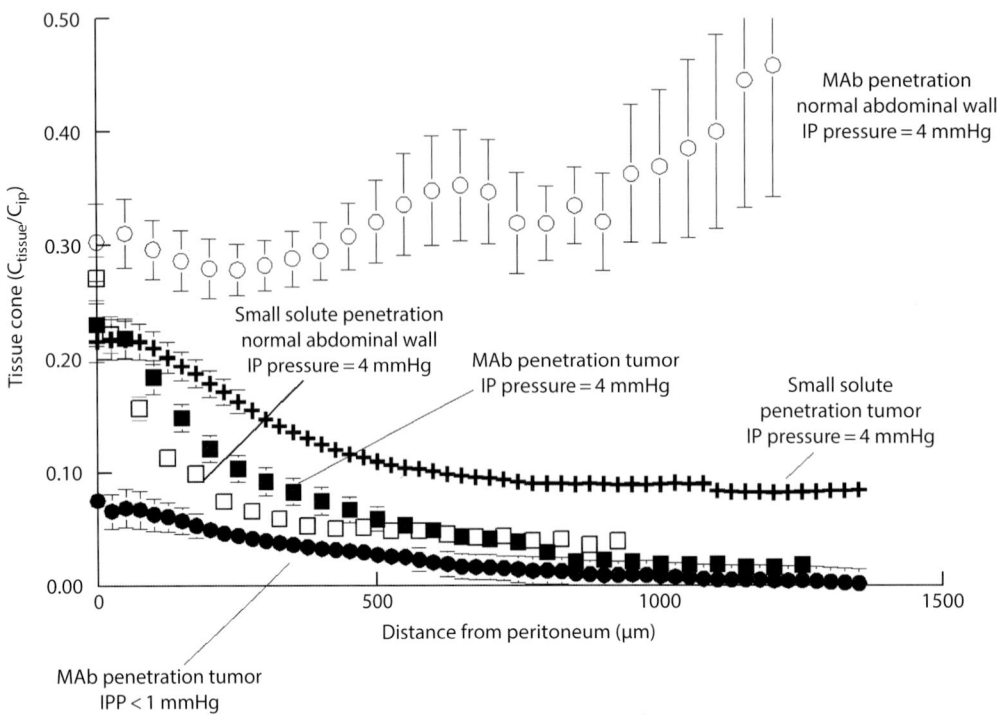

Figure 4.5 Comparison of penetration of small solute (mannitol or EDTA) or MAb (monoclonal antibody, Herceptin, Her2/neu) into normal tissue (open symbols) or SKOV3 xenograft nodule (closed symbols) located on the abdominal wall of the rat after 3 hours of treatment with a large intraperitoneal (IP) volume (IP pressure at 4 mmHg) or with a lower volume (IP pressure <1 mmHg). Mean ± SE concentrations vs. distance in microns from the peritoneal surface. (Replotted from Flessner, M.F. et al., *Am. J. Physiol.*, 273(6 Pt. 2), H2783, December 1997; Flessner, M.F. et al., *Am. J. Physiol.*, 248(3 Pt. 2), F425, March 1985; Choi, J. et al., *Clin. Cancer Res.*, 12(6), 1906, March 15, 2006; Flessner, M.F. et al., *J. Appl. Physiol.*, 97(4), 1518, October 2004; Flessner, M.F. et al., *Am. J. Physiol.*, 248(1 Pt. 2), H26, January 1985; Flessner, M.F. et al., *FASEB J.*, 4, A592, 1990.)

Antineoplastic agents will transport at faster rates through normal tissue due to increases in both diffusion and convection [42,45,112,146,149,151].

There exist remarkable differences between the *tumor microenvironment* and that of normal interstitium. Interstitial pressures in *normal tissue* are in the range of −2 to 0 mmHg [152,153]. This allows convection due to the hydrostatic pressure gradient from the solution in the cavity (3–10 mmHg) into the tissue, as illustrated in Figure 4.5 that portrays the concentration profiles of a small solute (mannitol) and a monoclonal antibody (MAb, Herceptin) in normal abdominal wall muscle and SKOV3 TNs in adjacent abdominal wall after 3 hours of a constant IP pressure of 4 mmHg or ~0 (<1) mmHg. As shown, the MAb penetration in normal abdominal wall can be quite high at 4 mmHg, while the penetration into the tumor is more limited. At lower pressures, the MAb concentrations in normal tissue or tumor are significantly lower, because macromolecules depend on convection (solvent drag) for transport. Small solute transport is dependent on diffusion and not as affected by convective force but will display higher concentration profiles in volume-expanded tumors (compare the small solute profiles in normal abdominal wall and the tumor). So why is the penetration of MAb so poor in the tumor at 4 mmHg in comparison with the normal tissue of the abdominal wall?

Studies of tumor interstitium show that the space between the cells is often markedly expanded in comparison to normal tissue [154]. A recent study in human ovarian carcinoma xenografts demonstrated an interstitial water space of two to three times that of normal muscle [148,155]. Gullino et al. have shown similar results in several tumors [154]. Thus, the high interstitial pressure results in an expanded interstitium, which would typically result in higher rates of diffusion and convection in normal tissue. However, the high interstitial pressure and intrinsic properties of the tumor interstitium resist any transfer of large molecules into the tumor [146,156–159]. On the other hand, smaller substances (MW < 500 Da) will diffuse into the tumor parenchyma in a fashion similar to normal tissue (see Figure 4.5) [145,148].

Interstitial pressures in tumors

In contrast to observations in normal tissue, several investigators have observed high interstitial pressures up to 45 mmHg in neoplastic tissue [147,156,157,160,161]. To deliver macromolecules by convection from the cavity into these tumors, the solution would have to attain a pressure greater than that of the tumor. The upper limit of pressure tolerated by an ambulatory patient is approximately 8–10 mmHg in the peritoneal cavity [62,147] and may limit the penetration of large solutes that depend on convection or solvent drag, if the tumor interstitium has a pressure higher than the IP pressure. In addition, steady IP pressures of >15 mmHg in a closed cavity may suppress the portal circulation [62]. Pressures of >20 mmHg may prevent the descent of the diaphragm [62] and compromise respiration. Therefore, an unanesthetized ambulatory patient will likely be unable to tolerate therapy, which depends on large volumes (>3–4 L) to produce high IP pressure. In the perioperative state, the pressure would also be limited by an open cavity or by the acutely placed catheters. If tumor interstitial pressures are higher than those that can be attained, macromolecular penetration and therefore therapy may be precluded. Anesthetized patients, who receive mechanical ventilation, may be able to tolerate higher levels of IP pressure, but the mesenteric circulation supplying the gut should be carefully monitored.

Microvascular barrier: Normal vs. tumor

Normal blood capillary endothelia are lined with a glycocalyx, which has been demonstrated to provide the endothelium with its barrier characteristics [162–165]. In portions of the interendothelial cleft, it is theorized that the glycocalyx is quite dense and only small molecules up to the size of insulin (~5500 Da) will typically pass through, while in other areas, a small number of gaps will have a less dense glycocalyx, which will permit protein leakage [160]. This provides the size-selective nature of the normal peritoneal barrier. However, inflammation or drugs such as adenosine [166] cause the elimination or degradation of the glycocalyx and an increase in the capillary permeability; the vessels of the normal peritoneum are likely affected during inflammation due to invasion by metastatic carcinoma [167]. Capillary permeability is markedly altered in neoplastic tissue, with typically a high permeability but a variable microvascular density [168,169]. Although detailed studies have not been carried out, all indications are that these highly permeable capillaries may be responsible for the rapid clearance of drugs into portions of the tumor from the systemic circulation [170]. While this can be an advantage in treatment of these tumors, the high pressures in the interstitium may actually result in difficulty in drug penetration [169,171]. The nature of angiogenic vessels is under scrutiny; these may not have the glycocalyx that lines the normal endothelium and provides much of the barrier to solute transfer [168,170–172]. Thus, many of the characteristics of these new vessels may be completely different from those of normal vasculature. In addition, the actual distribution of vessels is very irregular. In small (<1 cm diameter) ovarian xenografts, the vessels are located in the periphery of the tumor, which is expanding into the normal tissue [148]. The central part of the tumor may actually be necrotic and have no vasculature at all. Penetration to nonvascularized portions of the tumor is one of the problems of IV or IP administration. Targeting the vasculature simultaneously with IP

therapy may be a method of accessing these portions of the tumor and solving this problem.

Lymph drainage from the cavity is chiefly through the subdiaphragmatic lymphatics [160]. In normal conditions, the relaxation of the diaphragm will open specialized "stomata," which accept proteins, cells, and solution from the peritoneal cavity into the collecting lymphatics [31,32]. The subsequent contraction of the diaphragm will close the stomata and propel the material into the parasternal lymphatics and ultimately into the right or left lymph duct. Approximately 70%–80% of peritoneal lymph drainage occurs through this route [33]. Lymphatics from the viscera drain to the cisterna chyli at the base of the thoracic duct and ultimately into the left venous system [124].

With peritoneal carcinomatosis, the subdiaphragmatic *lymphatics* and the mesenteric lymphatics may be obstructed [173,174]. The obstruction produces severe ascites because the normal flow of fluid and proteins from the viscera into the peritoneal cavity cannot be cleared properly [36,174–176]. In addition, the lymphatics provide a route of metastasis to the remainder of the body, including the periaortic and thoracic nodes [177]; often supradiaphragmatic nodes are overwhelmed with tumor cells; and these same nodes then allow tumor cells to pass into the systemic circulation. However, if these pathways are still functional, IP therapy directly targets these routes of metastasis and is a direct route to the systemic circulation for all agents, particularly those with molecular sizes greater than that of albumin.

Summary of normal vs. neoplastic peritoneal barrier

The anatomic peritoneum is not a barrier to most drugs, including immunoglobulins. The mesothelial layer may be absent in a tumor implant on the peritoneum, and the vasculature and the microenvironment may be greatly altered. While viral vectors are totally absorbed in the normal mesothelium, its absence at a tumor surface may permit these very large particles (~900 kDa) to pass into the first few cell layers of the tumor; however, viral vectors will still have restricted movement in the tumor interstitium [146]. The tumor interstitium is markedly expanded and theoretically should promote high rates of diffusion and convection [146,148]. However, the high interstitial pressure and the tendency of flow from the center part of the tumor toward the periphery may cause a functional obstruction in the direction of the treatment drug originating from the peritoneum cavity [147,156,161,178]. In addition, there appear to be structural differences in the collagen matrix of the tumor interstitium that prevent significant convection and diffusion of negatively charged, macromolecular agents [146,159]. The tumor blood capillary and microcirculation are markedly abnormal in distribution and permeability characteristics [168,169,171]. Depending on the location and density of the tumor microvasculature, systemically administered drugs may rapidly distribute to perfused regions of the tumor but may not reach poorly vascularized locations altogether. Multiagent therapies that simultaneously attack the interstitium, vasculature, and peritoneal side of the tumor will therefore likely be more effective in remitting peritoneal carcinomatosis.

SUMMARY

IP chemotherapy should be considered as an alternative to IV therapy when the target is contained within the peritoneal cavity or within the adjacent tissue. A compartmental model has been used to formulate a mathematical scheme in order to evaluate the solute transport to specific tissue groups surrounding the cavity. Although the data to fully implement the model do not exist, a simplified version of the model with parameters derived from the literature can be used to solve for the steady-state concentrations in the peritoneal cavity and the plasma. The ratio of these two concentrations defines the regional advantage of IP therapy. Several applications of the theory are presented in order to illustrate the method in which IP therapy may be evaluated prior to use in patients. Application of the model to the treatment of metastatic carcinoma is complicated by major differences in the targeted tissue properties. Recent animal data are discussed to illustrate the challenges of IP chemotherapy and immunotherapy for cancer.

REFERENCES

1. Jones RB, Myers CE, Guarino AM, Dedrick RL, Hubbard SM, DeVita VT. High volume intraperitoneal chemotherapy ("belly bath") for ovarian cancer. *Cancer Chemotherapy and Pharmacology*. 1978;1:161.
2. Jones RB, Collins JM, Myers CE, Brooks AE, Hubbard SM, Balow JE et al. High volume intraperitoneal chemotherapy with methotrexate in patients with cancer. *Cancer Research*. 1981;41:55.
3. Speyer JL, Collins JM, Dedrick RL, Brennan MF, Buckpitt AR, Londer H et al. Phase I and pharmacological studies of 5-fluorouracil administered intraperitoneally. *Cancer Research*. 1980;40:567.
4. Speyer JL, Sugarbaker PH, Collins JM, Dedrick RL, Klecker RW, Myers CE. Portal levels and hepatic clearance of 5-fluorouracil after intraperitoneal administration in humans. *Cancer Research*. 1981;41:1916.
5. Markman M, Hakes T, Reichmann B, Hoskins W, Rubin S, Lewis JL. Intraperitoneal versus intravenous cisplatin-based therapy in small-volume residual refractory ovarian cancer: Evidence supporting an advantage for local drug delivery. *Regional Cancer Treatment*. 1990;3:10–2.
6. Markman M, Brady MF, Spirtos NM, Hanjani P, Rubin SC. Phase II trial of intraperitoneal paclitaxel in carcinoma of the ovary, tube, and peritoneum: A Gynecologic Oncology Group study. *Journal of Clinical Oncology*. 1998;16:2620–2624.
7. Barakat RR, Sabbatini P, Bhaskaran D, Revzin M, Smith A, Venkatraman E et al. Intraperitoneal chemotherapy for ovarian carcinoma: Results of long-term follow-up. *Journal of Clinical Oncology*. 2002;20:694–698.
8. Ozols RF, Young RC, Speyer JL. Phase I and pharmacological studies of adriamycin administered intraperitoneally to patients with ovarian cancer. *Cancer Research*. 1982;42:4265–4269.
9. Ozols RF, Young RC, Speyer JL, Waltz M, Collins JM, Dedrick RL et al. Intraperitoneal (IP) adriamycin (ADR) in ovarian carcinoma (OC). *Proceedings of American Society of Clinical Oncology*. 1980;21:425.
10. Ozols RF, Locker GY, Doroshow JH. Pharmacokinetics of adriamycin and tissue penetration in murine ovarian cancer. *Cancer Research*. 1979;39:3209–3214.
11. Gianni L, Jenkins JF, Greene RF, Lichter AS, Myers CE, Collins JM. Pharmacokinetics of the hypoxic radiosensitizers misonidazole and demethylmisonidazole after intraperitoneal administration in humans. *Cancer Research*. 1983;43:913–916.
12. Arbuck SG, Trave F, Douglas HO, Nava H, Zakrzewkski S, Rustum YM. Phase I and pharmacologic studies of intraperitoneal leucovorin and 5-fluorouracil in patients with advanced cancer. *Journal of Clinical Oncology*. 1986;4:1510–1517.
13. Markman M, Rowinsky E, Hakes T. Phase I trial of intraperitoneal taxol: A Gynecologic Oncology Group Study. *Journal of Clinical Oncology*. 1992;10:1485–1491.
14. Alberts DS, Liu PY, Hannigan EV, O'Toole R, Williams SD, Young JA et al. Intraperitoneal cisplatin plus intravenous cyclophosphamide versus intravenous cisplatin plus intravenous cyclophosphamide for stage III ovarian cancer. *New England Journal of Medicine*. 1996;335:1950–1955.
15. Muggia FM, Liu PY, Alberts DS. Intraperitoneal mitoxantrone or floxuridine: Effects on time-to-failure and survival in patients with minimal residual ovarian cancer after second-look laparotomy—A randomized phase II study by the Southwest Oncology Group. *Gynecologic Oncology*. 1996;61:395–402.
16. Goel R, Cleary SM, Horton C, Howell S. Effect sodium thiosulfate on the pharmacokinetics and toxicity of cisplatin. *Journal of the National Cancer Institute*. 1989;81:1552–1560.
17. Markman M, Walker JL. Intraperitoneal chemotherapy of ovarian cancer: A review, with a focus on practical aspects of treatment. *Journal of Clinical Oncology*. 2006;24:988–993.
18. Coccolini F, Gheza F, Lotti M, Virzi S, Iusco D, Ghermandi C et al. Peritoneal carcinomatosis. *World Journal of Gastroenterology*. November 7, 2013;19(41):6979–6994.

19. Elias D, Goere D, Dumont F, Honore C, Dartigues P, Stoclin A et al. Role of hyperthermic intraoperative peritoneal chemotherapy in the management of peritoneal metastases. *European Journal of Cancer.* January 2014;50(2):332–340.

20. Walker JL. Intraperitoneal chemotherapy requires expertise and should be the standard of care for optimally surgically resected epithelial ovarian cancer patients. *Annals of Oncology.* December 2013;24(Suppl. 10):x41–x45.

21. Avital I, Brucher BL, Nissan A, Stojadinovic A. Randomized clinical trials for colorectal cancer peritoneal surface malignancy. *Surgical Oncology Clinics of North America.* October 2012;21(4):665–688.

22. Eveno C, Goere D, Dartigues P, Honore C, Dumont F, Tzanis D et al. Ovarian metastasis is associated with retroperitoneal lymph node relapses in women treated for colorectal peritoneal carcinomatosis. *Annals of Surgical Oncology.* February 2013;20(2):491–496.

23. Ceelen WP. Current management of peritoneal carcinomatosis from colorectal cancer. *Minerva Chirurgica.* February 2013;68(1):77–86.

24. Yonemura Y, Ishibashi H, Canbay E, Sako S, Tsukiyama G, Mizumoto Y et al. Treatment results of diffuse malignant peritoneal mesothelioma. *Gan To Kagaku Ryoho.* November 2012;39(12):2416–2419.

25. Mi DH, Li Z, Yang KH, Cao N, Lethaby A, Tian JH et al. Surgery combined with intraoperative hyperthermic intraperitoneal chemotherapy (IHIC) for gastric cancer: A systematic review and meta-analysis of randomised controlled trials. *International Journal of Hyperthermia.* 2013;29(2):156–167.

26. Chua TC, Esquivel J, Pelz JO, Morris DL. Summary of current therapeutic options for peritoneal metastases from colorectal cancer. *Journal of Surgical Oncology.* May 2013;107(6):566–573.

27. Deraco M, Kusamura S, Laterza B, Favaro M, Fumagalli L, Costanzo P et al. Cytoreductive surgery and hyperthermic intra-peritoneal chemotherapy (HIPEC) in the treatment of pseudomyxoma peritonei: Ten years experience in a single center. *In Vivo.* November to December 2006;20(6A):773–776.

28. Allen L. On the penetrability of the lymphatics of the diaphragm. *Anatomical Record.* 1956;124:639–658.

29. Allen L, Weatherford T. Role of the fenestrated basement membrane in lymphatic absorption from the peritoneal cavity. *American Journal of Physiology.* 1959;197:551–554.

30. Leak LV, Rahil K. Permeability of the diaphragmatic mesothelium: The ultrastructural basis for 'stomata'. *American Journal of Anatomy.* 1978;151:557–594.

31. Bettendorf U. Electronmicroscopic studies on the peritoneal resorption of intraperitoneally injected latex particles via the diaphragmatic lymphatics. *Lymphology.* 1979;12:66–70.

32. Bettendorf U. Lymph flow mechanism of the subperitoneal diaphragmatic lymphatics. *Lymphology.* 1978;11:111–116.

33. Yoffey JM, Courtice FC. *Lymphatics, Lymph, and the Lymphomyeloid Complex,* London, U.K.: Academic, 1970.

34. Flessner MF, Parker RJ, Sieber SM. Peritoneal lymphatic uptake of fibrinogen and erythrocytes in the rat. *American Journal of Physiology.* 1983;244(1):H89–H96.

35. Abernathy NJ, Chin W, Hay JB, Rodela H, Oreopoulos DG, Johnston M. Lymphatic drainage of the peritoneal cavity in sheep. *American Journal of Physiology.* 1991;260:F353–F358.

36. Cavazzoni E, Bugiantella W, Graziosi L, Franceschini MS, Donini A. Malignant ascites: Pathophysiology and treatment. *International Journal of Clinical Oncology.* February 2013;18(1):1–9.

37. Flessner MF, Lofthouse J, Zakaria ER. Improving contact area between the peritoneum and intraperitoneal therapeutic solutions. *Journal of the American Society of Nephrology.* April 2001;12(4):807–813.

38. Flessner MF, Reynolds JC, Blasberg RG, Dedrick RL. Bidirectional peritoneal transport of IgG in rats: Tissue concentration profiles. *American Journal of Physiology.* 1992;263:F15–F23.

39. Flessner MF, Schwab A. Pressure threshold for fluid loss from the peritoneal cavity. *American Journal of Physiology.* February 1996;270(2 Pt. 2):F377–F390.

40. Pearson CM, Abramson DI. *Blood Vessels and Lymphatics,* New York: Academic, 1962.

41. Zakaria ER, Lofthouse J, Flessner MF. Effect of intraperitoneal pressures on tissue water of the abdominal muscle. 2000;F875–F885.

42. Zakaria ER, Lofthouse J, Flessner MF. In vivo effects of hydrostatic pressure on interstitium of abdominal wall muscle. *American Journal of Physiology.* February 1999;276(2 Pt. 2):H517–H529.

43. Flessner MF, Dedrick RL, Schultz JS. Exchange of macromolecules between peritoneal cavity and plasma. *American Journal of Physiology.* 1985;248:H15–H25.

44. Flessner MF, Dedrick RL, Schultz JS. A distributed model of peritoneal-plasma transport: Analysis of experimental data in the rat. *American Journal of Physiology.* March 1985;248(3 Pt. 2):F413–F424.

45. Flessner MF, Dedrick RL, Reynolds JC. Bidirectional peritoneal transport of immunoglobulin in rats: Tissue concentration profiles. *American Journal of Physiology.* July 1992;263(1 Pt. 2):F15–F23.

46. Flessner MF. Impact of the liver on peritoneal transport. *Peritoneal Dialysis International.* 1996;16(Suppl. 1):S205–S206.

47. Rubin J, Jones Q, Planch A, Stanak K. Systems of membranes involved in peritoneal dialysis. *Journal of Laboratory and Clinical Medicine.* 1987;110:448–453.

48. Esperanca MJ, Collins DL. Peritoneal dialysis efficiency in relation to body weight. *Journal of Pediatric Surgery.* 1966;1:162–169.

49. Dedrick RL. Interspecies scaling of regional drug delivery. *Journal of Pharmaceutical Sciences.* 1986;75:1047–1052.

50. Ludwig J. *Current Methods of Autopsy Practice,* Philadelphia, PA: WB Saunders, 1972.

51. Rubin J, Clawson M, Planch A, Jones Q. Measurements of peritoneal surface area in man and rat. *American Journal of the Medical Sciences.* 1988;295:453–458.

52. Rhodin JA. *Histology: A Text and Atlas,* New York: Oxford University Press, 1974.

53. DiFiore MSH. *Atlas of Human Histology,* Philadelphia, PA: Lea & Febiger, 1974.

54. Rubin J, Jones Q, Planch A, Rushton F, Bower JD. The importance of the abdominal viscera to peritoneal transport during peritoneal dialysis in the dog. *American Journal of the Medical Sciences.* 1986;292:203–208.

55. Vetterlein F, Schmidt G. Functional capillary density in skeletal muscle during vasodilation induced by isoprenaline and muscular exercise. *Microvascular Research.* 1980;20:156–164.

56. Guyton AC. *Textbook of Medical Physiology,* Philadelphia, PA: WB Saunders, 1981.

57. Mapleson WW. An electric analogue for uptake and exchange of inert gases and other agents. *Journal of Applied Physiology.* 1963;18:197–204.

58. Bonaccorsi A, Dejana E, Quintana A. Organ blood flow measured with microspheres in the unanesthetized rat: Effects of three room temperatures. *Journal of Pharmacological Methods.* 1978;1:321–328.

59. Grim E, Hamilton WF, Dow P. *Handbook of Physiology,* Washington, DC: American Physiological Society, 1963.

60. Chou CC, Grassmick B. Motility and blood flow distribution within the wall of the gastrointestinal tract. *American Journal of Physiology.* 1978;235:H34–3H9.

61. Aune S. Transperitoneal exchange: II. Peritoneal blood flow estimated by hydrogen gas clearance. *Scandinavian Journal of Gastroenterology.* 1970;5:99.

62. Flessner MF. *Transport of Water-Soluble Solutes Between the Peritoneal Cavity and Plasma in the Rat,* Ann Arbor, MI: University of Michigan, 1981.

63. Peters T, Potter R, Li X, He Z, Hoskins G, Flessner MF. Mouse model of foreign body reaction that alters the submesothelium and transperitoneal transport. *American Journal of Physiology: Renal Physiology.* January 2011;300(1):F283–F289.

64. Grzegorzewska AE, Moore HL, Nolph KD, Chen TW. Ultrafiltration and effective peritoneal blood flow during peritoneal dialysis in the rat. *Kidney International.* 1991;39:608–617.

65. Collins JM. Inert gas exchange of subcutaneous and intraperitoneal gas pockets in piglets. *Respiration Physiology.* 1981;46:391.

66. Kim M, Lofthouse J, Flessner MF. Blood flow limitations of solute transport across the visceral peritoneum. *Journal of the American Society of Nephrology.* 1997;8:1946–1950.

67. Demissachew H, Lofthouse J, Flessner MF. Tissue sources and blood flow limitations of osmotic water transport across the peritoneum. *Journal of the American Society of Nephrology.* February 1999;10(2):347–353.

68. Zakaria e, Carlsson O, Rippe B. Limitation of small-solute exchange across the visceral peritoneum: Effects of vibration. *Peritoneal Dialysis International.* 1997;17(1):72–79.

69. Erb RW, Greene JA, Weller JM. Peritoneal dialysis during hemorrhagic shock. *Journal of Applied Physiology.* 1967;22:131–135.

70. Rosengren BI, Rippe B. Blood flow limitation in vivo of small solute transfer during peritoneal dialysis in rats. *Journal of the American Society of Nephrology.* 2003;14:1599–2003.

71. Crandall LA, Barker SB, Graham DG. A study of the lymph flow from a patient with thoracic duct fistula. *Gastroenterology.* 1943;1:1040.

72. Morris B. The exchange of protein between the plasma and the liver and intestinal lymph. *Quarterly Journal of Experimental Physiology.* 1956;41:326–340.

73. Curto C, Itskov V, Morrison K, Roth Z, Walker JL. Combinatorial neural codes from a mathematical coding theory perspective. *Neural Computation.* July 2013;25(7):1891–1925.

74. O'Morchoe CCC, O'Morchoe DJ, Holmes MJ, Jarosz HM. Flow of renal hilar lymph during volume expansion and saline diuresis. *Lymphology.* 1978;11:27–31.

75. Shad H, Brechtelsbauer H. Thoracic duct lymph in conscious dog at rest and during changes of physical activity. *Pflügers Archiv: European Journal of Physiology.* 1978;367:235–240.

76. Tran L, Rodela H, Abernathy NJ, Johnston M. Lymphatic drainage of hypertonic solution from peritoneal cavity of anesthetized and conscious sheep. *Journal of Applied Physiology.* 1993;74:859–867.

77. Courtice FC, Simonds WJ, Steinbeck AW. Some investigations on lymph from a thoracic duct fistula in man. *Australian Journal of Experimental Biology and Medical Science.* 1951;29:201.

78. Twardowski ZJ, Prowant BF, Nolph KD. High volume, low frequency continuous ambulatory peritoneal dialysis. *Kidney International.* 1983;23:64–70.

79. Flessner MF, Lofthouse J, Williams A. Increasing peritoneal contact area during dialysis improves mass transfer. *Journal of the American Society of Nephrology.* 2001;12(10):2139–2145.

80. Chagnac A, Herskovitz P, Weinstein T, Elyashiv S, Hirsh J, Hamel I et al. The peritoneal membrane in peritoneal dialysis patients: Estimation of its functional surface area by applying stereologic methods to computerized tomography scans. *Journal of the American Society of Nephrology.* 1999;10:342–346.

81. Chagnac A, Herskovitz P, Ori Y, Weinstein T, Hirsh J, Katz M et al. Effect of increased dialysate volume on peritoneal surface area among peritoneal dialysis patients. *Journal of the American Society of Nephrology.* 2002;13:2554–2559.

82. Flessner MF, Lofthouse J, Zakaria ER. Improving contact area between the peritoneum and intraperitoneal therapeutic solutions. *Journal of the American Society of Nephrology.* 2001;12(4):807–813.

83. Hosie KB, Gilbert JA, Kerr DJ, Brown CB, Peers EM. Fluid dynamics in man of an intraperitoneal drug delivery solution: 4% icodextrin. *Drug Delivery.* 2001;8:9–12.

84. Van der Speeten K, Stuart OA, Sugarbaker PH. Pharmacology of perioperative intraperitoneal and intravenous chemotherapy in patients with peritoneal surface malignancy. *Surgical Oncology Clinics of North America.* October 2012;21(4):577–597.

85. Sugarbaker PH, Chang D, Stuart OA. Hyperthermic intraoperative thoracoabdominal chemotherapy. *Gastroenterology Research and Practice.* 2012;2012:623417.

86. Gilbert JA, Peers EM, Brown CB. IP drug delivery in cancer and aids, using Icodextrin. *Peritoneal Dialysis International.* 1999;19:S78.

87. Flessner MF. Small-solute transport across specific peritoneal tissue surfaces in the rat. *Journal of the American Society of Nephrology.* 1996;7:225–233.

88. Penzotti SC, Mattocks AM. Acceleration of peritoneal dialysis by surface active agents. *Journal of Pharmaceutical Sciences.* 1968;57:1192–1195.

89. Elias D, Bonnay M, Puizillou JM, Antoun S, Demirdjian S, El-Otmany A et al. Heated intra-operative intraperitoneal oxaliplatin after complete resection of peritoneal carcinomatosis: Pharmacokinetics and tissue distribution. *Annals of Oncology.* 2002;13:267–272.

90. Steller MA, Egorin MJ, Trimble EL, Bartlett DL, Suhowski EG, Alexander HR et al. A pilot phase I trial of continuous hyperthermic peritoneal perfusion with high-dose carboplatin as primary treatment of patients with small-volume residual ovarian cancer. *Cancer Chemotherapy and Pharmacology.* 1999;43:106–114.

91. vanRuth S, Mathot RA, Sparidans RW, Beijnen JH, Verwaal VJ, Zoetmulder FA. Population pharmacokinetics and pharmacodynamics of mitomycin during intraoperative hyperthermic intraperitoneal chemotherapy. *Clinical Pharmacokinetics.* 2004;43:131–143.

92. Witkamp AJ, deBree E, VanGoethem R, Zoetmulder FA. Rationale and techniques of intra-operative hyperthermic intraperitoneal chemotherapy. *Cancer Treatment Reviews.* 2001;27:365–374.

93. Jacquet P, Averbach A, Stephens AD, Stuart OA, Chang D, Sugarbaker PH. Heated intraoperative intraperitoneal mitomycin C and early postoperative intraperitoneal 5-fluorouracil: Pharmacokinetic studies. *Oncology.* 1998;55:130–138.

94. Gonzalez-Moreno S, Gonzalez-Bayon L, Ortega-Perez G. Hyperthermic intraperitoneal chemotherapy: Methodology and safety considerations. *Surgical Oncology Clinics of North America.* October 2012;21(4):543–557.

95. Fujiwara K, Nagao S, Aotani E, Hasegawa K. Principle and evolving role of intraperitoneal chemotherapy in ovarian cancer. *Expert Opinion on Pharmacotherapy.* September 2013;14(13):1797–1806.

96. Dedrick RL. Theoretical and experimental bases of intraperitoneal chemotherapy. *Seminars in Oncology.* 1985;12:1–6.

97. Krediet RT, Zemel D, Imholz AL, Koomen GC, Struijk DG, Arisz L. Indices of peritoneal permeability and surface area 19. *Peritoneal Dialysis International.* 1993;13(Suppl. 2):S31–S34.

98. Babb AL, Johansen PJ, Strand MJ, Tenckhoff H, Scribner BH. Bidirectional permeability of the human peritoneum to middle molecules. *Proceedings of the European Dialysis and Transplant Association.* 1973;10:247.

99. Keshaviah P, Emerson PF, Vonesh EF, Brandes JC. Relationship between body size, fill volume, and mass transfer area coefficient in peritoneal dialysis. *Journal of the American Society of Nephrology.* 1994;4:1820–1826.

100. Torres IJ, Litterst CI, Guarino AM. Transport of model compounds across the peritoneal membrane in the rat. *Pharmacology.* 1978;17:161–166.

101. Lewis C, Lawson N, Rankin EM et al. Phase I and pharmacokinetic study of intraperitoneal thioTEPA in patients with ovarian cancer. *Cancer Chemotherapy and Pharmacology.* 1990;26:283–287.

102. Wikes AD, Howell S. Pharmacokinetics of hexamethylmelamine administered via the ip route in and oil emulsion vehicle. *Cancer Treatment Reports.* 1985;69:657–662.

103. Hasovits C, Clarke S. Pharmacokinetics and pharmacodynamics of intraperitoneal cancer chemotherapeutics. *Clinical Pharmacokinetics.* April 1, 2012;51(4):203–224.

104. Van der Speeten K, Govaerts K, Stuart OA, Sugarbaker PH. Pharmacokinetics of the perioperative use of cancer chemotherapy in peritoneal surface malignancy patients. *Gastroenterology Research and Practice.* 2012;2012:378064.

105. Dedrick RL, Myers CE, Bungay PM, DeVita VT. Pharmacokinetic rationale for peritoneal drug administration in the treatment of ovarian cancer. *Cancer Treatment Reports*. 1978;62:1.

106. Pitts RF. *Physiology of the Kidney and Body Fluids*, Chicago, IL: Year Book Medical Publishers, 1963.

107. Lukas G, Brindle SD, Greongard P. The route of absorption of intraperitoneally administered compounds. *Journal of Pharmacology and Experimental Therapeutics*. 1971;178:562–566.

108. Collins JM, Dedrick RL, Flessner MF, Guarino AM. Concentration-dependent disappearance of fluorouracil from peritoneal fluid in the rat: Experimental observations and distributed modeling. *Journal of Pharmaceutical Sciences*. July 1982;71(7):735–738.

109. Gianola FJ, Sugarbaker P, Barofsky I, White DE, Myers CE. Toxicity studies of adjuvant intravenous versus intraperitoneal 5-FU in patients with advanced primary colon or rectal cancer. *American Journal of Clinical Oncology*. 1986;9:403–410.

110. Flessner MF, Dedrick RL, Schultz JS. A distributed model of peritoneal-plasma transport: Theoretical considerations. *American Journal of Physiology*. April 1984;246(4 Pt. 2):R597–R607.

111. Dedrick RL, Flessner MF, Collins JM, Schultz JS. Is the peritoneum a membrane? *American Society for Artificial Internal Organs Journal*. 1982;5:1–5.

112. Flessner MF, Lofthouse J, Zakaria e. In vivo diffusion of immunoglobulin G in muscle: Effects of binding, solute exclusion, and lymphatic removal. *American Journal of Physiology*. December 1997;273(6 Pt. 2):H2783–H2793.

113. Flessner MF. Transport of protein in the abdominal wall during intraperitoneal therapy. I. Theoretical approach. *American Journal of Physiology: Gastrointestinal and Liver Physiology*. August 2001;281(2):G424–G437.

114. Waniewski J, Dutka V, Stachowska-Pietka J, Cherniha R. Distributed modeling of glucose-induced osmotic flow. *Advances in Peritoneal Dialysis*. 2007;23:2–6.

115. Stachowska-Pietka J, Waniewski J, Flessner MF, Lindholm B. A distributed model of bidirectional protein transport during peritoneal fluid absorption. *Advances in Peritoneal Dialysis*. 2007;23:5–10.

116. Waniewski J, Stachowska-Pietka J, Flessner MF. Distributed modeling of osmotically driven fluid transport in peritoneal dialysis: Theoretical and computational investigations. *American Journal of Physiology: Heart and Circulatory Physiology*. 2009;296:H1960–H1968.

117. Baron MA. Structure of the intestinal peritoneum in man. *American Journal of Anatomy*. 1941;69:439–497.

118. Flessner MF, Dedrick RL, Reynolds JC. Bidirectional peritoneal transport of immunoglobulin in rats: Compartmental kinetics. *American Journal of Physiology*. February 1992;262(2 Pt. 2):F275–F287.

119. Rippe B, Stelin G, Ahlmen J, Maher JF, Winchester JF. *Frontiers in Peritoneal Dialysis,* New York: Field, Rich, 1986.

120. Heimburger O, Waniewski J, Werynski A, Park MS, Lindholm B. Lymphatic absorption in CAPD patients with loss of ultrafiltration capacity. PhD thesis. Stockholm, Sweden: Konogl Carolinska Medico Chirurgiska Institute; 1994. pp. 1–21.

121. Daugirdas JT, Ing TS, Gandhi VC, Hano JE, Chen WT, Yuan L. Kinetics of peritoneal fluid absorption in patients with chronic renal failure. *Journal of Laboratory and Clinical Medicine*. 1980;85:351–361.

122. Flessner MF. Peritoneal transport physiology: Insights from basic research. *Journal of the American Society of Nephrology*. August 1991;2(2):122–135.

123. Granger DN, Taylor AE. Effects of solute-coupled transport on lymph flow and oncotic pressures in the cat intestine. *American Journal of Physiology*. 1979;235:E429–E436.

124. Courtice FC, Steinbeck AW. Absorption of protein from the peritoneal cavity. *Journal of Physiology (London)*. 1951;114:336–355.

125. Flessner MF, Lofthouse J. An intact peritoneum is not necessary for osmotic flow from tissue to cavity. *Journal of the American Society of Nephrology*. 1998;9:191A.

126. Vazquez Vd, Stuart OA, Mohamed F, Sugarbaker P. Extent of parietal peritonectomy does not change intraperitoneal chemotherapy pharmacokinetics. *Cancer Chemotherapy Reports*. 2003;52:108–112.

127. Hekking LHP, Harvey VS, Havenith CEG, van den Born J, Beelen RHJ, Jackman RW et al. Mesothelial cell transplantation in models of acute inflammation and chronic peritoneal dialysis. *Peritoneal Dialysis International*. 2003;23:323–330.

128. Margetts PJ, Gyorffy S, Kolb M, Yu L, Hoff CM, Holmes CJ et al. Antiangiogenic and antifibrotic gene therapy in a chronic infusion model of peritoneal dialysis in rats. *Journal of the American Society of Nephrology*. 2002;13(3):721–728.

129. Margetts PJ, Kolb M, Galt T, Hoff CM, Shockley TR, Gauldie J. Gene transfer of transforming growth factor-beta1 to the rat peritoneum: Effects on membrane function. *Journal of the American Society of Nephrology*. 2001;12(10):2029–2039.

130. Jackman RW, Hoff CM, Shockley TR, Nagy JA. Adenovirus-mediated transfer of rat catalase cDNA into rat primary mesothelial cells confers increased resistance to oxidant-induced injury in vitro. *Journal of the American Society of Nephrology*. 1999;10:446A–447A.

131. Hoff CM, Piscopo D, Inman KL, Shockley TR. Adenovirus-mediated gene transfer to the peritoneal cavity. *Peritoneal Dialysis International*. 2000;20:128–136.

132. Alvarez RD, Curiel DT. A phase I study of recombinant adenovirus vector-mediated intraperitoneal delivery of herpes simplex virus thymidine kinase

(HSV-TK) gene and intravenous ganciclovir for previously treated ovarian and extraovarian cancer patients. *Human Gene Therapy.* 1997;8:597–613.

133. Mujoo K, Maneval DC, Anderson SC, Gutterman JU. Adenoviral-mediated p53 tumor suppressor gene therapy of human ovarian carcinoma. *Oncogene.* 1996;12:1617–1623.

134. Tong XW, Block A, Chen SH, Contact CF, Agoulnik I, Blankenburg K et al. In vivo gene therapy of ovarian cancer by adenovirus-mediated thymidine kinase gene transduction and ganciclovir administration. *Gynecologic Oncology.* 1996;61:175–179.

135. deForni M, Boneu A, Otal P, Martel P, Shubinski R, Bugat R et al. Anatomic changes in the abdominal cavity during intraperitoneal chemotherapy: Prospective study using scintigraphic peritoneography. *Bulletin du Cancer.* 1993;80:345–350.

136. Binder S, Lewis AL, Lohr JM, Keese M. Extravascular use of drug-eluting beads: A promising approach in compartment-based tumor therapy. *World Journal of Gastroenterology.* November 21, 2013;19(43):7586–7593.

137. De Smet L, Ceelen W, Remon JP, Vervaet C. Optimization of drug delivery systems for intraperitoneal therapy to extend the residence time of the chemotherapeutic agent. *Scientific World Journal.* 2013;2013:720858.

138. Reed RK, Rubin K, Wiig H, Rodt SA. Blockade of á 1-integrins in skin causes edema through lowering of interstitial fluid pressure. *Circulation Research.* 1992;71:978–983.

139. Rubin K, Sundberq C, Ahlen K, Reed RK, Mattale NG, Bert JL et al. Integrins: Transmembrane links between the extracellular matrix and the cell interior. In: Wayne D. Comper, ed., *Interstitium, Connective Tissue, and Lymphatics,* London, U.K.: Portland Press Ltd, 1995. pp. 29–40.

140. Rubin K, Gullberg D, Tomasini-Johansson B, Reed RK, Ryden C, Borg TK et al. Molecular recognition of the extracellular matrix by cell surface receptors. In: Wayne D. Comper, ed., *Extracellular Matrix,* Amsterdam, the Netherlands: Harwood Academic Publishers, 1996. pp. 262–309.

141. Laurent TC, Reed RK, McHale NG, Bert JL, Winlove CP, Laine GA. Structure of the extracellular matrix and the biology of hyaluronan. In: Wayne D. Comper, ed., *Interstitium, Connective Tissue, and Lymphatics,* London, U.K.: Portland Press, 1995. pp. 1–12.

142. Fraser JRE, Laurent TC, Comper WD. Hyaluronan. In: *Extracellular Matrix,* Amsterdam, the Netherlands: Harwood Academic Publishers, 1996. pp. 141–199.

143. Wiig H, DeCarlo M, Sibley L, Renkin EM. Interstitial exclusion of albumin in rat tissues measured by a continuous infusion method. *American Journal of Physiology.* 1992;263:H1222–H1233.

144. Wiig H, Kaysen GA, Al-Bander HA, DeCarlo M, Sibley L, Renkin EM. Interstitial exclusion of IgG in rat tissues estimated by continuous infusion. *American Journal of Physiology.* 1994;266:H212–H219.

145. Flessner MF, Fenstermacher JD, Dedrick RL, Blasberg RG. A distributed model of peritoneal-plasma transport: Tissue concentration gradients. *American Journal of Physiology.* March 1985;248(3 Pt. 2):F425–F435.

146. Choi J, Credit K, Henderson K, Deverkadra R, He Z, Wiig H et al. Intraperitoneal immunotherapy for metastatic ovarian carcinoma: Resistance of intratumoral collagen to antibody penetration. *Clinical Cancer Research.* March 15, 2006;12(6):1906–1912.

147. Flessner MF, Choi J, Credit K, Deverkadra R, Henderson K. Resistance of tumor interstitial pressure to the penetration of intraperitoneally delivered antibodies into metastatic ovarian tumor. *Clinical Cancer Research.* April 15, 2005;11(8):3117–3125.

148. Flessner MF, Choi J, He Z, Credit K. Physiological characterization of human ovarian cancer cells in a rat model of intraperitoneal antineoplastic therapy. *Journal of Applied Physiology.* October 2004;97(4):1518–1526.

149. Zakaria ER, Lofthouse J, Flessner MF. In vivo hydraulic conductivity of muscle: Effects of hydrostatic pressure. *American Journal of Physiology.* 1997;273:H2774–H2782.

150. Gotloib L, Mines M, Garmizo L, Varka I. Hemodynamic effects of increasing intra-abdominal pressure in peritoneal dialysis. *Peritoneal Dialysis Bulletin.* 1981;1:41–43.

151. Flessner MF. Intraperitoneal drug therapy: Physical and biological principles. *Cancer Treatment and Research.* 2007;134:131–152.

152. Wiig H, Reed RK, Aukland K. Micropuncture measurement of interstitial fluid pressure in rat subcutis and skeletal muscle: Comparison to the wick-in-needle technique. *Microvascular Research.* 1981;21:308–319.

153. Wiig H, Reed RK. Interstitial compliance and transcapillary Starling pressures in cat skin and skeletal muscle. *American Journal of Physiology.* 1985;248:H666–H673.

154. Gullino PM, Grantham FH, Smith SH. The interstitial water space of tumors. *Cancer Research.* 1965;25:727–731.

155. Butler TP, Grantham FH, Gullino PM. Bulk transfer of fluid in the interstitial compartment of mammary tumors. *Cancer Research.* 1975;35:3084–3088.

156. Boucher Y, Baxter LT, Jain RK. Interstitial pressure gradients in tissue-isolated and subcutaneous tumors: Implications for therapy. *Cancer Research.* 1990;50:4478–4484.

157. Boucher Y, Kirkwood JM, Opacic D, Desantis M, Jain RK. Interstitial hypertension in superficial metastatic melanomas in humans. *Cancer Research.* 1991;51:6691–6694.

158. Jain RK. Transport of molecules in the tumor interstitium: A review. *Cancer Research*. 1987;47:3039–3051.

159. Netti PA, Berk DA, Swartz MA, Grodzinsky AJ, Jain RK. Role of extracellular matrix assembly in interstitial transport in solid tumors. *Cancer Research*. 2000;60:2497–2503.

160. Flessner MF. The transport barrier in intraperitoneal therapy. *American Journal of Physiology*. March 2005;288(3):F433–F442.

161. Roh HD, Boucher Y, Kalnicki S, Buchsbaum R, Bloomer WD, Jain RK. Interstitial hypertension in carcinoma of uterine cervix in patients: Possible correlation with tumor oxygenation and radiation exposure. *Cancer Research*. 1991;51:6695–6698.

162. Vink H, Duling BR. Identification of distinct luminal domains for macromolecules, erythrocytes, and leucocytes within mammalian capillaries. *Circulation Research*. 1996;79:581–589.

163. Vink H, Duling BR. Capillary endothelial surface layer selectively reduces plasma solute distribution volume. *American Journal of Physiology: Heart and Circulatory Physiology*. 2000;278:H285–H289.

164. Fu B, Curry FE, Adamson RH, Weinbaum S. A model for interpreting the tracer labeling of interendothelial clefts. *Annals of Biomedical Engineering*. 1997;25:375–397.

165. Fu BM, Curry FE, Weinbaum S. A diffusion wake model for tracer ultrastructure-permeability studies in microvessels. *American Journal of Physiology*. 1995;269:H2124–H2140.

166. Platts SH, Duling BR. Adenosine A3 receptor activation modulates the capillary endothelial glycocalyx. *Circulation Research*. 2004;94:77–82.

167. Matsuki T, Duling BR. TNF-alpha increases entry of macromolecules into luminal endothelial cell glycocalyx. *Microcirculation*. 2000;7:411–418.

168. Leunig M, Yuan F, Menger MD, Boucher Y, Goetz AE, Messmer K et al. Angiogenesis, microvascular architecture, microhemodynamics, and interstitial fluid pressure during early growth of human adenocarcinoma LS174T in SCID mice. *Cancer Research*. 1992;52:6553–6560.

169. Nugent LJ, Jain RK. Plasma pharmacokinetics and interstitial diffusion of macromolecules in a capillary bed. *American Journal of Physiology*. 1984;246:H129–H137.

170. Yuan F, Leunig M, Berk DA, Jain RK. Microvascular permeability of albumin, vascular surface area, and vascular volume measured in human adenocarcinoma LS174T using dorsal chamber in SCID mice. *Microvascular Research*. 1993;45:269–289.

171. Gerlowski LE, Jain RK. Microvascular permeability of normal and neoplastic tissues. *Microvascular Research*. 1986;31:288–305.

172. Henry CBS, Duling BR. TNF-alpha increases entry of macromolecules into luminal endothelial cell glycocalyx. *American Journal of Physiology*. 2000;279:H2815–H2823.

173. Courtice FC, Steinbeck AW. The effects of lymphatic obstruction and of posture on absorption of protein from the peritoneal cavity. *Australian Journal of Experimental Biology and Medical Science*. 1951;29:451–458.

174. Dykes PW, Jones JH. Albumin exchange between plasma and ascites fluid. *Clinical Science*. 1964;34:185–197.

175. Graziosi L, Bugiantella W, Cavazzoni E, Donini A. Laparoscopic intraperitoneal hyperthermic perfusion in palliation of malignant ascites. Case report. *Giornale di Chirurgia*. May 2009;30(5):237–239.

176. Patriti A, Cavazzoni E, Graziosi L, Pisciaroli A, Luzi D, Gulla N et al. Successful palliation of malignant ascites from peritoneal mesothelioma by laparoscopic intraperitoneal hyperthermic chemotherapy. *Surgical Laparoscopy, Endoscopy & Percutaneous Techniques*. August 2008;18(4):426–428.

177. Rusznyák I, Földi M, Szabo G. *Lymphatics and Lymph Circulation*, London, U.K.: Pergamon Press, 1967.

178. Baxter LT, Jain RK. Transport of fluid and macromolecules in tumor. I. Role of interstitial pressure and convection. *Microvascular Research*. 1989;37:77–104.

179. Krediet RT, Struijk DG, Koomen GCM. Peritoneal transport of macromolecules in patients on CAPD. *Contributions to Nephrology*. 1991;89:161–174.

180. Flessner MF, Fenstermacher JD, Blasberg RG, Dedrick RL. Peritoneal absorption of macromolecules studied by quantitative autoradiography. *American Journal of Physiology*. January 1985;248(1 Pt. 2): H26–H32.

181. Flessner MF, Dedrick R, Reynolds J. Peritoneal tissue transport of IgG. *FASEB Journal*. 1990;4:A592.

Peritoneal Carcinomatosis: Basic mechanisms

5

Molecular biology of peritoneal carcinomatosis

RIOM KWAKMAN, NINA R. SLUITER, ERIENNE M.V. DE CUBA,
AND ELISABETH (LISETTE) A. TE VELDE

Selection of patients that will benefit most from current treatment is warranted. Prediction of biological behavior and response to treatment will help us in bringing the right treatment to the right patient, in this way providing a step toward personalized medicine. Assuming that the clinical phenotype of this disease is ultimately dictated by molecular mechanisms, characterization of these mechanisms might aid in predicting biological behavior.

In the basic pathogenesis of peritoneal carcinomatosis (PC), it is believed that peritoneal metastases arise per continuum, from free-floating cells in the peritoneal cavity that attach and grow to new metastases, whereas hepatic and lung metastases arise from hematogenous spread. Although definitive scientific evidence is lacking, we believe different molecular mechanisms result in peritoneal dissemination as compared to hematogenous dissemination. This is supported by the differences in microenvironment between liver and peritoneum. Liver metastases are marked by attachment to endothelium and survival in an oxygen-rich environment. However, the mesothelial lining of the peritoneum has other attachment molecules and is relatively less vascularized compared to hepatic tissue. Concordantly, cancer cells capable of developing liver metastases are believed to have a different molecular profile than tumor cells disseminating to the peritoneum.

This is further supported by evidence that not all patients with risk factors develop PC. Research has indicated that patients with stage T4 colorectal cancer (invasion beyond serosa) are at highest risk to develop PC, yet only a subset of these patients eventually develop PC [1]. Similarly, detecting cancer cells in peritoneal fluid is a risk factor for PC, but it is not unequivocal that these patients develop metastases [2]. It seems that cancer cells require specific capacities to disseminate to the peritoneum. It is reasonable to think that these specific capacities that mediate peritoneal metastasis are dictated by specific molecules and their function, and that these functions would be required during the multistep process that results in peritoneal dissemination.

On a molecular basis, the development of PC is divided into two phases. The first phase is when actual dissemination takes places. It involves the following steps [3]:

- Detachment from the primary tumor
- Anoikis evasion
- Motility in the peritoneal cavity
- Attachment to the mesothelium

The second phase occurs after the actual spread to the mesothelial lining of the peritoneal cavity. This is when the attached cells must create a microenvironment suitable for sustained growth and proliferation. These steps are adapted from the hallmarks of cancer as described by Hanahan and Weinberg [4]:

- Invasion beyond the mesothelium and basement membrane
- Sustaining proliferation and suppressing apoptosis
- Reprogramming of energy metabolism
- Evading immune destruction and hijacking inflammation
- Inducing angiogenesis

Considering the aforementioned list, we hypothesize that for metastasis to occur, the cancer cell needs to undergo several changes in its biology before it can readily spread to the peritoneum. These molecular changes and interactions as seen in PC will be discussed in this chapter. The detachment and attachment to the peritoneum is mostly facilitated by adhesion molecules and will only be discussed briefly as this is primarily covered in Chapter 7.

ATTACHMENT

Free-floating tumor cell spheroids must attach to the mesothelial lining of the peritoneum to gain access to nutrients and oxygen, which are not sufficiently provided in the peritoneal cavity. Transmembrane attachment molecules on the tumor cell scavenge proteins on the mesothelial cells for possible anchorage. Current candidates that have been shown to be able to mediate attachment are members of the integrin superfamily. Specifically, the α2 and β1 subunits have been shown to mediate peritoneal dissemination [5–9]. Integrins facilitate adhesion to extracellular matrix (ECM)-derived molecules such as laminin, fibronectin, vitronectin, and collagen I, which are also present on mesothelial cells [10,11]. A second molecule implicated in attachment is cluster of differentiation 44 (CD44). This molecule is recognized in several forms of PC [12,13]. CD44 binds to hyaluronan, a major constituent of ECM [14,15]. These molecular attachments might partly explain the preferential attachment to mesothelial-free surfaces of the peritoneum, such as milky spots in the omentum [16]. Furthermore, members of the immunoglobulin superfamily, such as intercellular adhesion molecule 1 and vascular cell adhesion molecule 1, are indicated in adhesion after surgery. Inflammation leads to upregulation of these molecules and might explain the worsened prognosis seen after surgery [17]. Other possible attachment molecules include blood group antigens (Sialyl Lewis X), mucins, and chemokine receptors [18].

MESOTHELIAL INVASION

The newly peritoneum-attached spheroid of tumor cells has the goal to proliferate, grow, invade, and metastasize, yet the current environment provides no tools for these goals. Attachment to the mesothelium provides poor anchorage as mesothelial cells protect the peritoneum from metastasis despite abundant attachment molecules [19]. Oxygen is only facilitated by diffusion, and the rapid proliferation and multiplication of cancer cells will quickly lead to necrosis in the absence of direct blood supply.

For metastases to grow and proliferate in the new environment, they must gain access to the submesothelial connective tissue (ECM) and create a tumor-friendly environment by recruitment of stromal cells that provide resources [20]. However, before angiogenesis can be induced and stromal factors can be used to sustain proliferation, the tumor cells must invade beyond the mesothelial layer and its basement membrane. Several mechanisms exist to mediate this step: destruction of the mesothelium and its basement membrane, diapedesis through the intercellular space, or expression of chemokines that induce mesothelial detachment [21]. The different processes of mesothelial invasion are depicted in Figure 5.1.

Research suggests that tumor spheroids are capable of exerting force on mesothelial cells and remove them from the underlying ECM. Ovarian cancer cells appear to promote adhesion disassembly of mesothelial–ECM adhesion, possibly by cleavage fibronectin by matrix metalloproteinase-2 (MMP-2) or MMP-9 [22]. Removal of mesothelial cells follows by attachment via integrin–fibronectin adhesions and force exertion in a talin I- and myosin-dependent manner, effectively creating a hole in the mesothelial layer [23]. Subsequent attachment to the underlying ECM is facilitated by the exposed matrix molecules and the more abundant attachment molecules of the tumor cells.

Current evidence in favor of the destruction of the mesothelial layer and basement membrane is derived from observations of apoptotic changes in mesothelial cells upon invasion of tumor cells. Such induced apoptosis might be facilitated by the Fas/Fas ligand pathway [24], the TNF-related apoptosis-inducing ligand (TRAIL) pathway, or other pathways leading to downstream caspase activation. In experimental models, gastric tumor cells have been shown to hijack the abundantly available macrophages in milky spots of the omentum by transforming their phenotype to the protumorigenic M2 subtype [25,26]. These macrophages in turn cause mesothelial apoptosis and augment the epithelial-to-mesenchymal transition by producing TGF-β [27]. This last step is required for the tumor–stroma interaction further described in the succeeding text.

Furthermore, many studies have found strong associations between MMPs and the development of PC. MMPs are responsible for breakdown of ECM lying deeper in the stroma, but also for molecules found in basement membranes. The peritoneal basement membrane is primarily composed of collagen I and fibronectin with a small layer of laminin and collagen IV [28]. Unsurprisingly, upregulation of MMP-7, a molecule which is responsible for cleavage of collagen, laminin, and fibronectin, has been linked to peritoneal dissemination in gastric cancer [29,30]. In colon cancer, MMP-9 has been linked to increased peritoneal metastases [31]. The transmembrane MMPs (membrane-type (MT)-MMPs) may form an even more important group of basement membrane cleaving proteins, as they are more easily targeted towards the collagen and fibronectin of the basement membrane rather than the soluble MMPs. MT1-MMP has been recognized as a critical mediator in both ovarian and gastric metastasis by cleavage of the collagen-rich basement membrane [8,32] and recently as important mediator in the shedding of the primary tumor [33]. MT1-MMP also has the capacity to activate MMP-2, which will result in further destruction of the basement membrane [34].

Another possible mode of invasion is the expression of molecules that alter mesothelial morphology and cause them to detach from the basement membrane. Research suggests that proinflammatory molecules such as TNF-α and interleukin-1beta (IL-1β) cause the mesothelial cells to become round and lose their cell–cell adhesions, leaving the underlying basement membrane or ECM exposed for attachment [35,36]. Conversely, attachment molecules of the integrin superfamily were upregulated on the surface mesothelial cells in response to TNF-α and could provide better attachment for homing tumor cells [37]. TNF-α can be highly expressed by tumor cells of ovarian and gastrointestinal origin and initiates invasion into the submesothelial stroma [38].

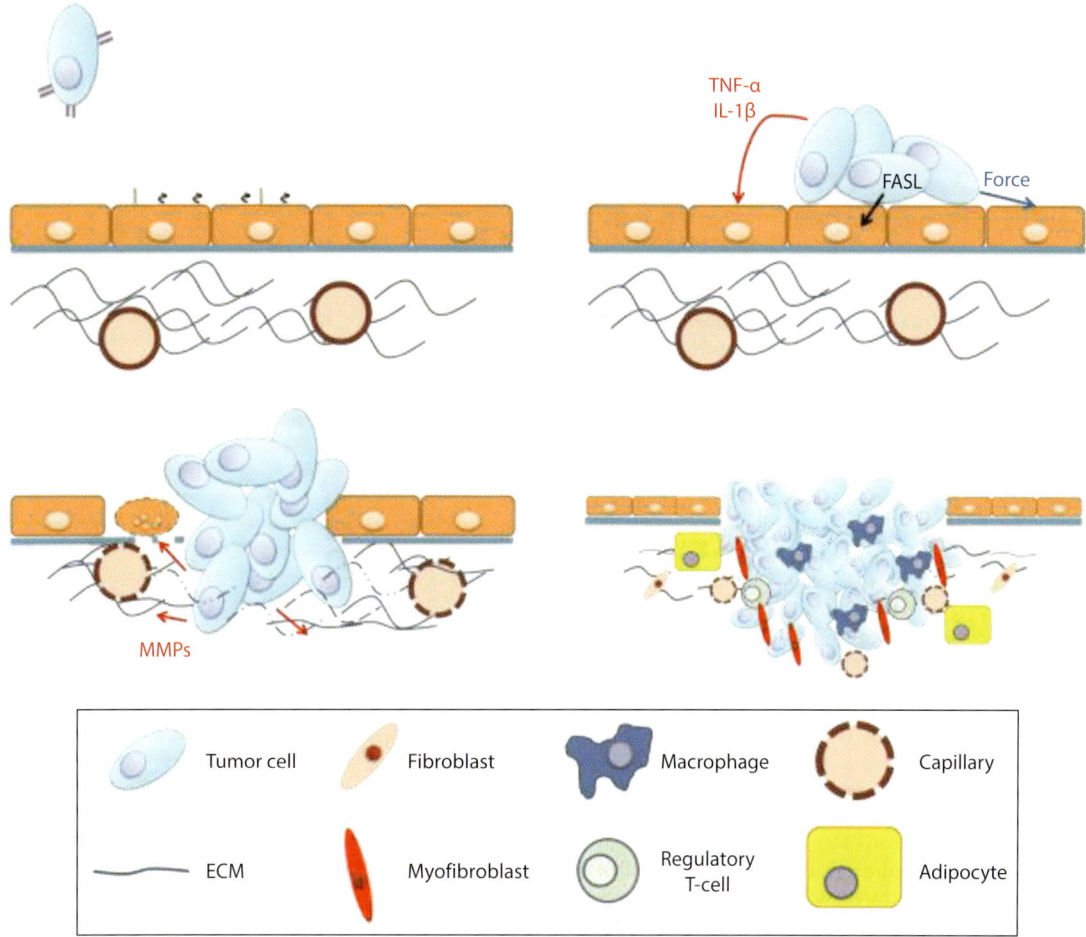

Figure 5.1 The multistep process of peritoneal metastasis. Tumor cells attach to the mesothelial lining by specific attachment molecules. Once attached, mesothelial invasion is facilitated by destruction of the mesothelial lining. ECM invasion is mediated by MMPs. Lastly, tumor cells attract stromal cells to provide proliferative signals.

PROLIFERATION

Cancer is defined by malignant cells with an unlimited dividing potential that fail to respond to apoptotic signals. Tumor cells that have nestled in the peritoneum exhibit an array of proliferative pathway dysregulation of intracellular proteins similar to that of their primary counterpart. For example, PC of colorectal origin often has Wnt pathway upregulation through *APC* deletion [39], ovarian carcinomas uniformly have a *TP53* mutation [40], and mucinous adenocarcinoma of the appendix often has *GNAS*, and *KRAS* mutations [41]. Common molecular deficits, such as *TP53* downregulation, are common among tumors disseminating to the peritoneum. However, the intracellular and autocrine proliferative and antiapoptotic signals are primarily based on the origin of the tumor rather than it being a common marker among all types of PC. The common factor in PC is defined by the environment the tumor cells disseminate to and their reaction to the new environment in order to sustain proliferation.

After adhesion to the mesothelial lining, tumor cells must migrate into the submesothelial matrix and recruit stromal cells to create a tumor–stromal interaction, which will facilitate proliferative signals, immune evasion, and inflammation.

Some MMPs, such as MMP-2 and MT1-MMP, more easily cleave ECM proteoglycans than basement membrane proteoglycans. Not only does this create space for invasion, but destruction of ECM will also release previously ECM-bound peptides, which function as proinflammatory and proliferative signals to the tumor cells. Moreover, MMPs have shown to exhibit a signaling function in the TNF cascade, adding immune response manipulation to their capacities [42]. MMPs are likely to be produced by both tumor cells and cancer-associated stromal cells.

The role of the tumor–stromal interaction in PC has recently been validated in several studies [43–45]. Coimplantation of peritoneally derived stromal cells at peritoneal metastatic sites results in more invasion and migration [44]. Cancer-associated stroma arises from transdifferentiation of fibroblasts, mesothelial cells, or even cancer cells to the tumor-associated myofibroblast [45,46]. This epithelial–mesenchymal transformation or transdifferentiation is driven by tumor-derived TGF-β [45] and PDGF [20] and activates the Smad4 pathway [46]. Subsequently, epithelial markers such as E-cadherin and cytokeratin are downregulated and mesenchymal markers

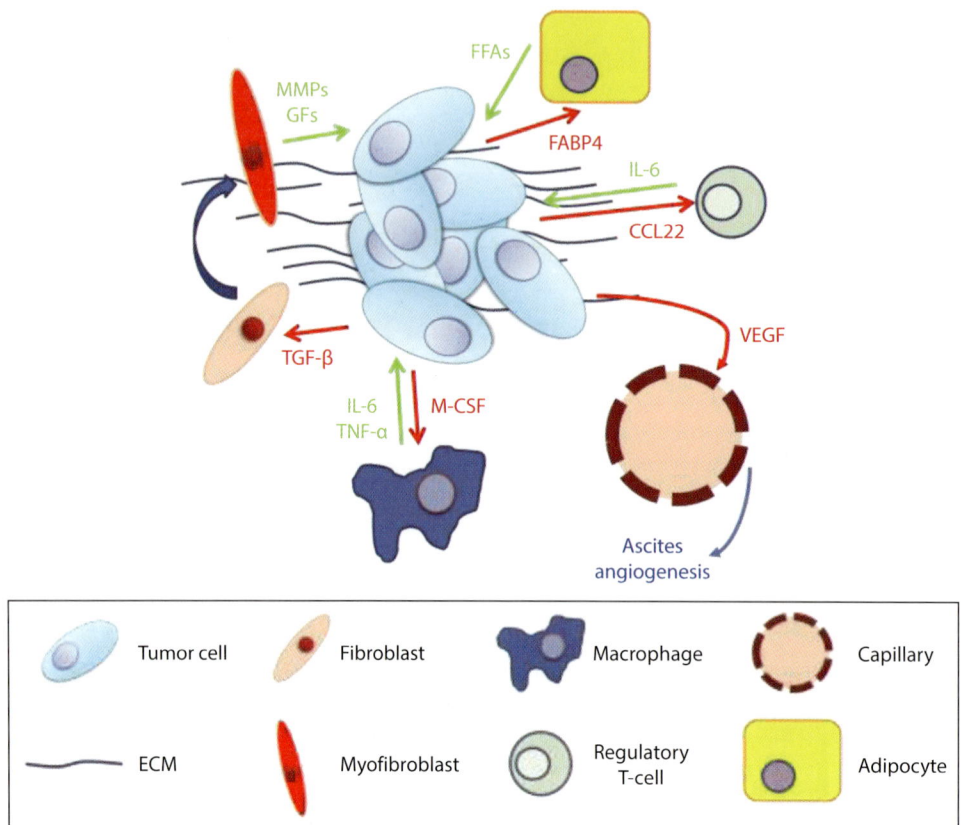

Figure 5.2 Tumors cells and their microenvironment. Tumor cells interact with several different cell types to sustain proliferation. ECM, extracellular matrix; MMP, matrix metalloproteinase; GF, growth factor; FFA, free fatty acid.

α-smooth muscle actin (α-SMA) and vimentin are upregulated [47]. The stromal myofibroblast are then instructed, possibly through IL-1β [48], to produce proinvasive and antiapoptotic molecules such as MMP-2, hepatocyte growth factor (HGF) [49], VEGF, IL-6, and IL-8 [48]. MMP-2 and MMP-9 are specifically produced by stromal cells, yet less produced by tumor cells in the setting of ovarian cancer. Tumor-associated stroma acquisition is displayed in Figure 5.2. Collectively, these findings have led to believe that tumor cells are dependent on stroma for proliferative signals. Crosstalk between tumor-associated stroma and tumor is a defining feature of PC. Possible disruption of the tumor–stroma crosstalk by pharmacological intervention is a novel treatment strategy that appears promising [50]. Tumor cells lacking molecules to attract and create stromal cells might explain why only a subset of tumors disseminates to the peritoneum in spite of abundant risk factors.

METABOLISM

Part of the hallmarks of cancer as described by Hanahan and Weinberg [4] includes the dysregulation and hijacking of the normal metabolism in order to not only sustain proliferation and cell division, but also to function in relatively hypoxic-ischemic conditions. Although much research on metabolism in cancer is available, very little knowledge exists on this process in PC. New research suggests tumor cells produce fatty acid binding protein 4 (FABP4) in the presence of omental or peritoneal adipocytes. Beta-adrenergic stimulation of adipocytes by a FABP4-mediated mechanism induces lipolysis in adipocytes and subsequent beta-oxidation provides free fatty acids. These free fatty acids are transported to the tumor cells, which require them for their high energy metabolism [51]. The exact mechanism of FABP4-mediated tumor–adipocyte fat transfer remains unknown.

INFLAMMATION AND EVADING IMMUNE DESTRUCTION

Inflammation is a state of an organ or tissue where the five cardinal signs of inflammation are present: rubor, calor, dolor, tumor, and functio laesa. Pathophysiologically, this is caused by a release of cytokines and inflammatory molecules, which results in increased vascular permeability, vasodilation, and edema. Although one is inclined to think that inflammation is the immune system's appropriate reaction to the tumor, cancer cells can harness the effects of inflammation to promote their own proliferation and nutrient supply. This is why inflammation has recently been put on the map as one of the new emerging hallmarks of cancer [4]. Already described in many types of cancer, inflammation is often seen in PC, which is why it is sometimes referred to as peritonitis carcinomatosa; cancerous inflammation of peritoneum. Patients with pseudomyxoma peritonei have higher levels of CRP in their blood than normal individuals, but a higher CRP is also linked to a higher chance of having ascites [52]. Patients with PC of colorectal origin have worse prognosis if presented with high CRP concentration [53].

On a molecular level, cytokines released in the process of inflammation are increasingly being linked to the development and invasiveness of PC. In the same study on pseudomyxoma peritonei (PMP), they showed that the concentration of IL-6 was a 200-fold higher in ascites compared to serum [52]. IL-6 was largely expressed by tumor-associated stroma cells, which provide antiapoptotic, protumorigenic, and angiogenic signals [54], possibly through an NFκB-mediated mechanism [55]. Importance of IL-6 has been shown in PMP, ovarian, and colorectal cancer [56]. Other molecules correlated to inflammation include IL-8, CC chemokine ligand (CCL)-2 and CCL-3 [52], IL-1β, and TNF-α [57], although the list is rapidly growing. Surprisingly, these molecules are not seen in inflammation by an external pathogen, suggesting a different cancer-mediated form of inflammation.

Next to production of chemokines by tumor–stroma cells that directly mediate inflammation, other chemokines are produced to attract certain types of inflammatory cells. Currently, the most investigated lymphocytes are the regulatory T-cells (Tregs). This subset of CD4+CD25+ T-cells exhibits immune modulating properties and is regarded as anti-inflammatory. In the case of PC, Tregs appear to downregulate the antitumor response. CCL22 (stromal-derived factor 1), produced by ovarian carcinoma, might be responsible for the recruitment of Tregs in peritoneal metastases [58]. These Tregs directly inhibit cytotoxic T-cells, which result in decreased levels of antitumorigenic chemokines such as IL-2 and interferon (IFN)-gamma. Tregs produce the chemokines IL-6, IL-10, and TNF-α to promote tumor proliferation [59]. Patients with increased levels of Tregs in their tumor have increased tumor load and decreased survival [58]. Also, when animals with PC are treated with monoclonal antibody to deplete Tregs, IFN-gamma increases, whereas IL-6 decreases, while tumor load decreases in treated animals [59]. The importance of Tregs is increasingly being recognized in PC of different origins [60,61]

Next to Tregs, macrophages are increasingly being recognized as protumorigenic. Macrophages can be subdivided into M1 and M2 macrophages. M1 macrophages are considered proinflammatory and important in infectious disease, whereas the M2 subtype is anti-inflammatory and implicated in cancer progression [62]. The M2 subtype can be recognized by surface markers such as CD163, CD204, and CD206. Macrophages are recruited as blood-derived monocytes by the chemoattractant CCL2 or monocyte chemotactic protein-1 (MCP-1). MCP-1 is readily overexpressed in ovarian carcinoma [63]. The M2 subtype can be induced by macrophage colony-stimulating factor and produces protumorigenic molecules such as IL-6 and TNF-α [64]. M2 macrophages also elicit angiogenic properties, as witnessed by increased endothelial tube formation in cultures with M2 macrophages [65], probably by expressing high levels of hypoxia-inducible factor 1α (HIF-1α) [66].

Moreover, even when encountering effective lymphocytes, tumor cells exhibit molecules to evade destruction by immune cells. Ovarian cells express programmed death-ligand 1 (PD-L1) when encountering lymphocytes, which downregulates the tumor cell lysis by cytotoxic T-cells [67]. This results in a loss of effective immune response and allows for uninhibited growth. PD-L1 is increased in hypoxic-ischemic conditions by upregulation through the production of HIF-1α [68]. HIF-1α, also implicated in angiogenesis, has the secondary property to induce macrophage transdifferentiation to the M2 subtype that further suppresses T-cell function [69].

The role of inflammation is also underlined in the case of surgery, when a large surgical wound causes the release of local and systemic inflammation mediators [70]. Surgery has been linked to increased PC on many occasions and is postulated to be mediated through inflammation and the surge of cytokines [31]. Surprisingly, this process seems irrespective of laparoscopic or open surgery yet may rather result from the pneumoperitoneum created during surgery, in open surgery exposure to air and in laparoscopic approach to carbon dioxide [71]. The effect of surgery on the peritoneum is further described in Chapter 9.

ANGIOGENESIS

By growing, the oxygen supply in each tumor nodule will gradually become insufficient for the tumor cells' hyperactive metabolism, and a state of hypoxia will occur. In this hypoxic state, the tumor cells will produce a variety of angiogenic factors leading to the activation of the angiogenic cascade. Such factors include HIF-1α [72,73] and IL-1 [74]. These factors cause angiogenesis through the VEGF pathway by inducing production of VEGF and promoting upregulation of VEGF receptors [75]. Sprouting of new vessels will occur to supply the tumor nodule, which in turn will start growing again, balancing between a state of hypoxia in which necrosis will occur and a state of proliferation. Molecules from the CXC family such as CXCR4 and CXCL12 synergize with VEGF to promote angiogenesis [76].

Furthermore, the production of VEGF-A will induce a locally increased vascular permeability, increasing nutrient supply to the tumor. Additionally, VEGF-A activates focal adhesion kinase, which destabilizes endothelial cell junctions by downregulating claudin 5 leading to malignant ascites [77,78]. Ascites per se further promotes metastasis though accumulation of nutrients and cytokines in the excessive peritoneal fluid and marks a poor prognosis [79,80]. It is perhaps the combination of angiogenesis and ascites formation that highlights the importance of VEGF in PC. VEGF overexpression is linked to decreased survival and ascites formation [78,81], yet microvessel density, a direct measurement of angiogenesis, is not linked to worsened survival [82].

Blocking of VEGF results in less ascites formation and less PC, leading to increased survival in patients. However, these effects appear modest and differ depending on the origin of PC.

VEGF-independent angiogenic mechanisms are increasingly being uncovered. HGF and insulin-like growth factor-binding protein 7 may induce angiogenesis through c-MET (hepatocyte growth factor receptor) activation of endothelial stem cells promoting sprouting and tube formation [83].

Vasohibin-2, unlike its homolog vasohibin-1, possesses angiogenic properties, which may be indicated in tumors producing little VEGF [84]. Whether this mechanism is truly VEGF-independent remains to be revealed. Also, proteins involved in the renin–angiotensin and kinin–kallikrein systems appear to mediate angiogenesis, vasodilation, and inflammation in PC [85]. Overall, the importance of angiogenesis and the molecular mechanisms in peritoneal dissemination are still a matter of debate.

CONCLUSION

Although science has recently started to uncover the basic pathophysiology of PC, current knowledge centers on therapy and early discovery of PC. However, expanding the knowledge on the molecular basics of PC is necessary to create insight into the mechanisms that lead to PC in order to search for improved therapeutic options. This chapter shows the molecular mechanisms we currently understand, yet we lack understanding of which molecular changes are pivotal and which are byproducts.

Molecular mechanisms in PC are covered in the multiple facets of cancer hallmarks. Peritoneal dissemination is a multistep process dictated by a variety of proteins implicated in attachment, matrix destruction, cell signaling, and immunomodulation. The new emerging hallmarks seem more implicated in PC than in other metastatic sites. According to current knowledge, tumor–stroma interaction through epithelial–mesenchymal transition of fibroblasts and inflammation or immunosuppression by chemokine production appear to be the drivers of peritoneal dissemination.

REFERENCES

1. Lemmens VE, Klaver YL, Verwaal VJ, Rutten HJ, Coebergh JW, de Hingh IH. Predictors and survival of synchronous peritoneal carcinomatosis of colorectal origin: A population-based study. *International Journal of Cancer.* 2011;128(11):2717–2725.

2. Lee IK, Kim do H, Gorden DL, Lee YS, Sung NY, Park GS et al. Prognostic value of CEA and CA 19–9 tumor markers combined with cytology from peritoneal fluid in colorectal cancer. *Annals of Surgical Oncology.* 2009;16(4):861–870.

3. de Cuba EM, Kwakman R, van Egmond M, Bosch LJ, Bonjer HJ, Meijer GA et al. Understanding molecular mechanisms in peritoneal dissemination of colorectal cancer: Future possibilities for personalised treatment by use of biomarkers. *Virchows Archiv: An International Journal of Pathology.* 2012;461(3):231–243.

4. Hanahan D, Weinberg RA. Hallmarks of cancer: The next generation. *Cell.* 2011;144(5):646–674.

5. Chen CN, Chang CC, Lai HS, Jeng YM, Chen CI, Chang KJ et al. Connective tissue growth factor inhibits gastric cancer peritoneal metastasis by blocking integrin alpha3beta1-dependent adhesion. *Gastric Cancer: Official Journal of the International Gastric Cancer Association and the Japanese Gastric Cancer Association.* 2014;17(3).

6. Fukuda K, Saikawa Y, Yagi H, Wada N, Takahashi T, Kitagawa Y. Role of integrin alpha1 subunits in gastric cancer patients with peritoneal dissemination. *Molecular Medicine Reports.* 2012;5(2):336–340.

7. Wagner BJ, Lob S, Lindau D, Horzer H, Guckel B, Klein G et al. Simvastatin reduces tumor cell adhesion to human peritoneal mesothelial cells by decreased expression of VCAM-1 and beta1 integrin. *International Journal of Oncology.* 2011;39(6):1593–600.

8. Sodek KL, Ringuette MJ, Brown TJ. MT1-MMP is the critical determinant of matrix degradation and invasion by ovarian cancer cells. *British Journal of Cancer.* 2007;97(3):358–367.

9. Sodek KL, Murphy KJ, Brown TJ, Ringuette MJ. Cell-cell and cell-matrix dynamics in intraperitoneal cancer metastasis. *Cancer Metastasis Reviews.* 2012;31(1–2):397–414.

10. Ahmed N, Riley C, Rice G, Quinn M. Role of integrin receptors for fibronectin, collagen and laminin in the regulation of ovarian carcinoma functions in response to a matrix microenvironment. *Clinical & Experimental Metastasis.* 2005;22(5):391–402.

11. Burleson KM, Casey RC, Skubitz KM, Pambuccian SE, Oegema TR, Jr., Skubitz AP. Ovarian carcinoma ascites spheroids adhere to extracellular matrix components and mesothelial cell monolayers. *Gynecologic Oncology.* 2004;93(1):170–181.

12. Zou L, Yi T, Song X, Li S, Wei Y, Zhao X. Efficient inhibition of intraperitoneal human ovarian cancer growth by short hairpin RNA targeting CD44. *Neoplasma.* 2014;61(3):274–282.

13. Nishii T, Yashiro M, Shinto O, Sawada T, Ohira M, Hirakawa K. Cancer stem cell-like SP cells have a high adhesion ability to the peritoneum in gastric carcinoma. *Cancer Science.* 2009;100(8):1397–1402.

14. Casey RC, Skubitz AP. CD44 and beta1 integrins mediate ovarian carcinoma cell migration toward extracellular matrix proteins. *Clinical & Experimental Metastasis.* 2000;18(1):67–75.

15. Tamada Y, Takeuchi H, Suzuki N, Aoki D, Irimura T. Cell surface expression of hyaluronan on human ovarian cancer cells inversely correlates with their adhesion to peritoneal mesothelial cells. *Tumour Biology: The Journal of the International Society for Oncodevelopmental Biology and Medicine*. 2012;33(4):1215–1222.

16. Clark R, Krishnan V, Schoof M, Rodriguez I, Theriault B, Chekmareva M et al. Milky spots promote ovarian cancer metastatic colonization of peritoneal adipose in experimental models. *The American Journal of Pathology*. 2013;183(2):576–591.

17. Ziprin P, Ridgway PF, Pfistermuller KL, Peck DH, Darzi AW. ICAM-1 mediated tumor-mesothelial cell adhesion is modulated by IL-6 and TNF-alpha: A potential mechanism by which surgical trauma increases peritoneal metastases. *Cell Communication & Adhesion*. 2003;10(3):141–154.

18. Sluiter NR, De Cuba EM, Kwakman R, Kazemier G, Meijer GA, Te Velde EA. Adhesion molecules in peritoneal metastases of colorectal cancer: Their function, prognostic relevance and therapeutic options. Submitted. 2015.

19. Kenny HA, Krausz T, Yamada SD, Lengyel E. Use of a novel 3D culture model to elucidate the role of mesothelial cells, fibroblasts and extra-cellular matrices on adhesion and invasion of ovarian cancer cells to the omentum. *International Journal of Cancer (Journal International du Cancer)*. 2007;121(7):1463–1472.

20. De Wever O, Mareel M. Role of tissue stroma in cancer cell invasion. *The Journal of Pathology*. 2003;200(4):429–447.

21. Jayne D. Molecular biology of peritoneal carcinomatosis. *Cancer Treatment and Research*. 2007;134:21–33.

22. Kenny HA, Kaur S, Coussens LM, Lengyel E. The initial steps of ovarian cancer cell metastasis are mediated by MMP-2 cleavage of vitronectin and fibronectin. *The Journal of Clinical Investigation*. 2008;118(4):1367–1379.

23. Iwanicki MP, Davidowitz RA, Ng MR, Besser A, Muranen T, Merritt M et al. Ovarian cancer spheroids use myosin-generated force to clear the mesothelium. *Cancer Discovery*. 2011;1(2):144–157.

24. Heath RM, Jayne DG, O'Leary R, Morrison EE, Guillou PJ. Tumour-induced apoptosis in human mesothelial cells: A mechanism of peritoneal invasion by Fas Ligand/Fas interaction. *British Journal of Cancer*. 2004;90(7):1437–1442.

25. Liu XY, Miao ZF, Zhao TT, Wang ZN, Xu YY, Gao J et al. Milky spot macrophages remodeled by gastric cancer cells promote peritoneal mesothelial cell injury. *Biochemical and Biophysical Research Communications*. 2013;439(3):378–383.

26. Sica A. Role of tumour-associated macrophages in cancer-related inflammation. *Experimental Oncology*. 2010;32(3):153–158.

27. Na D, Lv ZD, Liu FN, Xu Y, Jiang CG, Sun Z et al. Transforming growth factor beta1 produced in autocrine/paracrine manner affects the morphology and function of mesothelial cells and promotes peritoneal carcinomatosis. *International Journal of Molecular Medicine*. 2010;26(3):325–332.

28. Witz CA, Montoya-Rodriguez IA, Cho S, Centonze VE, Bonewald LF, Schenken RS. Composition of the extracellular matrix of the peritoneum. *Journal of the Society for Gynecologic Investigation*. 2001;8(5):299–304.

29. Yoshikawa T, Yanoma S, Tsuburaya A, Kobayashi O, Sairenji M, Motohashi H et al. Expression of MMP-7 and MT1-MMP in peritoneal dissemination of gastric cancer. *Hepato-Gastroenterology*. 2006;53(72):964–967.

30. Yonemura Y, Endou Y, Fujita H, Fushida S, Bandou E, Taniguchi K et al. Role of MMP-7 in the formation of peritoneal dissemination in gastric cancer. *Gastric Cancer: Official Journal of the International Gastric Cancer Association and the Japanese Gastric Cancer Association*. 2000;3(2):63–70.

31. Lee IK, Vansaun MN, Shim JH, Matrisian LM, Gorden DL. Increased metastases are associated with inflammation and matrix metalloproteinase-9 activity at incision sites in a murine model of peritoneal dissemination of colorectal cancer. *The Journal of Surgical Research*. 2013;180(2):252–259.

32. Nonaka T, Nishibashi K, Itoh Y, Yana I, Seiki M. Competitive disruption of the tumor-promoting function of membrane type 1 matrix metalloproteinase/matrix metalloproteinase-14 in vivo. *Molecular Cancer Therapeutics*. 2005;4(8):1157–1166.

33. Moss NM, Barbolina MV, Liu Y, Sun L, Munshi HG, Stack MS. Ovarian cancer cell detachment and multicellular aggregate formation are regulated by membrane type 1 matrix metalloproteinase: A potential role in I.p. metastatic dissemination. *Cancer Research*. 2009;69(17):7121–7129.

34. Strongin AY, Collier I, Bannikov G, Marmer BL, Grant GA, Goldberg GI. Mechanism of cell surface activation of 72-kDa type IV collagenase. Isolation of the activated form of the membrane metalloprotease. *The Journal of Biological Chemistry*. 1995;270(10):5331–5338.

35. Mochizuki Y, Nakanishi H, Kodera Y, Ito S, Yamamura Y, Kato T et al. TNF-alpha promotes progression of peritoneal metastasis as demonstrated using a green fluorescence protein (GFP)-tagged human gastric cancer cell line. *Clinical & Experimental Metastasis*. 2004;21(1):39–47.

36. Stadlmann S, Raffeiner R, Amberger A, Margreiter R, Zeimet AG, Abendstein B et al. Disruption of the integrity of human peritoneal mesothelium by interleukin-1beta and tumor necrosis factor-alpha. *Virchows Archiv: An International Journal of Pathology*. 2003;443(5):678–685.

37. Sandoval P, Jimenez-Heffernan JA, Rynne-Vidal A, Perez-Lozano ML, Gilsanz A, Ruiz-Carpio V et al. Carcinoma-associated fibroblasts derive from mesothelial cells via mesothelial-to-mesenchymal transition in peritoneal metastasis. *The Journal of Pathology*. 2013;231(4):517–531.

38. Balkwill F. Tumour necrosis factor and cancer. *Nature Reviews Cancer*. 2009;9(5):361–371.

39. Gryfe R, Swallow C, Bapat B, Redston M, Gallinger S, Couture J. Molecular biology of colorectal cancer. *Current Problems in Cancer*. 1997;21(5):233–300.

40. Cancer Genome Atlas Research N. Integrated genomic analyses of ovarian carcinoma. *Nature*. 2011;474(7353):609–615.

41. Alakus H, Babicky ML, Ghosh P, Yost S, Jepsen K, Dai Y et al. Genome-wide mutational landscape of mucinous carcinomatosis peritonei of appendiceal origin. *Genome Medicine*. 2014;6(5):43.

42. Stuelten CH, DaCosta Byfield S, Arany PR, Karpova TS, Stetler-Stevenson WG, Roberts AB. Breast cancer cells induce stromal fibroblasts to express MMP-9 via secretion of TNF-alpha and TGF-beta. *Journal of Cell Science*. 2005;118(Pt. 10):2143–2153.

43. Kojima M, Higuchi Y, Yokota M, Ishii G, Saito N, Aoyagi K et al. Human subperitoneal fibroblast and cancer cell interaction creates microenvironment that enhances tumor progression and metastasis. *PLOS ONE*. 2014;9(2):e88018.

44. Akagawa S, Ohuchida K, Torata N, Hattori M, Eguchi D, Fujiwara K et al. Peritoneal myofibroblasts at metastatic foci promote dissemination of pancreatic cancer. *International Journal of Oncology*. 2014;45(1):113–120.

45. Calon A, Espinet E, Palomo-Ponce S, Tauriello DV, Iglesias M, Cespedes MV et al. Dependency of colorectal cancer on a TGF-beta-driven program in stromal cells for metastasis initiation. *Cancer Cell*. 2012;22(5):571–584.

46. Lv ZD, Na D, Ma XY, Zhao C, Zhao WJ, Xu HM. Human peritoneal mesothelial cell transformation into myofibroblasts in response to TGF-ss1 in vitro. *International Journal of Molecular Medicine*. 2011;27(2):187–193.

47. Miao ZF, Zhao TT, Wang ZN, Miao F, Xu YY, Mao XY et al. Transforming growth factor-beta1 signaling blockade attenuates gastric cancer cell-induced peritoneal mesothelial cell fibrosis and alleviates peritoneal dissemination both in vitro and in vivo. *Tumour Biology: The Journal of the International Society for Oncodevelopmental Biology and Medicine*. 2014;35(4):3575–3583.

48. Schauer IG, Zhang J, Xing Z, Guo X, Mercado-Uribe I, Sood AK et al. Interleukin-1beta promotes ovarian tumorigenesis through a p53/NF-kappaB-mediated inflammatory response in stromal fibroblasts. *Neoplasia*. 2013;15(4):409–420.

49. Cai J, Tang H, Xu L, Wang X, Yang C, Ruan S et al. Fibroblasts in omentum activated by tumor cells promote ovarian cancer growth, adhesion and invasiveness. *Carcinogenesis*. 2012;33(1):20–29.

50. Ko SY, Naora H. Therapeutic strategies for targeting the ovarian tumor stroma. *World Journal of Clinical Cases*. 2014;2(6):194–200.

51. Nieman KM, Kenny HA, Penicka CV, Ladanyi A, Buell-Gutbrod R, Zillhardt MR et al. Adipocytes promote ovarian cancer metastasis and provide energy for rapid tumor growth. *Nature Medicine*. 2011;17(11):1498–1503.

52. Lohani K, Shetty S, Sharma P, Govindarajan V, Thomas P, Loggie B. Pseudomyxoma peritonei: Inflammatory responses in the peritoneal microenvironment. *Annals of Surgical Oncology*. 2014;21(5):1441–1447.

53. van de Poll MC, Klaver YL, Lemmens VE, Leenders BJ, Nienhuijs SW, de Hingh IH. C-reactive protein concentration is associated with prognosis in patients suffering from peritoneal carcinomatosis of colorectal origin. *International Journal of Colorectal Disease*. 2011;26(8):1067–1073.

54. Coward J, Kulbe H, Chakravarty P, Leader D, Vassileva V, Leinster DA et al. Interleukin-6 as a therapeutic target in human ovarian cancer. *Clinical Cancer Research: An Official Journal of the American Association for Cancer Research*. 2011;17(18):6083–6096.

55. Nishio H, Yaguchi T, Sugiyama J, Sumimoto H, Umezawa K, Iwata T et al. Immunosuppression through constitutively activated NF-kappaB signalling in human ovarian cancer and its reversal by an NF-kappaB inhibitor. *British Journal of Cancer*. 2014;110(12):2965–2974.

56. Belluco C, Nitti D, Frantz M, Toppan P, Basso D, Plebani M et al. Interleukin-6 blood level is associated with circulating carcinoembryonic antigen and prognosis in patients with colorectal cancer. *Annals of Surgical Oncology*. 2000;7(2):133–138.

57. Maccio A, Madeddu C. Inflammation and ovarian cancer. *Cytokine*. 2012;58(2):133–147.

58. Curiel TJ, Coukos G, Zou L, Alvarez X, Cheng P, Mottram P et al. Specific recruitment of regulatory T cells in ovarian carcinoma fosters immune privilege and predicts reduced survival. *Nature Medicine*. 2004;10(9):942–949.

59. Chen YL, Chang MC, Chen CA, Lin HW, Cheng WF, Chien CL. Depletion of regulatory T lymphocytes reverses the imbalance between pro- and anti-tumor immunities via enhancing antigen-specific T cell immune responses. *PLOS ONE*. 2012;7(10):e47190.

60. Yoneda A, Ito S, Susumu S, Matsuo M, Taniguchi K, Tajima Y et al. Immunological milieu in the peritoneal cavity at laparotomy for gastric cancer. *World Journal of Gastroenterology*. 2012;18(13):1470–1478.

61. Miselis NR, Lau BW, Wu Z, Kane AB. Kinetics of host cell recruitment during dissemination of diffuse malignant peritoneal mesothelioma. *Cancer Microenvironment: Official Journal of the International Cancer Microenvironment Society*. 2010;4(1):39–50.

62. Mantovani A, Schioppa T, Biswas SK, Marchesi F, Allavena P, Sica A. Tumor-associated macrophages and dendritic cells as prototypic type II polarized myeloid populations. *Tumori*. 2003;89(5):459–468.

63. Sica A, Saccani A, Bottazzi B, Bernasconi S, Allavena P, Gaetano B et al. Defective expression of the monocyte chemotactic protein-1 receptor CCR2 in macrophages associated with human ovarian carcinoma. *Journal of Immunology*. 2000;164(2):733–738.

64. Colvin EK. Tumor-associated macrophages contribute to tumor progression in ovarian cancer. *Frontiers in Oncology*. 2014;4:137.

65. Wang X, Zhao X, Wang K, Wu L, Duan T. Interaction of monocytes/macrophages with ovarian cancer cells promotes angiogenesis in vitro. *Cancer Science*. 2013;104(4):516–523.

66. Elbarghati L, Murdoch C, Lewis CE. Effects of hypoxia on transcription factor expression in human monocytes and macrophages. *Immunobiology*. 2008;213(9–10):899–908.

67. Abiko K, Mandai M, Hamanishi J, Yoshioka Y, Matsumura N, Baba T et al. PD-L1 on tumor cells is induced in ascites and promotes peritoneal dissemination of ovarian cancer through CTL dysfunction. *Clinical Cancer Research: An Official Journal of the American Association for Cancer Research*. 2013;19(6):1363–1374.

68. Barsoum IB, Smallwood CA, Siemens DR, Graham CH. A mechanism of hypoxia-mediated escape from adaptive immunity in cancer cells. *Cancer Research*. 2014;74(3):665–674.

69. Doedens AL, Stockmann C, Rubinstein MP, Liao D, Zhang N, DeNardo DG et al. Macrophage expression of hypoxia-inducible factor-1 alpha suppresses T-cell function and promotes tumor progression. *Cancer Research*. 2010;70(19):7465–7475.

70. Neuhaus SJ, Watson DI. Pneumoperitoneum and peritoneal surface changes: A review. *Surgical Endoscopy*. 2004;18(9):1316–1322.

71. Bergstrom M, Ivarsson ML, Holmdahl L. Peritoneal response to pneumoperitoneum and laparoscopic surgery. *The British Journal of Surgery*. 2002;89(11):1465–1469.

72. Nam SY, Ko YS, Jung J, Yoon J, Kim YH, Choi YJ et al. A hypoxia-dependent upregulation of hypoxia-inducible factor-1 by nuclear factor-kappaB promotes gastric tumour growth and angiogenesis. *British Journal of Cancer*. 2011;104(1):166–174.

73. Miyake S, Kitajima Y, Nakamura J, Kai K, Yanagihara K, Tanaka T et al. HIF-1alpha is a crucial factor in the development of peritoneal dissemination via natural metastatic routes in scirrhous gastric cancer. *International Journal of Oncology*. 2013;43(5):1431–1440.

74. Carmi Y, Voronov E, Dotan S, Lahat N, Rahat MA, Fogel M et al. The role of macrophage-derived IL-1 in induction and maintenance of angiogenesis. *Journal of Immunology*. 2009;183(7):4705–4714.

75. Sun W. Angiogenesis in metastatic colorectal cancer and the benefits of targeted therapy. *Journal of Hematology & Oncology*. 2012;5:63.

76. Kryczek I, Lange A, Mottram P, Alvarez X, Cheng P, Hogan M et al. CXCL12 and vascular endothelial growth factor synergistically induce neoangiogenesis in human ovarian cancers. *Cancer Research*. 2005;65(2):465–472.

77. Chen XL, Nam JO, Jean C, Lawson C, Walsh CT, Goka E et al. VEGF-induced vascular permeability is mediated by FAK. *Developmental Cell*. 2012;22(1):146–157.

78. Herr D, Sallmann A, Bekes I, Konrad R, Holzheu I, Kreienberg R et al. VEGF induces ascites in ovarian cancer patients via increasing peritoneal permeability by downregulation of Claudin 5. *Gynecologic Oncology*. 2012;127(1):210–216.

79. Senger DR, Galli SJ, Dvorak AM, Perruzzi CA, Harvey VS, Dvorak HF. Tumor cells secrete a vascular permeability factor that promotes accumulation of ascites fluid. *Science*. 1983;219(4587):983–985.

80. Kobold S, Hegewisch-Becker S, Oechsle K, Jordan K, Bokemeyer C, Atanackovic D. Intraperitoneal VEGF inhibition using bevacizumab: A potential approach for the symptomatic treatment of malignant ascites? *The Oncologist*. 2009;14(12):1242–1251.

81. Zebrowski BK, Yano S, Liu W, Shaheen RM, Hicklin DJ, Putnam JB, Jr. et al. Vascular endothelial growth factor levels and induction of permeability in malignant pleural effusions. *Clinical Cancer Research: An Official Journal of the American Association for Cancer Research*. 1999;5(11):3364–3368.

82. Sluiter N, De Cuba EM, Kwakman R, Meijerink WH, Delis-van Diemen PM, Coupé VM et al. Versican and VEGF expression levels are associated with survival after cytoreductive surgery and HIPEC. Submitted. 2015.

83. Winiarski BK, Wolanska KI, Rai S, Ahmed T, Acheson N, Gutowski NJ et al. Epithelial ovarian cancer-induced angiogenic phenotype of human omental microvascular endothelial cells may occur independently of VEGF signaling. *Translational Oncology*. 2013;6(6):703–714.

84. Takahashi Y, Koyanagi T, Suzuki Y, Saga Y, Kanomata N, Moriya T et al. Vasohibin-2 expressed in human serous ovarian adenocarcinoma accelerates tumor growth by promoting angiogenesis. *Molecular Cancer Research*. 2012;10(9):1135–1146.

85. Jiang J, Liu W, Guo X, Zhang R, Zhi Q, Ji J et al. IRX1 influences peritoneal spreading and metastasis via inhibiting BDKRB2-dependent neovascularization on gastric cancer. *Oncogene*. 2011;30(44):4498–4508.

6

Dissemination and adhesion of peritoneal cancer cells to the peritoneal wall

ELLY DE VLIEGHERE, MARC BRACKE, LAURINE VERSET, PIETER DEMETTER,
AND OLIVIER DE WEVER

INTRODUCTION

Peritoneal metastasis develops when cells from primary abdominal and pelvic tumors disseminate in the peritoneal cavity and eventually adhere to the peritoneal wall. Peritoneal metastasis is a stochastic event depending on optimal information and adhesive cues from the host tissue. As a first step, cancer cells detach from the primary tumor spontaneously or iatrogenically and are transported by the peritoneal fluid. This fluid is a suitable environment for disseminated cells to survive. For this reason, metastasis formation in the peritoneum is a more efficient process than its hematogenic counterpart. During a second step, these cells adhere to the peritoneal wall, while in a third step, they invade the stroma where they can proliferate and form a new colony of metastatic tumor cells [1,2] (Figure 6.1).

FREE CANCER CELLS IN THE PERITONEAL FLUID

The first step in the development of peritoneal metastasis is the detachment of cancer cells from the primary tumor. Spontaneous detachment is favored by interstitial pressure, osmotic pressure, and downregulation of cell–cell adhesion molecules [1]. Indeed, the cancer cells undergo an epithelial to mesenchymal transition (EMT) and downregulate their expression of different adhesion molecules (Table 6.1), e.g., E-cadherin, which is normally responsible for strong cell–cell contacts between epithelial cells [3]. Detachment allows cells to disseminate in the peritoneal cavity, and cells float in the ascitic fluid either as single cells or as multicellular aggregates [3]. So, ascites samples from ovarian cancer patients were shown to contain single cells and loose sheetlike or spheroid aggregates. Single cells show low levels of E-cadherin expression, while cells in the spheres express higher levels. The aggregates, however, are not purely composed of cancer cells (with markers such as CA125, EpCAM, and cytokeratin 7): also cancer-associated fibroblasts (CAFs), with their markers α-smooth muscle actin (α-SMA) and platelet-derived growth factor β-receptor (PDGFβ-R), are intermingled. Cancer stem cells (marker, Ocr-4) are present as well. The aggregation of cancer cells with other cells from the peritoneal fluid could help them to survive and avert anoikis [4,5].

Dissemination of cancer cells does not always occur spontaneously. Lloyd et al. [6] compared peritoneal lavages of 125 colorectal patients before and after resection and investigated the presence of free cancer cells. The postresection group showed 8% more positive patients than the preresection one, indicating that handling the tumor during resection as such can cause cancer cells to detach [6].

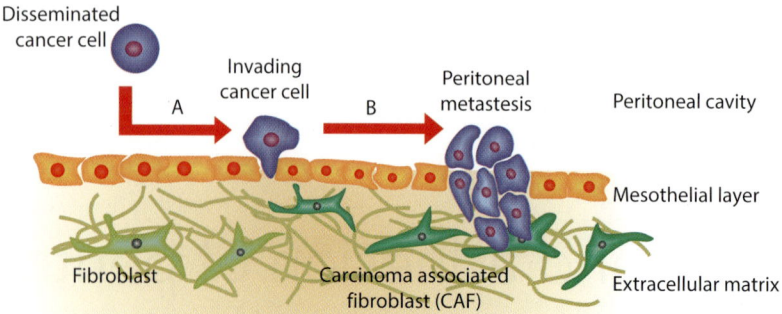

Figure 6.1 Peritoneal metastasis formation. Disseminated cancer cells in the peritoneal cavity adhere and break through the mesothelial layer (A) and infiltrate the extracellular matrix (B). Cancer cells activate fibroblasts to carcinoma-associated fibroblasts that modulate the ECM to a perfect cancer adhesion substrate.

Table 6.1 Adhesion molecules

Cancer cell	Cancer cell	Mesothelial cell	ECM	CAF
Ep CAM	Ep CAM			
N-Cad	E-Cad	N-Cad		N-Cad
P-Cad		P-Cad		
FGFR	N CAM			
$\alpha_x \beta_x$-Integrin complex		I CAM-1, V CAM-1, P CAM-1	Fibronectin, collagen type I/IV, vitronectin, laminin	
Sialophorin		I CAM-1		
CD44		Hyaluronate	Hyaluronate	
Hyaluronate		CD44		
Sialyl lex		E-selectin		
CA 125		Mesothelin		
MUC 16		Mesothelin		
L1		Neuropilin-1		
MT1-MMP			Collagen type I/III	

Sources: Ceelen, W.P. and Bracke, M.E., *Lancet Oncol.*, 10(1), 72, January 2009; Tamada, Y. et al., *Tumour Biol. J. Int. Soc. Oncodev. Biol. Med.*, 33(4), 1215, August 2012.

Note: A disseminated cancer cell can interact with the different layers of the peritoneal wall by various adhesion molecules expressed on the cellular matrix. Columns indicate different cell types and rows indicate interaction between adhesion molecules. ECM, extracellular matrix; Ep, I, V, and P CAM, epithelial, intracellular, vascular, and platelet cell adhesion molecule; N, P, and E-Cad, neural, placental, and epithelial cadherin; FGFR, fibroblast growth factor receptor; CD44, hyaluronate receptor; CA 125, cancer antigen 125; MUC 16, CA 125 positive mucin.

Because detachment is the first step of peritoneal metastasis, the detection of free cancer cells in the peritoneal fluid can be of predictive value. Bosanquet et al. [7] performed a meta-analysis of 12 studies that included 2580 colorectal cancer patients. In these studies, free cancer cells could be detected in 5%–40% of the peritoneal lavages before resection. The percentage of patients with free cancer cells, however, was highly dependent on the technique used. Three different methods were applied: cytopathology, immunocytochemistry, and polymerase chain reaction. The weighted means of these techniques were 8.4%, 28.3%, and 14.5%, respectively. Yet, each technique showed significantly higher mortality rates in the lavage-positive groups (odds ratio 4.02–6.57). So, the presence of disseminated cancer cells indicates a higher recurrence and poorer survival [7]. Similar results were published for other pelvic cancer patients [8–10]. Hara et al. [10] compared peritoneal lavage samples from gastric (24/132 positive lavages) and colorectal (29/126) cancer patients. The presence of free cancer cells in the samples was similar between different cancer types, but peritoneal recurrence rates were not. In this study, no patients with colorectal cancer showed peritoneal recurrence, while 10 of the gastric cancer group did. These results suggest that the rare peritoneal recurrence in colorectal patients is not due to a low incidence or a small number of intraperitoneal free cancer cells, but more likely reflects the relatively low peritoneal metastatic potential of colorectal cancer cells. So, besides the presence of free cancer cells, also their intrinsic metastatic capacity seems to determine peritoneal recurrence [10].

SPREADING OF CANCER CELLS BY THE PERITONEAL FLUID

Peritoneal recurrence can be local, i.e., at the site of the primary tumor, or disseminated in the peritoneal cavity. To understand why one tumor recurs locally while another spreads over the whole peritoneum, Carmignani et al. [11] prospectively examined the peritoneal metastatic spreading patterns of 129 patients with 5 different tumor types: pseudomyxoma peritonei, mucinous and nonmucinous colonic adenocarcinomas, ovarian carcinoma, and sarcoma. The peritoneal cavity was divided into 3 horizontal sectors, 9 regions, and 25 sites, and the incidence of tumor implants in these designated areas was reported. The study revealed that the presence of excess fluid (e.g., the abundant mucus ascites produced by mucinous adenocarcinoma) resulted in a more general distribution of cancer cells throughout the cavity. Distribution patterns were similar for all tumors with excess fluid, presumably because the free cancer cells had not adhered immediately, but had moved with the peritoneal fluid throughout the whole peritoneal cavity [11]. Physical forces such as gravity and diaphragm activity move the peritoneal fluid in a clockwise direction [12]. Furthermore, Carmignani et al. [11] found higher incidences of cancer implants on tissues known to absorb peritoneal fluid (diaphragm, *omentum majus*), on regions with slow peritoneal movement (*cul-de-sac* of Douglas) and on damaged tissues (surgery wounds) [11]. These sites offer longer contact periods between the cancer cells and the peritoneal wall or directly expose stroma to the cells (see the section "Adhesion to the Peritoneal Wall"). So, the distribution of cancer cells throughout the peritoneal cavity is mainly influenced by physical factors (amount and rheology of peritoneal fluid, absorption) rather than by biological factors (tumor type).

ADHESION TO THE PERITONEAL WALL

The normal peritoneum is composed of three layers: a single layer of flat mesothelial cells, a layer of submesothelial connective tissue (containing extracellular matrix [ECM]), and a layer of adipose tissue [13]. The superficial layer of mesothelial cells functions as a slippery, nonadhesive, and protective surface to facilitate organ movements [14]. Although this layer should prevent adhesion, a variety of different adhesion molecules can mediate the attachment of disseminated cancer cells (exposing integrin complexes, MUC 16, CD44, etc.) to the mesothelial cells (exposing ICAM-1, VCAM-1, mesothelin, hyaluronate, etc.) (Table 6.1) [1–3]. The expression of the adhesion molecules on the mesothelial cell surface is upregulated in case of inflammation after (surgical) trauma or under the influence of disseminated cancer cells [14]. Factors secreted by the cancer cells (TNF, INF-3) can indeed increase the levels of ICAM-1 and VCAM-1 on human mesothelial cells in culture [15]. Although adhesion molecules are responsible for the interaction between cancer cells and mesothelial cells, the actual degree of adhesion is not necessary related to the number of adhesion molecules expressed [14]. As an example, high CD44 expression levels are found in well-differentiated ovarian cancers with a favorable 5 years of overall survival rate. A study by Sillanpää et al. [16] analyzed 307 epithelial ovarian cancers: high levels of CD44 were found in 20% of the primary tumors, but only in 14% of the metastatic lesions. Furthermore, high expression levels of CD44 were associated with a 30% higher 5-year survival rate as compared to low expression levels [16].

A similar correlation was found for colon cancer patients [17]. In a group of ovarian cancer patients, high levels of hyaluronan expressed by the cancer cells were inversely correlated with the capacity to adhere to the peritoneum, although the mesothelium expressed high levels of its receptor CD44. High amounts of hyaluronan released from the cancer (or mesothelial) cells could block CD44 and thus inhibit adhesion to the peritoneal wall [18]. So, looking at the total level of CD44 might not be the best option for the assessment of prognosis. Considering the fact that CD44 has 19 isoforms, adhesion to the mesothelial layer could be facilitated by some specific isoforms [19]. However, it is probably not the ability to adhere to the mesothelial layer that makes free cancer cells metastatic, but rather the ability to break through the mesothelial layer (Figure 6.1) [20].

BREAKING THROUGH THE MESOTHELIAL LAYER

A surgical wound is known to be one of the first sites to be affected by peritoneal metastasis [11,21]. This was already described 100 years ago by Jones and Rous [22], who showed in mice experiments that cancer cells in the peritoneal cavity will preferentially adhere to the wounded peritoneal wall [22]. On this site, the mesothelial barrier is disrupted and the ECM exposed directly to the surface. Peritoneal metastasis can also manifest as small nodules that cover certain areas of the peritoneal wall. This pattern is called "milky spots," and originates from disseminated cancer cells attached to areas where the mesothelium was disrupted and the ECM was exposed [2]. Even when the peritoneum is healed and scar tissue is formed, cancer cells still prefer the wound site for metastasizing [22]. In agreement, molecules and signaling pathways involved in wound healing are also implicated in tumor growth, invasion, and metastasis. Wound healing starts with the inflammatory stage and the release of growth and chemotactic factors like PDGF, IGF-1, EFT, and TGF-β. This is followed by the proliferation stage characterized by fibroblast proliferation and ECM remodeling [23].

Histological analysis shows that mesothelial cells are absent between the peritoneal metastasis and the underlying matrix [24]. Experiments in vitro by Niedbala et al. [25] showed that human ovarian cancer cells, isolated from ascitic fluid, adhered more rapidly and firmer to ECM than to human mesothelial cells (isolated form ascites) or to plastic. When the system was agitated by a gyratory shaker at 125 rpm, the cancer cells could only attach to ECM coatings and to areas where the ECM was exposed in wounded mesothelium [25]. Kenny et al. [26] investigated the preferred substrates for ovarian cancer cell lines (SKOV3ip.1 and Hey A8) and cells isolated directly from patients. They found that ovarian cancer cells preferentially adhered to and invaded type I collagen, followed by type IV collagen, fibronectin, vitronectin, laminin 10, and laminin 1. While omental mesothelial cells inhibited adhesion, omental fibroblast induced adhesion and invasion [26]. All this suggest that even though the disseminated cancer cells can adhere to the protective mesothelial layer, their substrate of preference is the ECM. In accordance with those findings, Anttila et al. [27] showed that although CD44 was not a negative prognostic factor for survival, high levels of stromal hyaluronan were associated with poor differentiation, serous histological type, advanced stage, and large primary residual tumors, which resulted in poor survival [27].

Cancer cells that adhere to the mesothelial layer have to reach the underlying ECM to metastasize. There are two possible ways to achieve this: either the cancer cells adhere to the mesothelial layer first and invade toward the ECM later or the disseminated cells damage the protective mesothelial layer and adhere to the ECM immediately.

Adhesion to the mesothelial layer followed by invasion

Spheroids from ovarian carcinoma ascites can adhere to both mesothelial cells and ECM proteins [28,29]. Burleson et al. [20] allowed spheroids from seven ovarian cancer patients to adhere to a monolayer of human LP9 mesothelial cells. All spheroids adhered to the monolayer, but spheroids from two patients (and only 15% of these spheroids) had a more invasive phenotype and were able to break through the mesothelial monolayer and adhere to the plastic [20]. Adherence of ovarian cancer cells causes morphological changes in the mesothelial monolayer. Intracellular junctions are disrupted and this leads to cell retraction and exposes the underlying ECM [25]. Iwanicki et al. [29] has used a live, image-based model in vitro to monitor in real time the interaction between tumor spheroids and mesothelial cells. They revealed the phenomenon of "mesothelial clearance": the cancer cells first spread on top of the monolayer and subsequently penetrated the layer to trigger disruption of the adhesion of mesothelial cells to their underlying matrix. Migration of the cells ultimately led to mesothelial clearance. Ovarian cancer spheroids use integrin- and talin-dependent activation of myosin-generated force to "breach" and remove the mesothelial cell monolayer [29]. An alternative way to remove the mesothelial layer and to expose the ECM is to induce mesothelial apoptosis. Heath et al. [30] described that the colon cancer cell line SW40 adheres to human mesothelial cells and induces mesothelial cell shrinkage, nuclear fragmentation, and membrane blebbing, resulting in mesothelial apoptosis (confirmed by TUNEL assay) and the destruction of the protective mesothelial monolayer within hours after adding the cancer cells. In this model, the contact between the cancer and mesothelial cells is necessary. The authors suggest further that FasL/Fas signaling is responsible for triggering apoptosis. SW40 constitutively express Fas and FasL, while mesothelial cells only express Fas. However, after contact with SW40, FasL is upregulated in the mesothelial cells as well. Blocking with anti-FasL resulted in a reduction of mesothelial apoptosis [30].

Damaging the protective mesothelial layer before adhesion to the ECM

Kiyasu et al. [13] published a light and electron microscopy study of mesothelial cells from 34 gastric cancer patients. They noted morphological difference between cells from patients with and without peritoneal metastasis. Mesothelial cells differed between flat cells forming tight monolayers (no metastasis) and hemispherical shaped, disconnected cells (metastasis). Mesothelial cells exfoliated and ECM became visual between the cells. Cancer cells did not adhere to the mesothelial layer but to the exposed ECM. This suggests that the cancer cells first induce morphological changes in the mesothelial layer before adhering to the ECM [13]. These findings are a confirmation of laboratory animal experiments 50 years ago. Mice were inoculated intraperitoneally with murine Ehrlich ascites cancer cells. After 7 days morphological changes of the peritoneal wall were observed, after 8 days cancer cells adhered to the peritoneal wall, and 1 day later the peritoneal wall was infiltrated. This suggests that the mesothelial cell layer had altered and that the ECM was exposed before adherence of the cancer cells [31].

Disseminated cancer cells secrete a range of soluble factors that compromise the protective, antiadhesive mesothelial cell layer. Yashiro et al. [32] treated mice with intraperitoneal injection of conditioned medium (CM) of a gastric cancer cell line (OCUM-2MD3). The peritoneum of the treated mice showed hemispherical mesothelial cells that had lost tight cell–cell contacts [32]. Inflammatory cytokines secreted by disseminated cancer cells [1] and cytokines from inflammatory cells both contribute to the destruction of the mesothelial layer [33].

STROMA

Normal stroma

The ECM of the normal peritoneal stroma consists of large structural proteins (types I, III, and IV collagen, fibronectin, and laminin). These proteins are produced by fibroblasts and form the ideal substrate for a disseminated cell to adhere [1,25]. Integrin-mediated adhesion forms the primary cell-matrix adhesion mechanism. Integrin complexes are based on an α- and a β-subunit dimer. β_1-integrin can dimerize with α_1-, α_2-, α_3-, α_4-, α_5-, α_6-, or α_v-subunits (Table 6.2) [34]. The glycosylation pattern of the β_1-integrin subunit selects the α-subunit partner [35], and this α-subunit will on its turn determine the specificity and affinity of the binding to ECM proteins.

Tumor stroma

The tumor stroma differs from the normal stroma at several aspects. A fibronectin isoform, called oncofetal fibronectin (onfFN), is upregulated in tumor stroma, and the expression of this molecule correlates with metastatic

Table 6.2 Integrin complexes

Matrix molecule	Integrin complexes
Collagen type I	$\alpha_2\beta_1$
	$\alpha_1\beta_1, \alpha_3\beta_1$
Fibronectin	$\alpha_5\beta_1$
	$\alpha_3\beta_1, \alpha_4\beta_1, \alpha_v\beta_1$
Laminin	$\alpha_1\beta_1, \alpha_6\beta_1$
	$\alpha_2\beta_1$

Source: Albelda, S.M. and Buck, C.A., *FASEB J. Off. Publ. Fed. Am. Soc. Exp. Biol.*, 4(11), 2868, August 1990.

Note: Cancer cells adhere to the matrix molecules though there are several integrin complexes. Bold, the complex with the highest affinity.

implants in ovarian and colon cancers. The onfFN isoform may aid adhesion of the disseminated cancer cell to ECM [36,37]. There is a crosstalk between the peritoneal stroma and disseminated adhered cancer cells in the abdominal cavity. Cytokines and chemokines secreted by the cancer cell will change the local ecosystem to its own benefit. Matrix metalloprotease (MMP)-2 produced by ovarian cancer cells cleaves ECM proteins (fibronectin, vitronectin) into smaller fragments. The cancer cells adhere much stronger to smaller fragments using their fibronectin ($\alpha_5\beta_1$-integrin) and vitronectin ($\alpha_v\beta_3$-integrin)

receptors [3]. Furthermore, TGF-β, secreted by cancer cells, will lead to retraction of the mesothelial cells and activate tissue-resident fibroblasts (Figure 6.1) [38].

CAFs

Activated fibroblasts express high levels of α-SMA and are also called myofibroblasts, tumor-associated fibroblasts, or CAFs. CAFs are associated with advanced-stage disease and occurrence of lymph node metastases and omentum metastases (Figure 6.2) [39]. Jones and Rous [22] were probably the first to describe CAFs: experiments in mice showed that injuries to the submesothelial connective tissue greatly favored the lodging and growth of tumor fragments. They found that, as a reaction to the injury, the connective tissue showed a strong proliferation of fibroblast-like cells and that this "conditioned" stroma compared to nonconditioned stroma tumor made fragments more aggressive [22]. Fibroblasts and their activated counterparts modulate the stroma in physiological and pathological processes through both direct cell–cell contacts and their secretome [38]. De Boeck et al. [40] analyzed and compared the secretomes from mesenchymal stem cells (MSCs) treated or not with TGF-β (an activator of MSCs to generate CAFs). Some proteins were unique to CAFs: ECM components (e.g., TNC and several laminin subunits), proteases (e.g., MMP-2 and MMP-3),

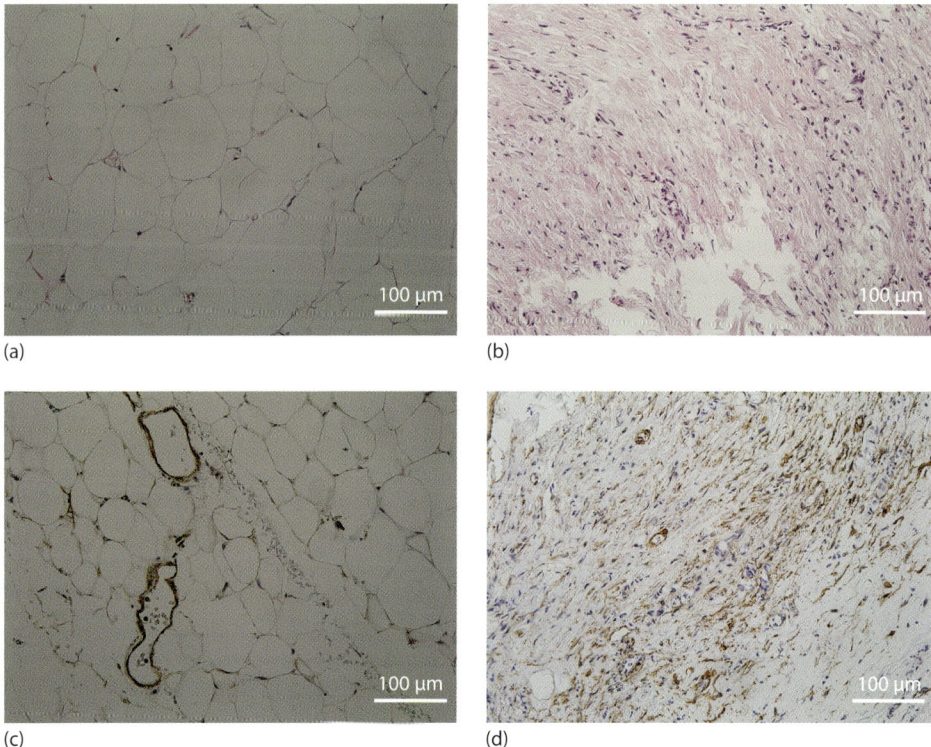

(a)　　　　(b)

(c)　　　　(d)

Figure 6.2 Histological images of peritoneal wall. **(a)** Hematoxyline and eosine (H&E) staining (200×), adipose tissue of a healthy peritoneum. **(b)** H&E staining (200×), peritoneal metastasis of a pancreas adenocarcinoma patient. **(c)** α-SMA staining (200×), adipose tissue of a healthy peritoneum; only pericytes are positive for α-SMA. **(d)** α-SMA staining (200×), peritoneal metastasis of a pancreas adenocarcinoma patient; pericytes and carcinoma-associated fibroblasts are positive for α-SMA.

chemokines and growth factors (e.g., SDF-1, hepatocyte growth factor [HGF], and EGF), and protease inhibitors (TIMP-4). When this secretome was offered to colon cancer cells (HCT8/E11) in vitro, cell invasion into a type I collagen gel was stimulated [40]. Cai et al. [41] compared the effects of normal fibroblasts and CAFs, both isolated from the omentum, on ovarian cancer cells (SK-OV-3) in a 3D model in vitro (mesothelial layer on top of a type I collagen gel with embedded fibroblast) and in an in vivo mouse model (IP injection of cancer cells with or without fibroblasts). They found that normal fibroblast was activated by SK-OV-3 via the secretion of TGF-β. The activated fibroblasts and the CAFs, in contrast to their normal counterparts, were able to promote adhesion and invasion of SK-OV-3 [41]. This was confirmed with ovarian cancer cells isolated from patients [39]. Adding an HGF-blocking antibody could partly counteract the effect of fibroblast activation [41]. HGF produced by the CAFs did not only help them to adhere to the ECM but also affected the integrity of the mesothelial monolayer. Mesothelial cells exposed to CM from peritoneal fibroblasts (NF-2P producing HGF, TGF-β, MMP-2, and MMP-9) rounded up and exfoliated from the peritoneum. Again, blocking HGF partly counteracted this effect [32]. CAFs also produce hyaluronan and high levels of this molecule in the stroma were associated with poor differentiation, serous histological type, advanced stage, and a large residual primary tumor volume, whereas it was not correlated with high CD44 expression on cancer cells [16,27].

The primary tumor and the metastatic lesions are not the only sites where CAFs can be found. Normal ovarian tissue is α-SMA negative (absence of CAFs), but CAFs can be detected in omental tissues of ovarian cancer patients without omental metastasis. This raises the possibility that cancer cells influence the omentum by CAF induction creating the perfect environment (soil) for the arriving cancer cells (seed) to metastasize [39]. The peritoneal fluid of 22 patients with advance disease stage also contained CAFs. Latifi et al. [5] collected cells out of spheroids from ovarian cancer ascites and described two types of cells. One cell type adhered and spread in culture conditions, while the other cells grew on top of each other. This latter type was considered as tumorigenic (E-cadherin, EpCam, and CA125, positive). The former, adherent type, however, showed a different expression pattern (CA125, negative; vimentin, MMP-2, and MMP-9, positive), and in combination with the fibroblastic phenotype, these cell could be considered as CAFs [5]. Wintzell et al. [4] came to the same conclusion. Ascites of 22 ovarian cancer patients contained single cells, loose sheetlike aggregates, and spheroids. The single cells and loose aggregates grow as monolayers when plated and were called M-type cells, whereas the spheroids remained as tight spheres even after agitation (S-type). S-type cells were E-cadherin positive and vimentin and α-SMA negative, while M-type cells were vimentin and α-SMA positive and E-cadherin negative [4]. The S-type cells were similar to the tumorigenic cells of the Latifi study, while the M-type cells can also be considered as CAFs. Presumably, ovarian cancer cells form spheroids in the peritoneal fluid to optimize their survival, and CAFs can help them to avoid anoikis.

ORIGIN OF CAFs AND THEIR PRECURSORS

The most obvious source of the CAFs in peritoneal metastasis is the *peritoneal fibroblast*. Yashiro et al. [32] described that after injection of CM from gastric cancer cells, enhanced proliferation of fibroblasts in the peritoneum was observed. Soluble factors secreted by the cancer cells were found to stimulate the fibroblast proliferation, even before cancer cells adhered to the peritoneal wall. Peritoneal fibroblasts could be activated by CM from colon cancer cells (HCT8/E11) to express α-SMA and become CAFs [32]. Fibroblast from the interlaying muscle tissue (mucosal fibroblasts), however, did not respond to CM of HCT8/E11. Histological analysis of colon peritoneal metastases showed fibrosis in the peritoneal layer with strong α-SMA staining in over 71% of the patients. In the same patients, only 21% had fibrosis in the deeper muscular layer. So, mucosal fibroblasts are probably not a source of CAFs [42]. Ko et al. [43] described that ovarian cancer cells that expressed HOXA9 induced normal peritoneal fibroblasts to express markers of CAFs through the secretion of TGF-β2. CAFs secrete on their turn TGF-β1 and TGF-β2 that enhance fibroblast activation via autocrine/paracrine loops. Furthermore, CAFs secrete IL-6 and SDF-1 to stimulate growth of cancer cells and IL-6 and VEGF to activate endothelial cells [43]. Ovarian cancer cells [41] and colon cancer cells [38] secrete TGF-β1 to activate fibroblasts: this results in paracrine phosphorylation of SMAD2 leading to α-SMA expression and to HGF and MMP-2 secretion [41]. TGF-β1 also creates CAFs through an autocrine loop. Lysophosphatidic acid (LPA) secreted by ovarian cancer cells stimulates TGF-β1 secretion in pre-CAFs leading to autocrine activation of SMAD2 [44]. CAFs can also be recruited from *adipose- and bone marrow–derived MSCs* by LPA, TGFβ1 and 2 secreted by cancer cells [38,43,44]. MSCs can also become activated to become carcinoma-associated MSCs (CA-MSCs). The cells remain multipotent, but stimulate cancer cells more than normal MSCs do. CA-MSCs are present in 90% of the ovarian cancer patients [45]. *Mesothelial cells* are another source of CAFs. The secretome of cancer cells changes the morphology of the mesothelial cells [32] and drives them into mesothelial to mesenchymal transition (MMT). Sandoval et al. [46] found WT1 (a mesothelial marker) to be present in the CAFs (α-SMA positive cells) in their peritoneal metastasis xenograft model. Cancer cell adhesion to the mesothelial layer after MMT was stimulated [46]. Although epithelial cancer cells may be a source of CAFs by EMT [38,47], Ko et al. [43] demonstrated using xenografts models that the CAFs in ovarian cancers did not derive from ovarian cancer cells. Indeed, in their xenograft mouse model with GFP-transfected ovarian cancer cells, all the CAFs (α-SMA positive cells) were GFP negative [43].

INVOLVEMENT OF OTHER CELL TYPES

CAFs are not the only cells in the tumor stroma that influence cancer cells. *Tumor-associated macrophages (TAMs)* play an important role in the tumor stroma. Ovarian cancer cells express monocyte chemoattractant protein-1 (MCP-1) and macrophage colony-stimulating factor to recruit monocytes and differentiate them into macrophages. IL-10, an TGF-β2 from ovarian cancer cells, can activate the macrophages to become TAMs. MCP-1 is also secreted by TAMs and CAFs creating an auto- and paracrine loop sustaining the TAM activation. TAMs produce, just like CAFs, MMPs helping the cancer cells to invade into the tumor stroma and are therefore associated with poor outcome for cancer patients [48]. Cancer cells and CAFs recruit and differentiate endothelial progenitors to *endothelial cells* by the secretion of SDF-1. The endothelial cells form new blood vessels stimulated by IL-6 and VEGF-A from CAFs. Angiogenesis supplies the newly formed metastases with oxygen and nutrition allowing them to grow. This is further aided by *adipocytes* via secretion of leptin and the transfer of lipids [48].

EXPERIMENTAL MODELS

Like for most experimental models, the trend holds that the more complex the model, the more it is patient relevant. However, complex models are generally low throughput, expensive, and labor intensive and sometimes rely on a more difficult readout. Many studies have been designed based on the assumption that peritoneal metastasis relies on cancer cell attachment to mesothelial cells. However, several other studies [22,25] indicated that cancer cells have a much greater affinity for the peritoneal ECM, which is consistent with the clinical pattern of metastatic spread [2]. Therefore, when investigating the adhesion of disseminated cancer cell to the peritoneal wall in vitro, a component of the ECM should be included. Type I collagen facilitates adhesion [26] and is quantitatively the main component of the ECM. So, the use of type I collagen or its degraded product (gelatin) is often the preferred component.

Cell lines versus cells isolated from patients

Cell lines have the advantage of being easy to handle, available in large numbers, and suitable for repeated experiments. But all cell lines can show artifacts resulting from long-time cell culture and possess a more homogeneous pheno-/genotype as compared to tumors, which often are very heterogeneous [49]. Therefore, it is recommended to use several cell lines [41,50]. Evidently, cells isolated from patients are closer to the in vivo situation and are heterogeneous. The procedure to isolate cells is more labor intensive and needs thorough characterization [25,26,30,51–53].

Cancer cells can be used as a single cell suspension or as cell spheroids. Spheroids can be isolated from ovarian cancer patients ascites directly [4,5] or can be generated from a single cell suspension by liquid gyrotory shaking [54] or culture on a nonadherent substrate [2,29].

ECM component

The ECM component can be offered as a coating on the bottom of a culture plastic well plate. Different components of the ECM can be used: type I/IV collagen, gelatin, fibronectin, vitronectin, and laminin [23,26,55]. These components can be used as pure substances or as mixtures and have the advantage to create a chemically well-defined matrix. To create a more complex coating, however, fibroblast monolayers are cultured for several days to deposit ECM molecules to the tissue culture plastic. After exposure of the cells to 0.02 M NH$_4$OH, the fibroblasts are removed without damaging the ECM matrix [25], and mesothelial cells can be seeded on top these matrices [29]. Coatings on glass coverslips are suitable for histology and immunostainings. For a 3D model, gels are used instead of coatings, since after fixation and paraffin embedding, histological sectioning is possible. Type I collagen as a 0.1% gel is often used as a model for ECM [54] and Matrigel for the basement membrane [32]. Inclusion of fibroblasts or CAFs will supply the gel with chemokines and growth factors [54]. The collagen texture in natural ECM is much denser than in the 0.1% gels. To create a denser gel, Jayne et al. [56] detached the gel with the fibroblasts from the plastic. After 7 days, the fibroblasts had contracted the collagen gel to a compact mass, and mesothelial cells were subsequentially seeded on top of contracted gel [56]. Similar effect can be created in the absence of fibroblast: Brown et al. [57] constituted the 0.1% gel in a mold and compressed the gel removing excessive water thereby creating a more dense gel. By weighing the gel, the new density can be calculated [57]. Yet, a perfect mimic of the peritoneal wall cannot be accomplished by in vitro adhesion assays. A fragment of the omentum can be used with or without enzymatic removal of the mesothelial cells [26]. Adhesion to the mesothelial cells in vivo is complicated due to the movement of the peritoneal fluid. This aspect can be mimicked by fluid agitation by placing the culture plate on a gyrotory shaker [25].

THERAPEUTIC IMPLICATIONS

Survival of the disseminated cancer cell in the peritoneal fluid and its adhesion to the peritoneal wall are the first steps in peritoneal metastasis development. If disseminated cancer cells fail to survive or if their adhesion to the peritoneal wall can be inhibited, peritoneal metastasis formation may be prevented after removal of the primary tumor.

Focal adhesion kinase (FAK) is a cytoplasmic protein tyrosine kinase associated with integrins and growth factor receptors. Elevated FAK expression correlates with poor survival in ovarian cancer patients [58]. FAK inhibition can lead to its relocalization to the nucleus and modulates gene expression and cell survival, affecting anchorage-independent ovarian carcinoma cell survival and growth. Ward et al. tested a small molecule FAK inhibitor (PF-271) that selectively prevents anchorage-independent cell growth by inhibition of FAK tyrosine (Y397) phosphorylation, resulting in increased tumor cell apoptosis and prevention of peritoneal metastasis in vitro and in vivo [58]. CD44 expression in cancer cells is not correlated with a bad prognosis. However, high expression of its ligand hyaluronate in the stroma is a poor prognosis marker [27]. Experimental data and correlative histological studies suggest CD44 as an interesting therapeutic drug candidate. Intraperitoneal injection of 36M2 positive cells (highly positive CD44 ovarian cancer cells) together with neutralizing monoclonal anti-CD44 inhibited the number of peritoneal implants by 70% without reducing the growth rate of tumors [50]. β1-integrin interacts with six divergent α-integrins covering the majority of ECM adhesion molecules (Table 6.2). Targeting β1-integrin for blocking adhesion is consequentially a logical approach in antiperitoneal metastasis therapy. Cheung et al. [55] blocked integrin adhesion in SK-OV-3 and Coav-3 by siRNA and blocking antibodies. Blocking β1-integrin inhibited adhesion of type I collagen, fibronectin, and laminin by 89%, while blocking α2-integrin decreased adhesion to type I collagen by 98%, and blocking α5 decreased adhesion to fibronectin by 94%. Inhibition of gonadotropin-releasing hormone receptor by siRNA (upstream of α2β1- and α5β1-integrin) in Coav-3 resulted in fewer peritoneal implants in a mouse model [55]. Cancer cells can adhere to mesothelial cells and to ECM via a wide range of adhesion molecules (Table 6.1), but do not form a homogeneous population: free cancer cells from similar tumor origin can use different molecular mechanisms to adhere. Besides this phenomenon, cancer cells show high phenotypic plasticity [49]. Blocking one adhesion molecule is inefficient; however, simultaneous targeting of several molecules could have a better result. Strobel et al. [50] combined neutralizing antibodies for β1-integrin and CD44 and found reduced adhesion of 36M2, CAOV-3, and SK-OV-3 ovarian cancer cells to human mesothelial cells compared to single antibody treatment [50].

CONCLUSION

Peritoneal metastasis is a multistep process requiring dynamic interactions between free cancer cells and the host tissue. A key characteristic is the intense communication of cancer cells with submesothelial CAFs. CAFs produce essential ECM molecules favoring adhesion and survival of cancer cells. A thorough molecular understanding of the molecular crosstalk and the adhesive mechanisms will lead to new therapeutic opportunities to prevent and to treat peritoneal metastatic disease.

REFERENCES

1. Ceelen WP, Bracke ME. Peritoneal minimal residual disease in colorectal cancer: Mechanisms, prevention, and treatment. *The Lancet Oncology*. January 2009;10(1):72–79.
2. Sodek KL, Murphy KJ, Brown TJ, Ringuette MJ. Cell-cell and cell-matrix dynamics in intraperitoneal cancer metastasis. *Cancer and Metastasis Reviews*. June 2012;31(1–2):397–414.
3. Lengyel E. Ovarian cancer development and metastasis. *The American Journal of Pathology*. September 2010;177(3):1053–1064.
4. Wintzell M, Hjerpe E, Lundqvist EA, Shoshan M. Protein markers of cancer-associated fibroblasts and tumor-initiating cells reveal subpopulations in freshly isolated ovarian cancer ascites. *BMC Cancer*. August 18, 2012;12:359.
5. Latifi A, Luwor RB, Bilandzic M, Nazaretian S, Stenvers K, Pyman J et al. Isolation and characterization of tumor cells from the ascites of ovarian cancer patients: Molecular phenotype of chemo-resistant ovarian tumors. *PLOS ONE*. October 8, 2012;7(10):e46858.
6. Lloyd JM, McIver CM, Stephenson SA, Hewett PJ, Rieger N, Hardingham JE. Identification of early-stage colorectal cancer patients at risk of relapse post-resection by immunobead reverse transcription-PCR analysis of peritoneal lavage fluid for malignant cells. *Clinical Cancer Research: An Official Journal of the American Association for Cancer Research*. January 15, 2006;12(2):417–423.
7. Bosanquet DC, Harris DA, Evans MD, Beynon J. Systematic review and meta-analysis of intraoperative peritoneal lavage for colorectal cancer staging. *The British Journal of Surgery*. June 2013;100(7):853–862.
8. Katsuragi K, Yashiro M, Sawada T, Osaka H, Ohira M, Hirakawa K. Prognostic impact of PCR-based identification of isolated tumour cells in the peritoneal lavage fluid of gastric cancer patients who underwent a curative R0 resection. *British Journal of Cancer*. August 20, 2007;97(4):550–556.
9. Broll R, Weschta M, Windhoevel U, Berndt S, Schwandner O, Roblick U et al. Prognostic significance of free gastrointestinal tumor cells in peritoneal lavage detected by immunocytochemistry and polymerase chain reaction. *Langenbeck's Archives of Surgery (Deutsche Gesellschaft fur Chirurgie)*. July 2001;386(4):285–292.

10. Hara M, Nakanishi H, Jun Q, Kanemitsu Y, Ito S, Mochizuki Y et al. Comparative analysis of intraperitoneal minimal free cancer cells between colorectal and gastric cancer patients using quantitative RT-PCR: Possible reason for rare peritoneal recurrence in colorectal cancer. *Clinical & Experimental Metastasis.* 2007;24(3):179–189.

11. Carmignani CP, Sugarbaker TA, Bromley CM, Sugarbaker PH. Intraperitoneal cancer dissemination: Mechanisms of the patterns of spread. *Cancer Metastasis Reviews.* December 2003;22(4):465–472.

12. Meyers MA. The spread and localization of acute intraperitoneal effusions. *Radiology.* June 1970;95(3):547–554.

13. Kiyasu Y, Kaneshima S, Koga S. Morphogenesis of peritoneal metastasis in human gastric cancer. *Cancer Research.* March 1981;41(3):1236–1239.

14. Mutsaers SE. Mesothelial cells: Their structure, function and role in serosal repair. *Respirology.* September 2002;7(3):171–191.

15. Jonjic N, Peri G, Bernasconi S, Sciacca FL, Colotta F, Pelicci P et al. Expression of adhesion molecules and chemotactic cytokines in cultured human mesothelial cells. *The Journal of Experimental Medicine.* October 1, 1992;176(4):1165–1174.

16. Sillanpää S, Anttila MA, Voutilainen K, Tammi RH, Tammi MI, Saarikoski SV et al. CD44 expression indicates favorable prognosis in epithelial ovarian cancer. *Clinical Cancer Research: An Official Journal of the American Association for Cancer Research.* November 1, 2003;9(14):5318–5324.

17. Nanashima A, Yamaguchi H, Sawai T, Yamaguchi E, Kidogawa H, Matsuo S et al. Prognostic factors in hepatic metastases of colorectal carcinoma: Immunohistochemical analysis of tumor biological factors. *Digestive Diseases and Sciences.* August 2001;46(8):1623–1628.

18. Tamada Y, Takeuchi H, Suzuki N, Aoki D, Irimura T. Cell surface expression of hyaluronan on human ovarian cancer cells inversely correlates with their adhesion to peritoneal mesothelial cells. *Tumour Biology: The Journal of the International Society for Oncodevelopmental Biology and Medicine.* August 2012;33(4):1215–1222.

19. Kim M, Rooper L, Xie J, Kajdacsy-Balla AA, Barbolina MV. Fractalkine receptor CX(3)CR1 is expressed in epithelial ovarian carcinoma cells and required for motility and adhesion to peritoneal mesothelial cells. *Molecular Cancer Research.* January 2012;10(1):11–24.

20. Burleson KM, Boente MP, Pambuccian SE, Skubitz AP. Disaggregation and invasion of ovarian carcinoma ascites spheroids. *Journal of Translational Medicine.* 2006;4:6.

21. Konigsrainer I, Zieker D, Beckert S, von Weyhern C, Lob S, Falch C et al. Local peritonectomy highly attracts free floating intraperitoneal colorectal tumour cells in a rat model. *Cellular Physiology and Biochemistry: International Journal of Experimental Cellular Physiology, Biochemistry, and Pharmacology.* 2009;23(4–6):371–378.

22. Jones FS, Rous P. On the cause of the localization of secondary tumors at points of injury. *The Journal of Experimental Medicine.* October 1, 1914;20(4):404–412.

23. Ceelen W, Pattyn P, Mareel M. Surgery, wound healing, and metastasis: Recent insights and clinical implications. *Critical Reviews in Oncology/Hematology.* January 2014;89(1):16–26.

24. Kenny HA, Nieman KM, Mitra AK, Lengyel E. The first line of intra-abdominal metastatic attack: Breaching the mesothelial cell layer. *Cancer Discovery.* July 2011;1(2):100–102.

25. Niedbala MJ, Crickard K, Bernacki RJ. Interactions of human ovarian tumor cells with human mesothelial cells grown on extracellular matrix. An in vitro model system for studying tumor cell adhesion and invasion. *Experimental Cell Research.* October 1985;160(2):499–513.

26. Kenny HA, Krausz T, Yamada SD, Lengyel E. Use of a novel 3D culture model to elucidate the role of mesothelial cells, fibroblasts and extra-cellular matrices on adhesion and invasion of ovarian cancer cells to the omentum. *International Journal of Cancer (Journal international du Cancer).* October 1, 2007;121(7):1463–1472.

27. Anttila MA, Tammi RH, Tammi MI, Syrjanen KJ, Saarikoski SV, Kosma VM. High levels of stromal hyaluronan predict poor disease outcome in epithelial ovarian cancer. *Cancer Research.* January 1, 2000;60(1):150–155.

28. Burleson KM, Casey RC, Skubitz KM, Pambuccian SE, Oegema Jr. TR, Skubitz AP. Ovarian carcinoma ascites spheroids adhere to extracellular matrix components and mesothelial cell monolayers. *Gynecologic Oncology.* April 2004;93(1):170–181.

29. Iwanicki MP, Davidowitz RA, Ng MR, Besser A, Muranen T, Merritt M et al. Ovarian cancer spheroids use myosin-generated force to clear the mesothelium. *Cancer Discovery.* July 2011;1(2):144–157.

30. Heath RM, Jayne DG, O'Leary R, Morrison EE, Guillou PJ. Tumour-induced apoptosis in human mesothelial cells: A mechanism of peritoneal invasion by Fas Ligand/Fas interaction. *British Journal of Cancer.* April 5, 2004;90(7):1437–1442.

31. Birbeck MS, Wheatley DN. An electron microscopic study of the invasion of ascites tumor cells into the abdominal wall. *Cancer Research.* May 1965;25:490–497.

32. Yashiro M, Chung YS, Inoue T, Nishimura S, Matsuoka T, Fujihara T et al. Hepatocyte growth factor (HGF) produced by peritoneal fibroblasts may affect mesothelial cell morphology and promote peritoneal dissemination. *International Journal of Cancer*. July 17, 1996;67(2):289–293.

33. Lopez-Novoa JM, Nieto MA. Inflammation and EMT: An alliance towards organ fibrosis and cancer progression. *EMBO Molecular Medicine*. September 2009;1(6–7):303–314.

34. Albelda SM, Buck CA. Integrins and other cell adhesion molecules. *FASEB Journal: Official Publication of the Federation of American Societies for Experimental Biology*. August 1990;4(11):2868–2880.

35. Guo HB, Lee I, Kamar M, Akiyama SK, Pierce M. Aberrant N-glycosylation of beta1 integrin causes reduced alpha5beta1 integrin clustering and stimulates cell migration. *Cancer Research*. December 1, 2002;62(23):6837–6845.

36. Menzin AW, Loret de Mola JR, Bilker WB, Wheeler JE, Rubin SC, Feinberg RF. Identification of oncofetal fibronectin in patients with advanced epithelial ovarian cancer: Detection in ascitic fluid and localization to primary sites and metastatic implants. *Cancer*. January 1, 1998;82(1):152–158.

37. Inufusa H, Nakamura M, Adachi T, Nakatani Y, Shindo K, Yasutomi M et al. Localization of oncofetal and normal fibronectin in colorectal cancer. Correlation with histologic grade, liver metastasis, and prognosis. *Cancer*. June 15, 1995;75(12):2802–2808.

38. De Wever O, Demetter P, Mareel M, Bracke M. Stromal myofibroblasts are drivers of invasive cancer growth. *International Journal of Cancer*. November 15, 2008;123(10):2229–2238.

39. Zhang Y, Tang H, Cai J, Zhang T, Guo J, Feng D et al. Ovarian cancer-associated fibroblasts contribute to epithelial ovarian carcinoma metastasis by promoting angiogenesis, lymphangiogenesis and tumor cell invasion. *Cancer Letters*. April 1, 2011;303(1):47–55.

40. De Boeck A, Hendrix A, Maynard D, Van Bockstal M, Daniels A, Pauwels P et al. Differential secretome analysis of cancer-associated fibroblasts and bone marrow-derived precursors to identify microenvironmental regulators of colon cancer progression. *Proteomics*. January 2013;13(2):379–388.

41. Cai J, Tang H, Xu L, Wang X, Yang C, Ruan S et al. Fibroblasts in omentum activated by tumor cells promote ovarian cancer growth, adhesion and invasiveness. *Carcinogenesis*. January 2012;33(1):20–29.

42. Kojima M, Higuchi Y, Yokota M, Ishii G, Saito N, Aoyagi K et al. Human subperitoneal fibroblast and cancer cell interaction creates microenvironment that enhances tumor progression and metastasis. *PLOS ONE*. February 4, 2014;9(2):e88018.

43. Ko SY, Barengo N, Ladanyi A, Lee JS, Marini F, Lengyel E et al. HOXA9 promotes ovarian cancer growth by stimulating cancer-associated fibroblasts. *The Journal of Clinical Investigation*. October 1, 2012;122(10):3603–3617.

44. Jeon ES, Moon HJ, Lee MJ, Song HY, Kim YM, Cho M et al. Cancer-derived lysophosphatidic acid stimulates differentiation of human mesenchymal stem cells to myofibroblast-like cells. *Stem Cells*. March 2008;26(3):789–797.

45. McLean K, Gong Y, Choi Y, Deng N, Yang K, Bai S et al. Human ovarian carcinoma-associated mesenchymal stem cells regulate cancer stem cells and tumorigenesis via altered BMP production. *The Journal of Clinical Investigation*. August 2011;121(8):3206–3219.

46. Sandoval P, Jimenez-Heffernan JA, Rynne-Vidal A, Perez-Lozano ML, Gilsanz A, Ruiz-Carpio V et al. Carcinoma-associated fibroblasts derive from mesothelial cells via mesothelial-to-mesenchymal transition in peritoneal metastasis. *The Journal of Pathology*. December 2013;231(4):517–531.

47. Xouri G, Christian S. Origin and function of tumor stroma fibroblasts. *Seminars in Cell & Developmental Biology*. February 2010;21(1):40–46.

48. Naora H. Heterotypic cellular interactions in the ovarian tumor microenvironment: Biological significance and therapeutic implications. *Frontiers in Oncology*. 2014;4:18.

49. Strauss R, Li ZY, Liu Y, Beyer I, Persson J, Sova P et al. Analysis of epithelial and mesenchymal markers in ovarian cancer reveals phenotypic heterogeneity and plasticity. *PLOS ONE*. 2011;6(1):e16186.

50. Strobel T, Cannistra SA. Beta1-integrins partly mediate binding of ovarian cancer cells to peritoneal mesothelium in vitro. *Gynecologic Oncology*. June 1999;73(3):362–367.

51. Beavis MJ, Williams JD, Hoppe J, Topley N. Human peritoneal fibroblast proliferation in 3-dimensional culture: Modulation by cytokines, growth factors and peritoneal dialysis effluent. *Kidney International*. January 1997;51(1):205–215.

52. Stylianou E, Jenner LA, Davies M, Coles GA, Williams JD. Isolation, culture and characterization of human peritoneal mesothelial cells. *Kidney International*. June 1990;37(6):1563–1570.

53. Yung S, Li FK, Chan TM. Peritoneal mesothelial cell culture and biology. *Peritoneal Dialysis International: Journal of the International Society for Peritoneal Dialysis*. March to April 2006;26(2):162–173.

54. De Wever O, Hendrix A, De Boeck A, Westbroek W, Braems G, Emami S et al. Modeling and quantification of cancer cell invasion through collagen type I matrices. *The International Journal of Developmental Biology*. 2010;54(5):887–896.

55. Cheung LW, Yung S, Chan TM, Leung PC, Wong AS. Targeting gonadotropin-releasing hormone receptor inhibits the early step of ovarian cancer metastasis by modulating tumor-mesothelial adhesion. *Molecular Therapy: The Journal of the American Society of Gene Therapy.* January 2013;21(1):78–90.

56. Jayne DG, O'Leary R, Gill A, Hick A, Guillou PJ. A three-dimensional in-vitro model for the study of peritoneal tumour metastasis. *Clinical & Experimental Metastasis.* 1999;17(6):515–523.

57. Brown RA, Wiseman M, Chuo CB, Cheema U, Nazhat SN. Ultrarapid engineering of biomimetic materials and tissues: Fabrication of nano- and microstructures by plastic compression. *Advanced Functional Materials.* November 2005;15(11):1762–1770.

58. Ward KK, Tancioni I, Lawson C, Miller NL, Jean C, Chen XL et al. Inhibition of focal adhesion kinase (FAK) activity prevents anchorage-independent ovarian carcinoma cell growth and tumor progression. *Clinical & Experimental Metastasis.* June 2013;30(5):579–594.

7

Genomic approaches to peritoneal carcinomatosis

HAROON A. CHOUDRY AND DAVID L. BARTLETT

CANCER GENOME

Cancers arise from the nonrandom accumulation of genomic aberrations that individually provide a varying degree of growth advantage to cells [1]. The acquisition of genomic alterations is facilitated by genomic instability, a process that drives tumor development by increasing the rate of spontaneous mutations in cells [2]. A vast majority of these genomic mutations are passenger mutations that do not affect tumor biology, while a small number of these genetic variants are driver mutations that confer a selective growth advantage to the cell. The genomic landscape for most cancers is characterized by frequent mutations in a handful of genes (mountains) and a low frequency of mutations in a larger set of genes (hills). The gene "mountains" are usually potent driver mutations that are important for initiation and progression of tumors, while the gene "hills" often contribute toward tumor phenotype, prognosis, drug response, and chemotherapy resistance. Based on comprehensive cancer genome analysis, including an aggregate of DNA sequencing, copy number analysis, RNA expression, and epigenetic profiling, it appears that approximately 50–100 cancer genes are involved in the initiation, progression, and maintenance of any particular cancer type. However, these cancer genes ("mountains" and "hills") converge on a limited number of signaling pathways that regulate core cellular processes, including cell fate, cell survival, and genome maintenance [3]. This implies that a common and limited set of cancer genes and pathways are responsible for most common forms of cancer. It would follow that the complex mutational landscape of the cancer genome is decipherable and targetable. The future of personalized cancer medicine lies in a genomic approach to deciphering the genetic changes underlying carcinogenesis.

CANCER GENOMICS

Cancer genomics refers to an unbiased and systematic analysis of the cancer genome in order to identify specific genetic loci that are recurrently altered in specific cancer types. These genetic alterations may include genomic loss or amplification, mutations in coding regions, chromosomal rearrangements, as well as aberrant methylation and expression profiles [4]. The goal of cancer genomics is to provide comprehensive characterization of driver mutations and the cancer genes that they alter in order to optimize strategies for cancer prevention, early detection, and therapy. In addition, cancer genomics facilitates cancer taxonomy through molecular signature-based classification, provides prognostic and predictive information, and helps identify targets for therapeutic intervention.

The complete sequencing of the normal human reference genome in 2003 under the auspices of the Human Genome Project paved the way for cancer genomics [5]. The initiation of The Cancer Genome Atlas (TCGA) project by the U.S. National Cancer Institute and the establishment of the International Cancer Genome Consortium in 2009, along with the concurrent emergence and evolution of massively parallel sequencing technology, made cancer genomics practical and feasible on a large scale [6]. Massively parallel sequencing allows an unbiased analysis of the cancer genome for both hypothesis generation and testing. Current massively parallel sequencing platforms are able to sequence more than 600 billion bases in a single run and allow comprehensive genomic analysis including single nucleotide variant, copy number variant (CNV) and structural variant (SV) analysis, RNA expression analysis, and epigenetic profiling at a reasonable cost. Furthermore, these approaches have the potential to identify subclonal genetic diversity within the population of cancer cells, with particular relevance to the detection of subclones carrying drug-resistance mutations [4].

Traditionally, low-throughput technologies like the Sanger sequencing, PCR-based restriction fragment length polymorphism, and fluorescence in situ hybridization assays have been the workhorses for genomic analysis in cancer. Currently, high-throughput next-generation sequencing technologies allow comprehensive profiling of all genomic alterations within the genome of cancer cells and have therefore been rapidly implemented for studying cancer genomics [7]. High-throughput cancer genotyping platforms, consisting of multiplexed assays and microarrays, are frequently used in clinical practice to identify known recurrent genetic alterations in tumors from different patients, thereby providing prognostic and predictive biomarkers and molecular targets for therapy. Similarly, comparative genomic hybridization arrays allow accurate high-throughput identification of genomic CNVs in cancer cells. High-throughput targeted genome sequencing platforms have allowed high-resolution focused sequencing of DNA regions of interest, such as the whole exome or the cancer genome with higher accuracy and reasonable cost, and are therefore increasingly being integrated into clinical practice. Finally, whole genome sequencing can identify any sequence variant within the entire genome in a high-throughput fashion. It is considered the unbiased "gold standard" since it provides information on structural and noncoding variants that cannot be captured from targeted genome sequencing. However, whole genome sequencing currently remains relatively expensive and time consuming for routine clinical application.

The field of cancer genomics is currently in its infancy and a number of challenges need to be addressed [7]. For example: (1) The detection of mutations with high accuracy against a background of sequencing errors, read-alignment inaccuracies, and tumor heterogeneity from subclonal variations remains challenging. (2) Correctly distinguishing driver mutations from passenger mutations has also been difficult. (3) Although a host of novel cancer genes effecting global processes (e.g., signaling pathways, cellular metabolism, epigenetics, chromatin biology, RNA transcript splicing, protein homeostasis, genomic integrity, telomere stability, and cell differentiation) have been identified, their precise connection to cancer remains obscure and the specific target(s) within these global processes that are disrupted by these newly discovered mutant genes have not been identified in a majority of tumors. (4) The majority of sequencing studies to date have been insufficiently powered and have lacked adequate depth of coverage to detect low-frequency candidate cancer genes (hills). (5) Numerical and structural chromosomal variations have been poorly studied to date given the paucity of whole genome sequencing studies; moreover, the specific genes affected by these chromosomal variations have not been identified in a majority of cancers. (6) The vast majority of mutations identified by whole genome sequencing are located outside the exome; however, the functional significance of this expansive noncoding component of the genome (>98%) remains uncharted.

Simultaneous advancement in bioinformatics tools has been essential for comprehensive analysis of the vast amount of genomic data that have been obtained through massively parallel sequencing. Computational analysis of this vast and exponentially increasing genomic data involves sequence alignment, detection of somatic mutations, and identification of significantly mutated genes [8]. However, bioinformatics technology has been lagging compared to the rapid advancement in genomic sequencing technology and has been the rate-limiting step in cancer genomics. A wide variety of algorithms and analysis software have been developed for identifying genetic changes responsible for tumor development, progression, metastasis, and recurrence. Most tools use either a composite statistical score or a formal probability test, although there also remain simple heuristic thresholds. However, their variant-calling accuracy and sensitivity needs improvement to optimally balance type I and II errors [8–10].

INTEGRATIVE GENOMICS

Although the discovery of a complete catalogue of genetic mutations is important in cancer research, the key to understanding cancer biology lies in performing an integrated analysis of these genetic changes in concert with epigenetic, transcriptional, and proteomic data within and across tumor specimens [11]. Genes and proteins function through interactions with other DNA, RNA, and proteins within a complex cellular signaling environment; therefore, integrative genomics is essential for identifying the crucial, rate-limiting molecular targets within this background of redundancy of pathways and heterogeneity of tumors. For example, genomic sequencing can identify SVs, but only by adding a technique that assesses RNA levels, such as RNA sequencing (RNA-seq), can it be determined whether structural variations affect the transcription levels of a gene. This also requires innovative bioinformatics strategies that facilitate data integration and interpretation from these various sequencing techniques. This comprehensive approach will enhance the goals of personalized cancer medicine centered on prevention, early detection, and therapy. Advancement in cancer profiling technology has rapidly identified novel molecular markers at the DNA, mRNA, microRNA, and protein levels effecting signaling pathways and cellular processes, while sophisticated mathematical and statistical techniques continue to be developed for the global and unbiased analysis, interpretation, and validation of biological data.

This era of cancer genomics is ushering in a paradigm shift away from large randomized trials that focus on group responses, toward the comprehensive analysis of a single patient's unique tumor and its altered pathways and processes. Ideally, integrative analysis should be able to provide a link between global genomic alterations and cancer-related pathways, improve disease classification based on molecular profiles, and provide prognostic and predictive information in a prospective manner. A variety of statistical methods and analytical tools have been developed with a varying ability to analyze these features. However, integrating genomic data are hindered by the current heterogeneity of experimental and analytical protocols, varying levels of data quality and the inadequacy of statistical methods like multiple-hypothesis testing. Multiple testing statistical method has been useful for identifying true positives in the context of a large number of statistical hypotheses and comparisons as occurs in 1D genomic studies; however, its utility is hampered in situations where families of tests are performed as is the case with multidimensional integrative genomics.

The evolution of high-throughput cancer genomics has highlighted the need for functional validation of the vast in silico findings (i.e., candidate cancer genes) in relevant living biological systems, as well as the development of adequate in vitro functional studies (e.g., siRNA screens, knock-in systems, and knockout systems) to determine their value as risk factors, predictive factors for therapeutic response, or therapeutic targets [9,12] Genomic information has facilitated the development of cDNA or open reading frame libraries for gain-of-function studies and libraries of RNAi for loss-of-function studies. However, experimental systems used for functional validation are highly variable in their efficiency and efficacy. While in vitro models (e.g., cell lines, tumor explants) are simpler and faster, in vivo models (e.g., tumor xenograft models and genetically engineered animal models) provide more clinically relevant biological information but require significantly higher resource and time investment.

PERSONALIZED CANCER MEDICINE

The ultimate aim of integrative cancer genomics is to be able to translate the comprehensive molecular knowledge of an individual patient's cancer into a strategy for cancer prevention, early detection, and curative therapy. Currently, a number of issues are hindering the translation of genomic information into personalized cancer medicine including an incomplete catalogue of genomic alterations in cancers and a lack of understanding of their biological consequences; significant inherent limitations in our bioinformatics tools as well as in vitro and in vivo experimental models to identify and validate candidate "driver mutations" and differentiate them from "passenger mutations"; and a lack of clarity of the complex interactions among the global genetic alterations especially when considering the specific context within which they are occurring, e.g., the tumor microenvironment and the cellular type and developmental stage.

Cancer research has evolved from the study of single genes or focused gene clusters toward high-throughput,

integrated analysis of the entire cancer genome, methylome, transcriptome, and proteome. Ultimately, a comprehensive molecular profile of the entire genome of each tumor will reveal the genetic profile responsible for its unique phenotype, prognosis, drug response, and chemotherapy resistance. In addition, cancer genomics will also become a key component of clinical trials to help stratify patients for enrollment and therapy based on their genetic profiles, e.g., KRAS mutation in patients with colon cancer indicates tumor responsiveness to anti-EGFR therapies; however, it is also a logical "inclusion biomarker" for the enrollment of patients likely to benefit from pharmacological inhibitors of the kinases MEK1 and MEK2 [4].

GENOMICS OF COLORECTAL CANCER

The vast majority of colorectal cancers (~70%) develop along a multistep sequence of genetic events ("conventional adenoma–carcinoma sequence") as proposed by Fearon and Vogelstein in 1990 [13]. Inactivating mutations of adenomatous polyposis coli (APC) tumor suppressor gene is an early rate-limiting step that initiates adenoma formation via the activation of WNT signaling. Subsequent progression to larger adenomas and carcinomas requires activating mutations of the proto-oncogene KRAS, loss of heterozygosity (LOH) at chromosome 18q (DCC, SMAD4, SMAD2, Cables genes), and inactivating mutations in TP53 tumor suppressor gene (chromosome 17p). Most colorectal cancers (~70%) also demonstrate chromosomal instability (CIN), characterized by extensive imbalance in chromosome number (aneuploidy) and LOH [14]. Although a direct link between CIN and the acquisition of mutations along the adenoma–carcinoma sequence has not been established, CIN is an early event during adenoma formation and is thought to facilitate tumorigenesis by increasing the cellular mutation rate

A minority of colorectal cancers (~30%) arise from serrated adenomas that characteristically demonstrate the CpG island methylator phenotype (CIMP) and mutations of the oncogene BRAF [15]. Hypermethylation of CpG dinucleotide clusters (CpG islands) within the promoter regions of tumor suppressor genes (e.g., p16INK4a and IGFBP7) synergizes with BRAF mutations to allow microsatellite stable (MSS) colorectal tumorigenesis along the "serrated adenoma pathway." CIMP-associated colorectal cancers are characterized by proximal tumor location, female gender, poor histologic differentiation, signet ring cell morphology, BRAF mutations, wild-type TP53, lack of CIN, and microsatellite instability (MSI) phenotype. Approximately half of all tumors with CIMP demonstrate MSI.

The MSI phenotype is associated with defective DNA mismatch repair enzymes and is characterized by a failure to correct random errors of replication at mono- and dinucleotide repeats within DNA sequences of target proto-oncogenes and tumor suppressor genes carrying such repetitive regions (e.g., CDC4, TGFβR2, BAX, IGF2R) [16]. The MSI phenotype is associated with proximal location, mucinous differentiation, KRAS mutations, wild-type TP53, lack of CIN, Crohn's-like lymphoid reaction, abundant tumor-infiltrating lymphocytes, tumor necrosis, and poor histologic differentiation. Approximately 15% of all colorectal cancers have MSI phenotype, and the majority of these are sporadic. Sporadic MSI-associated tumors with CIMP demonstrate loss of MLH1 mismatch repair gene expression through promoter methylation.

The discovery of these genomic instability pathways and the variety of specific genetic alterations in colorectal cancers has increased awareness of the tremendous diversity in these tumors. Elucidation of the molecular genetics/epigenetics of colorectal cancer has implications for tumor phenotyping, prognostication, and therapy. A variety of molecular classifications for CRC have been suggested, based on MSI/CIMP status, which provide a more robust understanding of carcinogenesis and the underlying heterogeneity of this complex disease [17,18]. Colorectal cancer patients with CIN phenotype and those with MSS-CIMP-BRAF-mutated tumors generally have a less favorable oncologic outcome compared to those that exhibit MSI. Tumors with MSI phenotype are less responsive to 5-FU chemotherapy and more sensitive to irinotecan, while CIN-associated tumors are intrinsically resistant to taxanes [19]. Small molecule inhibitors targeting molecular pathways for CIN have demonstrated antitumor activity in preclinical models and are being investigated in phase I and II trials for the treatment of solid malignancies [14]. Similarly, methylation is another potential therapeutic target that requires further research and development and would be applicable to the treatment of tumors developing along the serrated pathway. KRAS and BRAF mutations are currently being used in clinical practice to predict lack of response to epidermal growth factor receptor-specific antibodies cetuximab and panitumumab in patients with stage IV colorectal cancer.

Gene expression analysis has been used to classify colorectal cancer specimens into tumor subtypes with distinct prognostic and predictive characteristics. The 12-gene Oncotype DX Colon Cancer Recurrence Score Assay was developed using tumor gene expression data from patients with stage II and III colon cancer in four large independent development studies as a predictor of recurrence risk following surgical resection. Validation studies demonstrated significant association of the recurrence score with disease recurrence and survival irrespective of stage, mismatch repair status, patient age, tumor grade, lymph node involvement, and chemotherapy regimen. The recurrence score provides clinicians with a tool to better select patients that may derive a higher absolute benefit from adjuvant chemotherapy and avoid the unnecessary toxicity in those with low risk of disease recurrence [20,21]. Similarly, the 18-gene ColoPrint colon cancer prognostic classifier separates patients with stage II and III colon cancer into those with low or high risk for recurrence and identifies low-risk stage II patients that may be safely managed without adjuvant systemic chemotherapy, independent of conventional clinical and pathologic markers [22]. More recently, gene expression signatures have been used for molecular classification of colorectal cancers into distinct subtypes. Sadanandam et al. used microarray-based gene expression data to classify and validate primary colorectal cancer specimens into five molecular subtypes using independent gene expression data sets. Gene expression signatures from 786 genes identified 5 subtypes including goblet-like, inflammatory, enterocyte, stemlike, and transit-amplifying tumors. Patients with stem-cell subtype had the worst disease-free survival but benefited from adjuvant systemic chemotherapy, while those with transit-amplifying and goblet cell subtypes had the best disease-free survival but demonstrated detrimental effect from adjuvant systemic chemotherapy. The inflammatory subtypes frequently showed MSI phenotype, while a majority of transit-amplifying and stemlike subtypes were MSS. They also demonstrated a varying degree of responsiveness to cetuximab, conventional systemic chemotherapy, and MET inhibitors based on specific subtypes [23]. Similarly, Melo and colleagues identified and validated three colorectal subtypes using microarray-based gene expression profiling; subtype 1 (CCS1) correlated with CIN tumors; subtype 2 (CCS2) correlated with MSI-H/CIMP-H tumors; and subtype 3 (CCS3) correlated with sessile serrated adenomas demonstrating poor prognosis and lack of response to anti-EGFR therapy. The CCS3 subtype demonstrated upregulated epithelial–mesenchymal transition, matrix remodeling, cell migration, and transforming growth factor-β signaling that may explain the increased invasive and metastatic potential of these tumors and provide potential targets for therapy [24]. Finally, Marisa and colleagues identified and validated a six-subtype molecular classification system for colorectal cancers using a combination of microarray-based gene expression data and common DNA alterations (CIN, MSI, CIMP, KRAS, BRAF, and TP53) from a multicenter cohort of patients. Combination of the six subtypes into high-risk (subtypes C4 and C6) and low-risk (subtypes C1, C2, C3, and C5) categories demonstrated prognostic value, even after adjusting for stage and the prognostic classifier Oncotype DX Colon Cancer Recurrence Score Assay [25]. To date, no gene signature has been adopted in routine clinical practice for therapeutic decision making since reproducibility of their prognostic ability in independent data sets has been poor and their discriminative ability to accurately classify samples into high-risk and low-risk groups has been limited [26–28].

Genome-wide association studies (GWASs) have been useful for identifying commonly occurring low-penetrance genetic variants that are associated with increased hereditary risk of common cancers by comparing DNA variations in large cohorts of unrelated patient cases and controls [29,30]. This is important since only about 5% of colorectal cancer cases can be explained by rare, high-penetrance variants in susceptibility genes including APC in familial adenomatous polyposis syndrome, SMAD4 and BMPR1A in juvenile polyposis syndrome, LKB1/STK11 in Peutz–Jeghers syndrome, POLD1 and AXIN2 in familial colorectal cancer syndrome, MUTYH in MUTYH-associated polyposis, and DNA mismatch repair genes in Lynch syndrome. GWASs compare genetic variants between cases and controls in large populations using high-density SNP array-based genotyping and the annotated haplotype map of the human genome. Large-scale GWASs and meta-analyses have identified and validated common, low-risk variants in 20 genomic regions (colorectal susceptibility loci) as being responsible for the majority of the heritable risk of colorectal cancer [31,32].

Genomic sequencing studies have rapidly advanced our understanding of colorectal cancer genetics in the last decade. Initial large-scale Sanger sequencing of colorectal cancer specimens identified novel recurrently mutated genes, including PIK3CA, FBXW7, SMAD4, and EPHA3, in addition to the few well-known genes like APC, KRAS, and TP53 [33,34]. High-throughput sequencing technology has expanded the capacity for genomic research in a more efficient and cost-effective manner. TCGA network performed a comprehensive and integrated analysis of approximately 276 colorectal cancer samples analyzing exome sequence, DNA copy number alterations (using SNP arrays and whole genome sequencing), epigenetic data (using methylation arrays), and gene expression profiles (using mRNA arrays and RNA-seq) [35]. Based on genetic alterations, two distinct subgroups of colorectal cancers were identified; 16% of the cases were hypermutated (>12 mutations per Mb), while the majority were nonhypermutated. APC, TP53, and KRAS genes were more frequently mutated in nonhypermutated tumors, while BRAF and TGFBR2 were more frequent targets of mutation in hypermutated tumors. Hypermutated tumors were more likely to be right-sided, MSI-H, and hypermethylated (CIMP, MLH1 methylation) and lacked CIN. Common focal chromosomal amplifications were found at 17q (ERBB2), 8q (MYC), 11p (IGF2, miR-483), and 20q (HNF4A), while focal deletions were observed at chromosome 3p (FHIT), 18q (SMAD4), 5q (APC), and 10q (PTEN), among others. A novel recurrent fusion of NAV2-TCF7L1 was observed. Pathway analysis using the PARADIGM software platform demonstrated recurrent alterations in WNT (APC, CTNNB1, SOX9, TCF7L2, AXIN2, FBXW7, ARID1A, and FAM123B), MAPK (ERBB2/3, KRAS, NRAS, BRAF), PI3K (IGF2, IRS, PIK3CA, PIK3R1, PTEN), TGF-β (TGFBR1/2, ACVR2A, ACVR1B, SMAD2/3/4), and p53 (TP53, ATM) signaling pathways, hence providing potential targets for therapy. The authors demonstrated that activation of WNT signaling and inactivation of TGF-β

signaling occurred in almost all colorectal cancers leading to MYC-mediated tumorigenesis. Lee and colleagues used elastic-net regularized regression analysis of the integrated TCGA genomic data to identify and rank genes associated with advanced clinical stage (e.g., WRN, SYK, DDX5, ADRA2C, and GNAS) that may play a role in tumor progression and metastasis [36]. Using RNA-seq data, recurrent fusions of R-spondin family members RSPO2 with EIF3E and RSPO3 and PTPRK have been observed in 10% of colorectal cancer cases [37]. Whole genome sequencing has improved our ability to identify genomic SVs, for example, an in-frame gene fusion between VTI1A (coding for a v-SNARE protein that mediates fusion of intracellular vesicles within the Golgi complex) and TCF7L2 (coding for TCF4, a binding partner for β-catenin) in 3% of cases [38].

GENOMICS OF MUCINOUS APPENDICEAL CANCER

The molecular basis for the mucinous phenotype of mucinous appendiceal neoplasms and genetic aberrations underlying their malignant transformation are poorly understood. KRAS mutations have been demonstrated (40%–100%) and may increase mucin production and progression to pseudomyxoma peritonei [39–41]. GNAS gene mutations have been identified in 50% of low-grade mucinous appendiceal neoplasms and may be associated with mucin production through activated adenylyl cyclase activity. Concurrence of GNAS and KRAS oncogene mutations has also been implicated in mucinous appendiceal tumorigenesis [42]. Alteration in tumor suppressor gene TP53 expression has been demonstrated in 44% of patients, particularly in high-grade tumors [40,41]. Maheshwari and colleagues demonstrated LOH in 61% of patients with mucinous appendiceal neoplasms/ pseudomyxoma peritonei by analyzing polymorphic microsatellite markers associated with CMM/RIZ (cutaneous malignant melanoma/retinoblastoma protein-interacting zinc finger), VHL/OGG (von Hippel–Lindau tumor suppressor/8-oxoguanine DNA glycosylase), APC, MET, CDKN2A/p16 (cyclin-dependent kinase inhibitor 2A/p16 subunit of actin-related protein 2/3 complex), PTCH1, PTEN, DCC, and TP53 gene loci [43]. Alakus and colleagues used whole exome sequencing to perform comprehensive molecular profiling of mostly metastatic tissue from low-grade mucinous appendiceal neoplasms and validated their findings in a second cohort of patients [44]. They identified statistically significant, recurrent protein-altering mutations in 25 unique genes affecting RAS-PI3K-AKT, WNT, TGF-β, cAMP-PKA, DNA repair, and Hippo pathways, among others. They demonstrated clear differences in mutations and CNVs between low-grade mucinous appendiceal neoplasms and colorectal cancers; low-grade mucinous appendiceal neoplasms were less likely to have APC and TP53 mutations, demonstrated lower CNVs, and frequently had

GNAS (82%) and KRAS (91%) mutations. In addition, low-grade and high-grade mucinous appendiceal neoplasms demonstrated clear genetic differences; high-grade tumors had more frequent CNVs and TP53 mutations and lacked GNAS mutations but demonstrated activating mutations in PKA. Based on these genomic data, they hypothesized that KRAS mutations occur early in the course of tumorigenesis, additional GNAS mutations facilitate low-grade tumor formation, and activating PKA mutations along with p53 mutations drive high-grade mucinous appendiceal neoplasms. From a therapeutic standpoint, the high incidence of KRAS mutations in mucinous appendiceal neoplasms, especially low-grade tumors, provides a rational basis for the use of MEK inhibitors. Similarly, targeted agents against PI3K-AKT, WNT, TGF-β, and cAMP-PKA signaling pathways may be beneficial. Levine and colleagues performed gene expression profiling of metastatic peritoneal tissue from colon and predominantly low-grade appendiceal cancer cases [45]. They identified distinct genomic signatures separating low-risk appendiceal, high-risk appendiceal, and colorectal cancers, highlighting the fact that even within low-grade appendiceal tumors prognosis varied significantly. Genes associated with worse prognosis in the appendiceal tumors (high-risk appendiceal cancers) included mucin-related genes such as mucin 5, mucin 2, and trefoil factors 1 and 2. A high-risk genetic signature may help stratify patients with low-grade appendiceal tumors that would benefit from adjuvant systemic therapy. Gene set enrichment analysis identified the Src, TGF-β, and immune-related pathways as being differentially regulated in the high-risk appendiceal cancer patients, providing potential targets for therapy. A better understanding of these gene expression profiles would elucidate biologic processes and pathways associated with worse prognosis and chemotherapy resistance.

GENOMIC APPROACH TO PERITONEAL CARCINOMATOSIS

The identification of genetic alterations that specifically mediate metastasis has been elusive. Moreover, it remains unclear whether additional mutations are necessary to induce a metastatic phenotype beyond those alterations that are responsible for primary tumorigenesis [46]. However, tumors are genetically dynamic and demonstrate continuous acquisition of genetic alterations within the primary tumor and metastatic deposits as they evolve. Vermaat et al. demonstrated substantial genetic differences between primary colorectal cancers and their paired hepatic metastases and hypothesized that such genetic heterogeneity could be responsible for variable response to targeted therapies in the primary and metastatic lesions [47].

Therefore, comprehensive genomic analysis of the primary tumor as well as its metastatic lesions would be important to better understand tumor biology and identify relevant biomarkers for prognosis and therapy. The current era of cancer genomics and integrative genomic analysis promises to facilitate such an in-depth analysis of an individual tumor's genotype and therefore has the potential to make personalized cancer medicine a reality.

REFERENCES

1. Stratton MR, Campbell PJ, Futreal PA. The cancer genome. *Nature*. April 2009;458(7239):719–724.
2. Negrini S, Gorgoulis VG, Halazonetis TD. Genomic instability—An evolving hallmark of cancer. *Nature Reviews Molecular Cell Biology*. March 2010;11(3):220–228.
3. Vogelstein B, Papadopoulos N, Velculescu VE, Zhou S, Diaz LA Jr., Kinzler KW. Cancer genome landscapes. *Science*. March 2013;339(6127):1546–1558.
4. Garraway LA, Lander ES. Lessons from the cancer genome. *Cell*. March 2013;153(1):17–37.
5. International Human Genome Sequencing C. Finishing the euchromatic sequence of the human genome. *Nature*. October 2004;431(7011):931–945.
6. Wheeler DA, Wang L. From human genome to cancer genome: The first decade. *Genome Research*. July 2013;23(7):1054–1062.
7. Tran B, Dancey JE, Kamel-Reid S, McPherson JD, Bedard PL, Brown AM et al. Cancer genomics: Technology, discovery, and translation. *Journal of Clinical Oncology: Official Journal of the American Society of Clinical Oncology*. February 2012;30(6):647–660.
8. Ding L, Wendl MC, McMichael JF, Raphael BJ. Expanding the computational toolbox for mining cancer genomes. *Nature Reviews Genetics*. August 2014;15(8):556–570.
9. Chin L, Hahn WC, Getz G, Meyerson M. Making sense of cancer genomic data. *Genes & Development*. March 2011;25(6):534–555.
10. Raphael BJ, Dobson JR, Oesper L, Vandin F. Identifying driver mutations in sequenced cancer genomes: Computational approaches to enable precision medicine. *Genome Medicine*. 2014;6(1):5.
11. Kristensen VN, Lingjaerde OC, Russnes HG, Vollan HK, Frigessi A, Borresen-Dale AL. Principles and methods of integrative genomic analyses in cancer. *Nature Reviews Cancer*. May 2014;14(5):299–313.
12. Chin L, Andersen JN, Futreal PA. Cancer genomics: From discovery science to personalized medicine. *Nature Medicine*. March 2011;17(3):297–303.
13. Fearon ER. Molecular genetics of colorectal cancer. *Annual Review of Pathology*. 2011;6:479–507.
14. Pino MS, Chung DC. The chromosomal instability pathway in colon cancer. *Gastroenterology*. June 2010;138(6):2059–2072.

15. Leggett B, Whitehall V. Role of the serrated pathway in colorectal cancer pathogenesis. *Gastroenterology.* June 2010;138(6):2088–2100.

16. Boland CR, Goel A. Microsatellite instability in colorectal cancer. *Gastroenterology.* June 2010;138(6):2073–2087.e3.

17. Jass JR. Classification of colorectal cancer based on correlation of clinical, morphological and molecular features. *Histopathology.* January 2007;50(1):113–130.

18. Ogino S, Goel A. Molecular classification and correlates in colorectal cancer. *The Journal of Molecular Diagnostics.* January 2008;10(1):13–27.

19. Walther A, Johnstone E, Swanton C, Midgley R, Tomlinson I, Kerr D. Genetic prognostic and predictive markers in colorectal cancer. *Nature Reviews Cancer.* July 2009;9(7):489–499.

20. Gray RG, Quirke P, Handley K, Lopatin M, Magill L, Baehner FL et al. Validation study of a quantitative multigene reverse transcriptase-polymerase chain reaction assay for assessment of recurrence risk in patients with stage II colon cancer. *Journal of Clinical Oncology: Official Journal of the American Society of Clinical Oncology.* December 2011;29(35):4611–4619.

21. Yothers G, O'Connell MJ, Lee M, Lopatin M, Clark-Langone KM, Millward C et al. Validation of the 12-gene colon cancer recurrence score in NSABP C-07 as a predictor of recurrence in patients with stage II and III colon cancer treated with fluorouracil and leucovorin (FU/LV) and FU/LV plus oxaliplatin. *Journal of Clinical Oncology: Official Journal of the American Society of Clinical Oncology.* December 2013;31(36):4512–4519.

22. Salazar R, Roepman P, Capella G, Moreno V, Simon I, Dreezen C et al. Gene expression signature to improve prognosis prediction of stage II and III colorectal cancer. *Journal of Clinical Oncology: Official Journal of the American Society of Clinical Oncology.* January 2011;29(1):17–24.

23. Sadanandam A, Lyssiotis CA, Homicsko K, Collisson EA, Gibb WJ, Wullschleger S et al. A colorectal cancer classification system that associates cellular phenotype and responses to therapy. *Nature Medicine.* May 2013;19(5):619–625.

24. De Sousa EMF, Wang X, Jansen M, Fessler E, Trinh A, de Rooij LP et al. Poor-prognosis colon cancer is defined by a molecularly distinct subtype and develops from serrated precursor lesions. *Nature Medicine.* May 2013;19(5):614–618.

25. Marisa L, de Reynies A, Duval A, Selves J, Gaub MP, Vescovo L et al. Gene expression classification of colon cancer into molecular subtypes: Characterization, validation, and prognostic value. *PloS Medicine.* 2013;10(5):e1001453.

26. Nannini M, Pantaleo MA, Maleddu A, Astolfi A, Formica S, Biasco G. Gene expression profiling in colorectal cancer using microarray technologies: Results and perspectives. *Cancer Treatment Reviews.* May 2009;35(3):201–209.

27. Sanz-Pamplona R, Berenguer A, Cordero D, Riccadonna S, Sole X, Crous-Bou M et al. Clinical value of prognosis gene expression signatures in colorectal cancer: A systematic review. *PLOS ONE.* 2012;7(11):e48877.

28. Shibayama M, Maak M, Nitsche U, Gotoh K, Rosenberg R, Janssen KP. Prediction of metastasis and recurrence in colorectal cancer based on gene expression analysis: Ready for the clinic? *Cancers.* 2011;3(3):2858–2869.

29. Hirschhorn JN, Daly MJ. Genome-wide association studies for common diseases and complex traits. *Nature Reviews Genetics.* February 2005;6(2):95–108.

30. Wong SH, Sung JJ, Chan FK, To KF, Ng SS, Wang XJ et al. Genome-wide association and sequencing studies on colorectal cancer. *Seminars in Cancer Biology.* December 2013;23(6 Pt. B): 502–511.

31. Dunlop MG, Dobbins SE, Farrington SM, Jones AM, Palles C, Whiffin N et al. Common variation near CDKN1A, POLD3 and SHROOM2 influences colorectal cancer risk. *Nature Genetics.* July 2012;44(7):770–776.

32. Houlston RS, Cheadle J, Dobbins SE, Tenesa A, Jones AM, Howarth K et al. Meta-analysis of three genome-wide association studies identifies susceptibility loci for colorectal cancer at 1q41, 3q26.2, 12q13.13 and 20q13.33. *Nature Genetics.* November 2010;42(11):973–977.

33. Sjoblom T, Jones S, Wood LD, Parsons DW, Lin J, Barber TD et al. The consensus coding sequences of human breast and colorectal cancers. *Science.* October 2006;314(5797):268–274.

34. Wood LD, Parsons DW, Jones S, Lin J, Sjoblom T, Leary RJ et al. The genomic landscapes of human breast and colorectal cancers. *Science.* November 2007;318(5853):1108–1113.

35. Cancer Genome Atlas Network. Comprehensive molecular characterization of human colon and rectal cancer. *Nature.* July 2012;487(7407):330–337.

36. Lee H, Flaherty P, Ji HP. Systematic genomic identification of colorectal cancer genes delineating advanced from early clinical stage and metastasis. *BMC Medical Genomics.* 2013;6:54.

37. Seshagiri S, Stawiski EW, Durinck S, Modrusan Z, Storm EE, Conboy CB et al. Recurrent R-spondin fusions in colon cancer. *Nature.* August 2012;488(7413):660–664.

38. Bass AJ, Lawrence MS, Brace LE, Ramos AH, Drier Y, Cibulskis K et al. Genomic sequencing of colorectal adenocarcinomas identifies a recurrent VTI1A-TCF7L2 fusion. *Nature Genetics*. October 2011;43(10):964–968.

39. Kabbani W, Houlihan PS, Luthra R, Hamilton SR, Rashid A. Mucinous and nonmucinous appendiceal adenocarcinomas: Different clinicopathological features but similar genetic alterations. *Modern Pathology: An Official Journal of the United States and Canadian Academy of Pathology, Inc.* June 2002;15(6):599–605.

40. Shetty S, Thomas P, Ramanan B, Sharma P, Govindarajan V, Loggie B. KRAS mutations and p53 overexpression in pseudomyxoma peritonei: Association with phenotype and prognosis. *The Journal of Surgical Research*. March 2013;180(1):97–103.

41. Szych C, Staebler A, Connolly DC, Wu R, Cho KR, Ronnett BM. Molecular genetic evidence supporting the clonality and appendiceal origin of pseudomyxoma peritonei in women. *The American Journal of Pathology*. June 1999;154(6):1849–1855.

42. Nishikawa G, Sekine S, Ogawa R, Matsubara A, Mori T, Taniguchi H et al. Frequent GNAS mutations in low-grade appendiceal mucinous neoplasms. *British Journal of Cancer*. March 2013;108(4):951–958.

43. Maheshwari V, Tsung A, Lin Y, Zeh HJ 3rd, Finkelstein SD, Bartlett DL. Analysis of loss of heterozygosity for tumor-suppressor genes can accurately classify and predict the clinical behavior of mucinous tumors arising from the appendix. *Annals of Surgical Oncology*. December 2006;13(12):1610–1616.

44. Alakus H, Babicky ML, Ghosh P, Yost S, Jepsen K, Dai Y et al. Genome-wide mutational landscape of mucinous carcinomatosis peritonei of appendiceal origin. *Genome Medicine*. 2014;6(5):43.

45. Levine EA, Blazer DG 3rd, Kim MK, Shen P, Stewart JHt, Guy C et al. Gene expression profiling of peritoneal metastases from appendiceal and colon cancer demonstrates unique biologic signatures and predicts patient outcomes. *Journal of the American College of Surgeons*. April 2012;214(4):599–606; discussion-7.

46. Nguyen DX, Massague J. Genetic determinants of cancer metastasis. *Nature Reviews Genetics*. May 2007;8(5):341–352.

47. Vermaat JS, Nijman IJ, Koudijs MJ, Gerritse FL, Scherer SJ, Mokry M et al. Primary colorectal cancers and their subsequent hepatic metastases are genetically different: Implications for selection of patients for targeted treatment. *Clinical Cancer Research: An Official Journal of the American Association for Cancer Research*. February 2012;18(3):688–699.

8

Surgery, wound healing, and peritoneal minimal residual disease in colorectal cancer

WIM P. CEELEN

INTRODUCTION

Surgery is the mainstay of therapy in colorectal cancer (CRC), and complete (R0) resection represents the single most important determinant of cure. Recent data, however, suggest that surgical removal may in itself be associated with enhanced or accelerated growth of microscopic or macroscopic residual tumor [1]. The fact that surgical intervention may promote cancer growth has been observed since ancient times but has received little attention from clinicians [2].

This chapter provides an overview of the underlying mechanisms giving rise to accelerated tumor growth in the presence of microscopic residual disease, with an emphasis on peritoneal cancer recurrence. First, we describe the various mechanisms known to cause minimal residual disease (MRD) after open and laparoscopic surgery. Secondly, an overview is provided of the evidence supporting the hypothesis that (surgical) cancer removal creates a permissive environment enhancing residual tumor growth. Finally, potential preventive and therapeutic approaches are highlighted.

INCIDENCE AND RISK FACTORS OF PERITONEAL SPREAD FROM COLORECTAL CANCER

Tumor stage and biology

The epidemiology and risk factors for peritoneal spread in CRC are not well established. In retrospective single-center series, the reported incidence of peritoneal carcinomatosis (PC) is approximately 7% of patients at primary surgery and 4%–19% of patients during follow-up after curative surgery [3]. In a recent population-based cohort study from Stockholm County in Sweden, 4.8% of 11,124 CRC patients had PC as the first and only site of metastatic disease [4]. Results from this cohort study as well as those from a large CRC cohort study in the Netherlands have identified several independent clinicopathological risk factors for synchronous PC: colon versus rectal cancer, right colon cancer, T stage, N stage, emergency and irradical resection, younger age, and mucinous tumors [5]. Recent molecular research in a series of 524 CRC patients has indicated that those with BRAF mutant cancers (11%) are at higher risk of

Table 8.1 Incidence and prognostic significance of peritoneal involvement (pT4a) of the resected colorectal cancer specimen

Author	Year	N	Stage II	Stage III	Detection rate	Comments or conclusion
Shepherd [11]	1997	412	42%	52%	27%	Peritoneal involvement significantly associated with OS in multivariate analysis; present in 45 of 46 patients who developed peritoneal recurrence
Solomon [149]	1997	103	47%	53%	14.6%	Only the type of surgery predicted peritoneal involvement in univariate analysis; higher incidence in rectal procedures
Lennon [10]	2003	118	100%		13.6%	Peritoneal involvement significantly associated with 5-year survival in multivariate analysis
Baskaranathan [150]	2004	281	63%	37%	9.3%	Peritoneal involvement significantly associated with cancer-specific survival in multivariate analysis
Keshava [151]	2007	665	49.9%	50.1%	5.3%	Serosal involvement significantly associated with local recurrence and OS in multivariate analysis
Stewart [152]	2007	82	100%		22%	Serosal invasion associated with 5-year survival in univariate analysis

peritoneal metastasis (46% vs. 24%, P = 0.001) [6]. Possibly, peritoneal spread is driven by a specific set of molecular alterations that differs from systemic (hepatic) metastasis [7,8]. In a preliminary analysis, we compared gene expression between CRC liver metastases and isolated peritoneal metastases and found 179 genes related to immune response, cellular differentiation, epithelial to mesenchymal transition (EMT), and cell growth to be differentially expressed [9]. Pathway analysis showed that interleukin-6 (IL-6) and transforming growth factor-β (TGF-β) signaling were upregulated in peritoneal metastases. Taken together, these results suggest that peritoneal spread and progression of CRC is driven by a specific set of genetic alterations.

Mechanistically, peritoneal disease spread from CRC can be caused by direct invasion, perforation, or shedding of loose cells. Several clinical studies have demonstrated that tumors penetrating the entire bowel wall (T_3) and those infiltrating the abdominal wall or adjacent organs (T_4) are associated with both a worse prognosis and an increased risk of peritoneal recurrence [10–12].

Several clinical studies showed a significantly poorer outcome in CRC patients in whom visceral peritoneal invasion was identified (pT4a) on pathological examination of the resection specimen (Table 8.1). Similarly, spontaneous bowel perforation has been shown to represent an adverse prognostic event and more than doubles the risk of postoperative PC compared to nonperforated cancers [13–16].

Mechanisms of peritoneal spread

The first step in the cascade resulting in PC is liberation of tumor cells from the primary cancer mass. This process can occur spontaneously, or can be iatrogenically caused. Several mechanisms have been proposed to explain shedding of cells

from the surface of CRC. First, downregulation of cell–cell adhesion molecules, such as E-cadherin via the transcription factor TWIST, has been reported to promote cancer cell detachment [17,18]. Second, spontaneous shedding of loose cells is facilitated by the elevated interstitial fluid pressure (IFP) in most solid tumors [19]. This hydrodynamic property of malignant tissue is caused by rapid cellular proliferation, defective lymphatic drainage, fibrosis and contraction of the interstitial matrix, and increased osmotic pressure generated by anaerobic glycolysis and leakage of plasma proteins [20,21]. Viability studies have suggested that, in contrast to circulating tumor cells in the blood, bone marrow, or liver, loose intraperitoneal (IP) cells exhibit clear metastatic efficiency [22–24]. However, the population of loose IP cancer cells is likely heterogeneous with both invasive cells possessing a metastatic phenotype and noninvasive cells that are merely transported by the physiological lymph flow. Free cancer cells in the peritoneal cavity are subject to passive movement dictated by gravity and by the excursion of the diaphragm. As a result, a predictable path is usually followed toward the pelvis and from the pelvis, along the right paracolic gutter, toward the subdiaphragmatic space [25]. Similarly, the greater omentum is nearly always involved in colorectal PC despite the presence of numerous macrophages in the omental milky spots [26]. Possibly, adhesion of cancer cells to the omental surface is facilitated by the reduced flow and shear forces along the irregular omental surface. In addition, omental adipose stem cells and adipocytes have recently been identified to play a role in the preferential homing of tumor cells to the omentum [27].

Iatrogenic causes of peritoneal spread

Technical circumstances can give rise to a peritoneal recurrence. Obviously, this will be the case when an R1 or R2 resection is performed or when the tumor is inadvertently ruptured, opened, or cut into. This is well illustrated in rectal cancer surgery, where a clear relationship exists between incomplete resection (positive circumferential resection margin) and the development of a local recurrence [28,29]. Theoretically, tumor spill could also arise from a section of blood or lymph vessels with subsequent leakage. This concept was proven by Hansen et al., who detected tumor cells in the blood shed during cancer surgery in 57 out of 61 patients [30]. Importantly, the identified cancer cells demonstrated proliferation capacity, invasiveness, and tumorigenicity.

Local recurrence situated at port site or extraction site skin incisions has been a concern since the introduction of laparoscopic techniques in CRC [31,32]. The risk of port site metastasis (PSM) depends on the surgical technique, instrumentation and technology, and tumor biology. Grasping and manipulating the tumor with laparoscopic instruments are associated with tumor cell contamination of both the instruments and the trocars [33,34]. Also, aerosolization of particles and viable cells can occur during laparoscopy [35,36]. Champault et al. passed the gas escaping from pneumoperitoneum through a filter in nine patients undergoing various laparoscopic procedures for both benign and malignant disease [37]. The filters and tubing were subsequently washed or examined by electron microscopy, and in six of nine samples, viable cells (although no cancer cells) were identified. Aerosolization of tumor cells could in turn cause PSM by the so-called chimney effect, when the insufflation gas is allowed to escape through a skin incision or along a trocar [38,39]. However, Wittich et al. showed in a rat CRC model that the tumor load in the gas flow required to cause PSM is very high and therefore the clinical relevance of this mechanism is probably limited [40]. The increase in IP pressure associated with laparoscopy has been shown to promote tumor growth and invasiveness in a number of preclinical studies [41–43]. Paraskeva et al. found that exposure of a human colon cancer cell line to a laparoscopic environment significantly enhanced production of the proteases matrix metalloproteinase (MMP)-2 and MMP-9 and urokinase-type plasminogen activator (uPA); at the same time invasive capacity as measured with a Matrigel assay was also enhanced [44]. Similarly, Basson et al. noted that even a moderate increase in pressure stimulated malignant colonocyte adhesion by a cation-dependent β_1-integrin-mediated mechanism [45]. The same group showed that increased extracellular pressure in general stimulates colon cancer cell adhesion by activating focal adhesion kinase (FAK) and Src [46,47]. The increased intra-abdominal pressure may also alter the functional integrity of the mesothelial lining. In an animal model, Volz et al. performed scanning electron microscopy of the peritoneum after IP injection of 200,000 cells of a malignant melanoma followed by CO_2 pneumoperitoneum for 30 minutes [48]. In the group that underwent pneumoperitoneum, pronounced alterations of the peritoneum were evident and parts of the underlying basal lamina

were laid bare; tumor cells were noted to attach to the free basal lamina. Similar ultrastructural alterations of the peritoneum were noted by Rosario et al. and were more pronounced after CO_2 pneumoperitoneum compared to air insufflation [49]. Also, elevated IP pressures cause contraction of mesothelial cells resulting of increased exposure of extracellular matrix (ECM) binding sites [50]. Apart from the mechanical effects on the mesothelial structure, the acidification and dehydration associated with CO_2 gas inflation during laparoscopic surgery were shown to promote tumor growth and invasiveness in a number of preclinical studies [51,52]. Despite the concerns raised by these preclinical models, the incidence of PSMs has been noted to decrease with appropriate protective measures such as trocar fixation, adequate wound protection, and avoidance of desufflation through a skin incision. The results of recently completed large randomized trials comparing open with laparoscopic colectomy for cancer demonstrated that the overall rate of wound recurrence is low (<1%) and does not differ between the open and laparoscopic technique [53,54].

Clinical significance of free peritoneal cancer cells

Although established peritoneal metastases are found in only a limited percentage of patients undergoing surgery, it is likely that microscopic spread occurs much more frequently [55]. Several authors have studied the presence of free peritoneal cancer cells immediately before or after CRC resection and related their presence to local recurrence and survival (Table 8.2). Overall, the results of these studies suggest that microscopic peritoneal disease at the time of surgery represents a prognostic factor and thus a possible therapeutic target in resectable CRC. A similar conclusion was formulated by the authors of a recent meta-analysis showing that the presence of free peritoneal cancer cells before CRC resection was associated with a higher risk of overall recurrence (odds ratio 0.19–0.88) and local recurrence (odds ratio 0.21 0.82), while after resection, the presence of free cancer cells resulted in a significantly higher risk of overall recurrence (odds ratio 0.03–0.18) [56]. In parallel, in vitro studies and animal tumorigenicity assays have shown that exfoliated CRC cells have the potential to proliferate and invade [57,58].

Postoperative factors contributing to peritoneal recurrence

Clinical studies have shown that the development of an anastomotic leak following colonic surgery is associated with an increased likelihood of local recurrence and a significantly worse survival [59,60]. The underlying mechanisms are at present unclear. Possibly, at least part of this effect is explained by the fact that patients who leaked probably had a more difficult procedure due to larger or more advanced cancers. On the other hand, there is evidence that viable

Table 8.2 Incidence and prognostic significance of peritoneal free cancer cells in colorectal cancer

Author	Year	N	Method	Markers or antibodies	Detection rate	Comments or conclusion
Juhl [153]	1995	67	ICC	C1P83 (CEA), Ra96, CA19-9	27%	Positive ICC correlates with OS in univariate analysis
Hase [154]	1998	140	CYT	17-1A, C54-0, KI-1	16%	CYT positivity at the end of surgery predicts local recurrence
Schott [155]	1998	109	ICC	C1P83 (CEA), CA19-9, 17-1A, Ra96, C54-0, KI-1	31%	Positive ICC correlates with OS in univariate analysis
Wind [156]	1999	88	CYT		28%	Presence of CYT+ cells provides no prognostic information
Vogel [157]	2000	90	CYT and ICC[b]	HEA-125	47%	Positive ICC does not predict local recurrence or outcome
Vogel [158]	2001	135	ICC	C1P83 (CEA), Ra96, CA19-9	23%	Detection of IP tumor cells correlates with prognosis in univariate analysis. Worst prognosis in the presence of CEA-positive intraperitoneal cells
Broll [159]	2001	75[a]	ICC and RT-PCR	CEA	63%	CEA mRNA detection by RT-PCR not recommended due to high FP rate; presence of ICC + cells represents independent prognostic factor in multivariate analysis
Lucha [160]	2002	56	CYT		2%	Only 1 patient with + cytology
Aoki [161]	2002	20	RT-PCR	CEA, CK20	24%	Detection rate increased in parallel with invasion depth
Guller [162]	2002	39	qRT-PCR	CEA, CK20	28%	Presence of PCR+ cells associated with worse DFS and OS in multivariate analysis
Yamamoto [163]	2003	189	CYT	6%		Presence of CYT+ cells predicted peritoneal recurrence and represents an independent prognostic factor in multivariate analysis
Kanellos [164]	2003	110	CYT		20%	Presence of CYT+ cells predicts locoregional recurrence but not survival
Bosch [165]	2003	53	CYT and ICC	Ks20.8 (CK20), Ber-Ep4	17%	Presence of CYT and/or ICC+ cells in blood and peritoneal lavage fluid associated with DFS and OS in multivariate analysis
Lloyd [166]	2006	125	Immunobead RT-PCR	CK20, CEA, EphB4, LAMγ2, matrilysin	29%	Presence of PCR+ cells in postresection lavage fluid predicts DFS in multivariate analysis (stage I and II cancers)
Kanellos [167]	2006	95	CYT and CEA		26%	Presence of CYT+ cells and high peritoneal CEA level predicts recurrence but not OS
Gozalan [168]	2007	88	CYT		15%	Presence of CYT + cells did not predict locoregional or systemic recurrence and does not provide prognostic information
Hara [169]	2007	128	qRT-PCR	CEA, CK20	23%	Presence of PCR + cells is not an independent prognostic factor in multivariate analysis and does not predict peritoneal recurrence

(Continued)

Table 8.2 (*Continued*) Incidence and prognostic significance of peritoneal free cancer cells in colorectal cancer

Author	Year	N	Method	Markers or antibodies	Detection rate	Comments or conclusion
Kristensen [170]	2008	237	PCR for k-RAS mutation		8%	Mutated k-RAS in peritoneal lavage samples following rectal cancer resection. Is associated with worse OS
Noura [171]	2009	697	CYT		2.2%	Positive CYT is an independent prognosticator of cancer-specific survival and peritoneal recurrence
Fujii [172]	2009	298	CYT		6%	CYT status before resection does not affect survival or peritoneal recurrence

Notes: CYT, cytology; ICC, immunocytochemistry; RT-PCR, reverse transcriptase polymerase chain reaction; OS, overall survival; DFS, disease-free survival.
[a] Includes 17 stomach cancer and 9 pancreas cancer cases.
[b] In a subset of 36 patients.

cancer cells may be present at the site of the anastomosis at the time of surgery [57]. Moreover, the additional local and systemic inflammation associated with an anastomotic leak could affect the growth of residual cancer cells that otherwise would not have survived or proliferated [61–63].

Entrapment of malignant cells by exudated fibrin(ogen) has been proposed as a mechanism of tumor growth on surgical wounds including peritonectomized surfaces [64]. Indirect evidence supporting this hypothesis is the demonstrated ability of fibrin and fibrin matrices to bind to a variety of normal and cancer cell types via cell surface integrin and nonintegrin (VE-cadherin, intercellular adhesion molecule (ICAM) 1, P-selectin) receptors [65]. Moreover, other plasma proteins present in wound surface exudate such as fibronectin and vitronectin may act as bridging molecules between endothelial cells, smooth muscle cells, and cancer cells via the $\alpha_5\beta_1$ and $\alpha_v\beta_3$ receptors [66].

LINK BETWEEN PERITONEAL TUMOR GROWTH AND SURGERY

Removal of a primary cancer by surgery, radiotherapy, or other means can enhance the growth of residual tumor by two general mechanisms. First, the inflammatory process associated with a (surgical) wound enhances tumor growth. Second, the primary cancer produces a number of antiangiogenic and antiproliferative stimuli that keep secondary cancer foci in a state of dormancy; removal of the primary cancer will therefore reactivate growth and invasiveness.

Importance of inflammation induced by wound healing

Hundreds of molecules and their signaling pathways are implicated in tumor growth, invasion, and metastasis, regulating the activities of the cancer cells and their communication with the tumor-promoting host cells. Many of these host cells and molecules are found also in healing wounds. Since the histological observation of Rudolf Virchow in the nineteenth century of leukocytes within a tumor, the link

between inflammation and cancer has been firmly established. Tumors have been denoted as "wounds that do not heal" by Harold Dvorak in 1986 [67]. Inflammatory processes, acute and chronic, may play a pivotal role in tumor initiation, transformation, invasion, and metastasis [68]. Surgical tissue trauma is rapidly followed by a complex cascade of inflammatory signaling and activation of epithelial, endothelial, and inflammatory cells, platelets, and fibroblasts. The process of wound healing following tissue injury is traditionally divided into three overlapping stages. The first inflammatory stage is initiated immediately after wounding by blood coagulation and activation of platelets, which release growth and chemotactic factors such as platelet-derived growth factor (PDGF), insulin-like growth factor I (IGF I), epidermal growth factor (EGF), and transforming growth factor-β (TGF-β). In response to chemotactic factors, lymphocytes and polymorphonuclear leukocytes (PMN) enter the wound within hours, followed by monocytes that subsequently mature into wound macrophages. This is followed from day 3 to 4 onward by a proliferation stage, characterized by fibroblast proliferation, ECM remodeling, angiogenesis, and simultaneous phagocytosis of debris by macrophages. Proliferation of epidermal cells and formation of granulation tissue are followed by scar formation mediated by keratinocytes and fibroblasts. Recent research has identified several populations of epidermal stem cells that are activated during wound healing and participate in tissue repair [69,70]. Many of the growth factors, chemokines, and cytokines released in the wound healing process may promote tumor progression locally or at a distance (Table 8.3).

In preclinical models, IP tumor growth has been shown to be related to the presence and extent of peritoneal trauma [71,72]. Also, growth of intraperitoneally administered colon carcinoma cells was enhanced when they were injected together with lavage fluid from intra-abdominally traumatized animals [72]. The importance of timing of peritoneal wounding versus tumor injection was illustrated by a paper of Zeamari et al., who found that tumor growth in an artificially induced peritoneal wound was

Table 8.3 Similarities between wound healing and tumor growth

	Role in wound healing	Effects on tumor growth	References
Growth factors			
EGF family (EGF, TGF-α, HB-EGF, epiregulin, amphiregulin, neuregulin)	Reepithelialization; angiogenesis	Invasion and proliferation	[173,174]
FGF family (FGF-2, FGF-7, FGF-10)	Granulation tissue formation, tissue remodeling	Proliferation, differentiation, angiogenesis	[175,176]
TGF-β family (TGF-β1-3, BMP, activins)	Reepithelialization, angiogenesis, stimulates collagen production	EMT, carcinogenesis, invasion, metastasis	[177–179]
PDGF	Mitogenicity and chemotaxis of inflammatory cells, vessel maturation, reepithelialization	Autocrine stimulation of tumor and stroma angiogenesis	[180,181]
VEGF	Angiogenesis, lymphangiogenesis	Invasion, angiogenesis	[182,183]
IGF I and II	Angiogenesis, EC chemotaxis reepithelialization	Tumorigenesis, metastasis	[184,185]
CTGF	Cellular/ECM cross talk	Promotes cancer cell invasion and migration	[186,187]
HGF (SF)	Liver regeneration	Tumorigenesis, invasion, angiogenesis	[188,189]
Cytokines			
IL-1α, IL-1β	Fibroblast and neutrophil recruitment, reepithelialization	Proliferation, angiogenesis	[190,191]
IL-6	Fibroblast and neutrophil recruitment	Tumorigenesis, invasion, metastasis	[192,193]
TNF-α	Leukocyte infiltration	Proliferation, invasion, angiogenesis	[194,195]
Chemokines			
M-CSF (CSF-1)	Macrophage recruitment	Invasion, migration	[196,197]
GM-CSF	Neutrophil recruitment, keratinocyte proliferation	Proliferation, differentiation	[198,199]
MCP-1 (CCL2)	Recruitment of monocytes and T cells	Cancer growth and invasion	[200,201]
IL-8 (CXCL8)	Neutrophil recruitment; reepithelialization	Angiogenesis, proliferation, migration	[202,203]
GRO-α (CXCL1)	Neutrophil recruitment, keratinocyte proliferation	Invasion, tumorigenicity	[204,205]
SDF-1 (CXCL12)	Angiogenesis, lymphocyte recruitment	Angiogenesis, metastasis	[206,207]
GRO-β (CXCL2, MIP2α)	Epithelial proliferation	Recruitment of tumor-promoting leukocytes	[208,209]

Notes: EGF, epidermal growth factor; TGF, transforming growth factor; BMP, bone morphogenetic proteins; PDGF, platelet-derived growth factor; VEGF, vascular endothelial growth factor; IGF, insulin-like growth factor; EC, endothelial cells; CTGF, connective tissue growth factor; HGF, hepatocyte growth factor; SF, scatter factor; IL, interleukin; TNF, tumor necrosis factor; M-CSF, macrophage colony-stimulating factor; GM-CSF, granulocyte monocyte colony-stimulating factor; MCP, macrophage chemoattractant protein; IP, interferon-inducible protein; GRO, growth-related oncogene; SDF, stromal cell–derived factor; MIP, macrophage inflammatory protein.

much less pronounced when cells were injected 10 days after the wounding versus injection after 8 hours to 3 days [73]. Adhesion of tumor cells to the peritoneum has been linked to inflammatory mediators such as IL-1 beta, IL-6, tumor necrosis factor-α (TNF-α), and EGF [74,75]. Interestingly, use of an inhibitory monoclonal antibody against ICAM-1 attenuated the enhanced mesothelial adhesion mediated by IL-6 or TNF-α in an in vitro model [74]. Taken together, these findings illustrate the long-established link between wound healing–associated inflammation and cancer [76].

One of the chief inflammation effectors present in the healing wound are the *macrophages*. Traditionally, infiltration of tumor by leukocytes has been associated with a better outcome. Macrophages, however, produce an array of mediators that have been shown to potentially and in certain circumstances enhance tumor growth. Whether macrophages have a stimulatory or inhibitory effect on tumor growth clearly depends on the tumor microenvironment and the stroma involved. It has been suggested that macrophages present in the tumor nodules (tumor-associated macrophages [TAM]) are associated with a better survival, whereas macrophages present in the (submesothelial) stroma appear to enhance tumor progression [77]. Recently, stromal *fibroblasts* have been shown to enhance tumor growth by their production of growth factors, chemokines, and ECM facilitating the angiogenic recruitment of endothelial cells and pericytes. A subpopulation of myofibroblasts has been identified that secrete elevated levels of stromal cell–derived factor 1 (SDF-1), also called CXCL12, which plays a central role in the promotion of tumor growth and angiogenis [78–80].

Surgery and tumor dormancy

A second mechanism that can enhance residual tumor growth following surgical removal of a primary cancer is related to the concept of tumor dormancy [81]. It is known that many of the tumor cells that reach the peritoneal surfaces or the systemic circulation and invade distant organs will never develop into a clinical metastasis. This phenomenon is termed "metastatic inefficiency" and results from tumor dormancy characterized by prolonged survival without DNA replication (G0 arrest; Ki67 negative) [82]. As a result, these cells are resistant to therapy with cytotoxic drugs. Tumor dormancy is the result of a balance between proliferation and apoptosis [83]. Recent data indicate that primary tumors induce apoptosis in micrometastatic foci by the production of antiangiogenic agents such as thrombospondin-1, endostatin, and angiostatin [84–88]. Guba et al. showed in a mouse colon carcinoma model that the presence of a primary tumor significantly inhibited the development of liver metastasis by interfering with angiogenesis [89]. Conversely, removal of the primary tumor by surgery or irradiation resulted in activation and growth of dormant residual cancer by turning on the "angiogenic switch" in animal models [90,91]. Clinically, activation of dormant metastatic deposits was proposed as

the underlying mechanism to explain the existence of an early (after 18 months) peak in relapse frequency in breast cancer patients treated with surgery only [92].

A key step in the establishment of metastatic disease is the homing of disseminated tumor cells in the target tissue. As already clinically noted by Stephen Paget in the nineteenth century, metastatic growth can only be supported in the presence of a favorable microenvironment [93]. It has now been established that this microenvironment is "primed" by the primary tumor as a premetastatic niche before the actual arrival of the disseminated tumor cells [94]. Several growth factors and chemokines produced by the primary tumor are implicated in the formation of the premetastatic niche by the recruitment of bone marrow–derived cells (BMDCs) and by remodeling of the ECM [95]. Kaplan and coworkers demonstrated that VEGF-A and PlGF from the primary tumor recruit VEGFR1+ BMDCs to the premetastatic niche [96]. Other secreted factors shown to mediate BMDC recruitment to the premetastatic niche include osteopontin and tissue factor [97,98].

PREVENTION AND TREATMENT OF PERITONEAL TUMOR GROWTH

Reduction of surgical trauma

Surgical trauma may be prevented by physical measures such as the use of atraumatic gauze or nonpowdered gloves [72,99]. Compared to open surgery, the use of laparoscopic techniques minimizes peritoneal trauma and reduced tumor growth compared to open surgery in several animal models, a finding usually attributed to a difference in postoperative immune competence [100–102]. Sylla et al. studied splenic T cell gene expression following laparotomy versus CO_2 pneumoperitoneum in a mouse model and found that 177 genes were increased and 15 decreased at least twofold after laparotomy relative to pneumoperitoneum [103].

Peritoneal irrigation

Exfoliated cancer cells may be eradicated by irrigation of the peritoneal cavity, either mechanically or by using a tumoricidal solution. There is some evidence from preclinical studies that instillation of povidone–iodine (PVD) is beneficial [104]. Basha et al. showed that instillation of PVD was effective in preventing tumor take in a rat model when a limited tumor inoculum was used [105]. In an animal model of laparoscopy-assisted tumor splenectomy, abdominal irrigation with dilute PVD significantly reduced the number of animals with peritoneal implant metastases [106]. Many of the commonly used antiseptics, however, are known to be inactivated by the presence of blood [107]. Huguet et al. used distilled water to achieve osmotic lysis of cancer cells [108]. Complete lysis in vivo took significantly longer (more than 30 minutes) compared to in vitro instillation. Clinical studies using these approaches have not been reported, and potential toxicity of IP PVD should be kept in mind [109].

Intraperitoneal chemotherapy

The concept of IP chemotherapy was first proposed almost half a century ago [110]. It is based on spatial proximity on the one hand, administering active therapy at the location of the target tissue, and on the presence of the peritoneal–plasma barrier. The latter allows administering much higher drug doses IP with resulting increased cytotoxicity while limiting systemic side effects. In animal models of CRC, IP administration of chemotherapy successfully prevented tumor development following IP injection of cancer cells [111]. Several authors have studied adjuvant IP chemotherapy following surgery in an effort to reduce the risk of peritoneal recurrence. A small clinical study was reported by Sugarbaker and coworkers, who assigned 66 patients to receive either intravenous (IV) or IP 5-FU [112]. Although no difference in disease-free (DFS) or overall survival (OS) was noted, the risk of peritoneal recurrence was significantly lower in patients who underwent IP therapy (91% vs. 20%, P < 0.0001). Similar results were obtained by Scheithauer et al., who randomized 241 patients with resected stage III or T4N0M0 CRC to either IV 5-FU and levamisole or combined IV and IP 5-FU and leucovorin [113]. A significant improvement in DFS and OS was noted in stage III, but not in stage II patients. Compared with the IV alone group, patients who received combined IV and IP adjuvant therapy had a significantly lower risk of locoregional recurrence (21% vs. 7.6%, P = 0.005). Two other trials were unable to demonstrate any benefit associated with adjuvant IP chemotherapy in CRC. Vaillant and coworkers randomly allocated 267 stage II and III CRC patients to either surgery alone or surgery combined with intraoperative IV 5-FU and early postoperative IP 5-FU during 6 days [114]. Overall, the experimental therapy failed to improve DFS, OS, or the risk of peritoneal recurrence. An unplanned subgroup analysis of the data indicated a DFS benefit in patients with stage II disease. Similarly, the randomized trial by Nordlinger et al. failed to show any survival benefit of immediate postoperative regional chemotherapy (IP or intraportal 5-FU according to the treatment center) followed by IV 5-FU–based chemotherapy compared with IV chemotherapy alone in patients with resected stage II or III CRC [115]. No data on locoregional recurrence were reported from this trial. Taken together, the results suggest an effect of adjuvant IP chemotherapy on the risk of locoregional recurrence after resection of CRC. Further randomized trials combining IP with modern IV regimens are warranted.

Hyperthermic intraperitoneal chemoperfusion

Since the clinicopathological risk factors for developing peritoneal recurrence from CRC are well established, an appealing strategy consists of administering hyperthermic intraperitoneal chemoperfusion (HIPEC) before peritoneal metastasis is apparent. The potential of "prophylactic" HIPEC during a planned second look after resection and adjuvant chemotherapy of high-risk CRC was explored by Elias et al [116,117]. Interestingly, they found that 56% of these patients turned out to have macroscopic, although asymptomatic, peritoneal recurrence. All patients underwent HIPEC, irrespective of the presence of PC, and only 2 out of 41 patients developed peritoneal-only recurrence, while the total incidence of PC (with or without systemic recurrence) was 17%. Sammartino and coworkers reported the results of "prophylactic" omentectomy, oophorectomy, and appendectomy followed by HIPEC in 25 cT3/4N0M0 patients with mucinous or signet ring cell differentiation [118]. They found that, compared to a group of patients who underwent standard resection, the "prophylactic" approach resulted in a significantly lower risk of developing PC (4% vs. 22%, P < 0.05) and a significant gain in median DFS (36.8 vs. 21.9 months, P < 0.01), although OS was similar.

Based on these results, a multicenter prospective randomized trial (ProphyloChip, ClinicalTrials.gov ID: NCT01226394) is now active in France that compares regular follow-up with planned second look and HIPEC in patients at high risk of peritoneal recurrence (i.e., perforated tumors, minimal PC resected at the time of primary surgery, and ovarian [Krukenberg] metastases). A similar prospective randomized trial, comparing standard follow-up with mandatory second look and HIPEC 1 year after curative surgery of high risk CRC, was announced by the National Cancer Institute (ClinicalTrials.gov ID: NCT01095523) [119]. It seems, however, that this trial has been withdrawn. A prospective Italian randomized phase II trial started in April 2012 (ClinicalTrials.gov ID: NCT01628211) aims to compare standard follow-up with exploratory laparoscopy and debulking/HIPEC when PC is found in patients who underwent curative resection of a mucinous CRC.

Inhibition of the angiogenic switch and reversal of tumor dormancy

Since dormant cells are resistant to cytotoxic drugs, therapeutic efforts should be directed toward inhibiting angiogenesis and activation of dormant cancer populations possibly starting already before surgery. In preclinical models, maintenance drugs shown to suppress the metastatic phenotype include histone deacetylase inhibitors, NFκB inhibitors, MMP modifiers, or growth factor antagonists [120–123]. Coffey et al. showed that adjuvant administration of the phosphoinositide 3-kinase inhibitor LY294002 prolonged survival and significantly attenuated recurrent tumor growth in a murine model of cytoreduction of a flank tumor [124].

Inhibition of the postoperative inflammatory response

As discussed earlier, it has been realized that the mechanisms involved in postoperative wound healing may stimulate the growth of residual cancer cells [127–128]. One of the essential features of both wound healing and tumor growth is angiogenesis. Therefore, postoperative inhibition of angiogenesis may prevent the outgrowth of peritoneal residual cancer. Understandably, however, inhibition of VEGF in the postoperative setting carries the risk of anastomotic and wound healing complications [129]. Thus, in the National Surgical Adjuvant Breast and Bowel Project (NSABP) C-08 trial that compared adjuvant chemotherapy (FOLFOX6) with or without bevacizumab in stage II or III CRC, the proportion of wound complications (incisional hernia, wound dehiscence, and port site dehiscence) was significantly higher in patients who received bevacizumab (1.7% vs. 0.3%, P < 0.01) [130]. Alternatively, one may avoid or suppress the inflammatory response after surgery. In a mouse model, Roh et al. found that the selective cyclo-oxygenase-2 (Cox-2) inhibitor celecoxib had a significant inhibitory effect on tumor growth in the surgical wound when administered daily from 1 day before surgical wounding and tumor implantation [125,126]. Also, restoration of surgery-induced immunosuppression may prevent postoperative locoregional cancer growth [2,131]. Small clinical trials in CRC patients have shown that perioperative systemic administration using IL-2, GM-CSF, or interferon restores postoperative immune function [132–134]. However, their effect on postoperative recurrence or survival is not known. In line with the observed effects of bacterial LPS on tumor apoptosis, anti-LPS therapy using taurolidine abrogated the effects of surgical trauma on primary and metastatic tumor growth in a mouse melanoma model [135]. In CRC patients, preoperative administration of IL-2 significantly reduced postoperative VEGF production and at the same time inhibited the decline of the antiangiogenic cytokine IL-12 [133]. Helguera et al. studied the effects of cytokines fused to antibodies in mice receiving IP HER2/neu expressing tumors and found that combined administration of (1) anti-HER2/neu fused with IL-2 and (2) anti-HER2/neu fused with granulocyte macrophage colony-stimulating factor (GM-CSF) prevented tumor growth in 100% of animals [136]. In preclinical models, IP immunotherapy using cytokines, monoclonal antibodies, or radionuclide antibody conjugates has been successfully used to treat or prevent PC [137].

Inhibition of adhesion of free intraperitoneal cancer cells

Specific therapy targeting the various mechanisms of tumor–mesothelial interaction has been addressed in preclinical studies. One approach has been directed toward the binding sites of the ECM. Alkhamesi et al. showed that IP application of heparin caused a significant decrease in tumor cell adhesion accompanied by a decrease in ICAM-1 expression [138]. Expression of ICAM-1 is also blocked in vitro by the grape polyphenol, resveratrol [139]. Similarly, low-molecular-weight heparin significantly reduced tumor growth following laparoscopy in a rat CRC model [140]. Heparins also inhibit tumor-induced production of thrombin, fibrin, and tissue factor, all of which have been implicated in primary and metastatic tumor growth and block P- and L-selectin–mediated cell adhesion [141,142]. Alternatively, covering the ECM binding sites with a phospholipid emulsion reduced tumor–mesothelial cell adhesion in animal models [143]. Targeting of specific adhesion molecules such as integrins [144–146], L1 cell adhesion molecule [147], and JAM-C [148] with monoclonal antibodies has shown to be effective in preventing tumor adhesion and/or growth in preclinical models and may represent a future clinical therapeutic tool.

SUMMARY AND CONCLUSIONS

The presence or persistence of peritoneal cancer cells is associated with the histology and stage of the primary CRC, the completeness and quality of surgery, and postoperative events such as anastomotic leakage or entrapment of cells in exudating wound surfaces. At present, there is no clinical evidence that the use of laparoscopic techniques adversely influences the risk of peritoneal recurrence. The inflammatory process associated with surgery shares a number of central mediators and pathways with tumor growth and invasiveness. Both cellular components (mainly macrophages and fibroblasts) and humoral factors associated with inflammation have been shown to enhance tumor growth in numerous preclinical studies. Tumor foci at a distance from the main cancer are kept in a dormant state by a range of antiangiogenic mediators produced by the main cancer. Preclinical studies have shown that removal of the primary cancer reactivates proliferative and metastatic pathways in the residual tumor. Strategies proposed to prevent the presence or outgrowth of peritoneal MRD encompass avoidance of tumor spill and minimization of surgical trauma and related inflammation. Efforts to remove or kill free IP cells by local antiseptic or cytotoxic regimens have met only limited clinical success. Specific targeted therapy aimed at inhibiting the inflammatory response, tumor cell adhesion, or the metastatic phenotype of dormant cells appears promising in preclinical models and needs to be addressed in future clinical trials.

REFERENCES

1. Ceelen W, Pattyn P, Mareel M. Surgery, wound healing, and metastasis: Recent insights and clinical implications. *Critical Reviews in Oncology/Hematology.* 2014;89(1):16–26.
2. Coffey JC, Wang JH, Smith MJF, Bouchier-Hayes D, Cotter TG, Redmond HP. Excisional surgery for cancer cure: Therapy at a cost. *Lancet Oncology.* 2003;4(12):760–768.
3. Koppe MJ, Boerman OC, Oyen WJG, Bleichrodt RP. Peritoneal carcinomatosis of colorectal origin—Incidence and current treatment strategies. *Annals of Surgery.* 2006;243(2):212–222.
4. Segelman J, Granath F, Holm T, Machado M, Mahteme H, Martling A. Incidence, prevalence and risk factors for peritoneal carcinomatosis from colorectal cancer. *British Journal of Surgery.* 2012;99(5):699–705.

5. Lemmens VE, Klaver YL, Verwaal VJ, Rutten HJ, Coebergh JWW, de Hingh IH. Predictors and survival of synchronous peritoneal carcinomatosis of colorectal origin: A population-based study. *International Journal of Cancer*. 2011;128(11):2717–2725.

6. Tran B, Kopetz S, Tie J, Gibbs P, Jiang ZQ, Lieu CH, Agarwal A, Maru DM, Sieber O, Desai J. Impact of BRAF mutation and microsatellite instability on the pattern of metastatic spread and prognosis in metastatic colorectal cancer. *Cancer*. 2011;117(20):4623–4632.

7. Kleivi K, Lind GE, Diep CB, Meling GI, Brandal LT, Nesland JM, Myklebost O et al. Gene expression profiles of primary colorectal carcinomas, liver metastases, and carcinomatoses. *Molecular Cancer*. 2007;6:2.

8. Varghese S, Burness M, Xu H, Beresnev T, Pingpank J, Alexander HR. Site-specific gene expression profiles and novel molecular prognostic factors in patients with lower gastrointestinal adenocarcinoma diffusely metastatic to liver or peritoneum. *Annals of Surgical Oncology*. 2007;14:3460–3471.

9. Debergh I, Van Damme N, Peeters M, Van Hummelen P, Pattyn P, Ceelen W. Differential gene expression between metastatic colorectal tumours in liver and peritoneum. *British Journal of Surgery*. 2008;95(S6):13.

10. Lennon AM, Mulcahy HE, Hyland JMP, Lowry C, White A, Fennelly D, Murphy JJ, O'Donoghue DP, Sheahan K. Peritoneal involvement in stage II colon cancer. *American Journal of Clinical Pathology*. 2003;119(1):108–113.

11. Shepherd NA, Baxter KJ, Love SB. The prognostic importance of peritoneal involvement in colonic cancer: A prospective evaluation. *Gastroenterology*. 1997;112(4):1096–1102.

12. Ludeman L, Shepherd NA. Serosal involvement in gastrointestinal cancer: Its assessment and significance. *Histopathology*. 2005;47(2):123–131.

13. McArdle CS, McMillan DC, Hole DJ. The impact of blood loss, obstruction and perforation on survival in patients undergoing curative resection for colon cancer. *British Journal of Surgery*. 2006;93(4):483–488.

14. Komatsu S, Shimomatsuya T, Nakajima M, Amaya H, Kobuchi T, Shiraishi S, Konishi S, Ono S, Maruhashi K. Prognostic factors and scoring system for survival in colonic perforation. *Hepatogastroenterology*. 2005;52(63):761–764.

15. Chen HS, Sheen-Chen SM. Obstruction and perforation in colorectal adenocarcinoma: An analysis of prognosis and current trends. *Surgery*. 2000;127(4):370–376.

16. Cheynel N, Cortet M, Lepage C, Ortega-Debalon P, Faivre J, Bouvier AM. Incidence, patterns of failure, and prognosis of perforated colorectal cancers in a well-defined population. *Diseases of the Colon & Rectum*. 2009;52(3):406–411.

17. Terauchi M, Kajiyama H, Yamashita M, Kato M, Tsukamoto H, Umezu T, Hosono S et al. Possible involvement of TWIST in enhanced peritoneal metastasis of epithelial ovarian carcinoma. *Clinical & Experimental Metastasis*. 2007;24(5):329–339.

18. Kokenyesi R, Murray KP, Benshushan A, Huntley ED, Kao MS. Invasion of interstitial matrix by a novel cell line from primary peritoneal carcinosarcoma, and by established ovarian carcinoma cell lines: Role of cell-matrix adhesion molecules, proteinases, and E-cadherin expression. *Gynecologic Oncology*. 2003;89(1):60–72.

19. Hayashi K, Jiang P, Yamauchi K, Yamamoto N, Tsuchiya H, Tomita K, Moossa AR, Bouvet M, Hoffman RM. Real-time Imaging of tumor-cell shedding and trafficking in lymphatic channels. *Cancer Research*. 2007;67(17):8223–8228.

20. Rutz HP. Hydrodynamic consequences of glycolysis—Thermodynamic basis and clinical relevance. *Cancer Biology & Therapy*. 2004;3(9):812–815.

21. Heldin CH, Rubin K, Pietras K, Ostman A. High interstitial fluid pressure—An obstacle in cancer therapy. *Nature Reviews Cancer*. 2004;4(10):806–813.

22. Patel H, Le Marer N, Wharton RQ, Khan ZAJ, Araia R, Glover C, Henry MM, Allen-Marsh TG. Clearance of circulating tumor cells after excision of primary colorectal cancer. *Annals of Surgery*. 2002;235(2):226–231.

23. Tanida O, Kaneshima S, Iitsuka Y, Kuda H, Kiyasu Y, Koga S. Viability of intraperitoneal free cancer-cells in patients with gastric-cancer. *Acta Cytologica*. 1982;26(5):681–687.

24. Kodera Y, Yamamura Y, Shimizu Y, Torii A, Hirai T, Yasui K, Morimoto T, Kato T. Peritoneal washing cytology: Prognostic value of positive findings in patients with gastric carcinoma undergoing a potentially curative resection. *Journal of Surgical Oncology*. 1999;72(2):60–64.

25. Meyers MA. Distribution of intraabdominal malignant seeding—Dependency on dynamics of flow of ascitic fluid. *American Journal of Roentgenology*. 1973;119(1):198–206.

26. Oosterling SJ, van der Bij GJ, Bogels M, van der Sijp JRM, Beelen RHJ, Meijer S, van Egmond M. Insufficient ability of omental milky spots to prevent peritoneal tumor outgrowth supports omentectomy in minimal residual disease. *Cancer Immunology, Immunotherapy*. 2006;55(9):1043–1051.

27. Koppe MJ, Nagtegaal ID, de Wilt JH, Ceelen WP. Recent insights into the pathophysiology of omental metastases. *Journal of Surgical Oncology*. 2014.

28. Adam IJ, Mohamdee MO, Martin IG, Scott N, Finan PJ, Johnston D, Dixon MF, Quirke P. Role of circumferential margin involvement in the local recurrence of rectal cancer. *Lancet* 1994;344(8924):707–711.

29. Nagtegaal ID, Marijnen CA, Kranenbarg EK, van de Velde CJ, van Krieken JH, Pathology Review C, Cooperative clinical I. Circumferential margin involvement is still an important predictor of local recurrence in rectal carcinoma: Not one millimeter but two millimeters is the limit. *The American Journal of Surgical Pathology.* 2002;26(3):350–357.

30. Hansen E, Wolff N, Knuechel R, Ruschoff J, Hofstaedter F, Taeger K. Tumor-cells in blood shed from the surgical field. *Archives of Surgery.* 1995;130(4):387–393.

31. Savalgi RS. Port-site metastasis in the abdominal wall: Fact or fiction? *Seminars in Surgical Oncology.* 1998;15(3):189–193.

32. Ouellette JR, Ko AS, Lefor AT. The physiologic effects of laparoscopy: Applications in oncology. *Cancer Journal.* 2005;11(1):2–9.

33. Hewett PJ, Thomas WM, King G, Eaton M. Intraperitoneal cell movement during abdominal carbon dioxide insufflation and laparoscopy—An in vivo model. *Diseases of the Colon & Rectum.* 1996;39(10):S62–S66.

34. Reymond MA, Wittekind C, Jung A, Hohenberger W, Kirchner T, Kockerling F. The incidence of port-site metastases might be reduced. *Surgical Endoscopy—Ultrasound and Interventional Techniques.* 1997;11(9):902–906.

35. Mathew G, Watson DI, Ellis T, DeYoung N, Rofe AM, Jamieson GG. The effect of laparoscopy on the movement of tumor cells and metastasis to surgical wounds. *Surgical Endoscopy—Ultrasound and Interventional Techniques.* 1997;11(12):1163–1166.

36. Champault G, Catheline JM, Taffinder N, Ziol M. Laparoscopic surgery: Can smoke particles carry cells? *Annales de Chirurgie.* 1997;51(2):140–143.

37. Champault G, Taffinder N, Ziol M, Riskalla H, Catheline JMC. Cells are present in the smoke created during laparoscopic surgery. *British Journal of Surgery.* 1997;84(7):993–995.

38. Tseng LNL, Berends FJ, Wittich P, Bouvy ND, Marquet RL, Kazemier G, Bonjer HJ. Port-site metastases—Impact of local tissue trauma and gas leakage. *Surgical Endoscopy—Ultrasound and Interventional Techniques.* 1998;12(12):1377–1380.

39. Ikramuddin S, Ellison EC, Schirmer WJ, Lucas J, Melvin WS. The detection of aerosolized cells during laparoscopy. *Gastroenterology.* 1997;112(4):A1450.

40. Wittich P, Marquet RL, Kazemier G, Bonjer HJ. Port-site metastases after CO2 laparoscopy—Is aerosolization of tumor cells a pivotal factor? *Surgical Endoscopy—Ultrasound and Interventional Techniques.* 2000;14(2):189–192.

41. Jacobi CA, Wenger FA, Ordemann J, Gutt C, Sabat R, Muller JM. Experimental study of the effect of intra-abdominal pressure during laparoscopy on tumour growth and port site metastasis. *British Journal of Surgery.* 1998;85(10):1419–1422.

42. Gutt CN, Kim ZG, Hollander D, Bruttel T, Lorenz M. CO_2 environment influences the growth of cultured human cancer cells dependent on insufflation pressure. *Surgical Endoscopy—Ultrasound and Interventional Techniques.* 2001;15(3):314–318.

43. Wittich P, Steyerberg EW, Simons SHP, Marquet RL, Bonjer HJ. Intraperitoneal tumor growth is influenced by pressure of carbon dioxide pneumoperitoneum. *Surgical Endoscopy—Ultrasound and Interventional Techniques.* 2000;14(9):817–819.

44. Paraskeva PA, Ridgway PF, Jones T, Smith A, Peck DH, Darzi AW. Laparoscopic environmental changes during surgery enhance the invasive potential of tumours. *Tumor Biology.* 2005;26(2):94–102.

45. Basson MD, Yu CF, Herden-Kirchoff O, Ellermeier M, Sanders MA, Merrell RC, Sumpio BE. Effects of increased ambient pressure on colon cancer cell adhesion. *Journal of Cellular Biochemistry.* 2000;78(1):47–61.

46. Thamilselvan V, Basson MD. Pressure activates colon cancer cell adhesion by inside-out focal adhesion complex and actin cytoskeletal signaling. *Gastroenterology.* 2004;126(1):8–18.

47. Thamilselvan V, Basson MD. The role of the cytoskeleton in differentially regulating pressure-mediated effects on malignant colonocyte focal adhesion signaling and cell adhesion. *Carcinogenesis.* 2005;26(10):1687–1697.

48. Volz J, Koster S, Spacek Z, Paweletz N. The influence of pneumoperitoneum used in laparoscopic surgery on an intraabdominal tumor growth. *Cancer.* 1999;86(5):770–774.

49. Rosario MTA, Ribeiro U, Corbett CEP, Ozaki AC, Bresciani CC, Zilberstein B, Gama-Rodrigues JJ. Does CO_2 pneumoperitoneum alter the ultrastructure of the mesothelium? *Journal of Surgical Research.* 2006;133(2):84–88.

50. Volz J, Koster S, Spacek Z, Paweletz N. Characteristic alterations of the peritoneum after carbon dioxide pneumoperitoneum. *Surgical Endoscopy—Ultrasound and Interventional Techniques.* 1999;13(6):611–614.

51. Ridgway PF, Smith A, Ziprin P, Jones TL, Paraskeva PA, Peck DH, Darzi AW. Pneumoperitoneum augmented tumor invasiveness is abolished by matrix metalloproteinase blockade. *Surgical Endoscopy—Ultrasound and Interventional Techniques.* 2002;16(3):533–536.

52. Jacobi CA, Sabat R, Bohm B, Zieren HU, Volk HD, Muller JM. Pneumoperitoneum with carbon dioxide stimulates growth of malignant colonic cells. *Surgery.* 1997;121(1):72–78.

53. Lacy AM, Garcia-Valdecasas JC, Delgado S, Castells A, Taura P, Pique JM, Visa J. Laparoscopy-assisted colectomy versus open colectomy for treatment of non-metastatic colon cancer: A randomised trial. *The Lancet.* 2002;359(9325):2224–2229.

54. Nelson H, Sargent D, Wieand HS, Fleshman J, Anvari M, Stryker SJ, Beart RW et al. A comparison of laparoscopically assisted and open colectomy for colon cancer. *The New England Journal of Medicine*. 2004;350(20):2050–2059.

55. Ceelen WP, Bracke ME. Peritoneal minimal residual disease in colorectal cancer: Mechanisms, prevention, and treatment. *Lancet Oncology*. 2009;10(1):72–79.

56. Rekhraj S, Aziz O, Prabhudesai S, Zacharakis E, Mohr F, Athanasiou T, Darzi A, Ziprin P. Can intra-operative intraperitoneal free cancer cell detection techniques identify patients at higher recurrence risk following curative colorectal cancer resection: A meta-analysis. *Annals of Surgical Oncology*. 2008;15(1):60–68.

57. Fermor B, Umpleby HC, Lever JV, Symes MO, Williamson RCN. Proliferative and metastatic potential of exfoliated colorectal-cancer cells. *Journal of the National Cancer Institute*. 1986;76(2):347–349.

58. Skipper D, Cooper AJ, Marston JE, Taylor I. Exfoliated cells and invitro growth in colorectal-cancer. *British Journal of Surgery*. 1987;74(11):1049–1052.

59. Artinyan A, Orcutt ST, Anaya DA, Richardson P, Chen GJ, Berger DH. Infectious postoperative complications decrease long-term survival in patients undergoing curative surgery for colorectal cancer: A study of 12,075 patients. *Annals of Surgery*. 2015;261(3):497–505.

60. Krarup PM, Nordholm-Carstensen A, Jorgensen LN, Harling H. Anastomotic leak increases distant recurrence and long-term mortality after curative resection for colonic cancer: A nationwide cohort study. *Annals of Surgery*. 2014;259(5):930–938.

61. Balkwill F, Mantovani A. Inflammation and cancer: Back to virchow? *Lancet*. 2001;357(9255):539–545.

62. Abramovitch R, Marikovsky M, Meir G, Neeman M. Stimulation of tumour growth by wound-derived growth factors. *British Journal of Cancer*. 1999;79(9–10):1392–1398.

63. Hilmy M, Bartlett JMS, Underwood MA, McMillan DC. The relationship between the systemic inflammatory response and survival in patients with transitional cell carcinoma of the urinary bladder. *British Journal of Cancer*. 2005;92(4):625–627.

64. Ceelen WP, Morris S, Paraskeva P, Pattyn P. Surgical trauma, minimal residual disease and locoregional cancer recurrence. *Cancer Treatment and Research*. 2007;134:51–69.

65. Laurens N, Koolwijk P, De Maat MPM. Fibrin structure and wound healing. *Journal of Thrombosis and Haemostasis*. 2006;4(5):932–939.

66. Ikari Y, Yee KO, Schwartz SM. Role of alpha 5 beta 1 and alpha v beta 3 integrins on smooth muscle cell spreading and migration in fibrin gels. *Thrombosis and Haemostasis*. 2000;84(4):701–705.

67. Dvorak HF. Tumors: Wounds that do not heal. Similarities between tumor stroma generation and wound healing. *The New England Journal of Medicine*. 1986;315(26):1650–1659.

68. Grivennikov SI, Greten FR, Karin M. Immunity, inflammation, and cancer. *Cell*. 2010;140(6):883–899.

69. Taylor G, Lehrer MS, Jensen PJ, Sun TT, Lavker RM. Involvement of follicular stem cells in forming not only the follicle but also the epidermis. *Cell*. 2000;102(4):451–461.

70. Levy V, Lindon C, Zheng Y, Harfe BD, Morgan BA. Epidermal stem cells arise from the hair follicle after wounding. *The FASEB Journal*. 2007;21(7):1358–1366.

71. Eggermont AMM, Steller EP, Sugarbaker PH. Laparotomy enhances intraperitoneal tumor-growth and abrogates the antitumor effects of interleukin-2 and lymphokine-activated killer-cells. *Surgery*. 1987;102(1):71–78.

72. van den Tol RM, van Rossen EME, van Eijck CHJ, Bonthuis F, Marquet RL, Jeekel H. Reduction of peritoneal trauma by using nonsurgical gauze leads to less implantation metastasis of spilled tumor cells. *Annals of Surgery*. 1998;227(2):242–248.

73. Zeamari S, Roos E, Stewart FA. Tumour seeding in peritoneal wound sites in relation to growth-factor expression in early granulation tissue. *European Journal of Cancer*. 2004;40(9):1431–1440.

74. Ziprin P, Ridgway PF, Pfistermuller KLM, Peck DH, Darzi AW. ICAM-1 mediated tumor-mesothelial cell adhesion is modulated by IL-6 and TNF-alpha: A potential mechanism by which surgical trauma increases peritoneal metastases. *Cell Communication and Adhesion*. 2003;10(3):141–154.

75. van Rossen MEE, Hofland LJ, van den Tol MP, van Koetsveld PM, Jeekel J, Marquet RL, van Eijck CHJ. Effect of inflammatory cytokines and growth factors on tumour cell adhesion to the peritoneum. *The Journal of Pathology*. 2001;193(4):530–537.

76. Rowley DR. What might a stromal response mean to prostate cancer progression ? *Cancer and Metastasis Reviews*. 1998;17(4):411–419.

77. Dalgleish AG, O'Byrne K. Inflammation and cancer: The role of the immune response and angiogenesis. In: *The Link Between Inflammation and Cancer. Wounds that do not heal*, New York: Springer, 2006. p. 11.

78. Bhowmick NA, Neilson EG, Moses HL. Stromal fibroblasts in cancer initiation and progression. *Nature*. 2004;432(7015):332–337.

79. Orimo A, Gupta PB, Sgroi DC, Arenzana-Seisdedos F, Delaunay T, Naeem R, Carey VJ, Richardson AL, Weinberg RA. Stromal fibroblasts present in invasive human breast carcinomas promote tumor growth and angiogenesis through elevated SDF-1/CXCL12 secretion. *Cell*. 2005;121(3):335–348.

80. Kalluri R, Zeisberg M. Fibroblasts in cancer. *Nature Reviews Cancer.* 2006;6(5):392–401.

81. Demicheli R, Retsky MW, Hrushesky WJ, Baum M, Gukas ID. The effects of surgery on tumor growth: A century of investigations. *Annals of Oncology.* 2008;19(11):1821–1828.

82. Luzzi KJ, MacDonald IC, Schmidt EE, Kerkvliet N, Morris VL, Chambers AF, Groom AC. Multistep nature of metastatic inefficiency—Dormancy of solitary cells after successful extravasation and limited survival of early micrometastases. *The American Journal of Pathology.* 1998;153(3):865–873.

83. Wong CW, Lee A, Shientag L, Yu J, Dong Y, Kao G, Al-Mehdi AB, Bernhard EJ, Muschel RJ. Apoptosis: An early event in metastatic inefficiency. *Cancer Research.* 2001;61(1):333–338.

84. Oreilly MS, Holmgren L, Shing Y, Chen C, Rosenthal RA, Moses M, Lane WS, Cao YH, Sage EH, Folkman J. Angiostatin—A novel angiogenesis inhibitor that mediates the suppression of metastases by a Lewis lung-carcinoma. *Cell.* 1994;79(2):315–328.

85. Holmgren L, Oreilly MS, Folkman J. Dormancy of micrometastases—Balanced proliferation and apoptosis in the presence of angiogenesis suppression. *Nature Medicine.* 1995;1(2):149–153.

86. Cao Y, O'Reilly MS, Marshall B, Flynn E, Ji RW, Folkman J. Expression of angiostatin cDNA in a murine fibrosarcoma suppresses primary tumor growth and produces long-term dormancy of metastases (vol 101, pg 1055, 1998). *Journal of Clinical Investigation.* 1998;102(11):2031–2031.

87. Naumov GN, Bender E, Zurakowski D, Kang SY, Sampson D, Flynn E, Watnick RS et al. A model of human tumor dormancy: An angiogenic switch from the nonangiogenic phenotype. *Journal of the National Cancer Institute.* 2006;98(5):316–325.

88. Indraccolo S, Stievano L, Minuzzo S, Tosello V, Esposito G, Piovan E, Zamarchi R, Chieco-Bianchi L, Amadori A. Interruption of tumor dormancy by a transient angiogenic burst within the tumor microenvironment. *Proceedings of the National Academy of Sciences of the United States of America.* 2006;103(11):4216–4221.

89. Guba M, Cernaianu G, Koehl G, Geissler EK, Jauch KW, Anthuber M, Falk W, Steinbauer M. A primary tumor promotes dormancy of solitary tumor cells before inhibiting angiogenesis. *Cancer Research.* 2001;61(14):5575–5579.

90. Retsky M, Bonadonna G, Demicheli R, Folkman J, Hrushesky W, Valagussa P. Hypothesis: Induced angiogenesis after surgery in premenopausal node-positive breast cancer patients is a major underlying reason why adjuvant chemotherapy works particularly well for those patients. *Breast Cancer Research.* 2004;6(4):R372–R374.

91. Camphausen K, Moses MA, Beecken WD, Khan MK, Folkman J, O'Reilly MS. Radiation therapy to a primary tumor accelerates metastatic growth in mice. *Cancer Research.* 2001;61(5):2207–2211.

92. Baum M, Demicheli R, Hrushesky W, Retsky M. Does surgery unfavourably perturb the "natural history" of early breast cancer by accelerating the appearance of distant metastases? *European Journal of Cancer.* 2005;41(4):508–515.

93. Paget S. The distribution of secondary growths in cancer of the breast. *Lancet.* 1889;1:571–573.

94. Psaila B, Lyden D. The metastatic niche: Adapting the foreign soil. *Nature Reviews Cancer.* 2009;9(4):285–293.

95. Sleeman JP. The metastatic niche and stromal progression. *Cancer and Metastasis Reviews.* 2012;31(3–4):429–440.

96. Kaplan RN, Riba RD, Zacharoulis S, Bramley AH, Vincent L, Costa C, MacDonald DD et al. VEGFR1-positive haematopoietic bone marrow progenitors initiate the pre-metastatic niche. *Nature.* 2005;438(7069):820–827.

97. McAllister SS, Gifford AM, Greiner AL, Kelleher SP, Saelzler MP, Ince TA et al. Systemic endocrine instigation of indolent tumor growth requires osteopontin. *Cell.* 2008;133(6):994–1005.

98. Gil-Bernabe AM, Ferjancic S, Tlalka M, Zhao L, Allen PD, Im JH, Watson K et al. Recruitment of monocytes/macrophages by tissue factor-mediated coagulation is essential for metastatic cell survival and premetastatic niche establishment in mice. *Blood.* 2012;119(13):3164–3175.

99. van den Tol MP, Haverlag R, van Rossen MEE, Bonthuis F, Marquet RL, Jeekel J. Glove powder promotes adhesion formation and facilitates tumour cell adhesion and growth. *British Journal of Surgery.* 2001;88(9):1258–1263.

100. Allendorf JDF, Bessler M, Horvath KD, Marvin MR, Laird DA, Whelan RL. Increased tumor establishment and growth after open vs laparoscopic bowel resection in mice. *Surgical Endoscopy—Ultrasound and Interventional Techniques.* 1998;12(8):1035–1038.

101. Allendorf JDF, Bessler M, Horvath KD, Marvin MR, Laird DA, Whelan RL. Increased tumor establishment and growth after open vs laparoscopic surgery in mice may be related to differences in postoperative T-cell function. *Surgical Endoscopy—Ultrasound and Interventional Techniques.* 1999;13(3):233–235.

102. Carter JJ, Feingold DL, Kirman I, Oh A, Wildbrett P, Asi Z, Fowler R, Huang E, Whelan RL. Laparoscopic-assisted cecectomy is associated with decreased formation of postoperative pulmonary metastases compared with open cecectomy in a murine model. *Surgery.* 2003;134(3):432–436.

103. Sylla P, Nihalani A, Whelan RL. Microarray analysis of the differential effects of open and laparoscopic surgery on murine splenic T-cells. *Surgery.* 2006;139(1):92–103.

104. Pattana-Arun J, Wolff BG. Benefits of povidone-iodine solution in colorectal operations: Science or legend. *Diseases of the Colon & Rectum.* 2008;51(6):966–971.

105. Basha G, Ghirardi M, Geboes K, Yap SH, Penninckx F. Limitations of peritoneal lavage with antiseptics in prevention of recurrent colorectal cancer caused by tumor-cell seeding—Experimental study in rats. *Diseases of the Colon & Rectum.* 2000;43(12):1713–1718.

106. Lee SW, Gleason NR, Bessler M, Whelan RL. Peritoneal irrigation with povidone-iodine solution after laparoscopic-assisted splenectomy significantly decreases port-tumor recurrence in a murine model. *Diseases of the Colon & Rectum.* 1999;42(3):319–326.

107. Docherty JG, McGregor JR, Purdie CA, Galloway DJ, Odwyer PJ. Efficacy of tumoricidal agents in-vitro and in-vivo. *British Journal of Surgery.* 1995;82(8):1050–1052.

108. Huguet EL, Keeling NJ. Distilled water peritoneal lavage after colorectal cancer surgery. *Diseases of the Colon & Rectum.* 2004;47(12):2114–2119.

109. Keating JP, Neill M, Hill GL. Sclerosing encapsulating peritonitis after intraperitoneal use of povidone iodine. *ANZ Journal of Surgery.* 1997;67(10):742–744.

110. Weisberger AS, Levine B, Storaasli JP. Use of nitrogen mustard in treatment of serous effusions of neoplastic origin. *JAMA—Journal of the American Medical Association.* 1955;159(18):1704–1707.

111. Hribaschek A, Kuhn R, Pross M, Meyer F, Fahlke J, Ridwelski K, Boltze C, Lippert H. Intraperitoneal versus intravenous CPT-11 given intra- and postoperatively for peritoneal carcinomatosis in a rat model. *Surgery Today.* 2006;36(1):57–62.

112. Sugarbaker PH, Gianola FJ, Speyer JC, Wesley R, Barofsky I, Meyers CE. Prospective, randomized trial of intravenous versus intraperitoneal 5-fluorouracil in patients with advanced primary colon or rectal-cancer. *Surgery.* 1985;98(3):414–422.

113. Scheithauer W, Kornek GV, Marczell A, Karner J, Salem G, Greiner R, Burger D et al. Combined intravenous and intraperitoneal chemotherapy with fluorouracil plus leucovorin vs fluorouracil plus levamisole for adjuvant therapy of resected colon carcinoma. *British Journal of Cancer.* 1998;77(8):1349–1354.

114. Vaillant JC, Nordlinger B, Deuffic S, Arnaud JP, Pelissier E, Favre JP, Jaeck D et al. Adjuvant intraperitoneal 5-fluorouracil in high-risk colon cancer—A multicenter phase III trial. *Annals of Surgery.* 2000;231(4):449–456.

115. Nordlinger B, Rougier P, Arnaud JP, Debois M, Wils J, Ollier JC, Grobost O et al. Adjuvant regional chemotherapy and systemic chemotherapy versus systemic chemotherapy alone in patients with stage II–III colorectal cancer: A multicentre randomised controlled phase III trial. *Lancet Oncology.* 2005;6(7):459–468.

116. Elias D, Goere D, Di Pietrantonio D, Boige V, Malka D, Kohneh-Shahri N, Dromain C, Ducreux M. Results of systematic second-look surgery in patients at high risk of developing colorectal peritoneal carcinomatosis. *Annals of Surgery.* 2008;247(3):445–450.

117. Elias D, Honore C, Dumont F, Ducreux M, Boige V, Malka D, Burtin P, Dromain C, Goere D. Results of systematic second-look surgery plus HIPEC in asymptomatic patients presenting a high risk of developing colorectal peritoneal carcinomatosis. *Annals of Surgery.* 2011;254(2):289–293.

118. Sammartino P, Sibio S, Biacchi D, Cardi M, Accarpio F, Mingazzini P, Rosati MS, Cornali T, Di Giorgio A. Prevention of peritoneal metastases from colon cancer in high-risk patients: Preliminary results of surgery plus prophylactic HIPEC. *Gastroenterology Research and Practice.* 2012;2012:141585.

119. Ripley RT, Davis JL, Kemp CD, Steinberg SM, Toomey MA, Avital I. Prospective randomized trial evaluating mandatory second look surgery with HIPEC and CRS vs. standard of care in patients at high risk of developing colorectal peritoneal metastases. *Trials.* 2010;11:62.

120. Chiba T, Yokosuka O, Fukai K, Kojima H, Tada M, Arai M, Imazeki F, Saisho H. Cell growth inhibition and gene expression induced by the histone deacetylase inhibitor, trichostatin A, on human hepatoma cells. *Oncology.* 2004;66(6):481–491.

121. Greten FR, Eckmann L, Greten TF, Park JM, Li ZW, Egan LJ, Kagnoff MF, Karin M. IKK beta links inflammation and tumorigenesis in a mouse model of colitis-associated cancer. *Cell.* 2004;118(3):285–296.

122. Montel V, Kleeman J, Agarwal D, Spinella D, Kawai K, Tarin D. Altered metastatic behavior of human breast cancer cells after experimental manipulation of matrix metalloproteinase 8 gene expression. *Cancer Research.* 2004;64(5):1687–1694.

123. Weber KL, Doucet M, Price JE, Baker C, Kim SJ, Fidler IJ. Blockade of epidermal growth factor receptor signaling leads to inhibition of renal cell carcinoma growth in the bone of nude mice. *Cancer Research.* 2003;63(11):2940–2947.

124. Coffey JC, Wang JH, Smith MJF, Laing A, Bouchier-Hayes D, Cotter TG, Redmond HP. Phosphoinositide 3-kinase accelerates postoperative tumor growth by inhibiting apoptosis and enhancing resistance to chemotherapy-induced apoptosis. *The Journal of Biological Chemistry.* 2005;280(22):20968–20977.

125. Roh JL, Sung MW, Kim KH. Suppression of accelerated tumor growth in surgical wounds by celecoxib and indomethacin. *Head and Neck—Journal for the Sciences and Specialties of the Head and Neck.* 2005;27(4):326–332.

126. Roh JL, Sung MW, Park SW, Heo DS, Lee DW, Kim KH. Celecoxib can prevent tumor growth and distant metastasis in postoperative setting. *Cancer Research.* 2004;64(9):3230–3235.

127. Connolly EM, Harmey JH, O'Grady T, Foley D, Roche-Nagle G, Kay E, Bouchier-Hayes DJ. Cyclo-oxygenase inhibition reduces tumour growth and metastasis in an orthotopic model of breast cancer. *British Journal of Cancer.* 2002;87(2):231–237.

128. Harless WW. Revisiting perioperative chemotherapy: The critical importance of targeting residual cancer prior to wound healing. *BMC Cancer.* 2009;9:9.

129. McCormack PL, Keam SJ. Bevacizumab—A review of its use in metastatic colorectal cancer. *Drugs.* 2008;68(4):487–506.

130. Allegra CJ, Yothers G, O'Connell MJ, Sharif S, Colangelo LH, Lopa SH, Petrelli NJ et al. Initial safety report of NSABP C-08: A randomized phase III study of modified FOLFOX6 with or without bevacizumab for the adjuvant treatment of patients with stage II or III colon cancer. *Journal of Clinical Oncology.* 2009;27(20):3385–3390.

131. van der Bij GJ, Oosterling SJ, Beelen RHJ, Meijer S, Coffey JC, van Egmond M. The perioperative period is an underutilized window of therapeutic opportunity in patients with colorectal cancer. *Annals of Surgery.* 2009;249(5):727–734.

132. Mels AK, Muller MGS, van Leeuwen PAM, von Blomberg BME, Scheper RJ, Cuesta MA, Beelen RHJ, Meijer S. Immune-stimulating effects of low-dose perioperative recombinant granulocyte-macrophage colony-stimulating factor in patients operated on for primary colorectal carcinoma. *British Journal of Surgery.* 2001;88(4):539–544.

133. Brivio F, Lissoni P, Rovelli F, Nespoli A, Uggeri F, Fumagalli L, Gardani G. Effects of IL-2 preoperative immunotherapy on surgery-induced changes in angiogenic regulation and its prevention of VEGF increase and IL-12 decline. *Hepatogastroenterology.* 2002;49(44):385–387.

134. Oosterling SJ, Mels AK, Teunis BHG, van der Bij GJ, Tuk CW, Vuylsteke R, van Leeuwen PAM et al. Preoperative granulocyte/macrophage colony-stimulating factor (GM-CSF) increases hepatic dendritic cell numbers and clustering with lymphocytes in colorectal cancer patients. *Immunobiology.* 2006;211(6–8):641–649.

135. Da Costa ML, Redmond HP, Bouchier-Hayes DJ. Taurolidine improves survival by abrogating the accelerated development and proliferation of solid tumors and development of organ metastases from circulating tumor cells released following surgery. *Journal of Surgical Research.* 2001;101(2):111–119.

136. Helguera G, Rodriguez JA, Penichet ML. Cytokines fused to antibodies and their combinations as therapeutic agents against different peritoneal HER2/neu expressing tumors. *Molecular Cancer Therapeutics.* 2006;5(4):1029–1040.

137. Ströhlein M, Heiss M. Immunotherapy of peritoneal carcinomatosis. In: Ceelen W, ed., *Peritoneal Carcinomatosis: A Multidisciplinary Approach,* New York: Springer, 2007. pp. 483–491.

138. Alkhamesi NA, Ziprin P, Pfistermuller K, Peck DH, Darzi AW. ICAM-1 mediated peritoneal carcinomatosis, a target for therapeutic intervention. *Clinical & Experimental Metastasis.* 2005;22(6):449–459.

139. Park JS, Kim KM, Kim MH, Chang HJ, Baek MK, Kim SM, Do Jung Y. Resveratrol inhibits tumor cell adhesion to endothelial cells by blocking ICAM-1 expression. *Anticancer Research.* 2009;29(1):355–362.

140. Pross M, Lippert H, Misselwitz F, Nestler G, Kruger S, Langer H, Halangk W, Schulz HU. Low-molecular-weight heparin (reviparin) diminishes tumor cell adhesion and invasion in vitro, and decreases intraperitoneal growth of colonadeno-carcinoma cells in rats after laparoscopy. *Thrombosis Research.* 2003;110(4):215–220.

141. Niers TMH, Klerk CPW, DiNisio M, Van Noorden CJF, Buller HR, Reitsma PH, Richel DJ. Mechanisms of heparin induced anti-cancer activity in experimental cancer models. *Critical Reviews in Oncology Hematology.* 2007;61(3):195–207.

142. Borsig L. Antimetastatic activities of heparins and modified heparins. Experimental evidence. *Thrombosis Research.* 125:S66–S71.

143. Jansen M, Jansen PL, Otto J, Kirtil T, Neuss S, Treutner KH, Schumpelick V. The inhibition of tumor cell adhesion on human mesothelial cells (HOMC) by phospholipids in vitro. *Langenbeck's Archives of Surgery.* 2006;391(2):96–101.

144. Oosterling SJ, van der Bij GJ, Boegels M, ten Raa S, Post JA, Meijer GA, Beelen RHJ, van Egmond M. Anti-beta 1 integrin antibody reduces surgery-induced adhesion of colon carcinoma cells to traumatized peritoneal surfaces. *Annals of Surgery.* 2008;247(1):85–94.

145. Takatsuki H, Komatsu S, Sano R, Takada Y, Tsuji T. Adhesion of gastric carcinoma cells to peritoneum mediated by alpha 3 beta 1 integrin (VLA-3). *Cancer Research.* 2004;64(17):6065–6070.

146. Heyder C, Gloria-Maercker E, Hatzmann W, Niggemann B, Zanker KS, Dittmar T. Role of the beta(1)-integrin subunit in the adhesion, extravasation and migration of T24 human bladder carcinoma cells. *Clinical & Experimental Metastasis.* 2005;22(2):99–106.

147. Arlt MJE, Novak-Hofer I, Gast D, Gschwend V, Moldenhauer G, Grunberg J, Honer M, Schubiger PA, Altevogt P, Kruger A. Efficient inhibition of intra-peritoneal tumor growth and dissemination of human ovarian carcinoma cells in nude mice by anti-L1-cell adhesion molecule monoclonal antibody treatment. *Cancer Research.* 2006;66(2):936–943.

148. Lamagna C, Hodivala-Dilke KM, Imhof BA, Aurrand-Lions M. Antibody against junctional adhesion molecule-C inhibits angiogenesis and tumor growth. *Cancer Research.* 2005;65(13):5703–5710.

149. Solomon MJ, Egan M, Roberts RA, Philips J, Russell P. Incidence of free colorectal cancer cells on the peritoneal surface. *Diseases of the Colon & Rectum.* 1997;40(11):1294–1298.

150. Baskaranathan S, Philips J, McCredden P, Solomon MJ. Free colorectal cancer cells on the peritoneal surface: Correlation with pathologic variables and survival. *Diseases of the Colon & Rectum.* 2004;47(12):2076–2079.

151. Keshava A, Chapuis PH, Chan C, Lin BPC, Bokey EL, Dent OF. The significance of involvement of a free serosal surface for recurrence and survival following resection of clinicopathological stage B and C rectal cancer. *Colorectal Disease.* 2007;9(7):609–618.

152. Stewart CJR, Morris M, de Boer B, Iacopetta B. Identification of serosal invasion and extramural venous invasion on review of Dukes' stage B colonic carcinomas and correlation with survival. *Histopathology.* 2007;51(3):372–378.

153. Juhl H, Kalthoff H, Kruger U, Hennebruns D, Kremer B. Immunocytological detection of micrometastatic cells in gastrointestinal cancer-patients. *Zentralblatt für Chirurgie.* 1995;120(2):116–122.

154. Hase K, Ueno H, Kuranaga N, Utsunomiya K, Kanabe S, Mochizuki H. Intraperitoneal exfoliated cancer cells in patients with colorectal cancer. *Diseases of the Colon & Rectum.* 1998;41(9):1134–1140.

155. Schott A, Vogel I, Krueger U, Kalthoff H, Schreiber HW, Schmiegel W, Henne-Bruns D, Kremer B, Juhl H. Isolated tumor cells are frequently detectable in the peritoneal cavity of gastric and colorectal cancer patients and serve as a new prognostic marker. *Annals of Surgery.* 1998;227(3):372–379.

156. Wind P, Nordlinger B, Roger V, Kahlil A, Guin E, Parc R. Long-term prognostic value of positive peritoneal washing in colon cancer. *Scandinavian Journal of Gastroenterology.* 1999;34(6):606–610.

157. Vogel P, Ruschoff J, Kummel S, Zirngibl H, Hofstadter F, Hohenberger W, Jauch KW. Prognostic value of microscopic peritoneal dissemination—Comparison between colon and gastric cancer. *Diseases of the Colon & Rectum.* 2000;43(1):92–100.

158. Vogel I, Francksen H, Soeth E, Henne-Bruns D, Kremer B, Juhl H. The carcinoembryonic antigen and its prognostic impact on immunocytologically detected intraperitoneal colorectal cancer cells. *The American Journal of Surgery.* 2001;181(2):188–193.

159. Broll R, Weschta M, Windhoevel U, Berndt S, Schwandner O, Roblick U, Schiedeck THK, Schimmelpenning H, Bruch HP, Duchrow M. Prognostic significance of free gastrointestinal tumor cells in peritoneal lavage detected by immunocytochemistry and polymerase chain reaction. *Langenbecks Archives of Surgery.* 2001;386(4):285–292.

160. Lucha PA, Ignacio R, Rowley D, Francis M. The incidence of positive peritoneal cytology in colon cancer: A prospective randomized blinded trial. *The American Journal of Surgery.* 2002;68(11):1018–1021.

161. Aoki S, Takagi Y, Hayakawa M, Yamaguchi K, Futamura M, Kunieda K, Saji S. Detection of peritoneal micrometastases by reverse transcriptase-polymerase chain reaction targeting carcinoembryonic antigen and cytokeratin 20 in colon cancer patients. *Journal of Experimental & Clinical Cancer Research.* 2002;21(4):555–562.

162. Guller U, Zajac P, Schnider A, Bosch B, Vorburger S, Zuber M, Spagnoli GC et al. Disseminated single tumor cells as detected by real-time quantitative polymerase chain reaction represent a prognostic factor in patients undergoing surgery for colorectal cancer. *Annals of Surgery.* 2002;236(6):768–775.

163. Yamamoto S, Akasu T, Fujita S, Moriya Y. Long-term prognostic value of conventional peritoneal cytology after curative resection for colorectal carcinoma. *Japanese Journal of Clinical Oncology.* 2003;33(1):33–37.

164. Kanellos I, Demetriades H, Zintzaras E, Mandrali A, Mantzoros I, Betsis D. Incidence and prognostic value of positive peritoneal cytology in colorectal cancer. *Diseases of the Colon & Rectum.* 2003;46(4):535–539.

165. Bosch B, Guller U, Schnider A, Maurer R, Harder F, Metzger U, Marti WR. Perioperative detection of disseminated tumour cells is an independent prognostic factor in patients with colorectal cancer. *British Journal of Surgery.* 2003;90(7):882–888.

166. Lloyd JM, McIver CM, Stephenson SA, Hewett PJ, Rieger N, Hardingham JE. Identification of early-stage colorectal cancer patients at risk of relapse post-resection by immunobead reverse transcription-PCR analysis of peritoneal lavage fluid for malignant cells. *Clinical Cancer Research.* 2006;12(2):417–423.

167. Kanellos I, Zacharakis E, Kanellos D, Pramateftakis MG, Betsis D. Prognostic significance of CEA levels and positive cytology in peritoneal washings in patients with colorectal cancer. *Colorectal Disease.* 2006;8(5):436–440.

168. Gozalan U, Yasti AC, Yuksek YN, Reis E, Kama NA. Peritoneal cytology in colorectal cancer: Incidence and prognostic value. *The American Journal of Surgery.* 2007;193(6):672–675.

169. Hara M, Nakanishi H, Jun Q, Kanemitsu Y, Ito S, Mochizuki Y, Yamamura Y et al. Comparative analysis of intraperitoneal minimal free cancer cells between colorectal and gastric cancer patients using quantitative RT-PCR: Possible reason for rare peritoneal recurrence in colorectal cancer. *Clinical and Experimental Metastasis.* 2007;24(3):179–189.

170. Kristensen AT, Wiig JN, Larsen SG, Giercksky KE, Ekstrom PO. Molecular detection (k-ras) of exfoliated tumour cells in the pelvis is a prognostic factor after resection of rectal cancer? *BMC Cancer.* 2008;8:8.

171. Noura S, Ohue M, Seki Y, Yano M, Ishikawa O, Kameyama M. Long-term prognostic value of conventional peritoneal lavage cytology in patients undergoing curative colorectal cancer resection. *Diseases of the Colon & Rectum.* 2009;52(7):1312–1320.

172. Fujii S, Shimada H, Yamagishi S, Ota M, Kunisaki C, Ike H, Ichikawa Y. Evaluation of intraperitoneal lavage cytology before colorectal cancer resection. *International Journal of Colorectal Disease.* 2009;24(8):907–914.

173. Nanney LB. Epidermal and dermal effects of epidermal growth factor during wound repair. *Journal of Investigative Dermatology.* 1990;94(5):624–629.

174. Arteaga C. Targeting HER1/EGFR: A molecular approach to cancer therapy. *Seminars in Oncology.* 2003;30(3 Suppl. 7):3–14.

175. Powers CJ, McLeskey SW, Wellstein A. Fibroblast growth factors, their receptors and signaling. *Endocrine-Related Cancer.* 2000;7(3):165–197.

176. Daniele G, Corral J, Molife LR, de Bono JS. FGF receptor inhibitors: Role in cancer therapy. *Current Oncology Reports.* 2012;14(2):111–119.

177. Kane CJ, Hebda PA, Mansbridge JN, Hanawalt PC. Direct evidence for spatial and temporal regulation of transforming growth factor beta 1 expression during cutaneous wound healing. *Journal of Cellular Physiology.* 1991;148(1):157–173.

178. Heldin CH, Vanlandewijck M, Moustakas A. Regulation of EMT by TGFbeta in cancer. *FEBS Letters.* 2012;586(14):1959–1970.

179. Antsiferova M, Huber M, Meyer M, Piwko-Czuchra A, Ramadan T, MacLeod AS, Havran WL, Dummer R, Hohl D, Werner S. Activin enhances skin tumourigenesis and malignant progression by inducing a pro-tumourigenic immune cell response. *Nature Communications.* 2011;2:576.

180. Schneider L, Cammer M, Lehman J, Nielsen SK, Guerra CF, Veland IR, Stock C et al. Directional cell migration and chemotaxis in wound healing response to PDGF-AA are coordinated by the primary cilium in fibroblasts. *Cellular Physiology and Biochemistry.* 2010;25(2–3):279–292.

181. George D. Platelet-derived growth factor receptors: A therapeutic target in solid tumors. *Seminars in Oncology.* 2001;28(5 Suppl. 17):27–33.

182. Carmeliet P, Jain RK. Angiogenesis in cancer and other diseases. *Nature.* 2000;407(6801):249–257.

183. Wilgus TA, DiPietro LA. Complex roles for VEGF in dermal wound healing. *Journal of Investigative Dermatology.* 2012;132(2):493–494.

184. Aghdam SY, Eming SA, Willenborg S, Neuhaus B, Niessen CM, Partridge L, Krieg T, Bruning JC. Vascular endothelial insulin/IGF-1 signaling controls skin wound vascularization. *Biochemical and Biophysical Research Communications.* 2012;421(2):197–202.

185. Chitnis MM, Yuen JS, Protheroe AS, Pollak M, Macaulay VM. The type 1 insulin-like growth factor receptor pathway. *Clinical Cancer Research.* 2008;14(20):6364–6370.

186. Widgerow AD. Cellular/extracellular matrix crosstalk in scar evolution and control. *Wound Repair and Regeneration.* 2011;19(2):117–133.

187. Braig S, Wallner S, Junglas B, Fuchshofer R, Bosserhoff AK. CTGF is overexpressed in malignant melanoma and promotes cell invasion and migration. *British Journal of Cancer.* 2011;105(2):231–238.

188. Cecchi F, Rabe DC, Bottaro DP. Targeting the HGF/Met signalling pathway in cancer. *European Journal of Cancer.* 2010;46(7):1260–1270.

189. Conway K, Price P, Harding KG, Jiang WG. The molecular and clinical impact of hepatocyte growth factor, its receptor, activators, and inhibitors in wound healing. *Wound Repair and Regeneration.* 2006;14(1):2–10.

190. Hu Y, Liang D, Li X, Liu HH, Zhang X, Zheng M, Dill D et al. The role of interleukin-1 in wound biology. Part II: In vivo and human translational studies. *Anesthesia & Analgesia.* 2010;111(6):1534–1542.

191. Apte RN, Krelin Y, Song X, Dotan S, Recih E, Elkabets M, Carmi Y et al. Effects of micro-environment- and malignant cell-derived interleukin-1 in carcinogenesis, tumour invasiveness and tumour-host interactions. *European Journal of Cancer.* 2006;42(6):751–759.

192. Ashcroft GS, Masterson GR. Interleukin-6 and wound healing. *British Journal of Anaesthesia.* 1994;73(3):426.

193. Sansone P, Bromberg J. Targeting the interleukin-6/Jak/stat pathway in human malignancies. *Journal of Clinical Oncology.* 2012;30(9):1005–1014.

194. Ashcroft GS, Jeong MJ, Ashworth JJ, Hardman M, Jin W, Moutsopoulos N, Wild T et al. Tumor necrosis factor-alpha (TNF-alpha) is a therapeutic target for impaired cutaneous wound healing. *Wound Repair and Regeneration.* 2012;20(1):38–49.

195. Aggarwal BB, Gupta SC, Kim JH. Historical perspectives on tumor necrosis factor and its superfamily: 25 years later, a golden journey. *Blood.* 2012;119(3):651–665.

196. Wu L, Yu YL, Galiano RD, Roth SI, Mustoe TA. Macrophage colony-stimulating factor accelerates wound healing and upregulates TGF-beta1 mRNA levels through tissue macrophages. *Journal of Surgical Research.* 1997;72(2):162–169.

197. Hume DA, MacDonald KP. Therapeutic applications of macrophage colony-stimulating factor-1 (CSF-1) and antagonists of CSF-1 receptor (CSF-1R) signaling. *Blood.* 2012;119(8):1810–1820.

198. Bussolino F, Wang JM, Defilippi P, Turrini F, Sanavio F, Edgell CJ, Aglietta M, Arese P, Mantovani A. Granulocyte- and granulocyte-macrophage-colony stimulating factors induce human endothelial cells to migrate and proliferate. *Nature.* 1989;337(6206):471–473.

199. Hercus TR, Thomas D, Guthridge MA, Ekert PG, King-Scott J, Parker MW, Lopez AF. The granulocyte-macrophage colony-stimulating factor receptor: Linking its structure to cell signaling and its role in disease. *Blood.* 2009;114(7):1289–1298.

200. Lu Y, Cai Z, Galson DL, Xiao G, Liu Y, George DE, Melhem MF, Yao Z, Zhang J. Monocyte chemotactic protein-1 (MCP-1) acts as a paracrine and autocrine factor for prostate cancer growth and invasion. *Prostate.* 2006;66(12):1311–1318.

201. Low QE, Drugea IA, Duffner LA, Quinn DG, Cook DN, Rollins BJ, Kovacs EJ, DiPietro LA. Wound healing in MIP-1alpha(-/-) and MCP-1(-/-) mice. *The American Journal of Pathology.* 2001;159(2):457–463.

202. Rennekampff HO, Hansbrough JF, Kiessig V, Dore C, Sticherling M, Schroder JM. Bioactive interleukin-8 is expressed in wounds and enhances wound healing. *Journal of Surgical Research.* 2000;93(1):41–54.

203. Waugh DJ, Wilson C. The interleukin-8 pathway in cancer. *Clinical Cancer Research.* 2008;14(21):6735–6741.

204. Wen Y, Giardina SF, Hamming D, Greenman J, Zachariah E, Bacolod MD, Liu H et al. GROalpha is highly expressed in adenocarcinoma of the colon and down-regulates fibulin-1. *Clinical Cancer Research.* 2006;12(20 Pt. 1):5951–5959.

205. Li J, Thornhill MH. Growth-regulated peptide-alpha (GRO-alpha) production by oral keratinocytes: A comparison with skin keratinocytes. *Cytokine* 2000;12(9):1409–1413.

206. Toksoy A, Muller V, Gillitzer R, Goebeler M. Biphasic expression of stromal cell-derived factor-1 during human wound healing. *British Journal of Dermatology.* 2007;157(6):1148–1154.

207. Liekens S, Schols D, Hatse S. CXCL12-CXCR4 axis in angiogenesis, metastasis and stem cell mobilization. *Current Pharmaceutical Design.* 2010;16(35):3903–3920.

208. Jamieson T, Clarke M, Steele CW, Samuel MS, Neumann J, Jung A, Huels D et al. Inhibition of CXCR2 profoundly suppresses inflammation-driven and spontaneous tumorigenesis. *Journal of Clinical Investigation.* 2012;122(9):3127–3144.

209. Vandercappellen J, Van Damme J, Struyf S. The role of CXC chemokines and their receptors in cancer. *Cancer Letters.* 2008;267(2):226–244.

9

Role of the greater omentum in the pathogenesis of peritoneal carcinomatosis*

MANUEL J. KOPPE

INTRODUCTION

The greater omentum is a double-layered leaf of the peritoneum, attached to the greater curvature of the stomach as well as the transverse colon. Although it generally consists of fat, the omentum is commonly involved in peritoneal carcinomatosis in virtually every peritoneal surface malignancy. Therefore, it is usually partially or completely removed in debulking or cytoreductive surgery. In this chapter, after giving a short historical survey of the greater omentum from a cultural and surgical perspective, its macroscopic and microscopic anatomy will be reviewed in relation to its procancerous features. Further, the incidence of omental metastases and the role of omentectomy in cytoreductive surgery will be discussed.

HISTORICAL OVERVIEW OF THE GREATER OMENTUM IN MEDICINE

The etymologic background of the word omentum, allegedly, stems from ancient Egypt where the greater omentum was used to comprehend various omens from its form when mummifying human bodies [1]. In his Odyssey epic, Homer (eighth century BCE) may have mentioned its existence as a separate organ, describing the titan Tityus who was punished by Zeus who sent two vultures that, through a "net" (supposedly the omentum), ate his liver [2]. The surgical history

of the omentum has been recapitulated by Liebermann–Meffert [3]. A few historic facts or papers are worth summarizing. Briefly, in 1829, De Lamballe, a surgeon in the French army led by Napoleon, acknowledged the omentum as an organ that could seal off gastrointestinal perforations, thus saving the soldier's life by preventing peritonitis. Likewise, the American surgeon Nicholas Senn used the omentum to support intestinal anastomoses, in an effort to prevent fistulization. In the beginning of the twentieth century, Morison, a surgeon in Newcastle upon Tyne, called the omentum "the abdominal policeman" and compared its ability to move to places of inflammation that of a jellyfish [4]. A few decades later, the first papers were published on the surgical use of the greater omentum for the closure of vesicovaginal fistulas, as is practiced to date, and even for the treatment of ischemic heart disease [5]. In the late 1940s, Cannaday exploited the greater omentum as a pedicled flap, when he brought the omentum outside the abdominal cavity through a small midline laparotomy wound in order to cover an open underarm fracture in a young man. Ten days later he divided the arterial pedicle, leaving viable omental tissue ready for skin transplantation. Currently, the omentum is commonly used in surgical procedures to fill up areas at risk for postoperative infection, such as the pelvis after rectal surgery. In addition, it is frequently used in reconstructive operations of the abdominal or thoracic wall, especially when there is a chance of ischemia.

* This chapter is based on Koppe et al. Recent insights into the pathophysiology of omental metastases. *Journal of Surgical Oncology.* 2014;110(6):770–775. Permission for reuse of this article was granted by John Wiley & Sons, Inc.

MACROSCOPIC AND MICROSCOPIC ANATOMY OF THE OMENTUM IN RELATION TO ITS PROCANCEROUS CHARACTERISTICS

The greater omentum obtains its arterial blood supply from the right and left gastroepiploic arteries, which come off the gastroduodenal artery and splenic artery, respectively. It is attached to the greater curvature of the stomach and covers the lesser sac as it connects to the transverse colon. Frequently, a large portion of the dorsal part of the omentum adheres to the mesentery of the transverse colon. The greater omentum can be relatively large and may cover surface areas of up to 500 cm² [6].

Although the omentum largely consists of fat pads, some specific histological entities, known as the milky spots, are believed to be the immunological working units. These milky spots were first described by von Recklinghausen in 1863 [7] and named in "tâches laiteuses" 1874 by Ranvier [8], who studied the omentum in rabbits. In an autopsy study of six human fetuses between 20 and 40 weeks gestation, Krist et al. [9] observed small accumulations of cells, consisting of macrophages and lymphocytes in the omenta of all fetuses. Further, in three fetuses, older than 35 weeks of gestation, vascularized clusters of leucocytes, resembling true milky spots, were observed. It was concluded that milky spots are, indeed, specific structures in the omentum, formed between 20 and 35 weeks gestation in man. Figure 9.1 shows a representative example of a microscopic metastasis of adenocarcinoma in a milky spot.

The greater omentum carries a dense lymphatic network, which drains into the subpyloric nodes, and pathologists commonly identify lymph nodes in omental tissue. Microscopically, milky spots are aggregates of leucocytes, mostly macrophages and lymphocytes and have therefore been implicated as the working units of the greater omentum, clearing various kinds of particles from the abdominal cavity, including bacteria and tumor cells [10]. Indeed, there is an increase in the number of leucocytes in the milky spots and an increase in their size in response to intra-abdominal infectious stimuli [11]. Conversely, in a rat model, Agalar et al. showed that omentectomy resulted in a significant reduction of macrophages and a significant increase of lymphocytes in the peritoneal fluid, thus affecting and probably diminishing abdominal immunity [12].

In various animal models, it has been confirmed that, in the early stages of intraperitoneal dissemination, cancer cells preferentially localize to the milky spots of the omentum. For example, Lopes Cardozo et al. ascertained the pattern of dissemination of the colon carcinoma cells after intraperitoneal inoculation in rats and established the presence of tumor cells in omental milky spots within 4 hours thereafter [13]. Lately, several experimental studies were published that were specifically designed to investigate what attracts tumor cells to the greater omentum. Gerber et al. [14] studied the milky spots in intraperitoneal dissemination in various mouse models and cancer cell lines. Concurrent with the aforementioned observations, the cancer cells showed rather specific binding to the immune complexes. Interestingly, the authors postulate that the highly vascular microenvironment of the milky spots permits early survival of cancer cells, whereas the production of VEGF by mesothelial cells promotes angiogenesis, thus contributing to preferential tumor growth at the omentum. Nieman et al. [15] made an attempt to explain the preferential tumor growth in the omentum in ovarian cancer by focusing on the adipocytes. In a series of preclinical in vitro and in vivo studies, they found that the omental adipocytes contain specific fatty-acid-binding proteins (FABP4 proteins) that

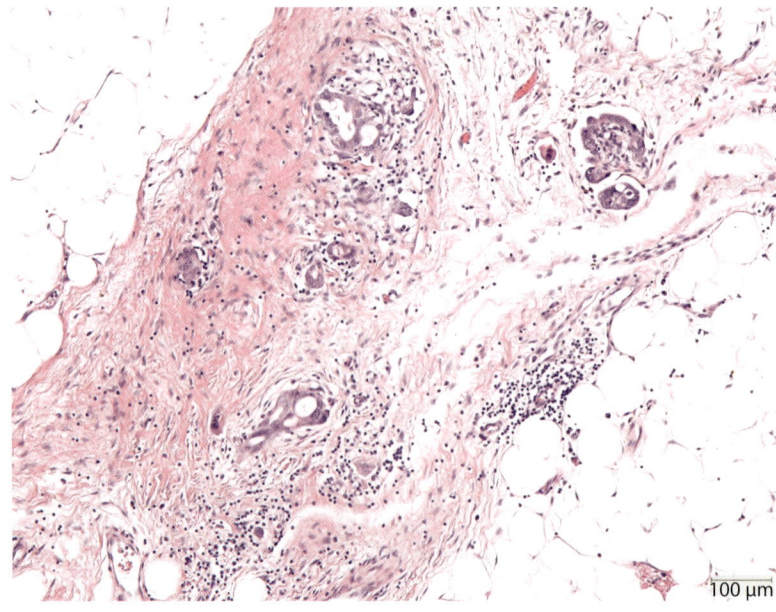

Figure 9.1 Hematoxylin and eosin (H&E) staining of human omentum, showing a metastatic deposit of colonic adenocarcinoma inside a milky spot (magnification 100×).

attract ovarian cancer cells, that these adipocytes form an energy source for the cancer cells, and that they are significantly more efficient in promoting invasive growth as compared to subcutaneous adipocytes.

These results corroborate those reported by Clarke et al. who studied the interaction of milky spots and adipose tissue in various mouse models using human and murine ovarian carcinoma cell lines and observed preferential colonization of tumor cells in the greater omentum, as opposed to other easily accessible fatty tissues in the abdomen, e.g., the mesentery and the gonadal fat pads [16]. In addition, in vitro studies showed that extracts of milky spots containing adipose tissue were able to induce tumor cell migration, to an extent 75% more than extracts from other fat tissues. Klopp et al. investigated the role of tumor-tropic mesenchymal progenitors, termed adipose stromal cells, in a subcutaneous tumor model of endometrial cancer [17]. Mesenchymal adipose stromal cells, derived from omentum, subcutaneous fat tissue, or the bone marrow and labeled with green or red fluorescent protein, were injected in the lower back of the animals and, interestingly, found to home to the subcutaneous xenografts but not to other organs, such as the liver or lungs. Furthermore, it was found that omental mesenchymal stromal cells secreted significantly higher levels of growth factors, including VEGF, as compared to subcutaneous stromal cells, and thus have distinct angiogenic effects, resulting in less central tumor necrosis and increased tumor cell proliferation. Similar results with regard to the homing of stromal cells to tumor xenografts were reported by Nowicka et al., who investigated the role of adipose stem cells in preclinical studies in ovarian cancer [18]. Interestingly, in that study, apart from preferential accumulating in intraperitoneal ovarian carcinoma xenografts, the omental stromal cells also contributed to an increased resistance to chemotherapy and radiotherapy of the tumor cells in vitro. In this regard, Zhang et al. studied the relevance of white adipose tissue in various mouse subcutaneous tumor models using several cancer cell lines [19,20]. It was demonstrated that the tumor cells themselves may be responsible for recruiting the endogenous adipose stem cells into the tumors and that these stem cells were able to differentiate into pericytes or adipocytes. Similar to the results reported by Klopp et al. [17], the blood vessel density was related to the presence of intratumoral adipocytes. In Table 9.1, the representative studies on the pathophysiology of omental metastases are summarized.

In conclusion, the homing to and the adhesion, survival, and growth of metastatic cancer cells in the omentum are most likely the result of a complex interaction between the tumor cells and the omental stroma.

FATE OF INTRAPERITONEALLY EXFOLIATED CANCER CELLS: SEED AND SOIL

There are two points in time during which intraperitoneal spread or seeding of gastrointestinal tumor cells to the omentum may occur [21]. First, intraperitoneal spread may

occur preoperatively as a result of full-thickness invasion of the bowel wall by an invasive cancer. Second, intraperitoneal spread may be induced iatrogenically during surgery, when in-transit tumor cells or emboli escape from dissected lymph vessels or the bowel lumen or reach the peritoneal cavity through blood spill from the surgical field. The reported incidence of peritoneal seeding during potentially curative surgery varies considerably, from 3% to up to 28%, which may reflect differences in procedures to discover cancer cells [22]. After reaching the peritoneal cavity, a tumor cell or embolus must then pass a series of steps before being able to give rise to metastatic tumor growth. Most likely these factors are similar to those concerning hematogenous metastatic cells and include survival in the peritoneal cavity (as opposed to the circulation), evasion of the immune system, reattachment to secondary sites, and the development of blood supply in order to provide for its metabolic needs (angiogenesis) [23,24]. Failure to complete any step of this metastatic cascade prohibits a cancer cell from evolving into a true metastasis. Due to the complexity of the metastatic process, most cancer cells will eventually not develop into metastases. This process is referred to as metastatic inefficiency and reflects a selection process separating the cells with true metastatic potential from those without [25,26].

Besides the preferential growth of tumor cells in the omentum, metastatic disease is frequently encountered on the diaphragm and in the paracolic gutters. This may be explained by the intra-abdominal flow of the peritoneal fluid, which is upward and caused by the breathing movements of the diaphragm [21]. Several authors have studied the metastatic pattern of cancers cells after intraperitoneal inoculation in animals and showed that these cells preferentially accumulate in the milky spots of the greater omentum as well as the lymphatic lacunae of the diaphragm [11,27]. Since at these sites in the peritoneal cavity the peritoneal fluid is absorbed, it has been hypothesized that tumor growth in the greater omentum or at the diaphragm could contribute to the subsequent development of malignant ascites [28]. Indeed, in extensive peritoneal carcinomatosis precluding complete or optimal surgical cytoreduction, a palliative omentectomy is frequently performed in order to reduce the production of debilitating ascites. The protein-rich ascites creates a fertile environment allowing tumor growth and permits the cancer cells to move freely throughout the abdominal cavity. Intraperitoneal dissemination of cancer cells may consequently contribute to a self-sustaining process of cancer growth.

INCIDENCE OF OMENTAL METASTASES AND THE VALUE OF OMENTECTOMY

In extensive peritoneal carcinomatosis, the greater omentum is almost invariably involved in virtually every malignancy giving rise to peritoneal surface disease. For this reason, omentectomy is routinely carried out as a standard operative procedure in cytoreductive surgery, also when it seems to be macroscopically normal. Data on the

Table 9.1 Representative publications on the pathophysiologic background of omental metastases

References	Model	Cell line(s) used	Most important findings
Lopes Cardozo et al. [13]	Syngeneic rat	CC-531 rat colon carcinoma	Preferential localization of tumor cells in the milky spots <4 hours after intraperitoneal inoculation.
Gerber et al. [14]	Syngeneic mouse	B16 mouse melanoma Line1 mouse lung carcinoma EMT6 mouse mammary carcinoma K1735.1 mouse melanoma ID8 mouse ovarian carcinoma	All tumor cell lines exhibited rapid and selective attachment to immune complexes on the omentum and mesentery. These immune complexes were characterized by a dense network of capillaries, possibly contributing to the survival of the cancer cells. Local production of VEGF-induced angiogenesis, conducive of continued tumor growth.
Niemann et al. [15]	In vitro studies Nude mouse	SKOV3ip1 human ovarian carcinoma	Adipocytes provide fatty acids for rapid tumor growth, thus functioning as energy reservoirs. Omental adipocytes were more efficient in promoting invasive tumor growth than subcutaneous adipocytes.
Clarke et al. [16]	Nude and syngeneic mouse In vitro studies	SKOV3ip1 human ovarian carcinoma HeyA8 human ovarian carcinoma CaOV3 human ovarian carcinoma ID8 mouse ovarian carcinoma	ID8, CaOV3, HeyA8, and SKOV3ip.1 preferentially lodge and grow in milky spot containing fat. There is an inverse relationship between metastatic burden and the adipocyte content of the omentum. In vitro studies indicated that the omentum secretes factors that enhance the preferential homing of tumor cells to the omentum.
Klopp et al. [17]	Nude mouse	Hec1a human endometrial carcinoma Human adipose stromal cells, derived from omentum, subcutaneous fat, or bone marrow	Human omental adipose stromal cells promoted tumor cell growth more potently than subcutaneous or bone marrow–derived adipose stromal cells. Human omental adipose stroma cells secrete higher levels of growth factors, e.g., VEGF, as compared to subcutaneous adipose stromal cells. Human omental adipose stroma cells showed preferential uptake to subcutaneous endometrial tumor xenografts.
Nowicka et al. [18]	In vitro studies Nude mouse	OVCA 429 human ovarian carcinoma OVCA 433 human ovarian carcinoma A2780 human ovarian carcinoma SKOV3 human ovarian carcinoma	Human omental adipose stem cells promoted ovarian cancer proliferation, migration, chemoresistance, and radiation resistance in vitro. Human omental adipose stem showed preferential uptake in intraperitoneal ovarian carcinoma xenografts after intraperitoneal administration.

incidence of microscopic metastases in macroscopically normal omentum, however, are lacking for gastrointestinal cancers. In ovarian cancer, known for its tendency to metastasize early to the peritoneum, the greater omentum is partially or completely removed for staging as well as therapeutic purposes. In a large series of 324 patients with ovarian cancer grossly confined to the pelvis, microscopic disease was found in only 7 out of 256 patients in whom an infracolic omentectomy was performed [29]. Furthermore, in only one patient (0.3%), the histological results of the random peritoneal biopsies and omentectomy led to a change in postoperative chemotherapeutic management. Arie et al. recently reviewed the literature with regard to the incidence of omental metastases in ovarian cancer and found that in early-stage ovarian cancer, i.e., disease limited to the pelvis, occult metastatic foci in the apparently normal omentum could be demonstrated in 0%–22% of patients [30,31]. The incidence of isolated omental involvement in apparently early-stage ovarian cancer ranged from 0% to 7%. The authors concluded that, because of the relatively low incidence of omental metastases in early-stage ovarian cancer and the efficacy of chemotherapy yet to be given, total omentectomy might not be necessary as a staging tool and random omental biopsies could be sufficient. Interestingly, the authors raise the question whether the role of the omentum is either valuable, absorbing and concentrating tumor cells, or detrimental, providing a shelter for tumor cells. It is postulated that an omentectomy should be postponed until macroscopic disease is present. Several experimental studies have been published, investigating the role of the omentum as well as the effect of omentectomy in early-stage peritoneal carcinomatosis. Yokoyama et al. [32] investigated the effects of omentectomy in rats with early-stage ovarian cancer and found that delaying omentectomy until the development of macroscopic disease, indeed, resulted in a significantly improved survival. These results indicate that the greater omentum may indeed have a beneficial role in the early stages of peritoneal seeding. In this regard, Oosterling et al. [33] tested the hypothesis that the greater omentum might have antitumor activity in a rat model of early-stage colorectal carcinomatosis. Simulating minimal residual disease by intraperitoneal injection of only 1.0×10^4 colon carcinoma cells, the authors found significantly less intraperitoneal tumor growth in rats that had previously undergone omentectomy. Prior omentectomy, however, did not affect tumor growth at other sites in the abdominal cavity, indicating that the greater omentum was not able to neutralize the small number of tumor cells, nor could it prevent or slow down tumor growth at other intraperitoneal sites in that animal model. In yet another rat model, Lawrance et al. [34] showed that omentectomy prior to intraperitoneal or intraluminal tumor cell inoculation significantly reduced tumor growth at bowel anastomoses. Weese et al. [35] studied the effect of the omentum on intraperitoneal tumor growth in a rat model of peritoneal carcinomatosis of colonic origin and found that omentectomy reduced the incidence of malignant small bowel

obstruction by more than 50%. Thus, the omentum and the milky spots have been implicated as initial sites of tumor growth after which secondary seeding occurs at sites of peritoneal trauma. The reported experimental results on the role of the omentum in the abdominal immune system against early peritoneal seeding of cancer cells, however, remain inconclusive.

Although the implementation of omentectomy as a routine procedure in ovarian cancer has resulted in some upward stage migration [29], there are no clinical studies on whether omentectomy contributes to the outcome of patients with peritoneal carcinomatosis. Furthermore, the extent of the omentectomy in ovarian cancer is under debate. Some argue that an infracolic omentectomy should always be done [36], while others believe that in case of a grossly normal omentum, only biopsies will be sufficient [30]. In patients with colorectal carcinomatosis, treated with cytoreductive surgery and hyperthermic intraperitoneal chemotherapy (HIPEC), usually a complete omentectomy is carried out. Here the greater omentum is dissected off transverse colon and the gastrocolic ligament, and the right and left gastroepiploic arteries up to the vasa brevia are resected. In this regard, it has been suggested that resection of the right gastroepiploic artery might be partially responsible for delayed gastric emptying, a common complication after cytoreductive surgery and HIPEC. However, Evers et al. [37] could not confirm this hypothesis in a randomized trial.

From a clinicopathological point of view, it should be noted that colorectal carcinomatosis differs from ovarian carcinomatosis in its sensitivity to systemic chemotherapy. Whereas ovarian cancer generally tends to respond well to intravenous chemotherapy, the response of colorectal carcinomatosis to systemic treatment is usually poor [38]. In this respect, the purpose of debulking surgery in ovarian cancer is to reduce the tumor burden to residual disease of <1 cm in diameter. In contrast, incomplete cytoreductive surgery in patients with colorectal carcinomatosis is associated with very poor survival [39]. Besides the poorer sensitivity of colorectal carcinomatosis to systemic chemotherapy, intraperitoneal recurrences after cytoreductive surgery and HIPEC are frequent [40] and associated with a dismal prognosis, supporting complete omentectomy. Still, the impact of complete omentectomy as a routine procedure in cytoreductive surgery for colorectal carcinomatosis on survival lacks scientific evidence and is only speculative.

CONCLUDING REMARKS

Because of its mitigating role in intra-abdominal inflammatory conditions, surgeons have learnt to appreciate the greater omentum as a valuable structure and use it as a well-vascularized organ for various surgical reconstructive operations. In peritoneal surface malignancy, however, preferential dissemination of cancer cells to the greater omentum remains an intriguing and worrying phenomenon, both from a clinical and pathological point of view. Being reproducible in virtually every animal model of peritoneal carcinomatosis, the milky spots have repeatedly been recognized as the first docking stations for tumor cells after intraperitoneal inoculation. Based on the available literature, it seems likely that this is related to the rich vascularization around the milky spots, permitting early survival of the cancer cells. The production of several growth factors, including VEGF, by the surrounding mesothelial cells, is likely to increase angiogenesis necessary for continued tumor growth. Recent research has indicated the mesenchymal adipose stem cells as well as the adipocytes, to play important roles in metastatic tumor growth in the omentum. The omental adipose stem cells are actively recruited into tumors, and seem to enhance the metastatic tumor growth, by the secretion of various growth factors, including VEGF, thereby increasing the formation of blood vessels. In addition, the omental adipocytes appear to function as caloric reservoirs for the growing omental tumor deposits. This is supported by the clinical observation of the so-called omental cake, where omental fat can be completely replaced by tumor in advanced stages of peritoneal carcinomatosis. Although most experimental studies on the pathophysiology of omental metastases were done using ovarian carcinoma cell lines, intuitively it seems plausible that the observed mechanisms also apply in other cancer types.

Whether the preferential homing of tumor cells to the omentum is primarily beneficial or eventually harmful still is subject of hypothesis. Similar to its mitigating role in intra-abdominal infection, the omentum might theoretically be a blessing in disguise, scavenging and concentrating tumor cells that might otherwise form metastatic deposits elsewhere in the peritoneal cavity or be shed in the circulation. In case of gross involvement of the greater omentum seen during cytoreductive surgery, omentectomy is obviously indicated. The high risk of omental recurrence favors complete omentectomy as opposed to partial omentectomy, especially in colorectal carcinomatosis, where systemic chemotherapy is less effective as compared to ovarian cancer. Whether the omentum should be partially or completely removed as a staging or therapeutic tool in peritoneal carcinomatosis could only be determined in a randomized trial. However, given the high incidence of intraperitoneal recurrence at other sites than the omentum after cytoreductive surgery in both colorectal and ovarian carcinomatosis, the theoretical difference in survival is likely to be small if not absent. Such a trial would need to have a noninferiority design and include a large number of patients and, therefore, seems only hypothetical. Therefore, whether omentectomy in cytoreductive surgery should be partial or complete will probably remain unknown.

ACKNOWLEDGMENT

Part of this study was supported by a grant from the Dutch Cancer Foundation (KWF), grant number KUN 2012-5377.

REFERENCES

1. Platell C, Cooper D, Papadimitriou JM, Hall JC. The omentum. *World Journal of Gastroenterology.* 2000;6:169–176.
2. Wobbes T, van Twisk R. The greater omentum, a much-used organ. *Nederlands Tijdschrift Geneeskunde.* 1988;132:248–251.
3. Liebermann DM, Kaufmann M. Utilization of the greater omentum in surgery: A historical review. *Netherlands Journal of Surgery.* 1991;43:136–144.
4. Morison R. Remarks on some functions of the omentum. *British Medical Journal.* 1906;1:76–78.
5. Davies DT, Mansell HE, O'Shaughnessy L. Surgical treatment of angina pectoris and allied conditions. *The Lancet.* 1938;231:1–11.
6. Liebermann-Meffert D. The greater omentum. Anatomy, embryology, and surgical applications. *Surgery Clinics of North America.* 2000;80:275–293, xii.
7. von Recklinghausen F. Über Eiter-Bindegewebskörperchen. *Virchows Arch Pathol Anat.* 1863;28:157–166.
8. Ranvier I. Du développement et de l'accroissement des vaisseaux sanguins. *Archives de Physiologie Normale et Pathologique.* 1874;6:429–449.
9. Krist LF, Koenen H, Calame W, van der Harten JJ, van der Linden JC, Eestermans IL et al. Ontogeny of milky spots in the human greater omentum: An immunochemical study. *Anatomical Record.* 1997;249:399–404.
10. Krist LF, Kerremans M, Broekhuis-Fluitsma DM, Eestermans IL, Meyer S, Beelen RH. Milky spots in the greater omentum are predominant sites of local tumour cell proliferation and accumulation in the peritoneal cavity. *Cancer Immunology, Immunotherapy.* 1998;47:205–212.
11. Shimotsuma M, Shields JW, Simpson-Morgan MW, Sakuyama A, Shirasu M, Hagiwara A et al. Morpho-physiological function and role of omental milky spots as omentum-associated lymphoid tissue (OALT) in the peritoneal cavity. *Lymphology.* 1993;26:90–101.
12. Agalar F, Sayek I, Cakmakci M, Hascelik G, Abbasoglu O. Effect of omentectomy on peritoneal defence mechanisms in rats. *European Journal of Surgery.* 1997;163:605–609.
13. Lopes Cardozo AM, Gupta A, Koppe MJ, Meijer S, van Leeuwan PA, Beelen RJ et al. Metastatic pattern of CC531 colon carcinoma cells in the abdominal cavity: An experimental model of peritoneal carcinomatosis in rats. *European Journal of Surgical Oncology.* 2001;27:359–363.
14. Gerber SA, Rybalko VY, Bigelow CE, Lugade AA, Foster TH, Frelinger JG et al. Preferential attachment of peritoneal tumor metastases to omental immune aggregates and possible role of a unique

vascular microenvironment in metastatic survival and growth. *American Journal of Pathology.* 2006;169:1739–1752.

15. Nieman KM, Kenny HA, Penicka CV, Ladanyi A, Buell-Gutbrod R, Zillhardt MR et al. Adipocytes promote ovarian cancer metastasis and provide energy for rapid tumor growth. *Nature Medicine.* 2011;17:1498–1503.

16. Clark R, Krishnan V, Schoof M, Rodriguez I, Theriault B, Chekmareva M et al. Milky spots promote ovarian cancer metastatic colonization of peritoneal adipose in experimental models. *American Journal of Pathology.* 2013;183:576–591.

17. Klopp AH, Zhang Y, Solley T, Amaya-Manzanares F, Marini F, Andreeff M et al. Omental adipose tissue-derived stromal cells promote vascularization and growth of endometrial tumors. *Clinical Cancer Research.* 2012;18:771–782.

18. Nowicka A, Marini FC, Solley TN, Elizondo PB, Zhang Y, Sharp HJ et al. Human omental-derived adipose stem cells increase ovarian cancer proliferation, migration, and chemoresistance. *PLOS ONE.* 2013;8:e81859.

19. Zhang Y, Daquinag AC, Amaya-Manzanares F, Sirin O, Tseng C, Kolonin MG. Stromal progenitor cells from endogenous adipose tissue contribute to pericytes and adipocytes that populate the tumor microenvironment. *Cancer Research.* 2012;72:5198–5208.

20. Zhang Y, Daquinag A, Traktuev DO, Amaya-Manzanares F, Simmons PJ, March KL et al. White adipose tissue cells are recruited by experimental tumors and promote cancer progression in mouse models. *Cancer Research.* 2009;69:5259–5266.

21. Sugarbaker PH. Observations concerning cancer spread within the peritoneal cavity and concepts supporting an ordered pathophysiology. *Cancer Treatment and Research.* 1996;82:79 100.

22. Koppe MJ, Boerman OC, Oyen WJ, Bleichrodt RP. Peritoneal carcinomatosis of colorectal origin: Incidence and current treatment strategies. *Annals of Surgery.* 2006;243:212–222.

23. Weiss L. Metastatic inefficiency: Intravascular and intraperitoneal implantation of cancer cells. *Cancer Treatment and Research.* 1996;82:1–11.

24. Weiss L. Inefficiency of metastasis from colorectal carcinomas. Relationship to local therapy for hepatic metastasis. *Cancer Treatment and Research.* 1994;69:1–11.

25. Wong CW, Lee A, Shientag L, Yu J, Dong Y, Kao G et al. Apoptosis: An early event in metastatic inefficiency. *Cancer Research.* 2001;61:333–338.

26. Sugarbaker PH. Metastatic inefficiency: The scientific basis for resection of liver metastases from colorectal cancer. *Journal of Surgical Oncology.* 1993;3(Suppl.):158–160.

27. Shimotsuma M, Shirasu M, Hagiwara A, Takahashi T. Role of omentum-associated lymphoid tissue in the progression of peritoneal carcinomatosis. *Cancer Treatment and Research.* 1996;82:147–154.

28. Adam RA, Adam YG. Malignant ascites: Past, present, and future. *Journal of the American College of Surgeons.* 2004;198:999–1011.

29. Lee JY, Kim HS, Chung HH, Kim JW, Park NH, Song YS. The role of omentectomy and random peritoneal biopsies as part of comprehensive surgical staging in apparent early-stage epithelial ovarian cancer. *Annals of Surgical Oncology.* 2014;21:2762–2766.

30. Arie AB, McNally L, Kapp DS, Teng NN. The omentum and omentectomy in epithelial ovarian cancer: A reappraisal: Part II—The role of omentectomy in the staging and treatment of apparent early stage epithelial ovarian cancer. *Gynecologic Oncology.* 2013;131:784–790.

31. Ben Arie A, McNally L, Kapp DS, Teng NN. The omentum and omentectomy in epithelial ovarian cancer: A reappraisal. Part I—Omental function and history of omentectomy. *Gynecologic Oncology.* 2013;131:780–783.

32. Yokoyama Y, Hirakawa H, Wang H, Mizunuma H. Is omentectomy mandatory in the operation for ovarian cancer? Preliminary results in a rat study. *European Journal of Obstetrics, Gynecology, and Reproductive Biology.* 2012;164:89–92.

33. Oosterling SJ, van der Bij GJ, Bogels M, van der Sijp JR, Beelen RH, Meijer S et al. Insufficient ability of omental milky spots to prevent peritoneal tumor outgrowth supports omentectomy in minimal residual disease. *Cancer Immunology, Immunotherapy.* 2006;55:1043–1051.

34. Lawrance RJ, Loizidou M, Cooper AJ, Alexander P, Taylor I. Importance of the omentum in the development of intra-abdominal metastases. *Brirish Journal of Surgery.* 1991;78:117–119

35. Weese JL, Ottery FD, Emoto SE. Does omentectomy prevent malignant small bowel obstruction? *Clinical & Experimental Metastasis.* 1988;6:319–324.

36. Trimbos JB, Vergote I, Bolis G, Vermorken JB, Mangioni C, Madronal C et al. Impact of adjuvant chemotherapy and surgical staging in early-stage ovarian carcinoma: European Organisation for Research and Treatment of Cancer-Adjuvant ChemoTherapy in Ovarian Neoplasm trial. *Journal of the National Cancer Institute.* 2003;95:113–125.

37. Evers DJ, Smeenk RM, Bottenberg PD, van Werkhoven ED, Boot H, Verwaal VJ. Effect of preservation of the right gastro-epiploic artery on delayed gastric emptying after cytoreductive surgery and HIPEC: A randomized clinical trial. *European Journal of Surgical Oncology.* 2011;37:162–167.

38. Hompes D, Aalbers A, Boot H, van Velthuysen ML, Vogel W, Prevoo W et al. A prospective pilot study to assess neo-adjuvant chemotherapy for unresectable peritoneal carcinomatosis from colorectal cancer. *Colorectal Disease.* 2014;16:O264–O272.

39. Verwaal VJ, van Tinteren H, van Ruth S, Zoetmulder FA. Predicting the survival of patients with peritoneal carcinomatosis of colorectal origin treated by aggressive cytoreduction and hyperthermic intraperitoneal chemotherapy. *British Journal of Surgery.* 2004;91:739–746.

40. Verwaal VJ, Boot H, Aleman BM, van Tinteren, Zoetmulder FA. Recurrences after peritoneal carcinomatosis of colorectal origin treated by cytoreduction and hyperthermic intraperitoneal chemotherapy: Location, treatment, and outcome. *Annals of Surgical Oncology.* 2004;11:375–379.

10

Lymphatic transport and the diaphragmatic stomata

KATHARINA G.M.A. D'HERDE

INTRODUCTION

The peritoneal cavity is connected to the retroperitoneum by a large anatomically continuous potential space, the subperitoneal space in between the inner surface of the peritoneum and the musculature of abdomen and pelvis and containing the vascular, nervous, and lymphatic systems that supply the viscera. It is known for over a century that particulate matter, injected into the peritoneal cavity, will rapidly pass through the mesothelial lining into the subperitoneal space containing an extensive lymphatic plexus [4].

Indeed drainage of fluid and cells in the peritoneal cavity is provided by lymphatic absorption starting at the lymphatic peritoneal stomata, i.e., openings in the peritoneal lining, while diffusive processes through the mesothelial epithelium have a minor role. Hence the lymphatic stomata are considered the main pathway for active drainage of intraperitoneal fluids and cells from the peritoneal cavity to the submesothelial lymphatic system [43]. This active lymphatic drainage is instrumental for setting the subatmospheric peritoneal liquid pressure.

In the clinic malignant ascites found in peritoneal carcinomatosis, it is in part due to lymphatic obstruction by tumor cells infiltrating the lymphatics [40].

As is the case for lymph vessels of other organs, the lymphatic system draining the peritoneal cavity transports fluid and other constituents of the lymph to the regional nodes and further on to the venous vasculature. In addition the peritoneal lymphatic system functions as an immunovascular organ. Recently, microarray analysis of various compartments of the rat peritoneal lymphatic system showed that the initial collecting prenodal lymphatics contain resident antigen presenting and processing cells confirming its important role in the immune system [8].

In this chapter we discuss the modalities of lymphatic drainage of the peritoneal cavity and look how in peritoneal carcinomatosis this elaborate peritoneal lymphatic system can be used to the benefit of the severely diseased patient, while in other circumstances it works disadvantageous for the patient.

THREEFOLD ORIGIN OF PERITONEAL CARCINOMATOSIS

The development of peritoneal carcinomatosis implies that tumors have acquired the ability for dissemination through a variety of means (discussed in Chapters 6 and 7) when they are not native to the peritoneal surface. Indeed three models explain the pathogenesis of peritoneal carcinomatosis:

(a) Dissemination of a primary tumor (gastrointestinal tumor [gastric, colon, colorectal, or appendiceal mucinous tumor], ovarian tumor, or extra-abdominal tumor [lung, breast, lymphoma]), (b) primary tumor from the peritoneum such as malign peritoneal mesothelioma, and (c) independent origins of primary tumor and peritoneal implants [20]. Once cancer cells are seeded in the peritoneal cavity, they spread to different regions of the abdomen and eventually the thorax based on three forces: gravity, peristaltic movement of the gastrointestinal tract, and negative pressure exerted during inspiration by diaphragm contractions. Common sites for intraperitoneal deposition of tumor are the Douglas pouch, the rectovesicular space, the right lower quadrant at the inferior junction of the small bowel mesentery, the right paracolic gutter, and the superior aspect of the sigmoid mesocolon [21]. Peritoneal carcinomatosis is regarded nowadays as a form of local rather than systemic spread [12], making it amenable to local control such as cytoreductive surgery combined with hyperthermic intraperitoneal chemotherapy (see Chapter 15) or other experimental intraperitoneal therapies (discussed in Chapters 30 through 35).

ROUTES OF DISSEMINATION OF A PRIMARY ABDOMINAL OR PELVIC TUMOR TO THE SUBPERITONEAL SPACE

Transmesothelial route: Contribution of active or passive gaps in the mesothelium

In the case of a transmesothelial route, either mesothelial cells expose the submesothelial basement membrane needed for adhesion of the tumor cell due to cytokine-mediated contraction of the lining mesothelial cells disabling the barrier function of the peritoneal lining [49] or the submesothelial basement membrane is exposed due to defects in the peritoneal lining caused by tumor-induced apoptosis of mesothelial cells by Fas ligand/Fas interaction [17].

Translymphatic route and the role of the lymphatic stomata

In the case of translymphatic dissemination, free peritoneal cancer cells gain access to subperitoneal lymphatic spaces through the so-called lymphatic stomata, round- or oval-shaped openings with variable diameter within an area of cuboidal-shaped mesothelial cells covered with microvilli and with connection to lymphatic capillaries. Importantly this dissemination type does not require proper invasion per se of the peritoneal and subperitoneal tissue and therefore would be established earlier in the metastatic process [49].

These interruptions in the continuity of the mesothelium have been subject of considerable debate since Von Recklinghausen [45] disclosed them at the diaphragmatic mesothelium using silver nitrate impregnation. Other light microscopical studies questioned the presence of the stomata and hypothesized that the discontinuities in the mesothelium were artifactual [19,30,41]. The latter implicated a myriad of mechanisms to explain the results of in vivo tracer studies, namely, passage of particulate matter through the mesothelial lining. They proposed intercellular and intracellular absorption, vital activity, phagocytosis, and diapedesis and accepted the concepts of osmosis and filtration pressure. Simplified, the peritoneum and

underlying lymphatic endothelium were thought to be anatomically closed but physiologically open [2]. Subsequently different groups confirmed the functionality of the openings in mesothelium with various tracers such as carbon particles, bacteria, spores of yeast and molds, erythrocytes of different species, polystyrene latex spherules, Indian ink, trypan blue, and unfiltered carmine solution [4,5,9,13,34]. Both the speed and the extent of the uptake of peritoneal fluid within the lymphatic system favor the concept of lymphatic stomata instead of a transcellular route or intercellular route as described under the Section "Transmesothelial Route: Contribution of Active or Passive Gaps in the Mesothelium." The diameter of the openings remained a point of discussion, but nowadays there is a general consent that the stomata have diameters up to 20 μm (for detailed references on this topic, see Michailova [31]).

LYMPHATIC STOMATA ARE NOT SOLELY CONFINED TO THE DIAPHRAGMATIC PARIETAL PERITONEUM

These lymphatic stomata, originally claimed to be exclusively restricted to the peritoneal surface of the diaphragm [22], called therefore diaphragmatic stomata, were later found at other parietal and visceral peritoneal surfaces and also in other body cavities [33,48]. The average distribution density of the lymphatic stomata varies according to the body cavity (peritoneal or pleural) and is congruent to the absorption capacity [23,35].

Their distribution is uneven appearing in clusters with 2–14 stomata per field as seen with scanning electron microscopy [35]. Besides their presence at the inferior surface of the diaphragm, they are also found at the greater omentum, the appendices epiploicae of the colon, the falciform ligament, the Douglas pouch, the broad ligament of the uterus, and the small bowel mesentery. Also at the pleural side of the diaphragm and in the pericardial cavity, their role in draining pleural and pericardial effusions is well documented [7,34,36]. Most studies today are devoted to the peritoneum covering the diaphragm, the omentum, and the ovaries. Recently, lymphatic stomata were disclosed by transmission electron microscopy in human testis tunica vaginalis [46] confirming early light microscopical findings of tunica vaginalis [3]. For a complete list of all locations of lymphatic stomata in different species, see Michailova et al. [32,33].

MORPHOLOGY OF THE LYMPHATIC STOMATA AND ASSOCIATED LYMPHATIC TISSUES

The lymphatic stomata, especially those situated within the omentum, the falciform ligament, and the Douglas pouch, are rich in the so-called milky spots, which are submesothelial lymphoid structures consisting in human of concentrations of macrophages and lymphocytes [50].

In this configuration macrophages of the milky spots are able to migrate through the lymphatic stomata to the peritoneal cavity in case of bacterial infection, and conversely free cancer cells have access through these peritoneal openings into the milky spots where they proliferate and induce angiogenesis or are killed by cytotoxic macrophages [6,44]. Thus the milky spots have a central role in the immunological barrier function of the peritoneal cavity. Furthermore, it was found in different animal models and humans that the lymphatic stomata situated in parietal and visceral peritoneum coincide with the maculae cribriformes, which are structures like sieves in the submesothelial collagen tissue [24,25,33].

Azzali [5] confirmed by 3D reconstructions of ultrathin serial sections the detailed morphology of the diaphragmatic stomata, the sieve-like structure in the connective tissue, and the continuity with lymphatic vessels.

The plexus organization of the connected submesothelial lymphatic system was elegantly visualized by light microscopy of in toto India ink stained lymphatics [15] and also by scanning electron microscopy of lymphatic corrosion casts [25].

A common finding when making abstraction of species differences and morphological discrepancies due to variations in the used techniques is the fact that functional continuity can be found between the mesothelium lining the peritoneal cavity and the lymphatic endothelium without intervening the basal lamina [1]. The subdiaphragmatic lymphatics seem to be quantitatively the most important pathway for lymph drainage of the peritoneal cavity in physiological conditions, but lymphatics of the visceral and parietal parts of the peritoneum also contribute especially when the peritoneal cavity is filled with large amounts of liquid [48]. The subdiaphragmatic lymphatics can dynamically adapt to the contraction or relaxation status of the diaphragm. Important for their function is the fact that the diameter of lymphatic stomata is variable in response to changing conditions and relies in part upon actin filaments. Although the cuboidal mesothelial cells surrounding the stomata display characteristics of high vital activity, it is clear that phagocytosis plays an insignificant role in lymph absorption processes.

Both cuboidal mesothelial processes and lymphatic endothelial flaps crisscrossing the lymphatic channels visualized via scanning and transmission electron microscopy approach were claimed to be involved in the necessary bicuspid valve function to ensure net unidirectional transport [42]. In the 3D reconstructed images of [5], no contribution of the mesothelial cells to the valves could be attributed. In a rat model intraperitoneal injection of near-infrared fluorescent tracer revealed the lymph nodes involved in the drainage of the peritoneal space; importantly this lymph node pattern is predictable so that the sentinel nodus concept can be applied [38].

Hence, visualization of sentinel nodi in case of peritoneal carcinomatosis would contribute to completeness of resection in case of cytoreductive surgery.

PATENCY OF LYMPHATIC STOMATA AFFECTING LYMPHATIC CONDUCTANCE IS REGULATED

Since the morphological discovery of the peritoneal stomata, the question arose whether the stomata are fixed openings or whether they are open only at certain circumstances representing a dynamic structure adaptive to physiological and pathological conditions. In this context it has been shown that stoma patency is modified passively in response to the contraction status of the diaphragm and increased abdominal pressure and actively by actin-mediated contraction of mesothelial cells bordering the stomata [35,42]. Furthermore, both diameter and average distribution of the lymphatic stomata can be increased experimentally in a mouse model by interfering with nitric oxide metabolism affecting the NO–cGMP–[Ca^{2+}] signaling pathway. NO generated by induced macrophages enlarge the lymphatic stomata and relax the lymphatic vessels, leading to enhanced absorption of ascites [14,26,27,47]. Compounds used in Chinese herbal medicine to treat ascites increase the concentration of endogenous NO thereby affecting absorption. Michailova [31] showed that under experimentally induced peritonitis, the number, diameter, and distribution of the lymphatic stomata were affected. This adaptation was explained by the increased abdominal pressure accompanying the peritonitis supporting an increased drainage by the diaphragm.

It is unclear from the literature so far whether the ultrastructural changes in the mesothelial cells lining the peritoneal cavity induced due to CO_2 pneumoperitoneum during laparoscopy [37,39] affect the function of the lymphatic stomata. In his context it is interesting to note that the concern that laparascopic resections for colon cancer had a worse prognosis compared to open surgery was not confirmed in a randomized controlled trial [11].

LYMPHATIC STOMATA AS A DOUBLE-EDGED SWORD

Transport of small solutes or macromolecules from the peritoneal cavity to the systemic circulation is hampered rather by the blood capillary wall and surrounding interstitium in the submesothelial tissue than by the one-layered mesothelium [10]. Indeed the peritoneal lining is not a significant barrier to solute and water transfer. Hence, fluid enters the vascular compartment by diffusion from the peritoneal compartment or indirectly as discussed earlier by absorption through the peritoneal lymphatic stomata. It is obvious that the lymphatic stomata provide a predominantly unidirectional route for cells and fluids that are beneficial for the patient. Indeed in case of intraperitoneal nutrition, intraperitoneal transfusion for the treatment of erythroblastosis fetalis [28], ascites elimination, and defense against peritonitis, the patency of the lymphatic stomata is crucial.

In the case of intraperitoneal chemotherapy in the treatment of peritoneal carcinomatosis, the goal is to maximize the concentration in the peritoneal cavity and subperitoneal tissue to treat metastasis without significant systemic toxicity [16]. It was demonstrated that for several chemotherapeutic molecules, the total drug exposure is greater for peritoneal fluid and regional lymphatics (reached through the lymphatic stomata) than for plasma [29]. It is likely that the combined action of high levels of chemotherapeutics in the peritoneal cavity and in the subperitoneal lymphatics is instrumental in the success of this adjuvant therapy for selected patients. On the other hand the lymphatic stomata potentially provide a means for dissemination of intraperitoneal free cancer cells, toxins, and microorganisms to the submesothelial tissue and lymph system. In case of peritoneal dialysis, the lymphatic uptake competes with the oppositely directed capillary ultrafiltration. Therefore, it is necessary to add drugs to the dialysate to contract the lymphatic stomata and reduce reabsorption. In studies of mesothelial cell transplantation to improve mesothelial repair after surgery, recurrent peritonitis, or peritoneal dialysis, it was shown that transplanted cells get trapped via the lymphatic stomata in the peritoneal lymphatics resulting in increased solutes and protein transport from the serum to the peritoneal cavity [18].

In conclusion research into the molecular mechanisms involved in the up- or downregulation of the lymph drainage pathway of the peritoneal cavity will have many clinical applications. Furthermore, we need to elucidate the mechanisms involved in the interaction between tumor cells, mesothelium, and macrophages of the milky spots and this in normal and pathological conditions.

REFERENCES

1. Abuhijleh MF, Habbal OA, Moqattash ST. The role of the diaphragm in lymphatic absorption from the peritoneal-cavity. *Journal of Anatomy.* 1995;186:453–467.
2. Allen L. On the penetrability of the lymphatics of the diaphragm. *Anatomical Record.* 1956;124(4):639–657.
3. Allen L. The lymphatics of the parietal tunica vaginalis propria of man. *Anatomical Record.* 1943;85(4):427–433.
4. Allen L. The peritoneal stomata. *Anatomical Record.* 1936;67:89–103.
5. Azzali G. The lymphatic vessels and the so-called "lymphatic stomata" of the diaphragm: A morphologic ultrastructural and three-dimensional study. *Microvascular Research.* 1999;57(1):30–43.
6. Beelen RHJ, Oosterling S, van Egmond M, van den Born J, Zareie M. Omental milky spots in peritoneal pathophysiology (spots before your eyes). *Peritoneal Dialysis International.* 2005;25:30–32.
7. Boulanger B, Yuan Z, Flessner M, Hay J, Johnston M. Pericardial fluid absorption into lymphatic vessels in sheep. *Microvascular Research.* 1999;57(2):174–186.
8. Bridenbaugh EA, Wang W, Srimushnam M, Cromer WE, Zawieja SD, Schmidt SE, Jupiter DC, Huang HC, Van Buren V, Zawieja DC. An immunological fingerprint differentiates muscular lymphatics from arteries and veins. *Lymphatic Research and Biology.* 2013;11(3):155–171.
9. Buxton BH, Torrey JC. Absorption from the peritoneal cavity. *Journal of Medical Research.* 1906;15:1–7.
10. Ceelen WP, Flessner MF. Intraperitoneal therapy for peritoneal tumors: Biophysics and clinical evidence. *Nature Reviews Clinical Oncology.* 2010;7(2):108–115.
11. Clinical Outcomes of Surgical Therapy Study Group. A comparison of laparoscopically assisted and open colectomy for colon cancer. *New England Journal of Medicine.* 2004;350(20):2050–2059.
12. Coccolini F, Gheza F, Lotti M, Virzi S, Iusco D, Ghermandi C, Melotti R, Baiocchi G, Giulini SM, Ansaloni L, Catena, F. Peritoneal carcinomatosis. *World Journal of Gastroenterology.* 2013;19(41):6979–6994.
13. Cunningham RS. The physiology of the serous membranes. *Physiological Reviews.* 1926;6:242–280.
14. Ding SP, Li JC, Xu J, Mao LG. Study on the mechanism of regulation on the peritoneal lymphatic stomata with Chinese herbal medicine. *World Journal of Gastroenterology.* 2002;8(1):188–192.
15. Durden C, Laslie M, Allen L. A method for injecting the lymphatics of serous cavities and for demonstrating a mechanism of lymphatic absorption. *Anatomical Record.* 1964;150(3):335–341.
16. Flessner MF. The transport barrier in intraperitoneal therapy. *American Journal of Physiology—Renal Physiology.* 2005;288(3):F433–F442.
17. Heath RM, Jayne DG, O'Leary R, Morrison EE, Guillou PJ. Tumour-induced apoptosis in human mesothelial cells: A mechanism of peritoneal invasion by Fas Ligand/Fas interaction. *British Journal of Cancer.* 2004;90(7):1437–1442.
18. Hekking LH, Zweers MM, Keuning ED, Driesprong BA, de Waart DR, Beelen RH, van den Born J. Apparent successful mesothelial cell transplantation hampered by peritoneal activation. *Kidney International.* 2005;68(5):2362–2367.
19. Kolossov A. Über die Struktur des Pleuroperitoneal- und Gefäßepithels (endothels). *Archiv für Mikroskopische Anatomie.* 1893;42:318–383.
20. Kusamura S, Baratti D, Zaffaroni N, Villa R, Laterza B, Balestra MR, Deraco M. Pathophysiology and biology of peritoneal carcinomatosis. *World Journal of Gastrointestinal Oncology.* 2010;2(1):12–18.
21. Le O. Patterns of peritoneal spread of tumor in the abdomen and pelvis. *World Journal of Radiology.* 2013;5(3):106–112.
22. Leak LV, Rahil K. Permeability of the diaphragmatic mesothelium. The ultrastructure basis for 'stomata'. *American Journal of Anatomy.* 1978;157:557–594.

23. Li J, Zhou J, Gao Y. The ultrastructure and computer imaging of the lymphatic stomata in the human pelvic peritoneum. *Annals of Anatomy.* 1997;179(3):215–220.

24. Li JC, Yu SM. Study on the ultrastructure of the peritoneal stomata in humans. *Acta Anatomica.* 1991;141(1):26–30.

25. Li JC, Zhao ZG, Zhou JL, Yu SM. A study of the three-dimensional organization of the human diaphragmatic lymphatic lacunae and lymphatic drainage units. *Annals of Anatomy (Anatomischer Anzeiger).* 1996;178(6):537–544.

26. Li YY, Li JC. Effects of nitric oxide on peritoneal lymphatic stomata and lymph drainage via NO-cGMP-Ca2+ pathway. *Sheng Li Xue Bao.* 2005;57(1):45–53.

27. Li YY, Li JC. Cell signal transduction mechanism for nitric oxide regulating lymphatic stomata and its draining capability. *Anatomical Record—Advances in Integrative Anatomy and Evolutionary Biology.* 2008;291(2):216–223.

28. Lin T, Shih J, Lin C, Lin S, Su Y, Lee C. Intraperitoneal and intracardiac transfusion of recurrent fetal erythroblastosis due to anti-M alloimmunization with unfavorable outcome. *Taiwanese Journal of Obstetrics & Gynecology.* 2012;51:253–255.

29. Lindner P, Heath D, Howell S, Naredi P, Hafstrom L. Vasopressin modulation of peritoneal, lymphatic, and plasma drug exposure following intraperitoneal administration. *Clinical Cancer Research.* 1996;2(2):311–317.

30. MacCallum WG. On the relation of the peritoneal cavity in the diaphragm and the mechanism of absorption of granular materials from the peritoneum. *Anatomischer Anzeiger.* 1903;13:157–159.

31. Michailova KN. Postinflammatory changes of the diaphragmatic stomata. *Annals of Anatomy (Anatomischer Anzeiger).* 2001;183(4):309–317.

32. Michailova KN, Usunoff KG. Serosal membranes (pleura, pericardium, peritoneum). Normal structure, development and experimental pathology. *Advances in Anatomy, Embryology, and Cell Biology.* 2006;183: i-vii, 1–144, back cover.

33. Michailova KN, Wassilev WA, Kuhnel W. Features of the peritoneal covering of the lesser pelvis with special reference to stomata regions. *Annals of Anatomy.* 2005;187(1):23–33.

34. Miura T, Shimada T, Tanaka K, Chujo M, Uchida Y. Lymphatic drainage of carbon particles injected into the pleural cavity of the monkey, as studied by video-assisted thoracoscopy and electron microscopy. *Journal of Thoracic and Cardiovascular Surgery.* 2000;120(3):437–447.

35. Negrini D, Mukenge S, Del Fabbro M, Gonano C, Miserocchi G. Distribution of diaphragmatic lymphatic stomata. *Journal of Applied Physiology (1985).* 1991;70(4):1544–1549.

36. Negrini D, Del Fabbro M. Subatmospheric pressure in the rabbit pleural lymphatic network. *Journal of Physiology.* 1999;520(3):761–769.

37. Neuhaus SJ, Watson DI. Pneumoperitoneum and peritoneal surface changes: A review. *Surgical Endoscopy.* 2004;18(9):1316–1322.

38. Parungo CP, Soybel DI, Colson YL, Kim SW, Ohnishi S, DeGrand AM et al. Lymphatic drainage of the peritoneal space: A pattern dependent on bowel lymphatics. *Annals of Surgical Oncology.* 2007;14(2):286–298.

39. Rosario MTA, Ribeiro U, Corbett CEP, Ozaki AC, Bresciani CC, Zilberstein B, Gama-Rodrigues JJ. Does CO_2 pneumoperitoneum alter the ultrastructure of the mesothelium? *Journal of Surgical Research.* 2006;133(2):84–88.

40. Sangisetty SL, Miner TJ. Malignant ascites: A review of prognostic factors, pathophysiology and therapeutic measures. *World Journal of Gastrointestinal Surgery.* 2012;4(4):87–95.

41. Tourneux F. Recherches sur L'Epithelium des Sereuses. *Journal of Anatomy & Physiology.* 1874;10:66–69.

42. Tsilibary EC, Wissig SL. Lymphatic absorption from the peritoneal cavity: Regulation of patency of mesothelial stomata. *Microvascular Research.* 1983;25(1):22–39.

43. Tsilibary EC, Wissig SL. Light and electron microscope observations of the lymphatic drainage units of the peritoneal cavity of rodents. *American Journal of Anatomy.* 1987;180(2):195–207.

44. Tsujimoto H, Takahashi T, Hagiwara A, Shimotsuma M, Sakakura C, Osaki K et al. Site-specific implantation in the milky spots of malignant cells in peritoneal dissemination: Immunohistochemical observation in mice inoculated intraperitoneally with bromodeoxyuridine-labelled cells. *British Journal of Cancer.* 1995;71:468–472.

45. Von Recklinghausen FD. Zur Fettresorbtion. *Virchows Archiv.* 1863;26:172–208.

46. Wang J, Ping Z, Jiang T, Yu H, Wang C, Chen Z, Zhang X, Xu D, Wang L, Li Z, Li JC. Ultrastructure of lymphatic stomata in the tunica vaginalis of humans. *Microscopy and Microanalysis.* 2013;19(6):1405–1409.

47. Wang ZB, Li M, Li JC. Recent advances in the research of lymphatic stomata. *Anatomical Record—Advances in Integrative Anatomy and Evolutionary Biology.* 2010;293(5):754–761.

48. Wassilev W, Wedel T, Michailova K, Kuhnel W. A scanning electron microscopy study of peritoneal stomata in different peritoneal regions. *Annals of Anatomy.* 1998;180(2):137–143.

49. Yonemura Y, Endou Y, Nojima M, Kawamura T, Fujita H, Kaji M et al. A possible role of cytokines in the formation of peritoneal dissemination. *International Journal of Oncology.* 1997;11(2):349–358.

50. Yonemura Y, Kawamura T, Bandou E, Tsukiyama G, Endou Y, Miura M. The natural history of free cancer cells in the peritoneal cavity. *Recent Results in Cancer Research.* 2007;169:11–23.

PART 3

Intraperitoneal Drug Therapy: Basic principles

11

Pharmacokinetics of intraperitoneal cytotoxic drug therapy

KURT VAN DER SPEETEN

INTRODUCTION

The peritoneal surface is an established failure site for digestive and gynecological malignancies, as well as the primary location for some tumors [1–6]. Historical attempts at cure with medical therapy alone or surgery alone have never resulted in long-term survival [3,5–10]. In the absence of systemic metastases, it was thought that disease confined to the peritoneum may be eradicated through optimal cytoreductive surgery (CRS) combined with intraperitoneal (IP) chemotherapy. Several Phase II and III trials have since demonstrated encouraging clinical results for this combined treatment modality [7,9–17]. The pharmacologic evidence in support of this approach is less established. This chapter aims to review the current pharmacokinetic data regarding IP (both normothermic and hyperthermic) chemotherapy following CRS in peritoneal surface malignancy patients.

PHARMACOLOGY

The pharmacology of IP chemotherapy can be subdivided into pharmacokinetics and pharmacodynamics. Whereas pharmacokinetics describes what the body does to the drug, pharmacodynamics looks at what the drug does to the body.

Pharmacokinetics of IP chemotherapy studies the alterations between the moment of administration of the IP chemotherapy and the cancer chemotherapy drug showing up at the level of the tumor nodule. As such, its basic denotation is a concentration over time graph. Pharmacodynamics subsequently looks into the effect of that cancer chemotherapy drug on the tumor. The corresponding illustration is an effect over concentration graph. This artificial division implies that no sound (clinical) conclusions can be based on pharmacokinetic data alone. Pharmacokinetic research seeks to deliver the chemotherapy in the most efficient way possible at the front door of the tumor.

DOSE INTENSIFICATION

The pharmacokinetic rationale of perioperative IP cancer chemotherapy is based on the dose intensification provided by the peritoneal plasma barrier [18]. From peritoneal dialysis research, Dedrick et al. [19] concluded that the peritoneal permeability of a number of hydrophilic anticancer drugs may be considerably less than the plasma clearance of the same drug after IP administration. The peritoneal clearance is inversely proportional to the square root of its molecular weight and results in a higher concentration in the peritoneal cavity than in the plasma after

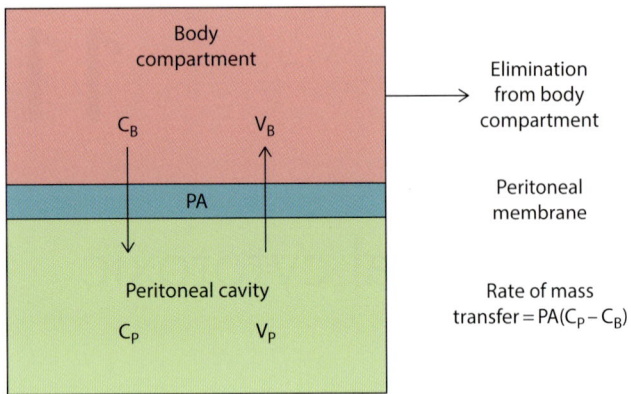

Figure 11.1 The traditional two-compartment model of peritoneal transport, transfer of a drug from the peritoneal cavity to the blood occurs across the "peritoneal membrane." The permeability-area product (PA) governs this transfer. PA is calculated by measuring the rate of drug disappearance from the cavity, which is divided by the overall concentration difference between the peritoneal cavity and the blood (or plasma). C_B, the free drug concentration in the blood (or plasma); V_B, volume of distribution of the drug in the body; C_P, the free drug concentration in the peritoneal fluid; V_P, volume of the peritoneal cavity. (Adapted from Dedrick, R.L. and Flessner, M.F., *J. Natl. Cancer Inst.*, 89(7), 480, 1997; Jackman, D.M., *Semin. Thorac. Cardiovasc. Surg.*, 21(2), 154, 2009.)

IP administration [20,21]. This dose intensification over the peritoneal membrane is nothing but an application of Fick's basic law of diffusion to transperitoneal transport. A simplified mathematical diffusion model considers the plasma to be a single compartment separated from another single compartment, the peritoneal cavity, by an effective membrane (Figure 11.1).

This results in the following equation:

$$\text{Rate of mass transfer} = PA(C_P - C_B)$$

where

PA is the permeability area (PA = effective peritoneal contact area A × permeability P)
C_P is the concentration in peritoneal cavity
C_B is the concentration in the blood [22]

This simple conceptual model indicates the importance of the effective contact area [23]. Although the equation permits calculation of the pharmacokinetic advantage, the model does not reveal anything about the specific penetration of the cancer chemotherapy drug into the tissue or tumor nodule [24], nor does it predict the value of the effective contact area. The model simply describes the transfer between two compartments. After CRS, this concentration difference increases the possibility of exposing residual tumor cells to high doses of chemotherapeutic agents with reduced systemic concentrations and lower systemic toxicity. This advantage is expressed by the area under the curve (AUC) ratios of IP versus plasma (IV) exposure.

PERITONEAL MEMBRANE

The rationale of administering chemotherapeutic drugs into the peritoneal cavity is based on the relative transport barrier formed by the tissue surrounding the peritoneal space. The peritoneum is a complex 3D organ covering the abdominopelvic organs and the abdominal wall and contains a potentially large space [25]. The initial description of the ultrastructure of the peritoneum in man was presented in 1941 by Baron [26]. The peritoneum consists of a monolayer of mesothelial cells supported by a basement membrane and five layers of connective tissue, which account for a total thickness of 90 μm. The connective tissue layers include interstitial cells and a matrix of collagen, hyaluronan, and proteoglycans. The cellular component consists of pericytes, parenchymal cells, and blood capillaries [25,27]. This complex is often referred to as the peritoneal membrane, and the description is a working model derived from research on the peritoneum as a dialysis membrane [28,29]. Contrary to intuitive thinking, the elimination of the mesothelial lining during peritonectomy procedures does not alter the pharmacokinetic properties of the peritoneum in the transport of chemotherapeutic agents from the peritoneal cavity to the plasma compartment. In a rodent model, Flessner et al. [30] demonstrated that neither removal of the stagnant fluid layer on the mesothelium nor removal of the mesothelial lining influences the mass transfer coefficient over the barrier. There is indirect evidence supporting this hypothesis in humans in that the extent of the parietal peritonectomy in peritoneal carcinomatosis (PC) patients does little to alter the IP chemotherapy pharmacokinetics of mitomycin C or 5-fluorouracil [31,32]. Extensive visceral peritonectomies seem to decrease peritoneal clearance of doxorubicin and mitomycin C [33,34]. Basic research indicates [22,28] that it is the submesothelial blood capillary wall and the surrounding interstitial matrix that are the principal barriers for clearance of molecules from the abdominopelvic space, not the mesothelial lining. Fluid enters the vascular compartment by diffusion from the peritoneal compartment or by absorption through the peritoneal lymphatic stomata, which are concentrated to the diaphragmatic surface [22,35–37]. Diffusion of fluid through the parietal peritoneum generally results in flow to the plasma compartment and drainage through the visceral peritoneum covering the surfaces of liver, spleen, stomach, small and large bowel, and mesentery is into the portal venous blood [25,27].

CANCER CHEMOTHERAPY DRUGS FOR INTRAPERITONEAL APPLICATION

IP application of a wide variety of cancer chemotherapy drugs was explored. The rationale for their administration was mostly based on the combination of extrapolation of data of systemic chemotherapy and perceived beneficial pharmacologic properties such as high molecular weight.

Table 11.1 summarizes the pharmacologic properties of the cancer chemotherapy drugs most frequently selected for IP application.

Table 11.1 Cancer chemotherapy drugs for intraperitoneal application

Drug	Type	Molecular weight (Da)	Dose	Exposure time	AUC ratio	Penetration depth	Thermal augmentation	Remarks
Cisplatin	Alkylator	300.1	50–250 mg/m²	30 minutes to 20 hours	7.8–21	1–5 mm	Yes	Dose-limiting nephrotoxicity
Carboplatin	Alkylator	371.25	200–800 mg/m²	30 minutes to 20 hours	1.9–10	0.5–9 mm	Yes	
Oxaliplatin	Alkylator	397.3	360–460 mg/m²	30 minutes to 20 hours	3.5–16	1–2 mm	Yes	Dextrose-based carrier
Melphalan	Alkylator	305.2	50–70 mg/m²	90–120 minutes	93		Yes	Rapid degradation
Mitomycin C	Antitumor antibiotic	334.3	15–35 mg/m²	90–150 minutes	10–23.5	2 mm	Yes	
Doxorubicin	Antitumor antibiotic	579.99	15–75 mg/m²	90 minutes	162–579	4–6-cell layers	Yes	
Docetaxel	Antimicrotubule agent	861.9	45–150 mg/m²	30 minutes to 23 hours	552	NA	Conflicting data	Cell-cycle-specific
Paclitaxel	Antimicrotubule agent	853.9	20 mg/m² to 180 mg total dose	30 minutes to 23 hours	1000	≥80 layers	Conflicting data	Cell-cycle-specific
5-Fluorouracil	Antimetabolite	130.08	650 mg/m² for 5 days (EPIC)	23 hours	250	0.2 mm	Yes, mild	Cell-cycle-specific
Gemcitabine	Antimetabolite	299.5	50–1000 mg/m²	60 minutes to 24 hours	500	NA	NA	Cell-cycle-specific
Pemetrexed	Antimetabolite	471.4	500 mg/m²	24 hours	19.2	NA	NA	Cell-cycle-specific

Cisplatin

Cisplatin (*cis*-diamminedichloroplatinum-III [CDDP]) is an alkylating agent that causes apoptotic cell death by formation of DNA adducts [38]. Both normothermic and hyperthermic IP applications have been explored in the treatment of ovarian cancer, gastric cancer, desmoplastic small round cell tumor, and peritoneal mesothelioma [13,16,17,39–42]. It is eliminated by renal excretion and consequently the main concern with its use is renal toxicity. Urano and coworkers showed an excellent in vitro and in vivo thermal augmentation of cisplatin [43]. The penetration of cisplatin into tumor nodules was studied by several groups. Los et al. for the first time described intratumoral distribution of cisplatin after IP administration and suggested that the advantage over IP versus IV administration was maximal in the first 1.5 mm [38]. Van de Vaart et al. investigated the cisplatin-induced DNA adduct formation and could measure this 3–5 mm into the tumor tissue [44]. Esquis et al. in an experimental model reported an enhanced cisplatin penetration when cisplatin was administered with increased pressure [45].

Carboplatin

Carboplatin ((1,1-cyclobutanedicarboxylate)platinum(II)) is a higher molecular weight platinum compound than cisplatin mainly explored for IP use in PC from ovarian origin [46–49]. Its main advantage is its decreased renal toxicity. In 1991, Los and coworkers compared carboplatin and cisplatin after IP administration in a rat model. They demonstrated that despite a clear pharmacokinetic advantage of IP carboplatin over cisplatin, its capacity to penetrate into peritoneal cancer nodules and tumor cells is far lower than that of cisplatin [50]. More recent pharmacokinetic data by Jandial et al. suggested the contrary [51]. This once again stresses the importance of tumor nodule characteristics (density, vascularity, etc.) in the final amount of chemotherapy reaching the tumor cells. Czejka et al. in a clinical study with normothermic carboplatin reported a relative bioavailability (calculated as AUC values), which was at least six times higher in the IP fluid than in the serum for 48 hours [52].

Oxaliplatin

Oxaliplatin (oxalato-1,2-diaminocyclohexane-platinum(II)) is a third-generation platinum complex with proven cytotoxicity in colon and appendiceal neoplasms [53]. In a dose escalation and pharmacokinetic study Elias et al. demonstrated that 460 mg/m² of oxaliplatin in 2 L/m² of chemotherapy solution over 30 minutes was well tolerated [54]. The low AUC ratio is compensated by the rapid absorption of the drug into the tissue. Most pharmacokinetics studies of IP oxaliplatin during hyperthermic intraperitoneal peroperative chemotherapy (HIPEC) have been based on the use of atomic absorption spectroscopy, an unselective analytical technique measuring the total platinum content [55,56]. This method will codetermine oxaliplatin and platinum-containing

cytotoxic and biologically inactive biotransformation products. Mahteme et al. in 2008 using a chromatographic technique demonstrated that the systemic exposure of oxaliplatin measured after HIPEC using a selective analytical technique is considerably lower than previously reported [57]. In contrast to cisplatin and mitomycin, traditionally, oxaliplatin is considered not stable in chloride-containing solutions. This necessitates a dextrose-based carrier, which may result in serious electrolyte disturbances and hyperglycemia during the intracavitary therapy [58]. Unknown to most, this degradation only accounts for 3% of the total amount at 30 minutes as when applied during HIPEC [59]. Oxaliplatin is subject to substantial heath augmentation [43,60].

Mitomycin C

Mitomycin C is an alkylating tumor antibiotic extracted from *Streptomyces* species, for which the most important mechanism of action is through DNA cross-linking. Although mitomycin C is not regarded as a prodrug, it is not active against cancerous tissue as the unchanged molecule. The drug is modified as it enters the cell into an active state [61]. It is inactivated by microsomal enzymes in the liver and is metabolized in the spleen and kidneys. Jacquet et al. reported a clear pharmacokinetic advantage after IP administration with an AUC IP/IV ratio of 23.5 [31]. It is used for PC from colorectal cancer, appendiceal cancer, ovarian cancer, and gastric cancer and for diffuse malignant peritoneal mesothelioma both as HIPEC and early postoperative intraperitoneal chemotherapy (EPIC) [9,10,31,34,62–64]. Barlogie et al. suggested in vitro thermal enhancement of mitomycin C [65]. Our pharmacokinetic data in 145 HIPEC patients suggest that the largest proportion (62%) of the total drug administered remained in the body at 90 minutes [34]. This is in line with similar findings by Jacquet et al. and van Ruth et al. [31,66]. The location and chemical state of this large amount of retained mitomycin C remains to be determined. Unfortunately, a reliable assay of tissue mitomycin C concentrations does not exist; determination of the anatomic site and anticancer activity of this large proportion of the total mitomycin C administered has not been determined. Controversies still exist regarding the proper dosimetry of the chemotherapy solution.

Doxorubicin

Doxorubicin or hydroxydaunorubicin (adriamycin) is an anthracycline antibiotic. Initial research categorized it as a DNA-intercalating drug. Triton et al. later demonstrated that the actual mechanism of action is a critical interaction of doxorubicin with the cell surface membrane [67,68]. Subsequently, Lane et al. reported this phenomenon to be temperature dependent [69]. Doxorubicin was considered a candidate for IP application based on its wide in vitro and in vivo activity against a broad range of malignancies, its slow clearance from the peritoneal compartment due to the high molecular weight of the hydrochloride salt, and its favorable AUC ratio of IP to intravenous concentration times of

230 [42,70–74]. The dose-limiting cardiotoxicity when administered IV can also be avoided. Pilati et al. suggested a mild hyperthermic augmentation based on increased drug uptake and sensitization of tumor cells (but not normal mucosal cells) to the cytotoxic effects of doxorubicin [75,76]. More recently pegylated liposomal doxorubicin has generated interest for HIPEC application due to its favorable pharmacokinetics [77,78]. Doxorubicin-based HIPEC has been used in peritoneal surface malignancy (PSM) from appendiceal, gastric, ovarian, and colon cancer, as well as in peritoneal mesothelioma.

Taxanes

Paclitaxel and docetaxel with their high molecular weight have a remarkable high AUC ratio of 853 and 861, respectively [79]. The taxanes stabilize the microtubule against depolymerization, thereby disrupting normal microtubule dynamics [80]. There is evidence supporting additional mechanisms of action [81]. They exert cytotoxic activity against a broad range of tumors. This translates itself into a clear pharmacokinetic advantage for IP administration [82]. The data regarding possible thermal augmentation of taxanes are conflicting [81]. Taxanes have been used in a neoadjuvant intraperitoneal and systemic chemotherapy (NIPS) setting as well as intraoperatively and postoperatively. Their cell-cycle-specific mechanism of action makes them a better candidate for repetitive application such as in EPIC, NIPS, or normothermic adjuvant postoperative IP chemotherapy. Novel formulations of taxanes aiming at an increased bioavailability are under investigation [83].

5-Fluorouracil

Since their introduction in 1957 by Heidelberger et al., the fluorinated pyrimidines have been successfully used for a wide variety of tumors and are still an essential component of all successful gastrointestinal cancer chemotherapy regimens [84,85]. This thymidylate synthase inhibitor binds covalently with the enzyme and prevents the formation of thymidine monophosphate, the DNA nucleoside precursor. Also 5-FU by its metabolites 5-fluoro-uridine diphosphate and 5-fluoro-uridine triphosphate gets incorporated in RNA, resulting in a second cytotoxic pathway. The action of 5-fluorouracil is therefore cell-cycle-specific. These characteristics limit the use of IP 5-fluorouracil to EPIC [86–89]. Minor augmentation of 5-fluorouracil by mild hyperthermia is reported [31]. 5-Fluorouracil is not chemically compatible with other drugs in a mixed solution for infusion or instillation.

Gemcitabine

Gemcitabine (2′,2′-difluorodeoxycytidine) is a pyrimidine analogue with a wide range of in vitro cytotoxic activity, particularly against pancreatic cancer. Pestieau et al. investigated the PK and tissue distribution of IP gemcitabine in a rat model [90]. The AUC ratio (IP/IV) after IP administration was 26.8 ± 5.8 and as such favorable for IP administration. Several investigators explored the use of both IP gemcitabine in both HIPEC and EPIC protocols for pancreatic and ovarian cancer [91–97].

Pemetrexed

Pemetrexed is multitargeted antifolate that belongs to the antimetabolites. It is an analogue of folic acid with cytotoxic activity against a variety of malignancies, especially mesothelioma, ovarian cancer and colon cancer. Significant survival improvement for patients with peritoneal and pleural mesothelioma after IV administration and favorable PK has generated interest in its IP application [98]. It acts mainly as a thymidylate synthase inhibitor but is also unique in terms of cellular transport and lipid solubility [99]. Pestieau et al. reported favorable IP PK with a 24-fold increase of peritoneal exposure after IP instillation when compared to IV administration [94]. It is currently under investigation for the IP treatment of peritoneal mesothelioma and ovarian cancer [100].

Melphalan

Melphalan (nitrogen mustard) is an alkylator with exceptional thermal enhancement [101,102]. Successful application of melphalan in other regional chemotherapy techniques such as isolated limb perfusion and isolated liver perfusion with high response rates generated interest for its potential IP administration [103–106].

Mild hyperthermia results in a remarkable increase in tissue absorption of the melphalan [107]. One environmental disadvantage is its rapid hydrolysis necessitating an operating room preparation of the IP solution and immediate application.

Its broad spectrum of cytotoxic activity has resulted in it being the prime choice of "salvage" cancer chemotherapy drug for repeat procedures.

PHARMACOLOGIC VARIABLES

Table 11.2 summarizes the most important pharmacokinetic and pharmacodynamic variables that characterize the pharmacology of IP chemotherapy. Unfortunately, this has resulted in a wide variability of cancer chemotherapy regimens applied during HIPEC and EPIC worldwide. A remarkable number of these IP chemotherapy regimens are based on little pharmacologic evidence supporting their application. Also, this substantially hampers evidence-based comparison of the regimens available. The concept of IP chemotherapy in PC patients after optimal CRS has been proven in phase II–III trials. Further

Table 11.2 Pharmacologic variables governing IP chemotherapy

Pharmacokinetic VR	Pharmacodynamic VR
Dose	Tumor nodule size
Volume	Density
Duration	Vascularity
Carrier solution	Interstitial fluid pressure
Pressure	Binding
Molecular weight	Temperature

improvement should come from both well-designed randomized trials and pharmacological guidance. There is an urgent need for standardization of the HIPEC and EPIC regimens based on structured pharmacokinetic research.

Carrier solution

Hypotonic, isotonic, and hypertonic solutions were explored with both low and high molecular weight chemotherapy molecules. Salt-based, dextrose-based, hetastarch, or icodextrin solutions have been used [108–113]. Also, stability of the chemotherapeutic agent in the chosen carrier should be considered [59]. The ideal carrier solution should enhance the exposure of the peritoneal surface and residual tumor cells to the chemotherapeutic agent. This is especially important in the setting of EPIC where maintenance of a high dwell volume of perfusate over a prolonged time period improves the distribution of the drug and the effectiveness of the treatment.

In a HIPEC setting with a relatively short dwell time, one could theoretically expect a pharmacodynamic advantage of a hypotonic carrier through the mechanism of increased tissue and tumor absorption. Contrary to experimental studies supporting this hypothesis, Elias et al. showed in humans no increase in tumor penetration. A concomitant high incidence (50%) of postoperative peritoneal bleeding and severe thrombocytopenia has contraindicated the further clinical use of hypotonic carriers [113].

Duration

A wide variation in the duration (ranging from 30 to 120 minutes) of HIPEC protocols are reported. The dose–response curves and their dependency on exposure time have been mathematically modeled by Gardner [114], and according to this model, a plateau in tumor cell kill will be reached, after which prolonged exposure time offers no further cytotoxic advantage. Theoretically, the most advantageous exposure time for cytotoxic effects in PC patients should be carefully weighed against systemic exposure and bone marrow toxicity and degradation processes. Duration of perioperative chemotherapy regimens should be pharmacology-driven and not arbitrary.

CONCENTRATION-BASED VERSUS BSA-BASED IP CHEMOTHERAPY

One of the most pressing issues needing resolution in IP chemotherapy is whether the dosimetry of the IP regimens should be body surface area (BSA) based versus concentration based. Most groups use a drug dose based on calculated BSA (mg/m²) in analogy to systemic chemotherapy regimens. Several groups reported a correlation between BSA and physiological functions (e.g., cardiac output, clearance) after systemic administration [115–118]. This resulted in a good prediction of systemic exposure after IV chemotherapy. Such correlation has not been substantiated after IP administration.

These regimens take BSA as a measure for the effective contact area = peritoneal surface area in the Dedrick formula.

Rubin et al. [115] demonstrate that there is an imperfect correlation between actual peritoneal surface area and calculated body surface area and there may be sex differences in peritoneal surface areas, which in turn affects absorption characteristics. The female has a 10% larger peritoneal surface in proportion to body size than the male [115,116]. There have been attempts to estimate the functional peritoneal surface area through applying stereologic methods to CT scans a by extrapolating data from cadaver measurements [117,118]. BSA-based IP chemotherapy will result in a fixed dose (BSA based) diluted in varying volumes of perfusate, that is, different concentrations depending on substantial differences in the body composition of patients and differences in the HIPEC technique (open vs. closed abdomen).

From the aforementioned Dedrick formula, we know that peritoneal concentration and not peritoneal dose is the driving diffusion force. The importance of this has been discussed by Elias et al. [55]. In a clinical investigation where 2, 4, and 6 L of chemotherapy solution was administered with a constant dose of chemotherapy solution, a more dilute IP chemotherapy concentration retarded the clearance of chemotherapy and resulted in less systemic toxicity [119]. Therefore, it can be assumed that by the diffusion model, less concentrated chemotherapy would penetrate less into the cancer nodules and into normal tissues. Concentration-based chemotherapy offers a more predictable exposure of the tumor nodules to the IP chemotherapy [120] and thus efficacy. Unfortunately, the prize to be paid for a better prediction of the efficacy of the IP chemotherapy is a high unpredictability of the plasmatic cancer chemotherapy levels and thus toxicity. Indeed, according to the aforementioned Dedrick formula of transport over the peritoneal membrane, an increase in the volume of concentration-based IP chemotherapy solution will cause an increase in both diffusion surface and the amount of drug transferred from peritoneal space to plasma. PK data in PSM patients substantiate this hypothesis. Figure 11.2 demonstrates that in 10 PSM patients with a markedly contracted abdomen and small filling volume during HIPEC with mitomycin C, there is statistically significant less transfer of the drug over the peritoneal membrane [34]. In contrast and clinically more important is the situation in PSM patients with preoperative abdominal distention due to ascites or mucus accumulation. Their significantly increased peritoneal surface area will result in higher plasmatic levels of the cancer chemotherapy drug and thus increased risk or toxicity.

TUMOR NODULE AS PHARMACOKINETIC ENDPOINT

Until recently, the pharmacologic efficacy of IP cancer chemotherapy protocols was assessed by looking at the pharmacokinetics of the IP and IV compartment. The efficacy of the IP protocol was then quantified by calculating the AUC ratio of the IP exposure over the AUC of the IV exposure. This takes not into account the important (pharmacodynamic) alterations taking place inside the tumor nodule. Figure 11.3 demonstrates that the

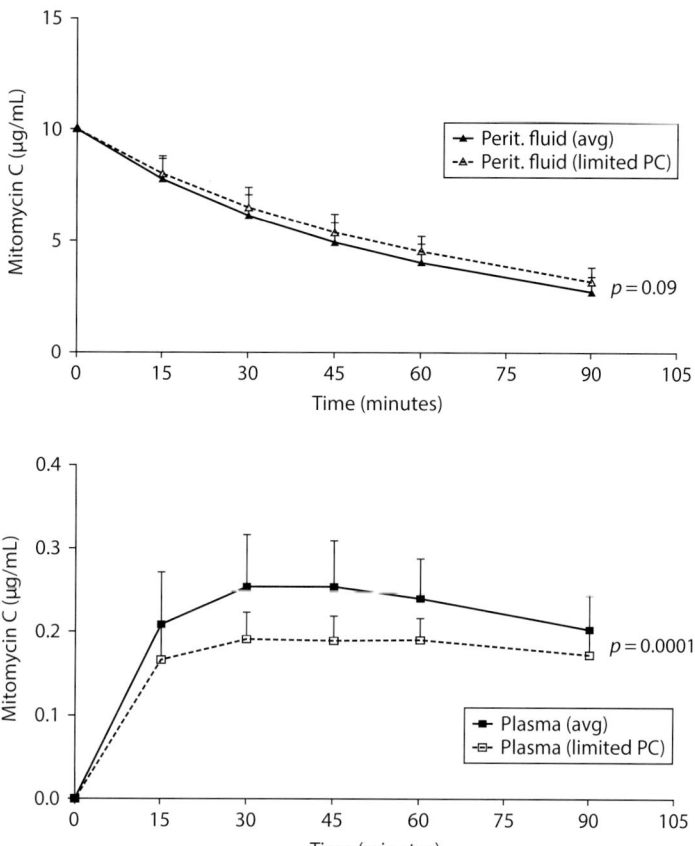

Figure 11.2 Study of a limited peritoneal space and its effect on pharmacokinetics of mitomycin C during HIPEC. The peritoneal fluid (top) and plasma (bottom) AUC are plotted in two groups of patients. One subgroup of 10 patients could receive into the intraperitoneal space only 65% or less of the total volume of chemotherapy solution. The concentrations of mitomycin C in this group were compared to the average of that in the 145 patients. With a limited peritoneal space, there is less mitomycin C absorbed into the plasma ($p = 0.0001$).

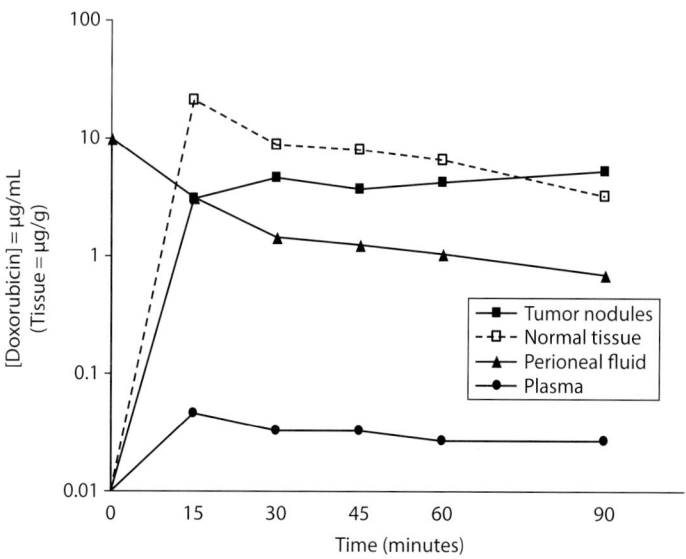

Figure 11.3 Doxorubicin concentrations in plasma, peritoneal fluid, tumor nodules, and normal adjacent tissues. (From Van der Speeten, K. et al., *Cancer Chemother. Pharmacol.*, 63(5), 799, 2009.)

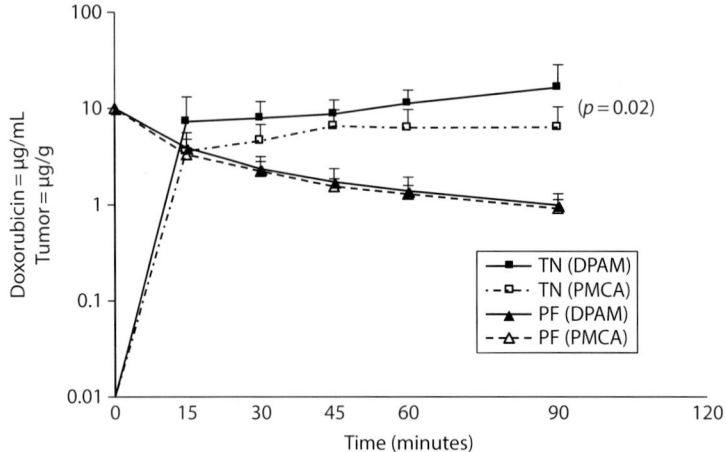

Figure 11.4 Doxorubicin levels in appendiceal tumor tissue showing PAM versus PMCA. Peritoneal fluid concentrations are also shown. TN, tumor nodule; PF, peritoneal fluid. (From Van der Speeten, K. et al., *Cancer Chemother. Pharmacol.*, 63(5), 799, 2009.)

pharmacodynamic event of doxorubicin binding to the tumor nodule results in higher intratumoral concentrations than can be predicted by the simple IP/IV pharmacokinetics. Another example of the equal importance of pharmacodynamics is shown in Figure 11.4. With identical pharmacokinetics the amount of doxorubicin showing up in the less dense diffuse peritoneal adenomucinosis subtype of appendiceal malignancy PC is statistically significantly lower than in the denser peritoneal mucinous carcinomatosis nodules [70]. The identical pharmacokinetic advantage (expressed as AUC IP/IV ratios) resulted in different drug levels according to the density of the tumor nodules: this stressed the importance of pharmacodynamic variables such as tumor nodule density, size, and vascularity. An increased awareness of the pharmacodynamic aspects of these treatment protocols has also been reported by Ceelen et al. [97]. Therefore, it was proposed that the tumor nodule was a more appropriate pharmacological endpoint than AUC ratios.

CONCLUSIONS

The last two decades saw the emergence of perioperative cancer chemotherapy protocols in the treatment of PC patients. This has resulted in remarkable clinical successes in contrast with prior failures. Now that the concept is proven, time has come to further improve the treatment protocols. Building more pharmacologic data on perioperative chemotherapy in PC patients should result in both more standardization and better clinical outcome.

REFERENCES

1. Brodsky JT, Cohen AM. Peritoneal seeding following potentially curative resection of colonic carcinoma: Implications for adjuvant therapy. *Diseases of the Colon and Rectum.* 1991;34(8):723–727.

2. Chu DZ, Lang NP, Thompson C, Osteen PK, Westbrook KC. Peritoneal carcinomatosis in nongynecologic malignancy. A prospective study of prognostic factors. *Cancer.* 1989;63(2):364–367.

3. Jayne DG, Fook S, Loi C, Seow-Choen F. Peritoneal carcinomatosis from colorectal cancer. *British Journal of Surgery.* 2002;89(12):1545–1550.

4. Sadeghi B, Arvieux C, Glehen O, Beaujard AC, Rivoire M, Baulieux J et al. Peritoneal carcinomatosis from non-gynecologic malignancies. *Cancer.* 2000;88(2):358–363.

5. Segelman J, Granath F, Holm T, Machado M, Mahteme H, Martling A. Incidence, prevalence and risk factors for peritoneal carcinomatosis from colorectal cancer. *The British Journal of Surgery.* 2012;99(5):699–705.

6. Shepherd NA, Baxter KJ, Love SB. The prognostic importance of peritoneal involvement in colonic cancer: A prospective evaluation. *Gastroenterology.* 1997;112(4):1096–1102.

7. Franko J, Shi Q, Goldman CD, Pockaj BA, Nelson GD, Goldberg RM et al. Treatment of colorectal peritoneal carcinomatosis with systemic chemotherapy: A pooled analysis of north central cancer treatment group phase III trials N9741 and N9841. *Journal of Clinical Oncology: Official Journal of the American Society of Clinical Oncology.* 2012;30(3):263–267.

8. Klaver YL, Simkens LH, Lemmens VE, Koopman M, Teerenstra S, Bleichrodt RP et al. Outcomes of colorectal cancer patients with peritoneal carcinomatosis treated with chemotherapy with and without targeted therapy. *European Journal of Surgical Oncology: The Journal of the European Society of Surgical Oncology and the British Association of Surgical Oncology.* 2012;38(7):617–623.

9. Verwaal VJ, Bruin S, Boot H, van Slooten G, van Tinteren H. 8-Year follow-up of randomized trial: Cytoreduction and hyperthermic intraperitoneal chemotherapy versus systemic chemotherapy in patients with peritoneal carcinomatosis of colorectal cancer. *Annals of Surgical Oncology*. 2008;15(9):2426–2432.

10. Verwaal VJ, van Ruth S, de Bree E, van Sloothen GW, van Tinteren H, Boot H et al. Randomized trial of cytoreduction and hyperthermic intraperitoneal chemotherapy versus systemic chemotherapy and palliative surgery in patients with peritoneal carcinomatosis of colorectal cancer. *Journal of Clinical Oncology: Official Journal of the American Society of Clinical Oncology*. 2003;21(20):3737–3743.

11. Glehen O, Gilly FN, Boutitie F, Bereder JM, Quenet F, Sideris L et al. Toward curative treatment of peritoneal carcinomatosis from nonovarian origin by cytoreductive surgery combined with perioperative intraperitoneal chemotherapy: A multi-institutional study of 1,290 patients. *Cancer*. 2010;116(24):5608–5618.

12. Chua TC, Moran BJ, Sugarbaker PH, Levine EA, Glehen O, Gilly FN et al. Early- and long-term outcome data of patients with pseudomyxoma peritonei from appendiceal origin treated by a strategy of cytoreductive surgery and hyperthermic intraperitoneal chemotherapy. *Journal of Clinical Oncology: Official Journal of the American Society of Clinical Oncology*. 2012;30(20):2449–2456.

13. Coccolini F, Cotte E, Glehen O, Lotti M, Poiasina E, Catena F et al. Intraperitoneal chemotherapy in advanced gastric cancer. Meta-analysis of randomized trials. *European Journal of Surgical Oncology: The Journal of the European Society of Surgical Oncology and the British Association of Surgical Oncology*. 2014;40(1):12–26.

14. Glehen O, Gilly FN, Arvieux C, Cotte E, Boutitie F, Mansvelt B et al. Peritoneal carcinomatosis from gastric cancer: A multi-institutional study of 159 patients treated by cytoreductive surgery combined with perioperative intraperitoneal chemotherapy. *Annals of Surgical Oncology*. 2010;17(9):2370–2377.

15. Markman M, Bundy BN, Alberts DS, Fowler JM, Clark-Pearson DL, Carson LF et al. Phase III trial of standard-dose intravenous cisplatin plus paclitaxel versus moderately high-dose carboplatin followed by intravenous paclitaxel and intraperitoneal cisplatin in small-volume stage III ovarian carcinoma: An intergroup study of the Gynecologic Oncology Group, Southwestern Oncology Group, and Eastern Cooperative Oncology Group. *Journal of Clinical Oncology: Official Journal of the American Society of Clinical Oncology*. 2001;19(4):1001–1007.

16. Armstrong DK, Bundy B, Wenzel L, Huang HQ, Baergen R, Lele S et al. Intraperitoneal cisplatin and paclitaxel in ovarian cancer. *The New England Journal of Medicine*. 2006;354(1):34–43.

17. Alberts DS, Liu PY, Hannigan EV, O'Toole R, Williams SD, Young JA et al. Intraperitoneal cisplatin plus intravenous cyclophosphamide versus intravenous cisplatin plus intravenous cyclophosphamide for stage III ovarian cancer. *The New England Journal of Medicine*. 1996;335(26):1950–1955.

18. Ceelen WP, Flessner MF. Intraperitoneal therapy for peritoneal tumors: Biophysics and clinical evidence. *Nature Reviews. Clinical Oncology*. 2010;7(2):108–115.

19. Dedrick RL, Myers CE, Bungay PM, DeVita VT Jr. Pharmacokinetic rationale for peritoneal drug administration in the treatment of ovarian cancer. *Cancer Treatment Reports*. 1978;62(1):1–11.

20. Flessner MF, Fenstermacher JD, Dedrick RL, Blasberg RG. A distributed model of peritoneal-plasma transport: Tissue concentration gradients. *The American Journal of Physiology*. 1985;248(3 Pt. 2):F425–F435.

21. Dedrick RL. Theoretical and experimental bases of intraperitoneal chemotherapy. *Seminars in Oncology*. 1985;12(3 Suppl. 4):1–6.

22. Flessner MF. The transport barrier in intraperitoneal therapy. *American Journal of Physiology—Renal Physiology*. 2005;288(3):F433–F442.

23. Flessner MF, Lofthouse J, Williams A. Increasing peritoneal contact area during dialysis improves mass transfer. *Journal of the American Society of Nephrology*. 2001;12(10):2139–2145.

24. Flessner MF. Intraperitoneal drug therapy: Physical and biological principles. *Cancer Treatment and Research*. 2007;134:131–152.

25. Michailova KN, Usunoff KG. Serosal membranes (pleura, pericardium, peritoneum). Normal structure, development and experimental pathology. *Advances in Anatomy, Embryology, and Cell Biology*. 2006;183:i–vii, 1–144, back cover.

26. Baron MA. Structure of the intestinal peritoneum in man. *American Journal of Anatomy*. 1941;69(3):439–497.

27. Nagy JA, Jackman RW. Anatomy and physiology of the peritoneal membrane. *Seminars in Dialysis*. 1998;11(1):49–56.

28. Flessner MF. Endothelial glycocalyx and the peritoneal barrier. *Peritoneal Dialysis International: Journal of the International Society for Peritoneal Dialysis*. 2008;28(1):6–12.

29. Anglani F, Forino M, Del Prete D, Ceol M, Favaro S. Molecular biology of the peritoneal membrane: In between morphology and function. *Contributions to Nephrology*. 2001(131):61–73.

30. Flessner M, Henegar J, Bigler S, Genous L. Is the peritoneum a significant transport barrier in peritoneal dialysis? *Peritoneal Dialysis International: Journal of the International Society for Peritoneal Dialysis.* 2003;23(6):542–549.

31. Jacquet P, Averbach A, Stephens AD, Stuart OA, Chang D, Sugarbaker PH. Heated intraoperative intraperitoneal mitomycin C and early postoperative intraperitoneal 5-fluorouracil: Pharmacokinetic studies. *Oncology.* 1998;55(2):130–138.

32. de Lima Vazquez V, Stuart OA, Mohamed F, Sugarbaker PH. Extent of parietal peritonectomy does not change intraperitoneal chemotherapy pharmacokinetics. *Cancer Chemotherapy and Pharmacology.* 2003;52(2):108–112.

33. Sugarbaker PH, Van der Speeten K, Anthony Stuart O, Chang D. Impact of surgical and clinical factors on the pharmacology of intraperitoneal doxorubicin in 145 patients with peritoneal carcinomatosis. *European Journal of Surgical Oncology: The Journal of the European Society of Surgical Oncology and the British Association of Surgical Oncology.* 2011;37(8):719–726.

34. Van der Speeten K, Stuart OA, Chang D, Mahteme H, Sugarbaker PH. Changes induced by surgical and clinical factors in the pharmacology of intraperitoneal mitomycin C in 145 patients with peritoneal carcinomatosis. *Cancer Chemotherapy and Pharmacology.* 2011;68(1):147–156.

35. Wang ZB, Li M, Li JC. Recent advances in the research of lymphatic stomata. *Anatomical Record.* 2010;293(5):754–761.

36. Wassilev W, Wedel T, Michailova K, Kuhnel W. A scanning electron microscopy study of peritoneal stomata in different peritoneal regions. *Annals of Anatomy (Anatomischer Anzeiger): Official Organ of the Anatomische Gesellschaft.* 1998;180(2):137–143.

37. Michailova K, Wassilev W, Wedel T. Scanning and transmission electron microscopic study of visceral and parietal peritoneal regions in the rat. *Annals of Anatomy (Anatomischer Anzeiger): Official Organ of the Anatomische Gesellschaft.* 1999;181(3):253–260.

38. Los G, Mutsaers PH, van der Vijgh WJ, Baldew GS, de Graaf PW, McVie JG. Direct diffusion of *cis*-diamminedichloroplatinum(II) in intraperitoneal rat tumors after intraperitoneal chemotherapy: A comparison with systemic chemotherapy. *Cancer Research.* 1989;49(12):3380–3384.

39. Conti M, De Giorgi U, Tazzari V, Bezzi F, Baccini C. Clinical pharmacology of intraperitoneal cisplatin-based chemotherapy. *Journal of Chemotherapy.* 2004;16(Suppl. 5):23–25.

40. Gladieff L, Chatelut E, Dalenc F, Ferron G. Pharmacological bases of intraperitoneal chemotherapy. *Bulletin du Cancer.* 2009;96(12):1235–1242.

41. Zivanovic O, Abramian A, Kullmann M, Fuhrmann C, Coch C, Hoeller T et al. HIPEC ROC I: A phase I study of cisplatin administered as hyperthermic intraoperative intraperitoneal chemoperfusion followed by postoperative intravenous platinum-based chemotherapy in patients with platinum-sensitive recurrent epithelial ovarian cancer. *International Journal of Cancer.* February 1, 2015;136(3):699–708.

42. Van der Speeten K, Stuart OA, Sugarbaker PH. Pharmacology of perioperative intraperitoneal and intravenous chemotherapy in patients with peritoneal surface malignancy. *Surgical Oncology Clinics of North America.* 2012;21(4):577–597.

43. Urano M, Kuroda M, Nishimura Y. For the clinical application of thermochemotherapy given at mild temperatures. *International Journal of Hyperthermia: The Official Journal of European Society for Hyperthermic Oncology, North American Hyperthermia Group.* 1999;15(2):79–107.

44. van de Vaart PJ, van der Vange N, Zoetmulder FA, van Goethem AR, van Tellingen O, ten Bokkel Huinink WW et al. Intraperitoneal cisplatin with regional hyperthermia in advanced ovarian cancer: Pharmacokinetics and cisplatin-DNA adduct formation in patients and ovarian cancer cell lines. *European Journal of Cancer.* 1998;34(1):148–154.

45. Esquis P, Consolo D, Magnin G, Pointaire P, Moretto P, Ynsa MD et al. High intra-abdominal pressure enhances the penetration and antitumor effect of intraperitoneal cisplatin on experimental peritoneal carcinomatosis. *Annals of Surgery.* 2006;244(1):106–112.

46. Suh DH, Kim JW, Kang S, Kim HJ, Lee KH. Major clinical research advances in gynecologic cancer in 2013. *Journal of Gynecologic Oncology.* 2014;25(3):236–248.

47. Barrios M, Diaz J, Schroeder E, Estape R, Angel K, Estape R. Combination intraperitoneal carboplatin and intravenous and intraperitoneal paclitaxel in the management of advanced-stage ovarian cancer. *Obstetrics and Gynecology.* 2014;123(Suppl. 1):90s.

48. Milczek T, Klasa-Mazurkiewicz D, Sznurkowski J, Emerich J. Regimens with intraperitoneal cisplatin plus intravenous cyclophosphamide and intraperitoneal carboplatin plus intravenous cyclophosphamide are equally effective in second line intraperitoneal chemotherapy for advanced ovarian cancer. *Advances in Medical Sciences.* 2012;57(1):46–50.

49. Morgan MA, Sill MW, Fujiwara K, Greer B, Rubin SC, Degeest K et al. A phase I study with an expanded cohort to assess the feasibility of intraperitoneal carboplatin and intravenous paclitaxel in untreated ovarian, fallopian tube, and primary peritoneal carcinoma: A Gynecologic Oncology Group study. *Gynecologic Oncology.* 2011;121(2):264–268.

50. Los G, Verdegaal EE, Mutsaers PA, McVie JG. Penetration of carboplatin and cisplatin into rat peritoneal tumor nodules after intraperitoneal chemotherapy. *Cancer Chemotherapy and Pharmacology.* 1991;28(3):159–165.

51. Jandial DD, Messer K, Farshchi-Heydari S, Pu M, Howell SB. Tumor platinum concentration following intraperitoneal administration of cisplatin versus carboplatin in an ovarian cancer model. *Gynecologic Oncology.* 2009;115(3):362–366.

52. Czejka M, Jager W, Schuller J, Teherani D. Pharmacokinetics of carboplatin after intraperitoneal administration. *Archiv der Pharmazie.* 1991;324(3):183–184.

53. Stewart JHt, Shen P, Russell G, Fenstermaker J, McWilliams L, Coldrun FM et al. A phase I trial of oxaliplatin for intraperitoneal hyperthermic chemoperfusion for the treatment of peritoneal surface dissemination from colorectal and appendiceal cancers. *Annals of Surgical Oncology.* 2008;15(8):2137–2145.

54. Elias D, Bonnay M, Puizillou JM, Antoun S, Demirdjian S, El OA et al. Heated intra-operative intraperitoneal oxaliplatin after complete resection of peritoneal carcinomatosis: Pharmacokinetics and tissue distribution. *Annals of Oncology: Official Journal of the European Society for Medical Oncology.* 2002;13(2):267–272.

55. Elias DM, Sideris L. Pharmacokinetics of heated intraoperative intraperitoneal oxaliplatin after complete resection of peritoneal carcinomatosis. *Surgical Oncology Clinics of North America.* 2003;12(3):755–769, xiv.

56. Ferron G, Dattez S, Gladieff L, Delord JP, Pierre S, Lafont T et al. Pharmacokinetics of heated intraperitoneal oxaliplatin. *Cancer Chemotherapy and Pharmacology.* 2008;62(4):679–683.

57. Mahteme H, Wallin I, Glimelius B, Pahlman L, Ehrsson H. Systemic exposure of the parent drug oxaliplatin during hyperthermic intraperitoneal perfusion. *European Journal of Clinical Pharmacology.* 2008;64(9):907–911.

58. De Somer F, Ceelen W, Delanghe J, De Smet D, Vanackere M, Pattyn P et al. Severe hyponatremia, hyperglycemia, and hyperlactatemia are associated with intraoperative hyperthermic intraperitoneal chemoperfusion with oxaliplatin. *Peritoneal Dialysis International: Journal of the International Society for Peritoneal Dialysis.* 2008;28(1):61–66.

59. Jerremalm E, Hedeland M, Wallin I, Bondesson U, Ehrsson H. Oxaliplatin degradation in the presence of chloride: Identification and cytotoxicity of the monochloro monooxalato complex. *Pharmaceutical Research.* 2004;21(5):891–894.

60. Piche N, Leblond FA, Sideris L, Pichette V, Drolet P, Fortier LP et al. Rationale for heating oxaliplatin for the intraperitoneal treatment of peritoneal carcinomatosis: A study of the effect of heat on intraperitoneal oxaliplatin using a murine model. *Annals of Surgery.* 2011;254(1):138–144.

61. Bachur NR, Gordon SL, Gee MV, Kon H. NADPH cytochrome P-450 reductase activation of quinone anticancer agents to free radicals. *Proceedings of the National Academy of Sciences of the United States of America.* 1979;76(2):954–957.

62. Fujita T, Tamura T, Yamada H, Yamamoto A, Muranishi S. Pharmacokinetics of mitomycin C (MMC) after intraperitoneal administration of MMC-gelatin gel and its anti-tumor effects against sarcoma-180 bearing mice. *Journal of Drug Targeting.* 1997;4(5):289–296.

63. Mohamed F, Cecil T, Moran B, Sugarbaker P. A new standard of care for the management of peritoneal surface malignancy. *Current Oncology.* 2011;18(2):e84–e96.

64. Levine EA, Stewart JHt, Shen P, Russell GB, Loggie BL, Votanopoulos KI. Intraperitoneal chemotherapy for peritoneal surface malignancy: Experience with 1,000 patients. *Journal of the American College of Surgeons.* 2014;218(4):573–585.

65. Barlogie B, Corry PM, Drewinko B. In vitro thermochemotherapy of human colon cancer cells with *cis*-dichlorodiammineplatinum (II) and mitomycin C. *Cancer Research.* 1980;40(4):1165–1168.

66. van Ruth S, Verwaal VJ, Zoetmulder FA. Pharmacokinetics of intraperitoneal mitomycin C. *Surgical Oncology Clinics of North America.* 2003;12(3):771–780.

67. Tritton TR. Cell surface actions of adriamycin. *Pharmacology & Therapeutics.* 1991;49(3):293–309.

68. Triton TR, Yee G. The anticancer agent adriamycin can be actively cytotoxic without entering cells. *Science.* 1982;217(4556):248–250.

69. Lane P, Vichi P, Bain DL, Tritton TR. Temperature dependence studies of adriamycin uptake and cytotoxicity. *Cancer Research.* 1987;47(15):4038–4042.

70. Van der Speeten K, Stuart OA, Mahteme H, Sugarbaker PH. A pharmacologic analysis of intraoperative intracavitary cancer chemotherapy with doxorubicin. *Cancer Chemotherapy and Pharmacology.* 2009;63(5):799–805.

71. Ozols RF, Young RC, Speyer JL, Sugarbaker PH, Greene R, Jenkins J et al. Phase I and pharmacological studies of adriamycin administered intraperitoneally to patients with ovarian cancer. *Cancer Research.* 1982;42(10):4265–4269.

72. Ozols RF, Locker GY, Doroshow JH, Grotzinger KR, Myers CE, Young RC. Pharmacokinetics of adriamycin and tissue penetration in murine ovarian cancer. *Cancer Research.* 1979;39(8):3209–3214.

73. Ozols RF, Locker GY, Doroshow JH, Grotzinger KR, Myers CE, Fisher RI et al. Chemotherapy for murine ovarian cancer: A rationale for ip therapy with adriamycin. *Cancer Treatment Reports.* 1979;63(2):269–273.

74. Nagai K, Nogami S, Egusa H, Konishi H. Pharmacokinetic evaluation of intraperitoneal doxorubicin in rats. *Die Pharmazie*. 2014;69(2):125–127.

75. Pilati P, Mocellin S, Rossi CR, Scalerta R, Alaggio R, Giacomelli L et al. Doxorubicin activity is enhanced by hyperthermia in a model of ex vivo vascular perfusion of human colon carcinoma. *World Journal of Surgery*. 2003;27(6):640–646.

76. Rossi CR, Foletto M, Mocellin S, Pilati P, De SM, Deraco M et al. Hyperthermic intraoperative intraperitoneal chemotherapy with cisplatin and doxorubicin in patients who undergo cytoreductive surgery for peritoneal carcinomatosis and sarcomatosis: Phase I study. *Cancer*. 2002;94(2):492–499.

77. Harrison LE, Bryan M, Pliner L, Saunders T. Phase I trial of pegylated liposomal doxorubicin with hyperthermic intraperitoneal chemotherapy in patients undergoing cytoreduction for advanced intra-abdominal malignancy. *Annals of Surgical Oncology*. 2008;15(5):1407–1413.

78. Salvatorelli E, De Tursi M, Menna P, Carella C, Massari R, Colasante A et al. Pharmacokinetics of pegylated liposomal doxorubicin administered by intraoperative hyperthermic intraperitoneal chemotherapy to patients with advanced ovarian cancer and peritoneal carcinomatosis. *Drug Metabolism and Disposition: The Biological Fate of Chemicals*. 2012;40(12):2365–2373.

79. Sugarbaker PH, Mora JT, Carmignani P, Stuart OA, Yoo D. Update on chemotherapeutic agents utilized for perioperative intraperitoneal chemotherapy. *The Oncologist*. 2005;10(2):112–122.

80. Rohena CC, Mooberry SL. Recent progress with microtubule stabilizers: New compounds, binding modes and cellular activities. *Natural Product Reports*. 2014;31(3):335–355.

81. de Bree E, Theodoropoulos PA, Rosing H, Michalakis J, Romanos J, Beijnen JH et al. Treatment of ovarian cancer using intraperitoneal chemotherapy with taxanes: From laboratory bench to bedside. *Cancer Treatment Reviews*. 2006;32(6):471–482.

82. Mohamed F, Sugarbaker PH. Intraperitoneal taxanes. *Surgical Oncology Clinics of North America*. 2003;12(3):825–833.

83. De Smet L, Ceelen W, Remon JP, Vervaet C. Optimization of drug delivery systems for intraperitoneal therapy to extend the residence time of the chemotherapeutic agent. *The Scientific World Journal*. 2013;2013:720858.

84. Heidelberger C, Chaudhuri NK, Danneberg P, Mooren D, Griesbach L, Duschinsky R et al. Fluorinated pyrimidines, a new class of tumour-inhibitory compounds. *Nature*. 1957;179(4561):663–666.

85. Muggia FM, Peters GJ, Landolph JR Jr. XIII International Charles Heidelberger Symposium and 50 Years of Fluoropyrimidines in Cancer Therapy Held on September 6 to 8, 2007 at New York University Cancer Institute, Smilow Conference Center. *Molecular Cancer Therapeutics*. 2009;8(5):992–999.

86. Wagner PL, Jones D, Aronova A, Shia J, Weiser MR, Temple LK et al. Early postoperative intraperitoneal chemotherapy following cytoreductive surgery for appendiceal mucinous neoplasms with isolated peritoneal metastasis. *Diseases of the Colon and Rectum*. 2012;55(4):407–415.

87. Yu W, Whang I, Chung HY, Averbach A, Sugarbaker PH. Indications for early postoperative intraperitoneal chemotherapy of advanced gastric cancer: Results of a prospective randomized trial. *World Journal of Surgery*. 2001;25(8):985–990.

88. Sugarbaker PH, Graves T, DeBruijn EA, Cunliffe WJ, Mullins RE, Hull WE et al. Early postoperative intraperitoneal chemotherapy as an adjuvant therapy to surgery for peritoneal carcinomatosis from gastrointestinal cancer: Pharmacological studies. *Cancer Research*. 1990;50(18):5790–5794.

89. Kwon OK, Chung HY, Yu W. Early postoperative intraperitoneal chemotherapy for macroscopically serosa-invading gastric cancer patients. *Cancer Research and Treatment: Official Journal of Korean Cancer Association*. 2014;46(3):270–279.

90. Pestieau SR, Stuart OA, Chang D, Jacquet P, Sugarbaker PH. Pharmacokinetics of intraperitoneal gemcitabine in a rat model. *Tumori*. 1998;84(6):706–711.

91. Ridwelski K, Meyer F, Hribaschek A, Kasper U, Lippert H. Intraoperative and early postoperative chemotherapy into the abdominal cavity using gemcitabine may prevent postoperative occurrence of peritoneal carcinomatosis. *Journal of Surgical Oncology*. 2002;79(1):10–16.

92. Sabbatini P, Aghajanian C, Leitao M, Venkatraman E, Anderson S, Dupont J et al. Intraperitoneal cisplatin with intraperitoneal gemcitabine in patients with epithelial ovarian cancer: Results of a phase I/II Trial. *Clinical Cancer Research: An Official Journal of the American Association for Cancer Research*. 2004;10(9):2962–2967.

93. Sugarbaker PH, Stuart OA, Bijelic L. Intraperitoneal gemcitabine chemotherapy treatment for patients with resected pancreatic cancer: Rationale and report of early data. *International Journal of Surgical Oncology*. 2011;2011:161862.

94. Tentes AA, Kyziridis D, Kakolyris S, Pallas N, Zorbas G, Korakianitis O et al. Preliminary results of hyperthermic intraperitoneal intraoperative chemotherapy as an adjuvant in resectable pancreatic cancer. *Gastroenterology Research and Practice*. 2012;2012:506571.

95. Kamath A, Yoo D, Stuart OA, Bijelic L, Sugarbaker PH. Rationale for an intraperitoneal gemcitabine chemotherapy treatment for patients with resected pancreatic cancer. *Recent Patents on Anti-Cancer Drug Discovery*. 2009;4(2):174–179.

96. Morgan RJ Jr., Synold TW, Xi B, Lim D, Shibata S, Margolin K et al. Phase I trial of intraperitoneal gemcitabine in the treatment of advanced malignancies primarily confined to the peritoneal cavity. *Clinical Cancer Research: An Official Journal of the American Association for Cancer Research.* 2007;13(4):1232–1237.

97. Ceelen WP, Påhlman L, Mahteme H. Pharmacodynamic aspects of intraperitoneal cytotoxic therapy. *Cancer Treatment Research.* 2007;134:195–214.

98. Jackman DM. Current options for systemic therapy in mesothelioma. *Seminars in Thoracic and Cardiovascular Surgery.* 2009;21(2):154–158.

99. Muhsin M, Gricks C, Kirkpatrick P. Pemetrexed disodium. *Nature Reviews Drug Discovery.* 2004;3(10):825–826.

100. Pestieau SR, Stuart OA, Sugarbaker PH. Multi-targeted antifolate (MTA): Pharmacokinetics of intraperitoneal administration in a rat model. *European Journal of Surgical Oncology: The Journal of the European Society of Surgical Oncology and the British Association of Surgical Oncology.* 2000;26(7):696–700.

101. Mohamed F, Marchettini P, Stuart OA, Urano M, Sugarbaker PH. Thermal enhancement of new chemotherapeutic agents at moderate hyperthermia. *Annals of Surgical Oncology.* 2003;10(4):463–468.

102. Mohamed F, Stuart OA, Glehen O, Urano M, Sugarbaker PH. Optimizing the factors which modify thermal enhancement of melphalan in a spontaneous murine tumor. *Cancer Chemotherapy and Pharmacology.* 2006;58(6):719–724.

103. Bijelic L, Sugarbaker PH, Stuart OA. Hyperthermic intraperitoneal chemotherapy with melphalan: A summary of clinical and pharmacological data in 34 patients. *Gastroenterology Research and Practice.* 2012;2012:827534.

104. Howell SB, Pfeifle CE, Olshen RA. Intraperitoneal chemotherapy with melphalan. *Annals of Internal Medicine.* 1984;101(1):14–18.

105. Piccart MJ, Abrams J, Dodion PF, Crespeigne N, Sculier JP, Pector JC et al. Intraperitoneal chemotherapy with cisplatin and melphalan. *Journal of the National Cancer Institute.* 1988;80(14):1118–1124.

106. Sardi A, Jimenez W, Nieroda C, Sittig M, Shankar S, Gushchin V. Melphalan: A promising agent in patients undergoing cytoreductive surgery and hyperthermic intraperitoneal chemotherapy. *Annals of Surgical Oncology.* 2014;21(3):908–914.

107. Glehen O, Stuart OA, Mohamed F, Sugarbaker PH. Hyperthermia modifies pharmacokinetics and tissue distribution of intraperitoneal melphalan in a rat model. *Cancer Chemotherapy and Pharmacology.* 2004;54(1):79–84.

108. Pestieau SR, Schnake KJ, Stuart OA, Sugarbaker PH. Impact of carrier solutions on pharmacokinetics of intraperitoneal chemotherapy. *Cancer Chemotherapy and Pharmacology.* 2001;47(3):269–276.

109. Mohamed F, Sugarbaker PH. Carrier solutions for intraperitoneal chemotherapy. *Surgical Oncology Clinics of North America.* 2003;12(3):813–824.

110. Mohamed F, Stuart OA, Sugarbaker PH. Pharmacokinetics and tissue distribution of intraperitoneal docetaxel with different carrier solutions. *The Journal of Surgical Research.* 2003;113(1):114–120.

111. Mohamed F, Marchettini P, Stuart OA, Yoo D, Sugarbaker PH. A comparison of hetastarch and peritoneal dialysis solution for intraperitoneal chemotherapy delivery. *European Journal of Surgical Oncology: The Journal of the European Society of Surgical Oncology and the British Association of Surgical Oncology.* 2003;29(3):261–265.

112. Kusamura S, Dominique E, Baratti D, Younan R, Deraco M. Drugs, carrier solutions and temperature in hyperthermic intraperitoneal chemotherapy. *Journal of Surgical Oncology.* 2008;98(4):247–252.

113. Elias D, El OA, Bonnay M, Paci A, Ducreux M, Antoun S et al. Human pharmacokinetic study of heated intraperitoneal oxaliplatin in increasingly hypotonic solutions after complete resection of peritoneal carcinomatosis. *Oncology.* 2002;63(4):346–352.

114. Gardner SN. A mechanistic, predictive model of dose-response curves for cell cycle phase-specific and -nonspecific drugs. *Cancer Research.* 2000;60(5):1417–1425.

115. Rubin J, Clawson M, Planch A, Jones Q. Measurements of peritoneal surface area in man and rat. *The American Journal of the Medical Sciences.* 1988;295(5):453–458.

116. Ates K, Erturk S, Nergisoglu G, Karatan O, Duman N, Erbay B et al. Sex-dependent variations in peritoneal membrane transport properties in CAPD patients. *Nephrology, Dialysis, Transplantation: Official Publication of the European Dialysis and Transplant Association—European Renal Association.* 1996;11(11):2375–2376.

117. Chagnac A, Herskovitz P, Weinstein T, Elyashiv S, Hirsh J, Hammel I et al. The peritoneal membrane in peritoneal dialysis patients: Estimation of its functional surface area by applying stereologic methods to computerized tomography scans. *Journal of the American Society of Nephrology.* 1999;10(2):342–346.

118. Albanese AM, Albanese EF, Mino JH, Gomez E, Gomez M, Zandomeni M et al. Peritoneal surface area: Measurements of 40 structures covered by peritoneum: Correlation between total peritoneal surface area and the surface calculated by formulas. *Surgical and Radiologic Anatomy.* 2009;31(5):369–377.

119. Sugarbaker PH, Stuart OA, Carmignani CP. Pharmacokinetic changes induced by the volume of chemotherapy solution in patients treated with hyperthermic intraperitoneal mitomycin C. *Cancer Chemotherapy and Pharmacology.* 2006;57(5):703–708.

120. Mas-Fuster MI, Ramon-Lopez A, Nalda-Molina R. Importance of standardizing the dose in hyperthermic intraperitoneal chemotherapy (HIPEC): A pharmacodynamic point of view. *Cancer Chemotherapy and Pharmacology.* 2013;72(1):273–274.

12

Tissue transport and pharmacodynamics of intraperitoneal chemotherapy

PIETER COLIN, FÉLIX GREMONPREZ, AND WIM P. CEELEN

INTRODUCTION

The pharmacokinetic rationale for intraperitoneal (IP) drug delivery is well characterized in terms of drug concentrations and their ratio in various bodily compartments. Depending on the physicochemical properties of the drug, the resulting ratio of peritoneal fluid/plasma area under the concentration over time curve (AUC) allows to deliver a high(er) IP dose while plasma exposure, and its associated toxicity, remains limited.

However, in order to exert their anticancer effects, drugs have to gain access to tumor cells by penetrating into tissue. The available data on tumor tissue distribution of cytotoxic drugs and their relation with antitumor efficacy are limited and mainly stem from in vitro multicellular models such as tumor spheroids (spherical tumor aggregates; diameter approximately 1 mm) and multilayered cell cultures [1,2]. Tissue penetration in these models is studied following incubation in a medium containing anticancer drugs, and generally the results show a very limited cytotoxic drug penetration. Limited tissue penetration is explained by a number of physical (high interstitial fluid pressure [IFP], dense extracellular matrix [ECM]) and chemical (binding, sequestration, metabolism, degradation) effects that prevent a drug from reaching an adequate number of target cells. As a consequence, the adverse properties of the tumor microenvironment are implicated in treatment resistance [3].

In animal and human studies, tissue penetration has been studied almost exclusively after systemic intravenous (IV) penetration. After IP instillation, tissue exposure is even more compromised by the (near) absence of vascular drug delivery. Very little is known on the dynamics of tissue drug transport after IP chemotherapy. In this chapter, we provide an overview of approaches that may enhance tissue penetration of IP chemotherapy. Also, we describe the use of pharmacodynamic modeling as a powerful tool to relate tissue drug concentrations to the exerted effects such as apoptosis.

TISSUE TRANSPORT OF INTRAPERITONEAL CHEMOTHERAPY: GENERAL MECHANISMS

The two main physical mechanisms of drug transport into tumor tissue are diffusion and convection. For small agents (MW < 6000 Da), transport occurs mainly by *diffusion*.

The rate of diffusive mass transport (DMT) can be described by the following equation [4]:

$$DMT = MTC * A (C_{per} - C_{pl})$$

where

    MTC represents the mass transfer coefficient that is related to the square root of the molecular weight of the agent

    A is the peritoneal contact area

    C_{per} and C_{pl} are the peritoneal and plasma concentrations, respectively

Large solutes such as proteins diffuse much more slowly, and their transport is typically governed by solvent drag or *convection*, driven by a pressure gradient (both osmotic and hydrostatic). The rate of solute convection (RSC) can be modeled as

$$RSC = K_T * C_{pl} * R_i * A * dP/dx$$

where

    K_T is the hydraulic conductivity of the tissue

    R_i is the fraction of drug that passes through the interstitial space at the same rate as the solvent

    dP/dx is the slope of the hydrostatic pressure profile in the tissue [5]

This pressure profile results from the difference between the IP pressure and the IFP within the tumor. Malignant tumors are characterized by a pathologically elevated IFP, which represents a barrier to convective drug transport [6]. Interestingly, in vivo experiments have shown that measures to reduce the IFP such as tumor decapsulation did not enhance tissue penetration of IP administered antibodies, suggesting that the structure of the intercellular matrix is the major resistance to macromolecular drug transport [7]. The efficacy of the drug ultimately depends on the intracellular concentrations that result from active and passive transport across the cell membrane. Recent evidence suggests that the copper transporter CTR1 mediates the transport of cisplatin into tumor cells and that exposure of the cell to cisplatin triggers downregulation of CTR1 [8,9]. In practice, the tumor penetration distance measured experimentally following IP drug delivery is limited, ranging from a few cell layers to a maximum of 3–5 mm [10–12]. After systemic administration, however, the penetration distance of extravasated drug has likewise been shown to be very limited [12]. In xenografts, the concentration of doxorubicin was shown to fall exponentially to half its (peri)vascular concentration after a distance of 40–50 μm [13].

In addition to direct transport from the peritoneal fluid into tumor tissue, other mechanisms affect tissue concentration. First, tumor capillaries may transport drug out of the tumor and lower tissue exposure, but the capillary network may also enhance drug delivery by the presence of a (although limited) plasma exposure. Second, the drug may penetrate peritoneal nodules not only from the peritoneal cavity but also from the invaded abdominal or organ wall through recirculation of systemically absorbed drug. As a result, the transport of cytotoxic drugs into peritoneal tumor nodules is influenced by a range of variables summarized in Figure 12.1.

APPROACHES TO INCREASE TUMOR DRUG PENETRATION

Increasing drug supply and contact time

Since tissue drug transport of most currently used chemotherapeutic agents is driven largely by passive diffusion, and thus by a concentration gradient, any increase in the peritoneal drug concentration is likely to enhance peritoneal tumor exposure. At the same time, numerous in vitro and in vivo experiments have demonstrated that the number of tumor cells killed correlates directly with the concentration of most chemotherapy drugs in the culture media. Conversely, a reduction in dose almost always results in a reduction in cure rate and response rate [14].

In addition to drug concentration, chemotherapy contact time (IP dwell time) is an important determinant of antitumor efficacy. In the setting of (hyperthermic) IP chemoperfusion, dwell times of 30–200 minutes are common, much shorter compared to the time frame used in in vitro cytotoxicity assays, which span 24–48 hours. Recent modeling data suggest that when exposure times are short (typically 30–90 minutes with HIPEC), increasing the concentration gradient will not always result in an equivalent tissue penetration. The dose–response curves and their dependency on exposure time have been theoretically modeled by Gardner [15]. Assuming a constant drug concentration throughout the exposure period, the survival fraction is described by

$$S = e^{-q * (1 - e^{-ay})}$$

where

    S is the survival fraction

    y is the drug concentration

    a is the level of drug resistance

    q is the exposure time in hours for non-cell cycle–specific drugs

From the resulting log dose–response curves, it becomes clear that a plateau in cell kill will be reached depending on the exposure time (Figure 12.2), as confirmed in various in vitro studies. This suggests that increasing the drug dose will not always compensate for a shorter exposure time. Similarly, the theoretical model of cisplatin pharmacodynamics proposed by El-Kareh and Secomb predicts that, at a given concentration, cisplatin cytotoxicity increases with exposure time [16]. These data suggest that exposure time is important and adds a theoretical argument for prolonged IP administration and for adding early postoperative IP

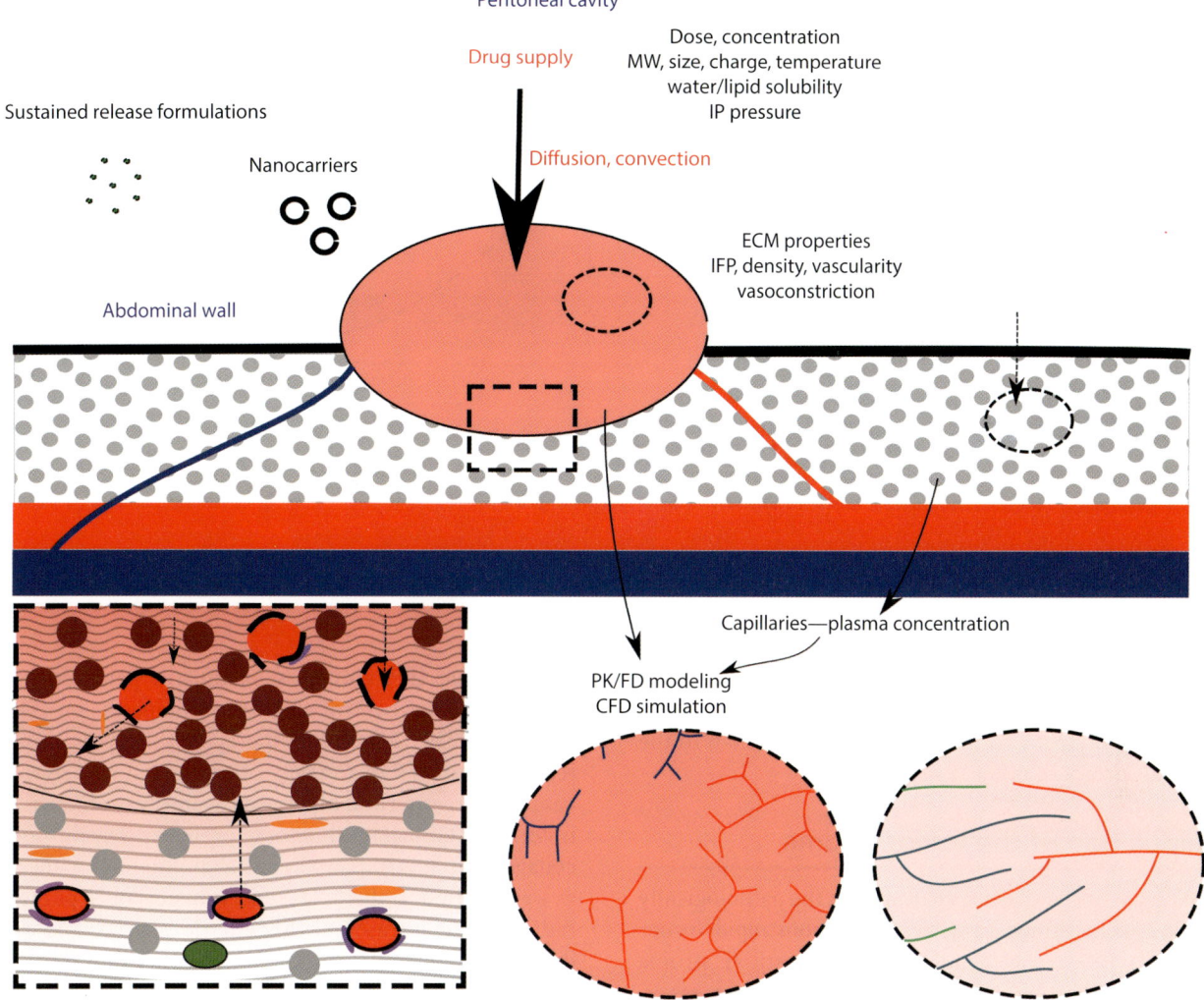

Figure 12.1 Overview of factors that affect tissue transport and penetration depth of IP chemotherapy. Drug transport is driven by diffusion (concentration gradient) and convection (pressure gradient). The transport rate is affected by the peritoneal dose and concentration, physicochemical properties of the drug (size, molecular weight [MW], water solubility), pharmaceutical formulation, and peritoneal cavity properties (IP pressure, temperature, and pH). Once taken up by the tissue, drug availability is affected by the properties of the ECM such as elevated IFP, high cellularity and collagen density, as well as vascular transport out of the tissue.

chemotherapy courses, especially when macroscopic tumor is left after cytoreduction.

Novel pharmaceutical formulations and carriers

None of the currently used chemotherapeutics were specifically designed, studied, or approved for the IP route of administration, and their use is "off label." Over the past few years, however, novel pharmaceutical carriers have been developed specifically aimed at IP delivery; these include microparticles, nanoparticles, liposomes, micelles, implants, and injectable depots [17]. The aim of these novel formulations is primarily to achieve improved IP retention of the agent, resulting in a sustained cytotoxic drug exposure. In addition, these carriers may enhance tumor penetration. In a recently reported mouse model of gastric cancer

peritoneal metastasis, a nanomicellar formulation of paclitaxel (PTX) resulted in higher PTX concentrations in tumor tissue and better antitumor efficacy compared to the traditional (Taxol™) formulation [18]. The reasons why nanomicellar particles penetrate more deeply into tumor tissue are unclear but may be related to their ability to penetrate cell membranes nonendocytically or to fuse with plasma membranes and enter the cytoplasm within a few minutes without bilayer disruption [19]. Similarly, a self- assembling telodendrimer nanoformulation of PTX achieved superior antitumor effects and deep tumor penetration in a mouse ovarian cancer model compared to Taxol™ and Abraxane™ at equivalent PTX doses [20]. Lu and coworkers developed PTX-loaded polymeric tumor-penetrating microparticles (TPM) and achieved superior tumor tissue penetration, long survival, and high cure rates in IP human ovarian and pancreatic tumor models [21,22]. The efficacy of TPM may

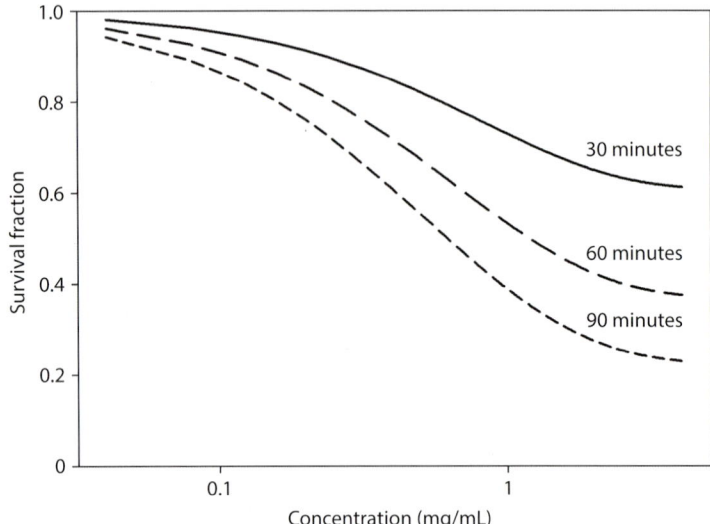

Figure 12.2 Theoretical calculation of the tumor survival fraction as a function of concentration of a non-cell cycle–specific cytotoxic drug and exposure time, based on the exponential kill model by Gardner [15]. Note that the plateau in cell kill depends on the exposure time.

be related to their preferential adherence to tumor tissue, resulting from interactions between poly(lactic-co-glycolic acid) (PLG) polymer and tumor surface, rather than to the peritoneal surface or other IP organs [23].

Manipulation of the tumor stroma

The main barrier for tissue penetration is the pathologically elevated IFP in tumor tissue resulting from rapid tumor cell proliferation, contraction of the interstitial stroma by activated fibroblasts, hyperpermeable microvessels, and deficient lymphatic drainage [6,24]. Pharmacological manipulation of the tumor microenvironment may improve systemic drug delivery [25]. We have recently demonstrated that, in a mouse colorectal carcinomatosis model, pretreatment with either bevacizumab or pazopanib significantly

lowers tissue IFP, enhances oxaliplatin penetration, and improves tumor control after IP chemoperfusion (Figures 12.3 and 12.4) [26]. Other therapies that were shown to reduce tumor IFP in a variety of preclinical models include vascular targeting and disrupting agents, vasodilators, antimitotics, TGF-beta inhibitors, proteases (hyaluronidase, collagenase), losartan, and epithelial junction opener JO-1 as well as physical therapies such as hyper- or hypothermia, radiotherapy, ultrasound, hyperbaric oxygen, and photodynamic therapy [27–30]. Cellular density may be reduced by sequential cell killing induced by "distribution enhancers" such as the taxanes. Preclinical studies have shown that pretreatment with PTX reduces tumor IFP, impairs tumor cellularity, and enhances drug delivery [31]. In the clinical setting, Taghian et al. measured tissue IFP and pO_2 before and after sequential PTX and doxorubicin in patients with

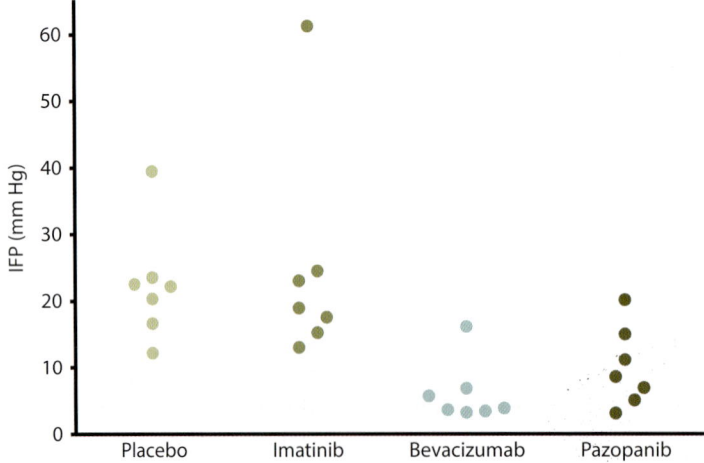

Figure 12.3 Effect of pharmacological intervention on IFP in a mouse isolated peritoneal tumor model. IFP was measured in vivo just before IP chemoperfusion with a Samba Preclin® sensor (Samba Sensors, Gothenburg, Sweden). Both bevacizumab and pazopanib groups had a significantly lower IFP (P = 0.0008; Kruskal–Wallis test).

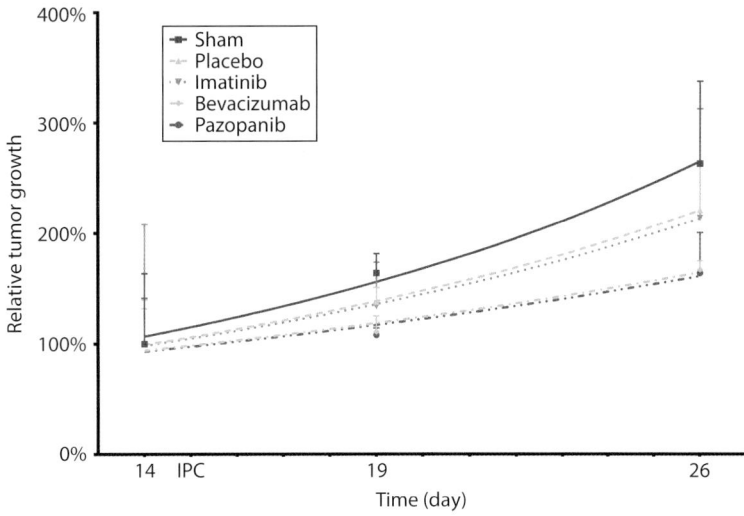

Figure 12.4 Effect of pharmacological manipulation of the tumor stroma on tumor growth delay (TGD). Exponential growth curves fitted to repeated tumor size measurements (T2 weighted MRI) of relative tumor size after IP chemoperfusion with oxaliplatin (P = 0.0006; nonlinear regression). Both bevacizumab and pazopanib groups are significantly different from sham. The bevacizumab group differs significantly from placebo.

breast cancer [32]. They found that PTX, but not doxorubicin, led to a significantly reduced tumor tissue IFP and increased pO_2, irrespective of size.

An alternative therapeutic target consists of the ATP-dependent drug transporters that confer cellular resistance to different cytotoxic agents [33]. In addition, modification of the pH of cellular organelles may prevent inactivation of sequestered basic drugs such as doxorubicin. This concept was recently demonstrated by Patel and coworkers, who showed that the proton pump inhibitor pantoprazole increased endosomal pH, increased nuclear uptake tissue penetration of doxorubicin in multilayered cell cultures, and led to increased growth delay in a mouse MCF7 xenograft model [34].

None of these agents or methods were, however, tested in the setting of IP drug delivery.

Hyperthermia

The potential of hyperthermia to enhance IP drug delivery is not well defined. Preclinical studies using murine colon, melanoma, and mammary tumors showed that whole body hyperthermia (39.5°C during 6 hours) lowers IFP, improves blood flow, and enhances the efficacy of radiotherapy [35]. Others, however, were unable to observe IFP lowering upon locoregional heating (41.8°C during 2 hours) in a glioma xenograft model [36]. Several authors have studied chemotherapy concentrations in tumor tissue after hyperthermic IP delivery. Los et al. found that, compared to normothermic administration, locoregional heating (41.5°C during 60 minutes) resulted in a fourfold increase in cisplatin tumor concentration in a rat CC531 colon carcinomatosis model [37]. Of note, plasma cisplatin levels were also significantly elevated after hyperthermic treatment, which raises the question whether the difference in tumor tissue drug concentration resulted from increased peritoneal to tumor transport or from increased systemic exposure. Later work by Zeamari and coworkers was unable to confirm the benefit of hyperthermia: mild hyperthermic perfusion with cisplatin (40°C during 90 minutes) did not improve drug uptake in small IP tumors in a rat model [38]. Similarly, Facy and colleagues did not find a significant difference in cisplatin concentration of ovarian peritoneal tumors in a rat model after normothermic or hyperthermic (42°C during 60 minutes) chemoperfusion [39]. These authors hypothesized that increased peritoneal drug clearance due to vasodilation and increased blood flow may explain the lack of benefit associated with hyperthermia.

Manipulation of peritoneal and tumor blood flow

Theoretically, tissue drug retention could be improved by vasoconstriction of the tumor capillary bed, preventing outward transport of the drug. The proof of principle in a pig model was described by Lindner et al., who noted a significant increase in peritoneal/plasma AUC ratio of IP carboplatin and etoposide following reduction of splanchnic circulation with an IV vasopressin analogue [40]. These observations were later confirmed in a rat model bearing syngeneic carcinomatosis [41]. In this model, IV vasopressin decreased peritoneal blood flow as measured indirectly with the Xe-133-clearance method; the presence of peritoneal carcinomatosis did not influence peritoneal blood flow or the effect of vasopressin. Mahteme et al. studied the uptake of radiolabeled 5-FU in a nude rat bearing human colorectal peritoneal nodules [42]. They found that tumor uptake was significantly higher after IP administration of the vasoconstrictive agent norbormide, which acts through modulation of calcium influx. Similar effects were found with epinephrine (adrenaline). Duvillard and coworkers found that concurrent IP administration of epinephrine leads to a 4- to 12-fold increase of platinum concentration in rat peritoneal tumors [43]. In addition, they noted that rats with nodules 1–2 mm in diameter, insensitive to IP cisplatin alone, were cured when the anticancer drug was combined with epinephrine. Based on these findings, early phase clinical studies were initiated. A phase I study of cytoreductive surgery (CRS) followed by IP instillation of 30 mg/L of cisplatin at 37°C and increasing concentrations of IP epinephrine showed that the recommended dose is 2 mg/L, the dose-limiting toxicity consisting of cardiac intolerance [44]. As expected, the coadministration of IP epinephrine resulted in a 60% decrease in the serum AUC of platinum. A population pharmacokinetic (PopPK) study from the same group based on samples from 55 patients, half of whom were treated with IP epinephrine, confirmed that epinephrine halves clearance between peritoneum and serum, increases the central volume of distribution of platinum, and enhances IP drug exposure [45]. Oman and coworkers reported a phase I/II study of IP 5-FU in 68 patients with unresectable pancreas cancer, 25% of whom were treated with concurrent IV vasopressin [46]. They found that IV vasopressin did not significantly decrease plasma 5-FU AUC but reduced C_{max} on day 2 of treatment. The overall efficacy of the treatment was low, with only 4% response and a median survival of 8 months.

Hypotonic carrier solutions

Preclinical IP chemotherapy models have shown that use of a hypotonic carrier solution increases cytotoxic drug uptake, presumably mediated by increased convective drug transport [47,48]. Clinical studies, however, did not substantiate the presumed advantage of hypotonic carrier solutions; moreover, troublesome toxicity was observed [49]. Wei and coworkers compared normal saline with HAES (isotonic 6% hydroxyethyl starch solution) as a carrier for IP 5-FU in healthy rats [50]. They observed increased peritoneal, portal vein, and normal tissue (gastric and colon) 5-FU concentrations with HAES.

Increased intra-abdominal pressure

Higher IP pressures could in theory improve convection-driven drug transport. Esquis et al. demonstrated in a rat carcinomatosis model that increasing the IP pressure (22 mm Hg during 1 hour) resulted in a significantly higher cisplatin penetration in tumor tissue and improved survival [51]. At the same time, they reported that a 40 mm Hg IP pressure during 2 hours was well tolerated in ventilated pigs. Similarly, Jacquet and coworkers found a significant enhancement of doxorubicin uptake in the abdominal wall and diaphragm of rats when the IP pressure was increased to 20–30 mm Hg [52]. Facy and colleagues studied the effect of moderately elevated IP pressure (25 cm H_2O or 18.3 mm Hg), created by a water column over the abdomen, on tissue distribution of IP oxaliplatin in healthy pigs [53].

They found that elevated IP pressure enhanced diffusion of the drug in both the visceral and parietal peritoneum; the combination with hyperthermia achieved the highest peritoneal tissue concentrations.

Interesting results were recently reported by Reymond and coworkers, who comprehensively studied the clinical effects of laparoscopically instilling low-dose chemotherapy as an aerosol (pressurized intraperitoneal aerosol chemotherapy [PIPAC]) in patients with advanced, unresectable carcinomatosis [54–57]. Following administration of a pressurized aerosol of CO_2 loaded with doxorubicin (1.5 mg/m²) and cisplatin (7.5 mg/m²) during 30 minutes at 12 mm Hg and 37°C, low systemic toxicities and excellent tissue penetration were observed. The interested reader is referred to Chapter 35 for a detailed overview of this promising technique.

PHARMACOKINETIC–PHARMACODYNAMIC MODELING

Rationale for PKPD modeling

Pharmacokinetic–pharmacodynamic (PKPD) modeling is recognized as a promising tool for quantitative decision making in oncology [58]. PKPD models that are constructed based on an in-depth understanding of the relationships between drug concentration (at the site of action) and treatment outcome are a valuable tool to optimize/individualize treatment regimens [59]. In oncology, where optimization of treatment regimens is hampered by the lack of easily obtainable measures of pharmacological effect and treatment response in terms of survival or progression-free survival is often highly variable, the implementation of model-based treatment regimens is an unmet need.

In the following sections, we will distinguish between different types of PKPD models. PopPK models are those that merely describe the pharmacokinetics and associated PK variability of a compound, whereas PKPD models expand on this concept and combine the PopPK modeling with relationships between secondary PK parameters (AUC_{24}, AUC_{inf}, etc.) and observable drug effects (toxicity, efficacy). Finally, PKPD models take into account the entire time course of drug concentrations and quantitatively link these (effect-site) concentrations to the drug action (i.e., target receptor binding and downstream processes). By simultaneously modeling PK and PD behavior of a compound, structural information is gained with respect to (1) the mechanisms responsible for the observed drug effects and (2) how variability in a patient cohort can impact the drug effects.

PopPK models in HIPEC therapy

Table 12.1 provides a summary of published models based on clinical data originating from HIPEC trials. In the HIPEC research field, PopPK models are most frequently encountered. These population-based pharmacokinetic models aim to describe the PK variability caused by the heterogeneity of the underlying physiological processes in the population,

Table 12.1 Summary of published models derived from HIPEC-related clinical trials

Drug	Type	PK observations	Covariate relationships	PD end points	Number of subjects	IP dose (mg/m^2)	Treatment duration	Temperature	References
Alkylating agents									
Mitomycin C	PKPD	Perfusate, plasma	Perfusate volume on V_{perf}, BSA on CL, and duration of surgery on V_2	WBC, PLAT	47	35 mg/m^2	90 minutes	40°C–41°C	[65]
	PopPK	Perfusate, plasma, urine	—	—	28	20 mg/m^2	60	37°C	[60]
Platinum compounds									
Cisplatin	PK	Perfusate, plasma, urine	—	—	16	60, 80, and 100 mg	NA	NA	[61]
	PK	Perfusate, plasma, plasma$_{unbound}$	Patient weight on V_{perf} plasma and intraperitoneal protein concentration on CL	—	31	30 mg/L	2 × 1 hour	37°C	[62]
	PKPD	Perfusate, plasma, plasma$_{unbound}$	Epinephrine use on CL_{IP} and V_1	Renal toxicity, in vitro IP target	27	30 mg/L	2 × 1 hour	37°C	[45,66]
Oxaliplatin	PK	Perfusate, plasma	—	—	24	180–230 mg/L	30 minutes	42°C	[63]
	PKPD	Perfusate, plasma	—	ANC	30	360 mg/m^2 in 2.5–6.0 L	30–60 minutes	42°C	[69]
	PKPD	Perfusate, plasma	CRS on neutropenia	ANC	84	360 mg/m^2 in 2.5–6.0 L	30–60 minutes	42°C	[64,68]

Notes: V_{perf}, volume of the perfusate compartment; BSA, body surface area, V_2, peripheral compartment volume; CL, plasma clearance; CL_{IP}, IP clearance (absorption from the abdominal cavity into the systemic circulation); V_1, central volume of distribution; WBC, white blood cells; PLAT, platelets; ANC, absolute neutrophil count.

such as renal function, plasma protein binding, or disease status. Through adequately designed clinical trials, the relationship between PK variability, resulting in (often uncontrolled) variability in (plasma) concentration time profiles, and patient characteristics is studied and integrated in pharmacostatistical models. These models provide a tool to researchers to better understand a compound's behavior during peroperative IP chemotherapy and aid in identifying the physiopathological parameters that affect drug exposure.

Several authors have developed PopPK models based on data from a cohort of patients treated with HIPEC using mitomycin C [60], cisplatin [61,62], or oxaliplatin [63]. These PopPK models mainly focus on describing (1) the uptake of the compound from the peritoneal cavity into the systemic circulation and (2) the plasma pharmacokinetics of the compound. Based on these models, it was estimated that the percentage of the administered dose that is absorbed from the peritoneal cavity is highly variable and compound-specific in HIPEC patients. Cerretani et al. [60] estimated that between 14% and 57% of a 20mg/m² dose of mitomycin C is absorbed into the systemic circulation following a 1 hour HIPEC treatment. For the platinum compounds, 15%–58% [61] and 40%–68% [63] have been reported for cisplatin and oxaliplatin, respectively.

Despite the high degree of variability that is observed for patients treated using HIPEC therapy, only a few studies succeeded in identifying patient/drug characteristics that could help in explaining or predicting this variability. For IP compartment volume, which is directly related to the systemic uptake of the drug from the abdominal cavity, correlations were shown with the type of drug formulation [64], patient weight [62], the perfusate volume [65], and the use of epinephrine [45]. Surprisingly, for plasma PK, a process that is normally well predicted from typical prognostic factors such as age, weight, and renal function, only plasma and IP protein levels [62] and body surface area (BSA) [65] were identified as prognostic factors in the prediction of cisplatin and mitomycin C clearance, respectively.

Although these PopPK models adequately describe the high degree of variability that is seen in plasma concentration time profiles following HIPEC treatment, the lack of inclusion of prognostic factors hampers the optimization of treatment regimens and precludes clinicians from using these models to predict the time course of drug concentrations in particular patients. Furthermore, in order to be able to evaluate currently used treatment protocols or evaluate newly optimized treatment strategies in silico, information with regards to the induced drug effects has to be included in these models.

PKPD and PKPD models in HIPEC therapy

Of the published models integrating PK and PD information, two are classified as PKPD models, i.e., linking secondary PK parameters to clinical end points and two classified as a PKPD model (Table 12.1).

Based on data from a clinical trial where a 90 minutes HIPEC treatment of mitomycin C was used at a dose of 35 mg/m², Van Ruth et al. [65] developed a PKPD model that predicted the percentage decrease in white blood cell counts and platelet counts from the mitomycin C plasma exposure (AUC$_\infty$). From their modeling efforts, based on the identified linear relationship between BSA and plasma clearance, the authors concluded that the currently used BSA-based dosing algorithm (35 mg/m²) appears reasonable. However, in order to further reduce the incidence of grade 3/4 leucopenia to a generally accepted rate of 10%, the authors cautiously suggested to lower the mitomycin C dose to 25 mg/m². Nevertheless, these conclusions might not extrapolate well to other centers due to the specific way of administration of mitomycin C at the author's institution (i.e., 50% of the dose is given at the start of the HIPEC and subsequently 25% is added at 30 and 60 minutes into the treatment).

A second series of PKPD models were published by Royer et al. [45,62,66,67] following several clinical investigations into the use of cisplatin via IP perfusion. In the studied clinical trials, cisplatin was administered at 37°C at a dose of 30 mg/L during a 1 hour IP perfusion. In a first analysis of their trial data, Royer et al. identified AUC$_{24h}$ to be significantly related to the incidence of renal toxicity (documented by an increase in serum creatinine) [66]. Using a chi-square test statistic, they identified 25 mg × h/L as an AUC$_{24h}$ cutoff to differentiate between patients at low and at high risk of renal toxicity. In a next step the authors integrated a previously determined threshold for maximum platinum-induced cytotoxicity in their analysis. Previously, it was shown, in a clonogenic assay using an OV-CAR-3 cell line, that the platinum concentration necessary to induce maximum in vitro cytotoxicity is 10 mg/L. Based on this consideration and their knowledge of the platinum concentrations in the perfusate during HIPEC, the authors decided to change their HIPEC protocols to a 2 × 1 hour perfusion instead of a 1 hour perfusion to optimize the time in which the perfusate concentration exceeds 10 mg/L.

In a subsequent follow-up study, Royer et al. modeled data from a clinical trial where patients were treated according to this new treatment protocol [62]. These data allowed them to identify IP and plasma protein concentrations as significant prognostic factors for systemic cisplatin clearance. Using Monte Carlo simulation, the authors developed a dosing nomogram to assist treating clinicians in selecting the most optimal IP cisplatin dose to be administered during IP perfusion. The nomogram allows for the evaluation of the percentage of patients that is expected to show an AUC$_{24h}$ > 25 mg × h/L with respect to the cisplatin dose within the perfusate and a patient's plasma protein level. Finally, Royer et al. developed a limited sampling strategy (LSS), i.e., a blood sampling schedule, that allows, after the cisplatin concentrations have been determined, to reliably estimate a patient's individual AUC$_{24h}$ from a few (4) concentration measurements. This LSS was later refined to accommodate the use of perfusion concentrations rather than plasma concentration in the assessment of a patient's individual PK parameters [45]. As the authors stated: "using these models, the impact of the dosing regimen on adverse effects and on platinum-related systemic toxicities may not only be evaluated, but also individually estimated."

In contrast to the work of Royer et al., Pérez-Ruixo et al. [68] and Valenzuela et al. [69] focused their attention toward the development of a PKPD model able to describe and predict neutrophil dynamics following HIPEC treatment with oxaliplatin. Based on earlier work from Friberg et al. [70], they developed a model integrating the underlying physiological process of granulopoiesis (i.e., neutrophil production, maturation, regulation, and elimination) and the effects of oxaliplatin on this process, thereby providing a quantitative framework to predict the hematotoxic effects of oxaliplatin after CRS and HIPEC treatment. Based on their modeling efforts, Valenzuela et al. [69] concluded that the maximum tolerated peritoneal oxaliplatin exposure (in terms of induction of neutropenia) is 120 mg × h/L and that

it is recommended to use granulocyte colony-stimulating factor (G-CSF) in prophylaxis for patients with an oxaliplatin exposure > 65 mg × h/L. However, these findings were later contradicted by Pérez-Ruixo et al.

Pérez-Ruixo et al. [68] further elaborated on these concepts and studied the neutrophil dynamics in different cohorts of patients who were treated with CRS with/without hyperthermic IP oxaliplatin (in two different carrier solutions). Through the design of their trials, the authors were able to discriminate the effects of CRS and HIPEC on the neutrophil dynamics. According to the model, a transient increase in the absolute neutrophil count (ANC) was induced by CRS in the immediate postoperative period (i.e., a neutrophilic effect mediated by systemic inflammatory processes) followed by a general neutropenic effect caused by the oxaliplatin administration. Based on an in silico

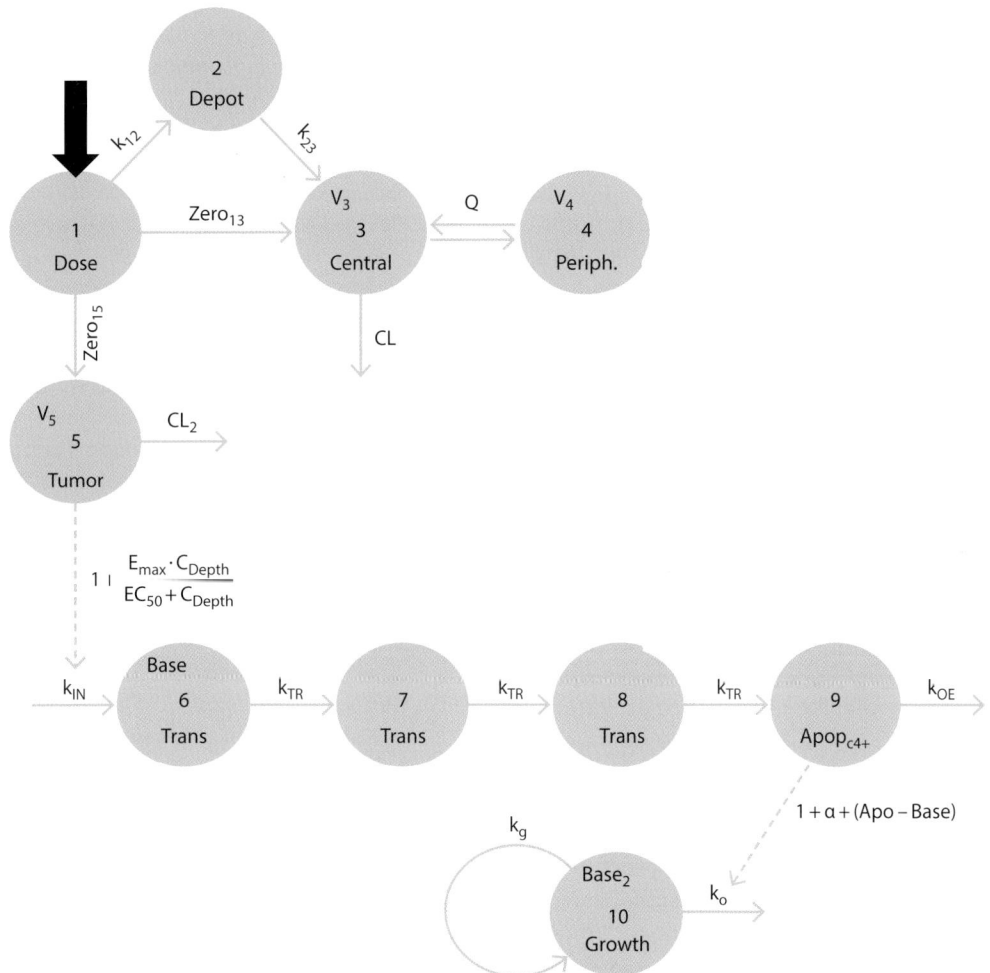

Figure 12.5 Overview of the structure of the final PKPD model to describe PTX PKPD following IPEC dosing of Taxol® in rats. The black arrow indicates the dose that is input into the peritoneal compartment (1). This compartment is reset 45 minutes after the start of the treatment. From the peritoneal compartment, PTX is directly absorbed via zero-order absorption into the plasma (3) and the tumor compartment (5). Toward the plasma, a parallel, first-order, absorption through a depot compartment (2) was used to describe the prolonged release of PTX into the plasma post treatment. Within the tumor compartment, the spatial distribution was modeled using an exponential decaying function. These concentrations were linked via an E_{max} model to a transduction model (6, 7, 8, 9) describing the onset of apoptosis (9) within the tumor tissue. Finally, the degree of apoptosis at ¼ of the tumor diameter was used to link to the observed inhibition of tumor growth dynamics (10) using a linear effect model. Observations were recorded in compartments 1, 3, 5, 9, and 10.

study into the interaction between treatment duration and perfusate concentration on the incidence of grade 4 neutropenia, the authors elegantly showed that higher doses than those evaluated to date (460 mg/m², corresponding to an initial concentration of 230 mg/L for a 2 L/m² volume of the carrier solution) could be used without substantially increasing the risk of severe neutropenia, thereby contradicting the earlier published results from Valenzuela et al.

All models published up until today focus on toxicity-related pharmacodynamic end points and dose optimization with respect to the avoidance of drug-related toxicity. Alternatively, efforts are directed toward the development of PKPD models that could be used to predict/increase efficacy (and decrease drug-related toxicities) in terms of tumor progression and inhibition of metastatic growth. In the preclinical setting, this type of models are currently being used (e.g., Colin et al. [71]) to guide the development of new drug formulations dedicated to the HIPEC setting. An overview of the final PKPD model structure used to describe PTX PKPD following IP perfusion of Taxol® in rats is shown in Figure 12.5. The PK part of the model includes perfusate, plasma, as well as tumor temporal/spatial kinetics following Taxol® dosing. The PKPD part of the model describes and accurately predicts the induction of apoptosis (measured within tumor tissue) and tumor growth inhibition as a function of the time course of intratumoral PTX concentrations following intraperitoneal chemoperfusion.

It is anticipated that translational PKPD modeling, aimed toward bridging between estimated drug effects in tumor xenograft models and the clinical setting, is the next step forward to gain more insight in the fundamental aspects of HIPEC pharmacotherapy. Finally, it is worthwhile pointing out that in the general oncology setting, this approach, first advocated by Rocchetti et al. [72], has been used successfully over the past few years for predicting the expected active dose in humans from animal studies.

SUMMARY AND CONCLUSIONS

Little is known on the mechanisms that govern drug transport after IP instillation. Several studies have shown that drug penetration is very limited (a few millimeters), and this may explain the relative frequent occurrence of treatment failure after IP chemotherapy. Various approaches have been tested aiming to enhance tissue penetration. These include the development of novel pharmaceutical formulations, manipulation of the tumor stroma, peritoneal wall vasoconstriction, and IP administration at elevated pressure or temperature. Only a few of these approaches have proved successful in the clinical setting.

Ultimately, antitumor efficacy depends on the induction of cancer cell death (apoptosis). PKPD models, which relate tissue drug concentrations to their cellular effect, hold considerable promise as a tool to describe and predict tumor growth inhibition following IP chemotherapy for peritoneal surface malignancy.

REFERENCES

1. Minchinton AI, Tannock IF. Drug penetration in solid tumours. *Nature Reviews Cancer.* 2006;6(8):583–592.
2. Tannock IF, Lee CM, Tunggal JK, Cowan DSM, Egorin MJ. Limited penetration of anticancer drugs through tumor tissue: A potential cause of resistance of solid tumors to chemotherapy. *Clinical Cancer Research.* 2002;8(3):878–884.
3. Tredan O, Galmarini CM, Patel K, Tannock IF. Drug resistance and the solid tumor microenvironment. *Journal of the National Cancer Institute.* 2007;99(19):1441–1454.
4. Dedrick RL, Flessner MF, Collins JM, Schultz JS. Is the peritoneum a membrane? *American Society for Artificial Internal Organs.* 1982;5:1–5.
5. Flessner MF, Dedrick RL, Schultz JS. A distributed model of peritoneal-plasma transport: Theoretical considerations. *American Journal of Physiology.* 1984;246:R597–R607.
6. Heldin CH, Rubin K, Pietras K, Ostman A. High interstitial fluid pressure—An obstacle in cancer therapy. *Nature Reviews Cancer.* 2004;4(10):806–813.
7. Flessner MF, Choi J, Credit K, Deverkadra R, Henderson K. Resistance of tumor interstitial pressure to the penetration of intraperitoneally delivered antibodies into metastatic ovarian tumors. *Clinical Cancer Research.* 2005;11(8):3117–3125.
8. Holzer AK, Samimi G, Katano K, Naerdemann W, Lin XJ, Safaei R, Howell SB. The copper influx transporter human copper transport protein 1 regulates the uptake of cisplatin in human ovarian carcinoma cells. *Molecular Pharmacology.* 2004;66(4):817–823.
9. Holzer AK, Katano K, Klomp LWJ, Howell SB. Cisplatin rapidly down-regulates its own influx transporter hCTR1 in cultured human ovarian carcinoma cells. *Clinical Cancer Research.* 2004;10(19):6744–6749.
10. Nederman T, Carlsson J. Penetration and binding of vinblastine and 5-fluorouracil in cellular spheroids. *Cancer Chemotherapy and Pharmacology.* 1984;13(2):131–135.
11. van de Vaart PJM, van der Vange N, Zoetmulder FAN, van Goethem AR, van Tellingen O, Huinink WWT, Beijnen JH, Bartelink H, Begg AC. Intraperitoneal cisplatin with regional hyperthermia in advanced ovarian cancer: Pharmacokinetics and cisplatin-DNA adduct formation in patients and ovarian cancer cell lines. *European Journal of Cancer.* 1998;34(1):148–154.
12. Gillern SM, Chua TC, Stojadinovic A, Esquivel J. KRAS status in patients with colorectal cancer peritoneal carcinomatosis and its impact on outcome. *American Journal of Clinical Oncology—Cancer Clinical Trials.* 2010;33(5):456–460.

13. Primeau AJ, Rendon A, Hedley D, Lilge L, Tannock IF. The distribution of the anticancer drug doxorubicin in relation to blood vessels in solid tumors. *Clinical Cancer Research*. 2005;11(24):8782–8788.

14. Lyman GH. Impact of chemotherapy dose intensity on cancer patient outcomes. *Journal of the National Comprehensive Cancer Network*. 2009;7(1):99–108.

15. Gardner SN. A mechanistic, predictive model of dose–response curves for cell cycle phase-specific and -nonspecific drugs. *Cancer Research*. 2000;60(5):1417–1425.

16. El-Kareh AW, Secomb TW. A mathematical model for cisplatin cellular pharmacodynamics. *Neoplasia*. 2003;5(2):161–169.

17. De Smet L, Ceelen W, Remon JP, Vervaet C. Optimization of drug delivery systems for intraperitoneal therapy to extend the residence time of the chemotherapeutic agent. *Scientific World Journal*. 2013;2013:720858.

18. Emoto S, Yamaguchi H, Kishikawa J, Yamashita H, Ishigami H, Kitayama J. Antitumor effect and pharmacokinetics of intraperitoneal NK105, a nano-micellar paclitaxel formulation for peritoneal dissemination. *Cancer Science*. 2012;103(7):1304–1310.

19. Goda T, Goto Y, Ishihara K. Cell-penetrating macromolecules: Direct penetration of amphipathic phospholipid polymers across plasma membrane of living cells. *Biomaterials*. 2010;31(8):2380–2387.

20. Xiao K, Luo JT, Fowler WL, Li YP, Lee JS, Xing L, Cheng RH, Wang L, Lam KS. A self-assembling nanoparticle for paclitaxel delivery in ovarian cancer. *Biomaterials*. 2009;30(30):6006–6016.

21. Lu Z, Tsai M, Lu D, Wang J, Wientjes MG, Au JLS. Tumor-penetrating microparticles for intraperitoneal therapy of ovarian cancer. *Journal of Pharmacology and Experimental Therapeutics*. 2008;327(3):673–682.

22. Lu Z, Tsai M, Wang J, Cole DJ, Wientjes MG, Au JLS. Activity of drug-loaded tumor-penetrating microparticles in peritoneal pancreatic tumors. *Current Cancer Drug Targets*. 2014;14(1):70–78.

23. Lu Z, Wang J, Wientjes MG, Au JL. Intraperitoneal therapy for peritoneal cancer. *Future Oncology*. 2010;6(10):1625–1641.

24. Padera TP, Stoll BR, Tooredman JB, Capen D, di Tomaso E, Jain RK. Pathology: Cancer cells compress intratumour vessels. *Nature*. 2004;427(6976):695.

25. Tailor TD, Hanna G, Yarmolenko PS, Dreher MR, Betof AS, Nixon AB, Spasojevic I, Dewhirst MW. Effect of pazopanib on tumor microenvironment and liposome delivery. *Molecular Cancer Therapeutics*. 2010;9(6):1798–1808.

26. Gremonprez F, Izmer A, Vanhaecke F, Ceelen W. Pharmacological modulation of tumor interstitial fluid pressure to enhance tissue penetration of intraperitoneal chemotherapy in a mouse colorectal carcinomatosis model. *Annals of Surgical Oncology*. 2014;21:S14–S15.

27. Provenzano PP, Cuevas C, Chang AE, Goel VK, Von Hoff DD, Hingorani SR. Enzymatic targeting of the stroma ablates physical barriers to treatment of pancreatic ductal adenocarcinoma. *Cancer Cell*. 2012;21(3):418–429.

28. Ariffin AB, Forde PF, Jahangeer S, Soden DM, Hinchion J. Releasing pressure in tumors: What do we know so far and where do we go from here? A review. *Cancer Research*. 2014;74(10):2655–2662.

29. Beyer I, Cao H, Persson J, Song H, Richter M, Feng Q, Yumul R et al. Coadministration of epithelial junction opener JO-1 improves the efficacy and safety of chemotherapeutic drugs. *Clinical Cancer Research*. 2012;18(12):3340–3351.

30. Chauhan VP, Martin JD, Liu H, Lacorre DA, Jain SR, Kozin SV, Stylianopoulos T et al. Angiotensin inhibition enhances drug delivery and potentiates chemotherapy by decompressing tumour blood vessels. *Nature Communications*. 2013;4:2516.

31. Moschetta M, Pretto F, Berndt A, Galler K, Richter P, Bassi A, Oliva P et al. Paclitaxel enhances therapeutic efficacy of the F8-IL2 immunocytokine to EDA-fibronectin-positive metastatic human melanoma xenografts. *Cancer Research*. 2012;72(7):1814–1824.

32. Taghian AG, Abi-Raad R, Assaad SI, Casty A, Ancukiewicz M, Yeh E, Molokhia P et al. Paclitaxel decreases the interstitial fluid pressure and improves oxygenation in breast cancers in patients treated with neoadjuvant chemotherapy: Clinical implications. *Journal of Clinical Oncology*. 2005;23(9):1951–1961.

33. Fuso Nerini I, Morosi L, Zucchetti M, Ballerini A, Giavazzi R, D'Incalci M. Intratumor heterogeneity and its impact on drug distribution and sensitivity. *Clinical Pharmacology & Therapeutics*. 2014;96(2):224–238.

34. Patel KJ, Lee C, Tan Q, Tannock IF. Use of the proton pump inhibitor pantoprazole to modify the distribution and activity of doxorubicin: A potential strategy to improve the therapy of solid tumors. *Clinical Cancer Research*. 2013;19(24):6766–6776.

35. Sen A, Capitano ML, Spernyak JA, Schueckler JT, Thomas S, Singh AK, Evans SS, Hylander BL, Repasky EA. Mild elevation of body temperature reduces tumor interstitial fluid pressure and hypoxia and enhances efficacy of radiotherapy in murine tumor models. *Cancer Research* 2011;71(11):3872–3880.

36. Hauck ML, Coffin DO, Dodge RK, Dewhirst MW, Mitchell JB, Zalutsky MR. A local hyperthermia treatment which enhances antibody uptake in a glioma xenograft model does not affect tumour interstitial fluid pressure. *International Journal of Hyperthermia*. 1997;13(3):307–316.

37. Los G, Sminia P, Wondergem J, Mutsaers PH, Havemen J, ten Bokkel Huinink D, Smals O, Gonzalez-Gonzalez D, McVie JG. Optimisation of intraperitoneal cisplatin therapy with regional hyperthermia in rats. *European Journal of Cancer*. 1991;27(4):472–477.

38. Zeamari S, Floot B, van der Vange N, Stewart FA. Pharmacokinetics and pharmacodynamics of cisplatin after intraoperative hyperthermic intraperitoneal chemoperfusion (HIPEC). *Anticancer Research*. 2003;23(2B):1643–1648.

39. Facy O, Radais F, Ladoire S, Delroeux D, Tixier H, Ghiringhelli F, Rat P, Chauffert B, Ortega-Deballon P. Comparison of hyperthermia and adrenaline to enhance the intratumoral accumulation of cisplatin in a murine model of peritoneal carcinomatosis. *Journal of Experimental & Clinical Cancer Research*. 2011;30:4.

40. Lindner P, Heath D, Howell S, Naredi P, Hafstrom L. Vasopressin modulation of peritoneal, lymphatic, and plasma drug exposure following intraperitoneal administration. *Clinical Cancer Research*. 1996;2(2):311–317.

41. Oman M, Tolli J, Naredi P, Hafstrom LO. Effect of carcinomatosis and intraperitoneal 5-fluorouracil on peritoneal blood flow modulated by vasopressin in the rat as measured with the Xe-133-clearance technique. *Cancer Chemotherapy and Pharmacology*. 2004;54(3):213–218.

42. Mahteme H, Sundin A, Larsson B, Khamis H, Arow K, Graf W. 5-FU uptake in peritoneal metastases after pretreatment with radioimmunotherapy or vasoconstriction: An autoradiographic study in the rat. *Anticancer Research*. 2005;25(2A):917–922.

43. Duvillard C, Benoit L, Moretto P, Beltramo JL, Brunet-Lecomte P, Correia M, Sergent C, Chauffert B. Epinephrine enhances penetration and anti-cancer activity of local cisplatin on rat sub-cutaneous and peritoneal tumors. *International Journal of Cancer*. 1999;81(5):779–784.

44. Guardiola E, Chauffert B, Delroeux D, Royer B, Heyd B, Combe M, Benoit L et al. Intraoperative chemotherapy with cisplatin and epinephrine after cytoreductive surgery in patients with recurrent ovarian cancer: A phase I study. *Anticancer Drugs*. 2010;21(3):320–325.

45. Royer B, Kalbacher E, Onteniente S, Jullien V, Montange D, Piedoux S, Thiery-Vuillemin A et al. Intraperitoneal clearance as a potential biomarker of cisplatin after intraperitoneal perioperative chemotherapy: A population pharmacokinetic study. *British Journal of Cancer*. 2012;106(3):460–467.

46. Oman M, Lundqvist S, Gustavsson B, Hafstrom L, Naredi P. Phase I/II trial of intraperitoneal 5-Fluorouracil with and without intravenous Vasopressin in non-resectable pancreas cancer. *Cancer Chemotherapy and Pharmacology*. 2005;56(6):603–609.

47. Kondo A, Maeta M, Oka A, Tsujitani S, Ikeguchi M, Kaibara N. Hypotonic intraperitoneal cisplatin chemotherapy for peritoneal carcinomatosis in mice. *British Journal of Cancer*. 1996;73(10):1166–1170.

48. Tsujitani S, Oka A, Kondo A, Katano K, Oka S, Saito H, Ikeguchi M, Maeta M, Kaibara N. Administration in a hypotonic solution is preferable to dose escalation in intraperitoneal cisplatin chemotherapy for peritoneal carcinomatosis in rats. *Oncology*. 1999;57(1):77–82.

49. Elias D, El Otmany A, Bonnay M, Paci A, Ducreux M, Antoun S, Lasser P, Laurent S, Bourget P. Human pharmacokinetic study of heated intraperitoneal oxaliplatin in increasingly hypotonic solutions after complete resection of peritoneal carcinomatosis. *Oncology*. 2002;63(4):346–352.

50. Wei ZG, Li GX, Huang XC, Zhen L, Yu J, Deng HJ, Qing SH, Zhang C. Pharmacokinetics and tissue distribution of intraperitoneal 5-fluorouracil with a novel carrier solution in rats. *World Journal of Gastroenterology*. 2008;14(14):2179–2186.

51. Esquis P, Consolo D, Magnin G, Pointaire P, Moretto P, Ynsa MD, Beltramo JL et al. High intra-abdominal pressure enhances the penetration and antitumor effect of intraperitoneal cisplatin on experimental peritoneal carcinomatosis. *Annals of Surgery*. 2006;244(1):106–112.

52. Jacquet P, Stuart OA, Chang D, Sugarbaker PH. Effects of intra-abdominal pressure on pharmacokinetics and tissue distribution of doxorubicin after intraperitoneal administration. *Anticancer Drugs*. 1996;7(5):596–603.

53. Facy O, Al Samman S, Magnin G, Ghiringhelli F, Ladoire S, Chauffert B, Rat P, Ortega-Deballon P. High pressure enhances the effect of hyperthermia in intraperitoneal chemotherapy with oxaliplatin: An experimental study. *Annals of Surgery*. 2012;256(6):1084–1088.

54. Tempfer CB, Celik I, Solass W, Buerkle B, Pabst UG, Zieren J, Strumberg D, Reymond MA. Activity of pressurized intraperitoneal aerosol chemotherapy (PIPAC) with cisplatin and doxorubicin in women with recurrent, platinum-resistant ovarian cancer: Preliminary clinical experience. *Gynecologic Oncology*. 2014;132(2):307–311.

55. Solass W, Kerb R, Murdter T, Giger-Pabst U, Strumberg D, Tempfer C, Zieren J, Schwab M, Reymond MA. Intraperitoneal chemotherapy of peritoneal carcinomatosis using pressurized aerosol as an alternative to liquid solution: First evidence for efficacy. *Annals of Surgical Oncology*. 2014;21(2):553–559.

56. Solass W, Giger-Pabst U, Zieren J, Reymond MA. Pressurized intraperitoneal aerosol chemotherapy (PIPAC): Occupational health and safety aspects. *Annals of Surgical Oncology*. 2013;20(11):3504–3511.

57. Blanco A, Giger-Pabst U, Solass W, Zieren J, Reymond MA. Renal and hepatic toxicities after pressurized intraperitoneal aerosol chemotherapy (PIPAC). *Annals of Surgical Oncology*. 2013;20(7):2311–2316.

58. Steimer JL, Dahl SG, De Alwis DP, Gundert-Remy U, Karlsson MO, Martinkova J, Aarons L et al. Modelling the genesis and treatment of cancer: The potential role of physiologically based pharmacodynamics. *European Journal of Cancer*. 2010;46(1):21–32.

59. Iyengar R, Zhao S, Chung SW, Mager DE, Gallo JM. Merging systems biology with pharmacodynamics. *Science Translational Medicine*. 2012;4(126):126–127.

60. Cerretani D, Nencini C, Urso R, Giorgi G, Marrelli D, De Stefano A, Pinto E, Cioppa T, Nastri G, Roviello F. Pharmacokinetics of mitomycin C after resection of peritoneal carcinomatosis and intraperitoneal chemohyperthermic perfusion. *Journal of Chemotherapy*. 2005;17(6):668–673.

61. Panteix G, Beaujard A, Garbit F, Chaduiron-Faye C, Guillaumont M, Gilly F, Baltassat P, Bressolle F. Population pharmacokinetics of cisplatin in patients with advanced ovarian cancer during intraperitoneal hyperthermia chemotherapy. *Anticancer Research*. 2002;22(2B):1329–1336.

62. Royer B, Jullien V, Guardiola E, Heyd B, Chauffert B, Kantelip JP, Pivot X. Population pharmacokinetics and dosing recommendations for cisplatin during intraperitoneal peroperative administration: Development of a limited sampling strategy for toxicity risk assessment. *Clinical Pharmacokinetics*. 2009;48(3):169–180.

63. Ferron G, Dattez S, Gladieff L, Delord JP, Pierre S, Lafont T, Lochon I, Chatelut E. Pharmacokinetics of heated intraperitoneal oxaliplatin. *Cancer Chemotherapy and Pharmacology*. 2008;62(4):679–683.

64. Perez-Ruixo C, Valenzuela B, Peris JE, Bretcha-Boix P, Escudero-Ortiz V, Farre-Alegre J, Perez-Ruixo JJ. Population pharmacokinetics of hyperthermic intraperitoneal oxaliplatin in patients with peritoneal carcinomatosis after cytoreductive surgery. *Cancer Chemotherapy and Pharmacology*. 2013;71(3):693–704.

65. van Ruth S, Mathot RA, Sparidans RW, Beijnen JH, Verwaal VJ, Zoetmulder FA. Population pharmacokinetics and pharmacodynamics of mitomycin during intraoperative hyperthermic intraperitoneal chemotherapy. *Clinical Pharmacokinetics*. 2004;43(2):131–143.

66. Royer B, Delroeux D, Guardiola E, Combe M, Hoizey G, Montange D, Kantelip JP, Chauffert B, Heyd B, Pivot X. Improvement in intraperitoneal intraoperative cisplatin exposure based on pharmacokinetic analysis in patients with ovarian cancer. *Cancer Chemotherapy and Pharmacology*. 2008;61(3):415–421.

67. Royer B, Guardiola E, Polycarpe E, Hoizey G, Delroeux D, Combe M, Chaigneau L et al. Serum and intraperitoneal pharmacokinetics of cisplatin within intraoperative intraperitoneal chemotherapy: Influence of protein binding. *Anticancer Drugs*. 2005;16(9):1009–1016.

68. Perez-Ruixo C, Valenzuela B, Peris JE, Bretcha-Boix P, Escudero-Ortiz V, Farre-Alegre J, Perez-Ruixo JJ. Neutrophil dynamics in peritoneal carcinomatosis patients treated with cytoreductive surgery and hyperthermic intraperitoneal oxaliplatin. *Clinical Pharmacokinetics*. 2013;52(12):1111–1125.

69. Valenzuela B, Nalda-Molina R, Bretcha-Boix P, Escudero-Ortiz V, Duart MJ, Carbonell V, Sureda M et al. Pharmacokinetic and pharmacodynamic analysis of hyperthermic intraperitoneal oxaliplatin-induced neutropenia in subjects with peritoneal carcinomatosis. *The AAPS Journal*. 2011;13(1):72–82.

70. Friberg LE, Henningsson A, Maas H, Nguyen L, Karlsson MO. Model of chemotherapy-induced myelosuppression with parameter consistency across drugs. *Journal of Clinical Oncology*. 2002;20(24):4713–4721.

71. Colin P, De Smet L, Vervaet C, Remon JP, Ceelen W, Van Bocxlaer J, Boussery K, Vermeulen A. A model based analysis of IPEC dosing of paclitaxel in rats. *Pharmaceutical Research*. 2014;31(10):2876–2886.

72. Rocchetti M, Simeoni M, Pesenti E, De Nicolao G, Poggesi I. Predicting the active doses in humans from animal studies: A novel approach in oncology. *European Journal of Cancer*. 2007;43(12):1862–1868.

13

Mathematical models of intraperitoneal drug delivery

JOANNA STACHOWSKA-PIETKA AND JACEK WANIEWSKI

INTRODUCTION

Mathematical models allow for the qualitative and quantitative description of the transport processes, resulting not only in better understanding of physiology but also in the prediction of local and global responses to therapy. The models may be helpful in the assessment of the applicability of treatment and its optimization. The mathematical description of the physiological processes yields also a quantitative estimation of treatment efficiency that can be verified in clinical and experimental studies. In the case of intraperitoneal therapies, it may provide an estimation of the penetration depth of the drug in the peritoneal tissue and its concentration in normal and neoplastic tissue [4,5,23,34,72,82,86]. It may help in the identification of the conditions that can improve the efficiency of the treatment as well as the estimation of the amount of therapeutic agent that is absorbed to the tissue and systemic circulation [20,22]. The effectiveness of the intraperitoneal therapy strongly depends on the target localization. The accessibility from the peritoneal cavity, distance for therapeutic agent to reach the target, therapeutic agent size, and transport characteristics of both target and drug determine the efficiency and utility of the intraperitoneal therapy [10,22,57].

The compartment or the so-called membrane modeling can be used for the estimation of the fluid and solute

flow between intraperitoneal fluid and blood circulation [80,81]. However, for the estimation of the absorption to the tissue and flows through the tissue, the spatial properties of the transport system must be taken into account and the so called spatially distributed approach should be used [15,22,72,73,82]. The distributed approach is used to provide detailed information on the peritoneal physiology and realistic description of the anatomy of the peritoneal transport system (PTS). It is based on the local tissue and microcirculatory physiology, and its parameters are derived from the local structure and properties of the tissue and microvasculature.

The first applications of the distributed model date back to the early 1960s and were limited to the diffusive solute transport. Piiper et al. studied the exchange of gases between blood and artificial gas pockets within the body [66]. The transport of gases between subcutaneous pockets and blood was studied in rats and piglets [12,79]. The exchange of heat and solutes between blood and tissue was investigated using distributed approach by Perl [64,65]. The first application of the distributed model for the description of the diffusive transport of small solutes was proposed by Patlak and Fenstermacher, in order to describe transport from cerebrospinal fluid to the brain [63]. Moreover, the diffusive delivery of drugs to the human bladder during intravesical chemotherapy, as well as from the skin surface to the dermis, was also experimentally studied in normal and tumor tissue providing the verification of the predictions from distributed approach [41,89,90].

The application of distributed models in intraperitoneal therapies was initiated in the early 1980s. The diffusive transport of gases between intraperitoneal pockets and blood was studied by Collins in 1981 [12]. In the peritoneal dialysis, the distributed approach was introduced by Dedrick, Flessner, and colleagues and applied to model the transport of small, middle, and macromolecules in animal studies and in patients on peritoneal dialysis [15,23,30,31,33,34]. The process of intraperitoneal drug delivery, especially for anticancer therapies, was also described using the distributed approach [13,20,23]. These models were applied for diffusive and convective peritoneal solute transport. Seames, Moncrief, and Popovich were the first who investigated osmotically driven fluid and solute transport during peritoneal dwell [69]. Their attempt was later disproved by animal experiments [21]. Further investigations by Leypoldt and Henderson were focused on solute transport driven by diffusion and ultrafiltration from blood and interactions of the solute with the tissue [54,56]. In another approach, the changes in the fluorouracil concentration within the tissue were studied experimentally and modeled taking into account local interactions of the solute with the tissue [13]. The distributed model of fluid absorption from the peritoneal cavity has been proposed by Stachowska-Pietka et al. [71,73]. The transport of IgG was modeled and studied experimentally by Flessner et al. [23,34]. The osmotically driven glucose transport was modeled by Cherniha, Waniewski, and coauthors [72,83]. A new attempt to apply distributed approach to model impact of chronic peritoneal inflammation from sterile solutions and structural changes within the tissue on the solute and water transport was undertaken recently by Flessner et al. [26]. In addition, convective and diffusive transport through the tumor tissue after intravascular injection has been studied theoretically and experimentally by Jain and coworkers [4,5,7,8,59].

In this chapter, we present a mathematical approach to describe peritoneal transport and some practical implications of the modeling for peritoneal chemotherapy. The spatially distributed mathematical model of fluid and solute transport through the peritoneal tissue is described and formulas for the estimation of the solute penetration depth derived from the model. A version of this model that is applied for a description of the transport in solid tumor is also discussed. Finally, the difference between transport parameters in the normal and neoplastic tissue and its consequences for the fluid and solute peritoneal transport are analyzed.

PERITONEAL TRANSPORT SYSTEM

Peritoneal fluid and solute exchange occurs in all the organs that surround the peritoneal cavity. Therapeutic agents may be transported to the tissue by diffusion or/and together with reabsorbed water from the peritoneal cavity. The tissue is perfused with blood and capillaries, and lymphatics are placed at different distance from the peritoneal surface. The bulk water flow drives drugs to the peritoneal tissue, where they interact with the tissue components to be slowly absorbed to the circulation by the local lymphatics and across the porous blood capillary wall.

The density of the capillary network and therefore blood and lymph flow rates depend on the organ, resulting in the differences in the PTS. Moreover, there are also differences in the effective area of the peritoneal surface that is in the contact with intraperitoneal fluid and through which drug uptake occurs. Due to diversity between the organs, four organ groups within the peritoneal tissue can be distinguished: diaphragm, abdominal wall, liver, and other viscera such as intestine, spleen, or stomach [20]. It has been shown that 10%–30% of total water absorption from the peritoneal cavity is caused by the direct lymph flow from the peritoneal cavity. The subdiaphragmatic lymphatics that are situated in diaphragm and open directly to the peritoneal cavity are responsible for 70%–80% of this direct lymph flow and are able to absorb even large particles up to the 25 µm of diameter [20]. Due to its localization, the transport in diaphragm is also strongly influenced by the respiration, which creates large, variable pressure gradient [20]. On the other hand, the high-pressure gradient that is exerted across the abdominal wall as well as the relatively small development of the lymphatics results in the fact that 40%–50% of total outflow from the peritoneal cavity enters this compartment making it the single largest recipient of the fluid [20]. The liver has been separated from the other viscera due to its role in the drug metabolism and also due to hepatic portal blood circulation that is different than in other organs [20].

Model concept and transport barriers

Typically, the distributed models are formulated for the plane tissue layer, and the transport within this tissue is considered in one dimension perpendicular to the tissue surface. This dimension, in the case of peritoneal transport, reflects distance in the tissue measured from the peritoneal surface. This theory can be easily extended to the 3D tissue.

The distributed approach takes into account the spatial distribution of the PTS components. This concept includes the spatial distribution of blood and lymph capillaries that are typically assumed to be uniformly distributed within the tissue. However, this simplifying assumption can in general be omitted, and the variability of the tissue space and structure can be taken into account. The interstitium that is treated as a deformable, porous medium is typically the most important transport pathway across the tissue [23,82]. In order to describe the distributed structure of PTS, the methods of partial differential equation should be applied. As a result, the changes in the spatial distribution of solutes and fluid in the tissue with time can be modeled.

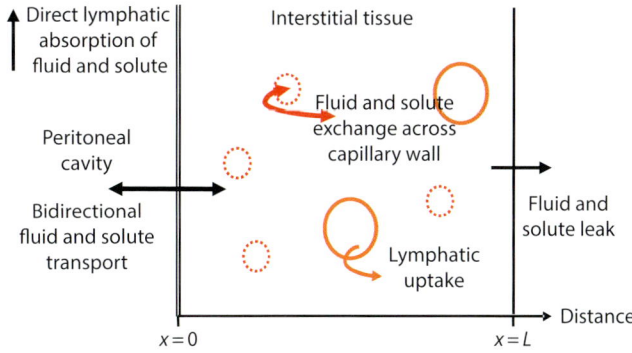

Figure 13.1 Fluid and solute transport pathways during intraperitoneal therapy.

Briefly, once water and solutes leave the peritoneal cavity and cross the anatomical peritoneum, they enter the adjacent tissue and penetrate to its interior. In the tissue, fluid and solute partly cross the heterosporous capillary wall and are washed out by the blood stream, whereas another fraction is absorbed from the tissue by local lymphatics. A part of the fluid and solute accumulates in the tissue. In some situations, a fraction of the fluid and solute flow can leave the tissue on its other side, as in the case of intestine or as in some experiments, when the impermeable outer surface (skin) was removed [21]. Figure 13.1 summarizes all described fluid and solute transport pathways.

Typically, two main transport barriers for bidirectional fluid and solute transport are considered in the distributed approach: the heterosporous capillary wall and interstitium. The experimental studies showed that interstitium, besides the capillary wall, seems to be the most important barrier for fluid and solute transport. In addition, Seames et al. considered the anatomic peritoneum to be a significant barrier and modeled it as a semipermeable membrane with the properties analogous to that of the endothelium [69]. They analyzed the combined transport of fluid and solutes such as blood urea nitrogen, creatinine, glucose, and inulin. They fitted the model to the data on intraperitoneal volume and solute concentrations in dialysate and blood and predicted negative values of interstitial hydrostatic pressure [69]. However, later studies by Flessner disproved this approach [21]. He found positive interstitial pressure profiles in the peritoneal layer, which observation demonstrated that peritoneum should not be considered as a significant barrier to water and solute transport [19,21]. In addition, the continuous profiles of labeled albumin and IgG across the peritoneum, decaying with the distance from the peritoneal cavity, were shown [29]. Moreover, it was shown that the transport of IgG from the peritoneal cavity into the adjacent tissue occurs at the same rate for either isotonic or hypertonic solution, and therefore its convective transport is not retarded by the ultrafiltration flow in the opposite direction [28].

Most of the fluid and solute transport during intraperitoneal therapy occurs through the tissue layer beneath the peritoneum. It is composed of the interstitium, which fills the extracellular space and forms connective and supporting tissue located outside the blood and lymphatics, capillaries, and parenchymal cells [2,92]. In general, for some solutes, the local cellular transport plays a secondary role if compared to the interstitial [1]. The exchange of the considered solutes (urea, creatinine, glucose, and albumin) between interstitium and cells (as muscle cells) was typically considered negligible compared to their exchange between blood and dialysis fluid during peritoneal dialysis [72,86]. Therefore, the transport through the cells (apart from the aquaporin mediated water transport across the endothelium) is typically not taken into account in the distributed modeling, and the attention is paid to the interstitial transport. However, for some solutes, the contribution of intracellular compartment into the peritoneal transport may be of clinical importance, as evidenced by potassium [11,84].

The capillaries play the main role in the microvascular exchange of fluid and solute between blood and tissue. It was established, on the basis of numerous experiments, that the capillary wall behaves functionally as a heterosporous structure. According to the pore theory, which was developed to model microvascular transport, three types of pore are considered: large pores (typically assumed radius 200–400 Å), small pores (usually modeled with radius 39–67 Å), and ultrasmall pores (also termed water channels, transcellular pores, or aquaporin channels). According to this concept, the small pores have the large total surface area and are the main routes for the transcapillary diffusive transport of small and middle-sized molecules (up to the size of inulin of 1.3 nm), whereas the transport of proteins is substantially restricted from the small pores. The large pores play the main role in the convective transport of macromolecules (especially proteins), whereas the ultrasmall pores are permeable only for water and help to shift efficiently water in response to osmotic and hydrostatic gradients across the capillary wall.

The lymphatic capillaries also participate in the local microvascular exchange. The major role of lymphatics is to return plasma proteins from extracellular space to the circulation and to help maintaining the interstitial fluid volume balance by the increase of lymph flow after the increase of interstitial volume and pressure. Lymphatic capillaries are thin-walled tubes with a diameter that is usually three to eight times larger than that of blood capillaries, but their number is usually smaller and differs between peritoneal organs [2,39,40]. Unlike the blood capillaries, they have irregular shape and may be constricted and dilated in different regions. However, experimental observations suggest "a relatively free communication between the interstitium and the initial lymphatics, leading to the concept that the lymphatics appear anatomically as well as physiologically to be an extension of the interstitial space in that fluid, electrolytes, proteins, and even particulate and cellular elements may freely enter the lymph capillaries" [2,88].

Major driving forces and transport processes

The infusion of fluid into the peritoneal cavity disturbs the local homeostasis and induces solute and water transport. The inflow of dialysis fluid changes the intraperitoneal fluid volume and increases intraperitoneal hydrostatic pressure (IPP). The hydrostatic pressure gradient between peritoneal cavity and underlying tissue layers results in the absorption of water from the peritoneal cavity (Figure 13.2). Additionally, when an osmotic agent is added to the infused fluid, it induces osmotic pressure gradient and the removal of water from the tissue and blood to the peritoneal cavity (Figure 13.2). This water flow driven by the osmotic pressure is typically called ultrafiltration.

The level of IPP depends not only on the amount of dialysis fluid infused but also on patient position and physical activity. The changes in IPP are proportional to the changes in the intraperitoneal volume [78]. Typically, infusion of 2 L increases IPP on average to 6.7 ± 0.8 mmHg (range 3.9–10.8 mmHg) in the supine position and to higher values in the upright position (12.6 ± 0.8 mmHg, range 9.2–15.2 mmHg) [47]. Twardowski et al. reported values at the highest point in the cavity from 2.5 mmHg (in supine position) to 7.5 mmHg (in sitting position) for 2 L of infused volume [78]. Another study by Twardowski et al. suggests that IPP may increase, even above 100 mmHg, due to patient's activity such as coughing, walking, and jogging [77]. The high variability in IPP measurements results partly from the intrapatient variability but also from the sensitivity of the method, especially the choice of the reference point. The lowest values of 2.5 mmHg were measured by Twardowski et al. in the supine position at the umbilicus level, whereas higher values of 7–13 mmHg were reported if the axillary line was used as the reference point [18,47].

The elevated IPP induces hydrostatic pressure-driven fluid absorption from the peritoneal cavity (c.f. Figure 13.2). Experiments in cats demonstrated that the fluid loss from the peritoneal cavity is directly proportional to the IPP for isotonic solution with and without 8% bovine serum albumin [99]. Similarly, a positive correlation between increased IPP and peritoneal fluid absorption rate was found in rats and in continuous ambulatory peritoneal dialysis patients [46,98]. Moreover, animal and clinical studies showed that fluid absorption is independent of fluid hypertonicity and therefore is not influenced by ultrafiltration to the peritoneal cavity [35,36,42,60]. There is strong evidence that fluid absorption from the peritoneal cavity involves two different pathways: direct lymphatic absorption, mainly by diaphragmatic lymphatic, and fluid absorption into the adjacent tissue. Typically, for the estimation of the peritoneal absorption and its components, the disappearance rate of macromolecular markers from the peritoneal cavity is used. This method is based on the fact that transport of macromolecules from the peritoneal cavity occurs without sieving. The typical value of the average fluid loss from the peritoneal cavity estimated by absorption of macromolecular markers in clinical studies amounts to 1.0–1.8 mL/min [43,46,85]. Slightly higher values of 2.34 ± 1.14 mL/min has been reported by Pannekeet et al. [62]. Substantially higher values of 4.5–5.0 mL/min were found in some patients on peritoneal dialysis with loss of ultrafiltration capacity [43,44]. Clinical studies showed that only about 10%–20% of total fluid absorption (loss) from the peritoneal cavity is due to direct lymphatic uptake, whereas the rest of the absorbed fluid takes part in the local exchange between peritoneal cavity and the surrounding tissue layers [43]. Animal studies suggested that elevation of IPP increases peritoneal absorption to the adjacent tissue, leaving direct lymphatic absorption, measured as the rate of radioisotopically labelled serum albumin (RISA) appearance in plasma, constant [98]. Therefore, fluid absorption by these two absorption pathways may be driven by different forces.

During intraperitoneal therapy, solutes can be transported by diffusion and/or convection in both directions, i.e., to and from the peritoneal cavity. The passive, diffusive transport is driven by the diffusive force created by the difference in solute concentration between dialysate in the peritoneal cavity and the surrounding tissue. The convective transport of solute is driven by water flow, which works as a vehicle to transport large molecules such as albumin and other proteins and drugs. Transport of low molecular weight (MW) solutes, i.e., with MW smaller than 600 Da, such as urea, creatinine, or glucose, occurs mainly due to diffusion, whereas convection is less important. For larger molecules, such as proteins, with MW higher than 40,000 Da, convection is the dominant mechanism of transport, although diffusive transport is also of some importance [34,55]. For solutes with MW in the range from 600 to 40,000 Da, both transport components, diffusive and convective, are important. Finally, independently of the size, solutes are also directly absorbed from the peritoneal cavity by lymphatic uptake of dialysate that occurs without sieving. The components of peritoneal solute transport and driving forces are presented schematically in Figure 13.3.

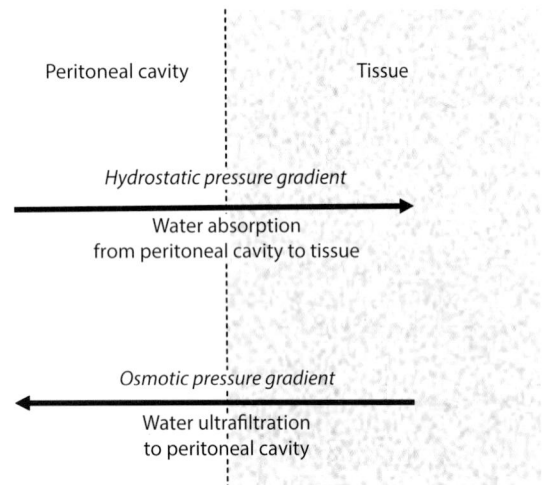

Figure 13.2 The major driving forces and directions of fluid transport between peritoneal cavity and tissue during intraperitoneal therapy.

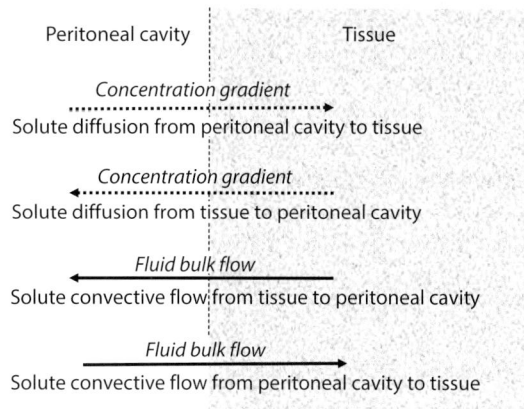

Figure 13.3 The components of peritoneal solute transport between peritoneal cavity and tissue and driving forces during intraperitoneal therapy.

FLUID AND SOLUTE TRANSPORT THROUGH THE PERITONEAL TISSUE

Based on the principles of physiology, a mathematical model of fluid and solute transport can be derived. It considers spatial propagation of fluid and solute as a function of the distance from the peritoneal cavity. Therefore, it can be applied for the description of the transport from the peritoneal cavity through the surrounding normal or tumor tissue (with modifications on the differences in the values of the transport parameters). Additional simplification of this model, typically applied for the description of the transport within the tumor, will be presented in the next section.

Modeling of fluid transport

Peritoneal transport of water is of a great importance in intraperitoneal therapies especially because of its role in the convective uptake of therapeutic agent. Increase of IPP (caused by fluid infusion) would result in the water absorption to surrounding tissue layers, causing local increase of tissue hydration and interstitial pressure. In addition, in the case of hypertonic solution such as glucose 1.36%, osmotic pressure gradient is created that induces local vasodilation and fluid flow from blood and tissue to the peritoneal cavity. This water inflow into the peritoneal cavity may counteract the drug uptake, which occurs in the opposite direction, especially for the high glucose concentration fluids such as glucose 3.86%. On the other hand, increase of vasodilation caused by high glucose concentrations in the infused fluid may enhance the drug uptake from the peritoneal cavity to blood. However, in the case of glucose 1.36% solution, osmotic gradient is relatively small and quickly disappears, and therefore during the rest time of the treatment, bulk fluid absorption from the peritoneal cavity plays major role in drugs uptake. Therefore, in the following consideration, the effect of osmotic gradient in the dialysate will not be taken into account.

The fluid space within the interstitium can be described using the *interstitial fluid void volume ratio*, θ, further in the

text called the void volume, which is defined as the fraction of the interstitial space that is available for interstitial fluid. Typically, at physiological equilibrium, this value remains around 15%–18% [67,97]. The changes in the void volume during the treatment reflect the changes in the tissue hydration. The local tissue hydration changes during the treatment due to the fluid flow through the interstitium (j_V) and local microvascular exchange through the blood capillaries q_V^{cap} and lymphatics (q_L). Based on the volume balance of the interstitium, this can be formulated as follows [73]:

$$\frac{\partial \theta}{\partial t} = -\frac{\partial j_V}{\partial x} + q_V^{cap} - q_L \qquad (13.1)$$

where

$\partial\theta/\partial t$ describes the changes in the void volume during the treatment

j_V is the fluid flux through the interstitium in the direction perpendicular to the peritoneal surface (in mL/min/cm²)

q_V^{cap} is the rate of the fluid flow into the tissue across the blood capillary wall (in 1/min)

q_L is the rate of local lymphatic flow (1/min)

x is the distance measured from the peritoneal surface (in cm)

t is time (in seconds)

Note that in the fact, changes in the tissue hydration depend on its compliance (defined as the ratio of the change in the interstitial fluid volume to the corresponding change in the interstitial pressure) and on the interstitial pressure changes in time, i.e., $\partial\theta/\partial t = (d\theta/dP)\cdot(\partial P/\partial t)$, where P is the interstitial hydrostatic pressure (in mmHg).

According to Darcy's law, fluid flux through the interstitium is proportional to the local tissue hydraulic conductivity, K, and local interstitial hydrostatic pressure gradient, $\partial P/\partial x$ [23,73]. Therefore,

$$j_V = -K \cdot \frac{\partial P}{\partial x} \qquad (13.2)$$

It has been shown that hydraulic conductivity of the tissue (K in cm²/min/mmHg) follows the changes in the tissue hydration and increases almost linearly in response to the increased interstitial pressure [96].

For the calculation of the microvascular fluid exchange between blood capillaries and tissue, pores or membrane approach (Starling's law) can be applied. According to both approaches, the fluid flow across the capillary wall, q_V^{cap}, is driven by the hydrostatic pressure difference and the sum of osmotic pressure differences that are exerted across the capillary wall. It can be formulated for the membrane or single pore approach as $q_V^{cap} = L_p a(P_B - P) - L_p a \sum_{S=1,...,N} \sigma_S^{cap} \cdot RT \cdot (C_{B,S} - C_S)$, where P_B and $C_{B,S}$ are blood capillary hydrostatic pressure and solute S concentration, respectively, typically assumed to be constant, C_S is the solute S concentration in the interstitial fluid, $L_p a$ is the capillary wall hydraulic conductance (L_p) times capillary surface area density per unit volume of wet tissue (in 1/min/mmHg), and σ_S^{cap} is the capillary wall reflection coefficient, and RT is the gas constant R times temperature T (in K). For isotonic fluid solutions, no vasodilatory effect is observed, and parameters for the capillary wall, $L_p a$ and σ_S^{cap}, can be assumed constant and their values estimated from experimental data or calculated according to the three-pore model. Note that from the van't Hoff law the solute concentration difference can be transformed to the osmolality difference. In this case,

$$q_V^{cap} = L_p a (P_B - P) - L_p a \sigma_S^{cap} \cdot (\Pi_B - \Pi) \qquad (13.3)$$

where Π_B and Π are blood and tissue osmotic pressures, respectively (in mmHg). In the case of the three-pore approach, fluid flow across the capillary wall should be calculated separately for each pore type and later summed up. In addition, one may assume for simplicity that osmotic (especially oncotic) pressure in the tissue, Π, depends on the interstitial fluid volume ratio θ and can be calculated as $\Pi = \Pi_0 \theta_0 / \theta$, where subscript "0" means the value of the function at time $t = 0$, i.e., in the state of physiological equilibrium. This functional relationship describes the effect of the dilution of interstitial fluid due to the inflow of protein-free dialysis fluid and the expansion of the interstitial fluid volume ratio.

The rate of lymphatic absorption can be assumed constant. However, animal experiments have been shown that when the tissue hydration and interstitial pressure increase, then the rate of lymphatic absorption tend to increase proportionally to the increase in P, in order to prevent creation of local edema [6,9]. Therefore, in general, the lymph flow can be described as a function of interstitial pressure given by $q_L = q_{L0} + q_{L1}(P - P_0)$, where q_{L0} is the rate of lymphatic absorption in the normal physiological equilibrium in the tissue, q_{L1} describes the sensitivity of lymphatic absorption for the increase in hydrostatic pressure, and P_0 denotes the interstitial pressure above which the increase of lymphatic absorption occurs. Some authors consider the rate of lymphatic absorption as proportional to the pressure difference between interstitium and lymphatics. In this case, lymph flow is described by $q_L = q_{L1}(P - P_L)$. Note that at the steady state there should be no net fluid flux across the tissue, $\partial j_V / \partial x = 0$, and therefore microvascular exchange across the capillary wall should be counterbalanced by the local lymphatic absorption. This would allowed for the calculation of q_{L0} or P_L, respectively, depending on the approach [4,73].

Modeling of solute transport

Experimental studies showed that distribution of the solute macromolecules in the interstitium can be restricted to even 50% of fluid distribution volume θ. The fraction of solute interstitial void volume, θ_S, i.e., the fraction of interstitial fluid void volume effectively available to the solute S,

depends on the solute molecular size and, in the case of large macromolecules, can be significantly smaller than that for fluid. Therefore, in general, $\theta_S \leq \theta$. The value of $\theta_S = 0.05\theta$ was measured experimentally and considered for the simulation of IgG transport by Flessner [23,34]. The solute concentration in the interstitial fluid depends on the solute flux through the tissue (j_S), on the restricted microvascular exchange across the capillary wall (q_S^{cap}), and the solute lymphatic absorption ($C_S q_L$). For some solutes, it might be also decreased by the rate at which the free molecule is binding (specific or nonspecific) to proteins or other tissue components (R_{bind}), on the rate at which solute is metabolized by the cells (R_{metab}), and finally on the tissue generation rate of solute S (R_{gen}). Therefore, in general, the solute concentration profiles within the tissue can be derived from the equation on the local solute mass balance as [23,72]

$$\frac{\partial(\theta_S \cdot C_S)}{\partial t} = -\frac{\partial j_S}{\partial x} + q_S^{cap} - C_S q_L - R_{bind} - R_{metab} + R_{gen} \qquad (13.4)$$

where

θ_S is the fraction of solute void volume

C_S is the free solute concentration in the interstitial fluid (in mmol/mL)

j_S is the solute flux across the tissue in the direction perpendicular to the peritoneal surface (in mmol/min/cm^2)

q_S^{cap} is the rate of solute inflow to the tissue across the blood capillary wall (in mmol/min/mL)

Note that in this case, C_S denotes free solute concentration in the interstitial fluid void volume, whereas in experiments, the solute concentration in the tissue is often expressed as the total amount of labeled solute per unit volume of the tissue and therefore should be recalculated to the real values in the interstitial fluid.

The diffusive transport of solute depends on the local concentration gradient, whereas fluid flux across the tissue induces convective transport of the solute. Therefore, the general equation for the solute flux across the tissue can be formulated as follows [23,70,72]:

$$j_S = -D_S \frac{\partial C_S}{\partial x} + \left(1 - \sigma_S^T\right) \cdot j_V \cdot C_S \qquad (13.5)$$

where

D_S is the diffusivity of solute S in the tissue (in cm^2/min)

σ_S^T is the tissue reflection coefficient of solute S

j_V is the fluid flux through the tissue

Note that changes in the tissue hydration may influence diffusive properties of the solute in the tissue, so in general, D_S should be considered as θ or P dependent. Moreover, in some applications, parameter $1 - \sigma_S^T$ is called the sieving coefficient or the retardation factor as it represents the ratio of solute to solvent velocity, and in applications to solid tumor, is typically assumed to be equal to 1.

The microvascular exchange of solute across the blood capillary wall can be calculated according to the three-pore or membrane approach. In both cases, solute flux across the capillary wall driven by the solute concentration difference between blood and tissue, $C_{B,S} - C_S$, and by the convective fluid flow across capillary wall, q_V^{cap}, should be considered, with appropriate formulas for the specific blood capillary wall transport parameters. The net solute inflow to the tissue across the blood capillary wall can be calculated as follows:

$$q_S^{cap} = p_S a(C_{B,S} - C_S) + \left(1 - \sigma_S^{cap}\right) q_V^{cap}[(1-f)C_{B,S} + f \cdot C_S]$$

(13.6)

where

$p_S a$ is the diffusive permeability of solute S across the capillary wall (in 1/min)

σ_S^{cap} is the capillary wall reflection coefficient for solute S

f is the weighting factor within the range from 0 to 1, which in general can be calculated from the fluid flow across the capillary wall according to the formula for the Peclet number [82]

If the three-pore model is applied and the heterosporous structure of the capillary wall is taken into consideration, the corresponding convective fluxes through each type of pore should be considered. Moreover, due to the lack of vasodilation caused by hypertonicity of the intraperitoneal fluid, $p_S a$ can be considered as constant.

Note that

$$\frac{\partial(\theta_S C_S)}{\partial t} = \theta_S \cdot \frac{\partial C_S}{\partial t} + \frac{\partial(\theta_S)}{\partial t} C_S$$

Therefore, Equation 13.4 can be transformed to the equation for the time evolution of solute concentration

$$\theta_S \cdot \frac{\partial C_S}{\partial t} = -\frac{\partial j_S}{\partial x} - \frac{\partial(\theta_S)}{\partial t} C_S + q_S^{cap} - C_S q_L - R_{bind} - R_{metab} + R_{gen}$$

Initial and boundary conditions

Typically, the distributed model of peritoneal transport of fluid and solutes is considered in a tissue that surrounds peritoneal cavity and which has at least partial contact with intraperitoneal fluid. If the tissue is in equilibrium before fluid infusion into the peritoneal cavity, as it happens in many applications, then the interstitial hydrostatic pressure at $t = 0$ is assumed to be equal to 0 ($P(0,x) = P_0 = 0$). Moreover, the initial solutes concentration in the interstitium is typically assumed to be homogeneous: $C_S(0,x) = C_{0,S}$. In addition, the initial existence of homeostasis in the tissue requires equilibration of each solute concentration between blood and tissue (with respect to the sieving effect across the capillary wall). In particular, for a therapeutic agent that is not present in the interstitium

before a treatment, one should assume that $C_S(0,x) = 0$. Note that these assumptions might not be correct in the case of continuously repeated treatment.

After fluid infusion into the peritoneal cavity, the solute concentration in the interstitial fluid and interstitial hydrostatic pressure equilibrate with intraperitoneal fluid on the peritoneal surface of the tissue. The permeability of the peritoneal surface and the ability of fluid and solute for equilibration imply that at the peritoneal surface (for $x = 0$) the hydrostatic pressure should be equal to the hydrostatic pressure in the peritoneal cavity, P_D, ($P(t,0) = P_D(t)$), and solutes concentration at the peritoneal surface should equilibrate with its concentration in intraperitoneal fluid, $C_{D,S}$, ($C_S(t,0) = C_{D,S}(t)$) at any time t of the treatment.

The condition for fluid and solute transport on the other boundary of the tissue layer is strongly related to the tissue type, i.e., to its geometry and to the existence of the contacts with dialysate or another medium. In the applications of the distributed model for the peritoneal transport, the transport within the abdominal wall limited by the skin is considered as an example. In this case, the boundary conditions at $x = x_{MAX}$ state that there is no fluid and solute flux across the external layer, i.e., $j_V(t,x_{MAX}) = 0$ and $j_S(t,x_{MAX}) = 0$ at any time t. This implies Neumann boundary conditions, which should be fulfilled at $x = x_{MAX}$, such as $\partial P/\partial x(t,x_{MAX}) = 0$ and $\partial C_S/\partial x(t,x_{MAX}) = 0$. If the tissue is permeable also at the other boundary, then $P(t,x_{MAX}) = P_{x_{MAX}}(t)$ and $C_S(t,x_{MAX}) = C_{x_{MAX},S}(t)$ at any treatment time t, where $P_{x_{MAX}}(t)$ and $C_{x_{MAX},S}(t)$ are the hydrostatic pressure and solute concentration at the other boundary. This situation occurs, for example, when the tissue is in contact with dialysate from both sides, as it is in the case for mesentery, omentum, liver, and pancreas, or when the tissue is bathed by the other solution on the side opposite to the peritoneal surface, as in the case of the gut mucosa.

Effective penetration depth of solutes to the tissue

The effective transport parameters, which characterize the net peritoneal solute transport as assessed using the measurements in the peritoneal cavity, can be estimated from the distributed models under additional assumptions. The theoretical formulas can be derived based on the local physiological parameters, indicating impact of each transport barrier in the estimated value of the overall parameter. The following discussion is separated according to the solute mass and transport processes involved, because of the differences in the formulas. Note that in the case of convective or diffusive–convective transport, additionally, description of fluid transport is necessary.

In the distributed model, the solute flow from the peritoneal cavity to the tissue across the peritoneal surface is given by $A \cdot j_S$ at $x = 0$, where A denotes the area of the contact between the peritoneum and fluid in which the therapeutic agent is diluted (in cm²). It can be shown that in this case, $A \cdot j_S(x=0) = effKBD_S(C_{D,S} - \kappa C_{B,S}) + (1-\sigma_S^T)A \cdot j_V((1-f)C_{D,S} - f\kappa C_{B,S})$, where $C_{D,S}$ and $C_{B,S}$ are the solute S concentrations in peritoneal cavity and in the blood, respectively,

$$effKBD_S = A\sqrt{D_S\left(Cl_{TB} + q_L\right)} \qquad (13.7)$$

is the effective diffusive mass transfer parameter (in mL/min), $\kappa = Cl_{BT,S}/(Cl_{TB,S}+q_L)$, $Cl_{BT,S} = p_Sa + (1-\sigma_S^{cap})q_V^{cap}f$ is unidirectional clearance (per unit tissue volume) for transport from blood to tissue, and $Cl_{TB,S} = p_Sa + (1-\sigma_S^{cap})q_V^{cap}(1-f)$ is unidirectional clearance for transport from tissue to blood. The parameter κ describes the ratio of the equilibrium concentration of the solute in the tissue over its concentration in blood and $q_S^{cap} = Cl_{BT,S}C_{B,S} - Cl_{TB,S}C_S$. For the simplicity reason, the formula for $effKBD_S$ has been presented neglecting impact of R_{bind}, R_{metab}, and R_{gen}. However, it can be easily extended for these effects by adding the corresponding rate in expression for $effKBD_S$, for example, assuming $R_{bind} = r_{bind}C_S$, one would get that $effKBD_S = A\sqrt{D_S(Cl_{TB} + q_L + r_{bind})}$.

Let us assume that steady state for solute transport has been reached in the sufficiently thick and homogeneous tissue, and that all the transport parameters are constant, including fluid flow. Under these conditions, the following estimations for the effective transport can be derived.

DIFFUSIVE TRANSPORT THROUGH THE TISSUE

Let us consider a special case in which diffusive transport through the tissue prevails over convective one. Note that this does not exclude convective transport across the capillary wall, which may occur especially for the large MW solutes such as proteins. Neglecting convective flows in equations for solute transport through the tissue, one would obtain in this case that solute flow from the peritoneal cavity to the tissue is equal to $effKBD_S(C_{D,S}-\kappa C_{B,S})$, and that diffusive mass transfer parameter for the solute transport between peritoneal cavity and blood circulation is equal to $effKBD_S = A\sqrt{D_S(p_Sa+q_L)}$. It can be shown that the penetration depth for diffusive transport through the tissue can be estimated for solute S as [82]

$$\Lambda_{Dif,S} = A\frac{D_S}{effKBD_S} = \sqrt{\frac{D_S}{Cl_{TB,S}+q_L}} \qquad (13.8)$$

For small solutes, the diffusive transport prevails also across the capillary wall and $p_Sa \gg q_L$. Dedrick et al. have shown that in this case, diffusive penetration depth is equal to [15]:

$$\Lambda_{Dif,S} = \sqrt{\frac{D_S}{p_Sa}} \qquad (13.9)$$

CONVECTIVE TRANSPORT THROUGH THE TISSUE

For large macromolecules (larger than albumin) such as specific antibodies, convective transport through the tissue prevails diffusive. In the case of pure convective transport,

it can be shown that, at the steady state and for constant j_V, the effective penetration depth for solute S to the tissue can be calculated as [82]

$$\Lambda_{Conv,S} = \frac{\left(1-\sigma_S^T\right)j_V}{Cl_{TB,S}+q_L} \qquad (13.10)$$

DIFFUSIVE–CONVECTIVE TRANSPORT

The aforementioned formulas were simplifications of the general description of diffusive–convective solute transport by assuming that only one component prevails. However, for some solutes, such simplifications are not valid. In particular, for middle MW solutes, both transport processes should be considered. In this case, the penetration depth to the solute can be estimated, assuming constant j_V through the tissue, as the combination of the diffusive and convective penetration depth, $\Lambda_{Dif,S}$ and $\Lambda_{Conv,S}$, respectively, according to the following formula [82]:

$$\Lambda_S = \frac{\Lambda_{Dif,S}^2}{\sqrt{\Lambda_{Dif,S}^2 + \Lambda_{Conv,S}^2/4} - \Lambda_{Conv,S}/2} \qquad (13.11)$$

where $\Lambda_{Dif,S}$ and $\Lambda_{Conv,S}$ are given by Equations 13.9 and 13.10, respectively.

MODELING OF TRANSPORT IN SOLID TUMORS

There are different types of therapeutic agents that can be used depending on the cancer disease, tumor location, treatment, and administration type. For example, in chemotherapy, molecules or microparticles can be used, whereas in immunotherapy, molecules such as antibodies or even cells such as activated lymphocytes are applied. In spite of the differences between therapeutic agents, the major driving forces and transport barriers in the solid tumor remain similar to those in normal tissue even though their parameters are often altered. The nonuniform blood supply and interstitial pressure distribution may result in the strong spatial variation of the therapeutic agent delivery to solid tumors.

Based on the perfusion rates, four different regions may be distinguished in a solid tumor starting from the center: an avascular, necrotic region, a seminecrotic region, a stabilized microcirculation region, and an advancing front. It has been shown that blood flow rate in the first two regions are very low, whereas the remaining two nonnecrotic outer regions contain fast dividing cells and have large blood supply that can be even higher than in the surrounding normal tissue [49]. In addition to the heterogeneous blood flow, elevated interstitial pressure plays crucial roles in tumor transport. It results in the reduction of the transcapillary pressure difference for the microvascular exchange of water and solute and induces the outward fluid flow through the interstitium toward the outer edges of the tumor and into the nearby normal tissue. Therefore, macromolecules have to overcome this outward fluid flow to be delivered to the tumor from the surrounding medium (tissue, peritoneal fluid, etc.). In the tissue, lymphatics take up extravascular macromolecules as well as the excess water from the interstitial space. On the contrary, typically no functional lymphatics within the tumor are present, and even if some lymphatics develop in solid tumors, they mostly collapse. The more specific details concerning transport parameters and local geometry will be presented in the section "Transport parameters for normal and neoplastic tissue."

Typically, in mathematical models, it is assumed that a tumor is spherical, and transport over the length scale of the tumor radius is considered. Moreover, it is typically assumed that physiological transport parameters, such as hydraulic conductivity, are independent of the time, because the timescale for transport is smaller than the timescale for tumor growth. Most of the mathematical models of transport in tumors were devoted to describe experiments in which drugs were administered intravenously. In this case, the blood capillary wall is considered as the first transport barrier to be crossed, and then drugs penetrated normal and tumor tissue. The equations presented in the previous section on mathematical modeling are also valid for the transport in the tumors and can be rewritten to the spherical geometry.

Fluid transport is solid tumor

In the spherical system of coordinates, r denotes the radial distance from the center of the system, and φ and ϕ denote polar and azimuthal angles, respectively. If one considers the tumor as a sphere, then, due to symmetry, the transport equations and their solutions are functions of r only. The presented model in the succeeding text is based on such an assumption [4].

The transport of fluid through the tumor interstitium can be described by Darcy's law for fluid flux in a porous medium as

$$j_V = -K \cdot \frac{\partial P}{\partial r} \qquad (13.12)$$

where

K denotes, similar as before, hydraulic conductivity of the interstitium (in cm²/min/mmHg)
P is the interstitial pressure (in mmHg)
r is the radical position (in cm)

Note that in this case, interstitial pressure is a function of time t and radical position r.

At the steady state, no changes in the tissue hydration are observed, and therefore fluid flux through the tissue should be equilibrated by the local microvascular exchange and lymphatic drainage in the outer tumor regions. However, in the necrotic core, no fluid flux should be observed. This can be formulated as follows:

$$\frac{\partial j_V}{\partial r} = q_V^{cap} - q_L \quad \text{for } r \geq R_N$$
$$\frac{\partial j_V}{\partial r} = q_V^{cap} = q_L = 0 \quad \text{for } r < R_N$$
$$(13.13)$$

where

R_N is the radius of necrotic core (in cm)
q_V^{cap} denotes fluid flux across the blood capillary wall to the interstitium given by Equation 13.3
q_L denotes volumetric flow into the lymphatics, if present

Let us assume that lymphatic absorption is described as $q_L = L_{PL}a_L(P - P_L)$, where $L_{PL}a_L$ is hydraulic conductance of the lymphatic wall times lymphatics surface area density per unit volume of wet tissue and P_L is the hydrostatic pressure in the lymphatics (in mmHg). It can be shown that if one additionally assumes that all the transport parameters are constant, one would obtain from Equation 13.13 that

$$\frac{1}{r^2}\frac{\partial}{\partial r}\left(r^2\frac{\partial P}{\partial r}\right) = \frac{\alpha^2}{R^2}(P - P_{SS}) \qquad (13.14)$$

where

$r = R$ is the outer edge of the tumor
$\alpha = R\sqrt{(L_P a + L_{PL}a_L)/K}$

$P_{SS} = (L_P a P_e + L_{PL}a_L P_L)/(L_P a + L_{PL}a_L)$ is the steady-state interstitial pressure such that microvascular flow across the blood capillary wall is balanced by the lymphatic absorption, and effective pressure P_e is such a pressure, which would yield zero net fluid flux across the blood capillary wall and is equal to $P_e = P_B - \sigma_S^{cap} \cdot (\Pi_B - \Pi)$ (por. Equation 13.3)

Due to the symmetry, no flux boundary condition is assumed at the center of the tumor that gives $j_{V,tumor}|_{r=0}$ and therefore $\partial P/\partial r = 0$ for $r = 0$. At the outer edge of the solid tumor (at $r = R$), two types of boundary conditions are possible. In the case of isolated tumor, when the surrounding tumor pressure is fixed, one may assume that pressure is the same as the surrounding pressure P_{outer}, i.e., $P|_{r=R} = P_{outer}$. However, if the tumor is surrounded by the normal tissue, pressure decreases smoothly over a distance, and it should be assumed that $j_{V,tumor}|_{r=R^-} = j_{V,normal}|_{r=R^+}$ and $P|_{r=R^-} = P|_{r=R^+}$.

Solute transport in solid tumor

Transport of solutes through the tumor tissue can be described using the same principles as for normal tissue (see the section "Peritoneal transport system") with the parameters for neoplastic tissue. In addition, if one considers tumor as a sphere, the axisymmetric transport can be considered with respect to the radial position, r. In this case, the interstitial transport of solute is typically described as

$$\frac{\partial(\theta_S C_S)}{\partial t} = -\frac{\partial j_S}{\partial r} + q_S^{cap} - C_S q_L - R_{bind} - R_{metab} + R_{gen} \quad (13.15)$$

where C_S is the free solute concentration in the interstitial fluid (in g/mL). Under the assumption of the constant parameters, at the steady state, this would lead to

$$0 = D_S \frac{1}{r^2} \frac{\partial}{\partial r} \left(r^2 \frac{\partial C_S}{\partial r} \right) - \left(1 - \sigma_S^T\right) \frac{1}{r^2} \frac{\partial(r^2 j_V C_S)}{\partial r}$$
$$+ q_S^{cap} - C_S q_L - R_{bind} - R_{metab} + R_{gen}$$

Typically, it is assumed that for tumor tissue $\sigma_S^T = 0$ in the expression for j_S, which means that the retardation factor that represents solute to fluid velocity is equal to 1.

Due to the symmetry, no flux boundary condition should be assumed at the center of the tumor given by $j_{S,tumor}\big|_{r=0} = 0$, where $r = 0$ denotes center of the tumor. Analogous to the fluid transport, two types of boundary conditions are possible at the outer edge of the solid tumor (at $r = R$). In particular, in the case of normal tissue, which surrounds solid tumor, one should assume that $j_{S,tumor}\big|_{r=R^-} = j_{S,normal}\big|_{r=R^+}$ and $C_S\big|_{r=R^-} = C_S\big|_{r=R^+}$.

TRANSPORT PARAMETERS FOR NORMAL AND NEOPLASTIC TISSUE

In order to apply the mathematical models presented in the previous sections, one needs more information concerning characteristics of the system that would be modeled and, in particular, the transport parameters that should be applied. However, although the number of clinical and experimental studies concerning tumor is growing, not much is known concerning tumor physiology in relation to intraperitoneal therapy. Most experimental and theoretical studies considered large tumors, which however are typically removed before the intraperitoneal chemotherapy [25,57].

Two types of factors have impact on the effectives of the intraperitoneal therapy. First type of factor is related to the composition and volume of the fluid that is infused to the peritoneal cavity. The pressure and concentration gradients between peritoneal cavity and the surrounding tissue layers are created and directly influence the effectiveness of therapy. The details concerning driving forces and relation between intraperitoneal volume and pressure were already presented in the section "Peritoneal transport system." The second type of factor, which is those related to the local physiological parameters, is presented in the succeeding text, with special attention focused on the differences between normal and neoplastic tissue.

Transport through the interstitium

In general, tumor interstitium is composed of the same elements as the normal tissue; however, their share in the creation of the interstitial matrix is different, resulting in the differences in the transport properties of the tissue. The interstitium of the tumor tissue is more disorganized than in the normal tissue and has the so-called reactive stroma [93]. It was found that in the tumor tissue, the number of fibroblasts is increased, as well as the density of the capillaries, type I collagen, and fibrin deposition [93]. In addition, experimental studies showed increased amount of collagens, proteoglycans, and glycosaminoglycans in tumor tissue that are presumably responsible for the resistance to fluid and macromolecular motion in the interstitium [50,93]. This, as well as the vascular differences (presented later on), would result in the alteration of the local transport properties of the interstitium. Both hydraulic conductivity of the tissue, K, and solute diffusivity in the tissue, D_S, are determined by the structure and composition of interstitium as well as properties of the solute and directly related to the solute transport through the tissue. In general, K corresponds to the water bulk flow that drives macromolecular convective flow, whereas D_S is related to the solute transport by diffusion. In normal tissue, the span range of K is of four orders magnitude, differing among tissue from high values in lung tissue, to low one in subcutaneous tissue [52]. In addition, experimental studies showed that tissue hydraulic conductivity increase linearly (above some threshold value) with the increase of tissue hydration and interstitial pressure [96]. Based on the animal experiments, one can assume for abdominal wall muscle that $K = a_0$ for interstitial pressure $P < b_0$ and $K = a_0 + a_1(P - b_0)$ for $P \geq b_0$, where the level of basal tissue hydraulic conductivity $a_0 = 0.9 \cdot 10^{-5}$ cm^2/min/mmHg, sensitivity of tissue hydraulic conductivity to increase in $P = a_1 = 0.56 \cdot 10^{-5}$ cm^2/min/mmHg^2, and the interstitial pressure level above which tissue hydraulic conductivity increases is $b_0 = 1.2$ mmHg [96]. In some theoretical studies, direct dependence of hydraulic conductivity on the tissue hydration was taken into account as $K = 5.13 \cdot 10^{-5} \cdot \theta$ cm^2/min/mmHg^2. Swabb and colleagues measured hydraulic conductivity in both normal and neoplastic tissue [75]. They reported values of fivefold higher in rat hepatoma than in normal subcutaneous tissue ($24.8 \cdot 10^{-7}$ and $5.1 \cdot 10^{-7}$ cm^2/min/mmHg, respectively). Higher values for colon adenocarcinoma were reported by Boucher et al., $1.0 \cdot 10^{-5}$ and $1.4 \cdot 10^{-5}$ cm^2/min/mmHg, for in vivo and in vitro experiments, respectively [8].

Due to the structure and composition of the interstitium, some parts of the tissue are excluded for the solute transport through the tissue. This fact, as well as the torturous pathway of solute transport and its charge, would result in the retardation of the solute diffusion through the tissue and, in consequence, would reduce the solute diffusivity in the tissue on one to two orders of magnitude (to that in water). The experimental studies suggest that solute diffusivity in the tumor is also lower than in water, but of order magnitude higher than in normal tissue [38,50,61]. Gerlowski et al. measured values of $D_S = 0.048 \cdot 10^{-8}$ and $D_S = 1.3 \cdot 10^{-8}$ cm²/s for IgG transport in normal and tumor tissue, respectively [38].

Microvascular exchange

Although the tumor vasculature originates from the host vasculature, its spatial organization and properties are different. It was shown that the fractal dimension and minimum path lengths of the tumor vasculature are different from the normal one [3,37,49]. In normal muscle tissue, blood vessels are oriented parallel, whereas in the tumor vasculature, they are chaotically organized, with uneven and dilated vessels that can create the local self-loops [17]. In addition, there are many smaller avascular spaces between vessels and only few large ones [3], which results in the creation of regions with flow-limited transport and reduced flow with lower pO_2 and pH in the tumor center [3,49]. Moreover, experimental studies showed that the velocity of red blood cells is no longer related to the vessel diameter [49]. Fluctuations in the blood flow, with random periods of flow reduction, stasis, followed by resumption of flow (sometimes in the opposite direction) were found in tumor vessels [49,50]. Typically, it is assumed that the average capillary surface area, a, is higher in tumor that in normal tissue and equal to 200 and 70 cm^{-1}, respectively [4,5]. Besides the spatial heterogeneity, ultrastructural studies in human and animal tumors showed that tumor vessels have wide interendothelial junctions, large number of fenestrate and transendothelial channels, and discontinuous or absent basement membrane [48]. These result in the higher values of p_S and L_P in tumor than in the normal (skin or muscle) tissue [50]. The blood vessels are more leaky to fluid and macromolecules, and microvascular exchange is lower for large tumors compared to smaller ones [5]. Gerlowski and Jain found effective capillary wall permeability of dextran 150,000 higher by 7.8 times in neoplastic than normal tissue [38]. In particular, they referred p_S values of $4.4 \cdot 10^{-8}$ and $34.4 \cdot 10^{-8}$ cm/min, for normal and tumor tissue, respectively [38]. Typically, the values of hydraulic conductance of blood capillary wall ranges between $3.5 \cdot 10^{-5}$ and $10 \cdot 10^{-5}$ mL/mmHg/min/g [14,58,82,87]. However, higher values of $L_P a$ around $15 \cdot 10^{-5}$ or even $40 \cdot 10^{-5}$ mL/mmHg/min/g and higher, possibly related to the increased tissue perfusion, were also reported [68,87]. Based on the fact that large molecules are transported across the capillary wall mostly by convection, and that effective permeability of the capillary wall is proportional to the hydraulic conductance of blood vessels, Baxter and Jain assumed values of $L_P a$ 7.8 times higher in tumor than in the normal tissue, having $11.7 \cdot 10^{-4}$ mL/mmHg/min/g for tumor tissue [4,5].

The net fluid exchange across the microvascular wall is driven by the hydrostatic and colloid osmotic pressure difference acting across the capillary wall (Equation 13.3). However, although the Starling principles are valid for both normal and tumor tissue, there are substantial differences in the values of those pressures. The altered effective permeability of the capillary wall and the lack of lymphatics in tumor tissue result in the higher colloid osmotic pressure and therefore reduced oncotic pressure difference across the capillary wall in tumors. Typically, values of 20–26 and 5–15 mmHg are assumed in plasma and normal tissue, respectively [4,23,50,73]. Stohrer et al. measured values of 20 and 8.2 mmHg in plasma and subcutaneous tissue, respectively [74]. In contrast, experimental studies showed that in tumor, interstitial colloid osmotic pressure, Π_i, tends to be higher than in the subcutaneous tissue and often not significantly different from the corresponding plasma values. Stohrer et al. measured oncotic pressure in tumor and found values similar to that in plasma in the case of rhabdomyosarcoma (24.2 mmHg), squamous cell carcinoma (19.9 mmHg), and cell lung carcinoma (21.1 mmHg). Lower value of 16.7 mmHg was reported for colon adenocarcinoma [74]. Similar values were also measured in rats by Wiig et al. in chemically induced mammary carcinoma [91]. However, not only the colloid osmotic pressure and protein concentration in the interstitial fluid in tumor are higher but there is also a different protein composition in the interstitial fluid. In both studies, concentration of proteins with $MW < 25$ kDa was significantly (two- to four-fold) higher than in plasma. For proteins with MW in the range 25–75 kDa and larger, the concentration in interstitial fluid was similar or slightly lower (for $MW > 75$ kDa) to that in plasma and higher than in the subcutaneous tissue.

The infusion of fluid into the peritoneal cavity induces fluid absorption into the adjacent tissue. This leads to the increase of tissue hydration and interstitial pressure in a layer close to the peritoneal cavity, as predicted by the numerical simulations and experimental data (Figure 13.4). The tissue layer close to peritoneal cavity with almost double increase of interstitial fluid void volume over its physiological level of 18% (indicating maximal tissue hydration in this layer (c.f. Figure 13.4) can possibly expand deeper to the tissue depending on the composition and volume of the infused fluid and the length of treatment. In tumor tissue, the hydrostatic pressure gradient across the capillary wall has the major role, since the colloid osmotic pressure difference is substantially reduced compared to normal tissue. Indirect studies suggest decreased P_B, whereas direct measurements in sandwich tumors suggest rather similar pressure at the arterial side and lower pressure at venous side in tumor vessels. For the purpose of modeling, the average plasma hydrostatic pressure is often applied, assumed by Baxter and Jain to be constant and equal to 15.6 mmHg based on the measurements by Brace and Guyton [4,5]. Similar value of 14.6 mmHg has been assumed by Flessner as suggested by Levick [23,53]. The tumor interstitial pressure was measured and studied extensively. Whereas typically interstitial pressure remains slightly negative or close to zero, many solid tumors showed an increased interstitial hydrostatic pressure that may create significant obstacle for tumor treatment [45]. This values may even exceed 20 mmHg, as it is in the case of cervical carcinomas (23–30 mmHg),

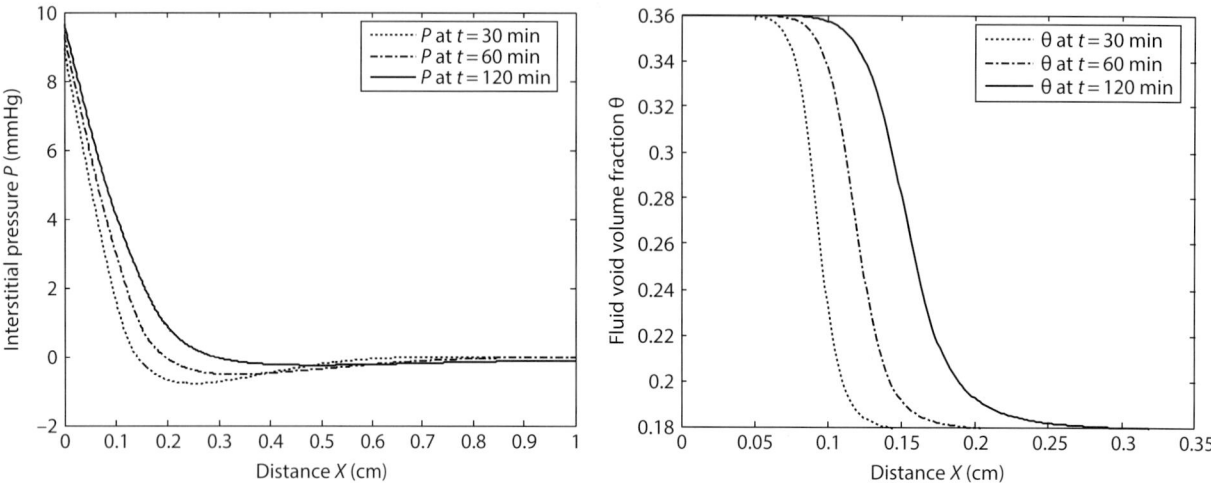

Figure 13.4 The numerical simulations of interstitial hydrostatic pressure and tissue hydration (interstitial fluid void volume ratio) profiles at time t = 30, 60, and 120 minutes after infusion of fluid to the peritoneal cavity as a function of distance from the peritoneal cavity. Simulation was done based on the mathematical model from [72] for the assumed intraperitoneal volume of 2.4 L of hypertonic fluid with glucose 3.86%.

some breast carcinomas (29 mmHg), or renal cell carcinomas (38 mmHg) [49,50]. Moreover, Boucher et al. showed that interstitial pressure rises proportionally to the tumor growth [7], which remains in agreement with the older studies [94,95]. The higher value of interstitial pressure correlates with the reduction of the tumor blood flow and development of necrosis [50]. In addition, experimental and theoretical studies showed that tumor interstitial pressure profiles are not homogeneous. These results indicate that P_i is elevated throughout the tumor and drops sharply at the tumor periphery or to the surrounding tissue [4,7,50]. Experimental studies in rats suggest that maximal interstitial value is reached within less than 1 mm distance from the periphery, with almost uniform pressure in the deeper parts of the solid tumor [7,24]. In an experimental study, Netti and colleagues showed that P_i in the center of isolated tumor would follow the changes in the arterial pressure with the time delay of 11 seconds, and with delay of 1500 seconds in the case of cessation of tumor blood flow [59]. Moreover, theoretical studies by Baxter and Jain suggest that the time needed for interstitial pressure to reach plateau is shorter for larger values of parameter α^2 in Equation 13.14, which depends on the tumor radius and the ratio of hydraulic conductance of capillaries to the hydraulic conductivity of the interstitium [4,5]. Similar dependence was obtained experimentally for small (<0.6 g) and large tumors (>1.2 g).

If the interstitial pressure, in normal tissue that surrounds tumor, is lower than tumor interstitial pressure, the pressure gradient toward normal tissue regions would be created, inducing fluid flow outward the tumor. The radially outward velocity of interstitial fluid flow of 0.1–0.2 μm/s at the periphery of isolated tumor could be of the order of magnitude lower for tumors situated in the subcutaneous or muscle tissue [4]. The macromolecule that enters the tissue from the peritoneal cavity has to overcome this fluid outflow from the tumor, in order to penetrate the deeper part of the tumor.

PERITONEAL TRANSPORT OF SOLUTES TO NORMAL AND TUMOR TISSUE

In neoplastic tissue alterations of the interstitium structure, the microvascular exchange and the lymphatic absorption hinder effective penetration of therapeutic agents into the tumor tissue from blood and surrounding medium. Although the transport parameters in neoplastic tissue (such as K, D_S) are elevated, high-pressure gradient (especially in large tumors) prevents solute transport into the tumor. In most tissues, once the solute gets through the normal tissue to the tumor surface, it has to overcome the high interstitial pressure gradient and fluid outflow from the tumor, to enter and penetrate tumor tissue. However, in some cases, the penetration of a drug to the tumor may be more effective than to normal tissue as it was observed by Wientjes et al. [89]. They studied penetration of mytomycin C in dog and in human bladder to both normal and neoplastic tissue. They found concentration of mytomycin C two- to threefold higher in tumor than in normal tissue. Moreover, they showed that mytomycin C was able to penetrate deeper parts of the tumor bladder than for normal tissue [89]. The increase of hydrostatic pressure in the peritoneal cavity or in the bladder results in the following increase of interstitial pressure in the tissue layers close to the cavity [73]. This might decrease fluid outflow from the tumor or even change the direction of fluid flow, especially in the case of small tumors, which have lower interstitial pressures.

Once a therapeutic agent is infused to the peritoneal cavity, the concentration gradient is created, and it diffuses to the surrounding tissue layers. The monotonically decreasing profile of solute concentration in the interstitial fluid as a function of the distance from the peritoneal cavity may be observed [25,27]. Similarly, steep decreases with the distance profiles of monoclonal antibody (MAb) and [14C]

Table 13.1 Estimated penetration depths for different transport processes for normal and tumor tissue for the assumed fluid absorption from the peritoneal cavity equal to 1 and 0.1 mL/min, respectively

Peritoneal fluid absorption solute	Normal tissue 1 mL/min			Tumor tissue 0.1 mL/min		
	Λ_{Dif} (mm)	Λ_{Conv} (mm)	Λ (mm)	Λ_{Dif} (mm)	Λ_{Conv} (mm)	Λ (mm)
Glucose	0.260	0.039	0.280	0.162	0.000	0.162
Mytomycin C	0.269	0.053	0.297	0.168	0.001	0.168
β_2-Microglobulin	1.415	0.628	1.764	0.432	0.009	0.436
Albumin	0.243	3.314	3.332	0.701	0.176	0.795
IgG	0.081	3.842	3.844	1.752	2.703	3.564

Note: The estimations were done according to formulas given in Equations 13.8 through 13.11 for the assumed transport parameters (see text).

mannitol were observed experimentally in a solid tumor transplanted to the rat abdominal wall [25,27]. Moreover, similar to normal tissue, deeper penetration of smaller molecule (mannitol) into tumor tissue and its leveling concentration in the central region of tumor was observed [25].

In the case of larger molecules, bulk fluid flow plays crucial role in their convective transport through the tissue. The fluid penetration depth from the peritoneal cavity depends on the pressure gradients between peritoneal cavity and surrounding tissue layers. The numerical simulation suggests that fluid penetrates only 0.2–0.3 cm of the human abdominal wall [86], Figure 13.4. Swartz and colleagues found penetration of 0.2 cm of normal and 0.1 cm in the case of edematous mouse tail [76]. In the case of tumor tissue, smaller penetration of less than 0.08 cm was found in experiments in rats [7]. Flessner and colleagues measured peritoneal absorption rate of the labeled albumin for different tissue types [32]. They found highest and relatively constant concentration in the parietal tissue (anterior abdominal wall and the diaphragm) and lower decreasing profiles in visceral tissue [32]. The almost flat solute tissue concentration profile suggests equilibration of the albumin concentration between peritoneal cavity and parietal tissue. However, this might not be the case in humans since their abdominal wall is much thicker, as predicted by the numerical studies. Moreover, the experimental studies on the peritoneal transport of IgG indicate that, although large molecules are transported through the tissue mainly due to convection, their diffusive transport is not negligible [34]. Estimated solute penetration depth for normal and tumor tissue are presented in Table 13.1. The estimations were done according to the formulas given in Equations 13.8 through 13.11 and based on the experimental data as presented in the previous section, assuming fluid absorption from the peritoneal cavity equal to 1 mL/min (in normal tissue), and of order magnitude lower in neoplastic tissue (caused by the alteration of the pressure gradients), effective area of the contact between the peritoneum and fluid equal to 0.6 cm². The pore model with parameters taken from [82] was applied assuming no lymphatic absorption and 7.8 times higher values of $L_p a$ and $p_s a$ in tumor tissue [38]. Tissue diffusivities of small solutes were calculated from their diffusivity in water, corrected by factor 0.053 for normal tissue diffusivity, and by 0.16 in the

case of neoplastic tissue. Tissue diffusivity of solutes larger than β_2-microglobulin was calculated according to the formulas from [61] for normal and tumor tissue.

In general, the uptake of therapeutic agents from the peritoneal cavity can be influenced by the amount and composition of infused fluid. In normal tissue, the increase of fluid volume results in the elevation of the intraperitoneal pressure, which in consequence increases water absorption from the peritoneal cavity to the normal tissue. Similar results were observed in the case of tumor tissue [25]. Elevation of IgG concentration in tumor tissue within the distance 0.6 cm from the peritoneal cavity was observed after increase of intraperitoneal pressure [25]. The increase over six times in intraperitoneal pressure (from less than 1 mmHg to over 6 mmHg) results in the almost threefold increase in tumor IgG concentration close to the peritoneal cavity. In addition, intraperitoneal fluid osmolality creates additional osmotic force that would move water back to the peritoneal cavity. In normal tissue, the osmotic flow would decrease net water absorption from the peritoneal cavity decreasing solute uptake. The corresponding difference in the interstitial concentration of ^{125}I-MAb 96.5 was observed within the distance of 0.6 cm from the peritoneal cavity [27]. However, in the tumor tissue, no such an effect was observed except at the peritoneal surface [27].

SUMMARY

The process of penetration of fluid and solutes into perfused tissue may be theoretically described by the spatially distributed mathematical model [15,72,73,86]. Many theoretical, experimental, and clinical studies were devoted to the exchange of solutes between blood and peritoneal fluid, mostly in the context of peritoneal dialysis [15,23,30,31,33,34,72]. These, as well as other studies on transport systems in different organs, demonstrated the usefulness of the model [12,41,63,79,89,90]. However, its applications for cancers in the peritoneal cavity are mostly limited and focused on large solid tumors [4,5,27]. The same distributed model was also applied for the analysis of the transport of macromolecules (as monoclonal antibodies) from blood to solid tumors [4,5]. The studies on the penetration of drugs into the small and possibly avascular tumors are still lacking.

The studies on the neoplastic tissue and its vasculature showed many changes in the tissue structure and the forces driving the transport of fluid and macromolecules (as the Starling forces) [24,25,27,49,50]. Nevertheless, the same mathematical model may be applied for both normal and neoplastic tissue with the modified parameters and boundary conditions. The model can comprise the description of low molecular cytostatic drugs (as mytomycin), which are transported mainly by diffusion, and macromolecules (as monoclonal antibodies) and nanoparticles that are transported mainly by convection with interstitial fluid bulk flow [23,24,27,51,57,72].

The experimental and theoretical studies suggest rather low penetration of macromolecules into the large solid tumors because of high interstitial pressure that can be similar or higher than that in the peritoneal cavity after infusion of 2 L of dialysis fluid [16,18,24,25,27,47]. Therefore, the effect of monoclonal antibodies may be expected mostly on the peritoneal surface of the tumor. In contrast, small cytostatic drugs may penetrate deeper into the small avascular and large solid tumors.

REFERENCES

1. Aukland K, Nicolaysen G. Interstitial fluid volume: Local regulatory mechanisms. *Physiological Reviews.* 1981;61:556–643.
2. Aukland K, Reed RK. Interstitial-lymphatic mechanisms in the control of extracellular fluid volume. *Physiological Reviews.* 1993;73:1–78.
3. Baish JW, Gazit Y, Berk DA, Nozue M, Baxter LT, Jain RK. Role of tumor vascular architecture in nutrient and drug delivery: An invasion percolation-based network model. *Microvascular Research.* 1996;51:327–346.
4. Baxter LT, Jain RK. Transport of fluid and macro-molecules in tumors. I. Role of interstitial pressure and convection. *Microvascular Research.* 1989;37:77–104.
5. Baxter LT, Jain RK. Transport of fluid and macro-molecules in tumors. II. Role of heterogeneous perfusion and lymphatics. *Microvascular Research.* 1990;40:246–263.
6. Bert JL, Perce RH. The interstitium and microvas-cular exchange. In: Renkin EM, Michel CC, eds., *Handbook of Physiology. The Cardiovascular System. IV Microcirculation*, Bethesda, MD: American Physiological Society, 1984. pp. 521–547.
7. Boucher Y, Baxter LT, Jain RK. Interstitial pres-sure gradients in tissue-isolated and subcutaneous tumors: Implications for therapy. *Cancer Research.* 1990;50:4478–4484.
8. Boucher Y, Brekken C, Netti PA, Baxter LT, Jain RK. Intratumoral infusion of fluid: Estimation of hydrau-lic conductivity and implications for the delivery of therapeutic agents. *British Journal of Cancer.* 1998;78:1442–1448.
9. Casley-Smith JR. A model of the factors affecting interstitial volume in oedema. Part I: Hierarchies, some new factors and their equations. *Biorheology.* 1992;29:535–548.
10. Ceelen WP, Flessner MF. Intraperitoneal therapy for peritoneal tumors: Biophysics and clinical evidence. *Nature Reviews Clinical Oncology.* 2010;7:108–115.
11. Coester AM, Struijk DG, Smit W, de Waart DR, Krediet RT. The cellular contribution to effluent potassium and its relation to free water transport during peritoneal dialysis. *Nephrology Dialysis Transplantation.* 2007;22:3593–3600.
12. Collins JM. Inert gas exchange of subcutaneous and intraperitoneal gas pockets in piglets. *Respiration Physiology.* 1981;46:391–404.
13. Collins JM, Dedrick RL, Flessner MF, Guarino AM. Concentration-dependent disappearance of fluoro-uracil from peritoneal fluid in the rat: Experimental observations and distributed modeling. *Journal of Pharmaceutical Sciences.* 1982;71:735–738.
14. Crone C, Levitt DG. Capillary permeability to small solutes. In: Renkin EM, Michel CC, eds., *Handbook of Physiology, Section 2, Cardiovascular System,* vol. IV, Bethesda, MD: American Physiological Society, 1984. pp. 411–461.
15. Dedrick RL, Flessner MF, Collins JM, Schultz JS. Is the peritoneum a membrane? *ASAIO Journal.* 1982;5:1–8.
16. Dejardin A, Robert A, Goffin E. Intraperitoneal pressure in PD patients: Relationship to intraperi-toneal volume, body size and PD-related complica-tions. *Nephrology, Dialysis, Transplantation: Official Publication of the European Dialysis and Transplant Association—European Renal Association.* 2007;22:1437–1444.
17. Dreher MR, Liu W, Michelich CR, Dewhirst MW, Yuan F, Chilkoti A. Tumor vascular permeability, accu-mulation, and penetration of macromolecular drug carriers. *Journal of the National Cancer Institute.* 2006;98:335–344.
18. Durand PY, Chanliau J, Gamberoni J, Hestin D, Kessler M. Routine measurement of hydrostatic intraperitoneal pressure. *Advances in Peritoneal Dialysis.* 1992;8:108–112.
19. Flessner M, Henegar J, Bigler S, Genous L. Is the peritoneum a significant transport barrier in peri-toneal dialysis? *Peritoneal Dialysis International.* 2003;23:542–549.
20. Flessner MF. Intraperitoneal chemotherapy. In: Khanna R, Krediet RT, eds., *Nolph and Gokal's Textbook of Peritoneal Dialysis*, New York: Springer, 2009. pp. 861–883.
21. Flessner MF. Osmotic barrier of the parietal peritoneum. *American Journal of Physiology.* 1994;267:F861–F870.
22. Flessner MF. The transport barrier in intraperitoneal therapy. *American Journal of Physiology—Renal Physiology.* 2005;288:F433–F442.

23. Flessner MF. Transport of protein in the abdominal wall during intraperitoneal therapy. I. Theoretical approach. *American Journal of Physiology: Gastrointestinal and Liver Physiology*. 2001;281:G424–G437.

24. Flessner MF, Choi J, Credit K, Deverkadra R, Henderson K. Resistance of tumor interstitial pressure to the penetration of intraperitoneally delivered antibodies into metastatic ovarian tumors. *Clinical Cancer Research*. 2005;11:3117–3125.

25. Flessner MF, Choi J, He Z, Credit K. Physiological characterization of human ovarian cancer cells in a rat model of intraperitoneal antineoplastic therapy. *Journal of Applied Physiology (1985)*. 2004;97:1518–1526.

26. Flessner MF, Choi J, Vanpelt H, He Z, Credit K, Henegar J, Hughson M. Correlating structure with solute and water transport in a chronic model of peritoneal inflammation. *American Journal of Physiology—Renal Physiology*. 2006;290:F232–F240.

27. Flessner MF, Dedrick RL. Monoclonal antibody delivery to intraperitoneal tumors in rats: Effects of route of administration and intraperitoneal solution osmolality. *Cancer Research*. 1994;54:4376–4384.

28. Flessner MF, Dedrick RL, Reynolds JC. Bidirectional peritoneal transport of immunoglobulin in rats: Compartmental kinetics. *American Journal of Physiology*. 1992;262:F275–F287.

29. Flessner MF, Dedrick RL, Reynolds JC. Bidirectional peritoneal transport of immunoglobulin in rats: Tissue concentration profiles. *American Journal of Physiology*. 1992;263:F15–F23.

30. Flessner MF, Dedrick RL, Schultz JS. A distributed model of peritoneal-plasma transport: Analysis of experimental data in the rat. *American Journal of Physiology*. 1985;248:F413–F424.

31. Flessner MF, Dedrick RL, Schultz JS. A distributed model of peritoneal-plasma transport: Theoretical considerations. *American Journal of Physiology*. 1984;246:R597–R607.

32. Flessner MF, Fenstermacher JD, Blasberg RG, Dedrick RL. Peritoneal absorption of macromolecules studied by quantitative autoradiography. *American Journal of Physiology*. 1985;248:H26–H32.

33. Flessner MF, Fenstermacher JD, Dedrick RL, Blasberg RG. A distributed model of peritoneal-plasma transport: Tissue concentration gradients. *American Journal of Physiology*. 1985;248:F425–F435.

34. Flessner MF, Lofthouse J, Zakaria el R. In vivo diffusion of immunoglobulin G in muscle: Effects of binding, solute exclusion, and lymphatic removal. *American Journal of Physiology*. 1997;273:H2783–H2793.

35. Flessner MF, Parker RJ, Sieber SM. Peritoneal lymphatic uptake of fibrinogen and erythrocytes in the rat. *American Journal of Physiology*. 1983;244:H89–H96.

36. Flessner MF, Schwab A. Pressure threshold for fluid loss from the peritoneal cavity. *American Journal of Physiology*. 1996;270:F377–F390.

37. Gazit Y, Berk DA, Leunig M, Baxter LT, Jain RK. Scale-invariant behavior and vascular network formation in normal and tumor tissue. *Physical Reviews Letters*. 1995;75:2428–2431.

38. Gerlowski LE, Jain RK. Microvascular permeability of normal and neoplastic tissues. *Microvascular Research*. 1986;31:288–305.

39. Gnepp DR. Lymphatics. In: Staub NC, Taylor AE, eds., *Edema*, Raven Press: New York, 1984. pp. 263–298.

40. Granger DN, Laine GA, Barnes GE, Lewis RE. Dynamics and control of transmicrovascular fluid exchange. In: Staub NC, Taylor AE, eds., *Edema*, Raven Press: New York, 1984. pp. 189–228.

41. Gupta E, Wientjes MG, Au JL. Penetration kinetics of 2′,3′-dideoxyinosine in dermis is described by the distributed model. *Pharmaceutical Research*. 1995;12:108–112.

42. Heimbürger O, Waniewski J, Werynski A, Lindholm B. A quantitative description of solute and fluid transport during peritoneal dialysis. *Kidney International*. 1992;41:1320–1332.

43. Heimbürger O, Waniewski J, Werynski A, Park MS, Lindholm B. Lymphatic absorption in CAPD patients with loss of ultrafiltration capacity. *Blood Purification*. 1995;13:327–339.

44. Heimbürger O, Waniewski J, Werynski A, Tranaeus A, Lindholm B. Peritoneal transport in CAPD patients with permanent loss of ultrafiltration capacity. *Kidney International*. 1990;38:495–506.

45. Heldin CH, Rubin K, Pietras K, Ostman A. High interstitial fluid pressure—An obstacle in cancer therapy. *Nature Reviews Cancer*. 2004;4:806–813.

46. Imholz AL, Koomen GC, Struijk DG, Arisz L, Krediet RT. Effect of an increased intraperitoneal pressure on fluid and solute transport during CAPD. *Kidney International*. 1993;44:1078–1085.

47. Imholz AL, Koomen GC, Voorn WJ, Struijk DG, Arisz L, Krediet RT. Day-to-day variability of fluid and solute transport in upright and recumbent positions during CAPD. *Nephrology Dialysis Transplantation*. 1998;13:146–153.

48. Jain RK. Transport of molecules across tumor vasculature. *Cancer and Metastasis Reviews*. 1987;6:559–593.

49. Jain RK. Transport of molecules, particles, and cells in solid tumors. *Annual Review of Biomedical Engineering*. 1999;1:241–263.

50. Jain RK. Vascular and interstitial barriers to delivery of therapeutic agents in tumors. *Cancer and Metastasis Reviews*. 1990;9:253–266.

51. Jain RK, Stylianopoulos T. Delivering nanomedicine to solid tumors. *Nature Reviews Clinical Oncology*. 2010;7:653–664.

52. Levick JR. Flow through interstitium and other fibrous matrices. *Quarterly Journal of Experimental Physiology.* 1987;72:409–437.

53. Levick JR. Revision of the Starling principle: New views of tissue fluid balance. *Journal of Physiology.* 2004;557:704.

54. Leypoldt JK. Interpreting peritoneal membrane osmotic reflection coefficients using a distributed model of peritoneal transport. *Advances in Peritoneal Dialysis.* 1993;9:3–7.

55. Leypoldt JK, Blindauer KM. Convection does not govern plasma to dialysate transport of protein. *Kidney International.* 1992;42:1412–1418.

56. Leypoldt JK, Henderson LW. The effect of convection on bidirectional peritoneal solute transport: Predictions from a distributed model. *Annals of Biomedical Engineering.* 1992;20:463–480.

57. Lu Z, Wang J, Wientjes MG, Au JL. Intraperitoneal therapy for peritoneal cancer. *Future Oncology.* 2010;6:1625–1641.

58. Michel CC. Fluid movements through capillary walls. In: Renkin EM, Michel CC, eds., *Handbook of Physiology, Section 2, Cardiovascular System*, vol. IV, Bethesda, MD: American Physiological Society, 1984. pp. 375–409.

59. Netti PA, Baxter LT, Boucher Y, Skalak R, Jain RK. Time-dependent behavior of interstitial fluid pressure in solid tumors: Implications for drug delivery. *Cancer Research.* 1995;55:5451–5458.

60. Nolph KD, Mactier R, Khanna R, Twardowski ZJ, Moore H, McGary T. The kinetics of ultrafiltration during peritoneal dialysis: The role of lymphatics. *Kidney International.* 1987;32:219–226.

61. Nugent LJ, Jain RK. Extravascular diffusion in normal and neoplastic tissues. *Cancer Research.* 1984;44:238–244.

62. Pannekeet MM, Imholz AL, Struijk DG, Koomen GC, Langedijk MJ, Schouten N, de Waart R, Hiralall J, Krediet RT. The standard peritoneal permeability analysis: A tool for the assessment of peritoneal permeability characteristics in CAPD patients. *Kidney International.* 1995;48:866–875.

63. Patlak CS, Fenstermacher JD. Measurements of dog blood-brain transfer constants by ventriculocisternal perfusion. *American Journal of Physiology.* 1975;229:877–884.

64. Perl W. An extension of the diffusion equation to include clearance by capillary blood flow. *Annals of the New York Academy of Sciences.* 1963;108:92–105.

65. Perl W. Heat and matter distribution in body tissues and the determination of tissue blood flow by local clearance methods. *Journal of Theoretical Biology.* 1962;2:201–235.

66. Piiper J, Canfield RE, Rahn H. Absorption of various inert gases from subcutaneous gas pockets in rats. *Journal of Applied Physiology.* 1962;17:268–274.

67. Reed RK, Wiig H. Compliance of the interstitial space in rats. I. Studies on hindlimb skeletal muscle. *Acta Physiologica Scandinavica.* 1981;113:297–305.

68. Rippe B, Kamiya A, Folkow B. Simultaneous measurements of capillary diffusion and filtration exchange during shifts in filtration-absorption and at graded alterations in the capillary permeability surface area products (PS). *Acta Physiologica Scandinavica.* 1978;104:318–336.

69. Seames EL, Moncrief JW, Popovich RP. A distributed model of fluid and mass transfer in peritoneal dialysis. *American Journal of Physiology.* 1990;258:R958–R972.

70. Stachowska-Pietka J, Waniewski J. Distributed models of peritoneal transport. In: Krediet RT, ed., *Progress in Peritoneal Dialysis*, Rijeka, Croatia: InTech, 2011. pp. 23–48.

71. Stachowska-Pietka J, Waniewski J, Flessner M, Lindholm B. A mathematical model of peritoneal fluid absorption in the tissue. *Advances in Peritoneal Dialysis.* 2005;21:9–12.

72. Stachowska-Pietka J, Waniewski J, Flessner MF, Lindholm B. Computer simulations of osmotic ultrafiltration and small-solute transport in peritoneal dialysis: A spatially distributed approach. *American Journal of Physiology—Renal Physiology.* 2012;302:F1331–F1341.

73. Stachowska-Pietka J, Waniewski J, Flessner MF, Lindholm B. Distributed model of peritoneal fluid absorption. *American Journal of Physiology: Heart and Circulatory Physiology.* 2006;291:H1862–H1874.

74. Stohrer M, Boucher Y, Stangassinger M, Jain RK. Oncotic pressure in solid tumors is elevated. *Cancer Research.* 2000;60:4251–4255.

75. Swabb EA, Wei J, Gullino PM. Diffusion and convection in normal and neoplastic tissues. *Cancer Research.* 1974;34:2814–2822.

76. Swartz MA, Kaipainen A, Netti PA, Brekken C, Boucher Y, Grodzinsky AJ, Jain RK. Mechanics of interstitial-lymphatic fluid transport: Theoretical foundation and experimental validation. *Journal of Biomechanics.* 1999;32:1297–1307.

77. Twardowski ZJ, Khanna R, Nolph KD, Scalamogna A, Metzler MH, Schneider TW, Prowant BF, Ryan LP. Intraabdominal pressures during natural activities in patients treated with continuous ambulatory peritoneal dialysis. *Nephron.* 1986;44:129–135.

78. Twardowski ZJ, Prowant BF, Nolph KD, Martinez AJ, Lampton LM. High volume, low frequency continuous ambulatory peritoneal dialysis. *Kidney International.* 1983;23:64–70.

79. Van Liew HD. Coupling of diffusion and perfusion in gas exit from subcutaneous pocket in rats. *American Journal of Physiology.* 1968;214:1176–1185.

80. Waniewski J. Mathematical modeling of fluid and solute transport in hemodialysis and peritoneal dialysis. *Journal of Membrane Science.* 2006;274:24–37.

81. Waniewski J. Peritoneal fluid transport: Mechanisms, pathways, methods of assessment. *Archives of Medical Research*. 2013;44:576–583.

82. Waniewski J. Physiological interpretation of solute transport parameters for peritoneal dialysis. *Journal of Theoretical Medicine*. 2001;3:177–190.

83. Waniewski J, Dutka V, Stachowska-Pietka J, Cherniha R. Distributed modeling of glucose-induced osmotic flow. *Advances in Peritoneal Dialysis*. 2007;23:2–6.

84. Waniewski J, Heimburger O, Werynski A, Lindholm B. Paradoxes in peritoneal transport of small solutes. *Peritoneal Dialysis International*. 1996;16(Suppl. 1):S63–S69.

85. Waniewski J, Heimbürger O, Werynski A, Lindholm B. Simple models for fluid transport during peritoneal dialysis. *The International Journal of Artificial Organs*. 1996;19:455–466.

86. Waniewski J, Stachowska-Pietka J, Flessner MF. Distributed modeling of osmotically driven fluid transport in peritoneal dialysis: Theoretical and computational investigations. *American Journal of Physiology: Heart and Circulatory Physiology*. 2009;296:H1960–H1968.

87. Watson PD. Permeability of cat skeletal muscle capillaries to small solutes. *American Journal of Physiology*. 1995;268:H184–H193.

88. Wiederhielm CA, Weston BV. Microvascular, lymphatic, and tissue pressures in the unanesthetized mammal. *American Journal of Physiology*. 1973;225:992–996.

89. Wientjes MG, Badalament RA, Wang RC, Hassan F, Au JL. Penetration of mitomycin C in human bladder. *Cancer Research*. 1993;53:3314–3320.

90. Wientjes MG, Dalton JT, Badalament RA, Drago JR, Au JL. Bladder wall penetration of intravesical mitomycin C in dogs. *Cancer Research*. 1991;51:4347–4354.

91. Wiig H, Aukland K, Tenstad O. Isolation of interstitial fluid from rat mammary tumors by a centrifugation method. *American Journal of Physiology: Heart and Circulatory Physiology*. 2003;284:H416–H424.

92. Wiig H, Gyenge C, Iversen PO, Gullberg D, Tenstad O. The role of the extracellular matrix in tissue distribution of macromolecules in normal and pathological tissues: Potential therapeutic consequences. *Microcirculation*. 2008;15:283–296.

93. Wiig H, Tenstad O, Iversen PO, Kalluri R, Bjerkvig R. Interstitial fluid: The overlooked component of the tumor microenvironment? *Fibrogenesis Tissue Repair*. 2010;3:12.

94. Wiig H, Tveit E, Hultborn R, Reed RK, Weiss L. Interstitial fluid pressure in DMBA-induced rat mammary tumours. *Scandinavian Journal of Clinical & Laboratory Investigation*. 1982;42:159–164.

95. Young JS, Lumsden CE, Stalker AL. The significance of the tissue pressure of normal testicular and of neoplastic (Brown-Pearce carcinoma) tissue in the rabbit. *Journal of Pathology and Bacteriology*. 1950;62:313–333.

96. Zakaria el R, Lofthouse J, Flessner MF. In vivo hydraulic conductivity of muscle: Effects of hydrostatic pressure. *American Journal of Physiology*. 1997;273:H2774–H2782.

97. Zakaria ER, Lofthouse J, Flessner MF. In vivo effects of hydrostatic pressure on interstitium of abdominal wall muscle. *American Journal of Physiology*. 1999;276:H517–H529.

98. Zakaria ER, Rippe B. Peritoneal fluid and tracer albumin kinetics in the rat. Effects of increases in intraperitoneal hydrostatic pressure. *Peritoneal Dialysis International*. 1995;15:118–128.

99. Zink J, Greenway CV. Control of ascites absorption in anesthetized cats: Effects of intraperitoneal pressure, protein, and furosemide diuresis. *Gastroenterology*. 1977;73:1119–1124.

PART 4

Surgical Techniques for Intraperitoneal Drug Delivery

14

Management of peritoneal metastases using cytoreductive surgery and perioperative chemotherapy

PAUL H. SUGARBAKER

INTRODUCTION

Successful treatment of peritoneal metastases (PM) requires a comprehensive management plan that utilizes systemic chemotherapy, cytoreductive surgery (CRS), and perioperative chemotherapy. Proper patient selection is mandatory. Complete resection of all visible malignancy is essential for treatment of peritoneal surface malignancy to result in long-term survival. Up to five parietal peritonectomy procedures and several visceral resections must be utilized to adequately resect all visible evidence of disease. Their utilization depends on the distribution and extent of invasion of the malignancy disseminated within the peritoneal space. Normal peritoneum is not excised, only that which is implanted by cancer.

In an attempt to preserve this surgical complete response, perioperative chemotherapy is used. Drugs may be used intraperitoneally (IP) with heat or intravenously (IV) targeted to peritoneal surfaces by the hyperthermia. The goal is to destroy the last cancer cell that is present within the abdomen and the pelvis.

PATIENT SELECTION USING QUANTITATIVE PROGNOSTIC INDICATORS

The greatest impediments to lasting benefits from CRS and perioperative chemotherapy are improper patient selection and intraoperative or postoperative adverse events. A great number of patients with advanced intra-abdominal disease may be treated with only a few to minimal benefit. Excluding pseudomyxoma peritonei and other minimally aggressive tumors, extensive CRS and aggressive IP chemotherapy is not likely to produce a lasting benefit in patients with advanced disease.

In general, long-term benefit is expected with low-grade minimally aggressive PM even if the disease extent is extremely large. For high-grade invasive peritoneal metastatic disease, long-term benefit is expected with small extent of disease. Rapid recurrence of peritoneal surface cancer combined with progression of systemic disease is likely to interrupt long-term survival in these patients. Patients most likely to benefit have minimal peritoneal surface disease and an absence of systemic metastases so that complete cytoreduction can occur. Uniform access of peritoneal surfaces to chemotherapy is required so that complete eradication of cancer cells and minute cancer nodules is possible. In the natural history of PM, early initiation of treatment has a great bearing on the benefits achieved. Treatment of asymptomatic patients with small volume peritoneal surface malignancy must be the goal for the combined treatment.

Prognostic indicators of peritoneal surface malignancy

In the past, PM was considered to be a uniformly fatal disease process. The only assessment used was either carcinomatosis *present* with a presumed fatal outcome or carcinomatosis *absent* with curative treatment options available. Currently, there are four important clinical assessments of PM that need to be used to select patients who are most likely to benefit from treatment protocols. These are (1) the histopathology to assess the invasive character of the malignancy, (2) the preoperative computed tomography (CT) scan of the abdomen and pelvis, (3) the peritoneal cancer index (PCI), and (4) the completeness of cytoreduction (CC) score.

Histopathology to assess the invasive character of the malignancy

The biological aggressiveness of a peritoneal surface malignancy, as estimated by its histopathology, will have profound influence on its treatment options. Noninvasive tumors such as pseudomyxoma peritonei showing adenomucinosis or peritoneal mesothelioma with nuclear diameter less than 31 millimicrons may have extensive spread on peritoneal surfaces and yet be completely resectable by peritonectomy procedures. Also, these noninvasive malignancies are extremely unlikely to metastasize to the lymph nodes or to the liver and other systemic sites. Therefore, protocols for CRS and IP chemotherapy may have a curative intent in patients with a large mass of widely disseminated pseudomyxoma peritonei and well-differentiated peritoneal mesothelioma [1,2]. Also, some low-grade sarcomas despite extensive disease progression may be aggressively treated with cure as a goal using CRS and IP chemotherapy [3]. Pathology review and an assessment of the invasive or nonaggressive nature of a malignancy are essential to treatment planning [4].

Preoperative CT scan with oral and intravenous contrast

The preoperative CT scan of the chest, abdomen, and pelvis may be of great value in planning treatments for peritoneal surface malignancy. Systemic metastases can be clinically excluded and direct extension into the pleural space ruled out. Unfortunately, the CT scan should be regarded as an inaccurate test by which to quantitate intestinal-type (nonmucinous) adenocarcinoma PM [5]. The malignant tissue progresses on the peritoneal surfaces and its shape conforms to the normal contours of the abdominopelvic structures. This is quite different from the metastatic process in the liver or lung that progresses as 3D tumor nodules and can be accurately assessed by CT.

In contrast, the CT scan has been of great help in locating and quantitating mucinous adenocarcinoma within the peritoneal cavity [6]. These tumors produce large volumes of mucoid material that is readily distinguished by shape and by density from normal structures. Using two distinctive radiologic criteria, those patients with a high likelihood for complete cytoreduction can be selected from those with nonresectable malignancy. This keeps patients who are unlikely to benefit from undergoing cytoreductive surgical procedures from which little or no benefit occurs. The two radiologic criteria found to be most useful are (1) segmental obstruction of the small bowel and (2) the presence of tumor nodules greater than 5 cm in diameter on the small bowel surfaces or directly adjacent to the small bowel mesentery of the jejunum and upper ileum.

These two criteria reflect radiologically the biology of the mucinous adenocarcinoma. Obstructed segments of the bowel signal an invasive character of malignancy on small bowel surfaces that would be unlikely to be completely cytoreduced. Extensive mucinous cancer on the small bowel or small bowel mesentery indicates that the mucinous cancer is no longer redistributed [7]. This means that the small bowel surfaces or small bowel mesentery will have residual disease after cytoreduction because these surfaces cannot be cleared by peritonectomy procedures.

The CT scan is also of great help in the identification of nodules of recurrent sarcoma and sarcomatosis. The recurrences on peritoneal surfaces are nodular and the result of fibrin entrapment of traumatically disseminated sarcoma cells. In a CT scan with maximal filling of the bowel with oral contrast, even small 1 cm nodular sarcoma recurrences are imaged [8].

Yan and coworkers used a composite analysis of two radiologic features to select patients for cytoreduction for peritoneal mesothelioma. The concerning radiologic features they identified were >5 cm tumor mass in the epigastric region and loss of normal architecture of the small bowel and its mesentery. None of the patients with these radiologic features had an adequate cytoreduction. Patients

who lacked these two preoperative CT scan findings had a 94% probability of an adequate cytoreduction [9].

Peritoneal cancer index

The third assessment of peritoneal surface malignancy is the PCI. This is a clinical integration of both peritoneal implant size and distribution of nodules on the peritoneal surface (Figure 14.1). It should be used as part of the decision-making process at two different times. Preoperatively, the CT can be used to estimate the PCI (CT-PCI). Then, as the abdomen and pelvis are explored, an intraoperative CT is determined. To arrive at a score, the size of IP nodules must be assessed. The lesion size (LS) score should be used. An LS-0 score means that no malignant deposits are visualized. An LS-1 score signifies tumor nodules less than 0.5 cm present. The number of nodules is not scored, only the size of the largest nodule. An LS-2 score signifies tumor nodules between 0.5 and 5.0 cm present. LS-3 signifies tumor nodules greater than 5.0 cm in any dimension present. If there is a confluence or layering of tumor, the LS is scored as 3.

In order to assess the distribution of peritoneal surface disease, the abdominopelvic regions are utilized. For each of these 13 regions, an LS score is determined. The summation of the LS score in each of the 13 abdominopelvic regions is the PCI for that patient. A maximal score is 39 (13 × 3).

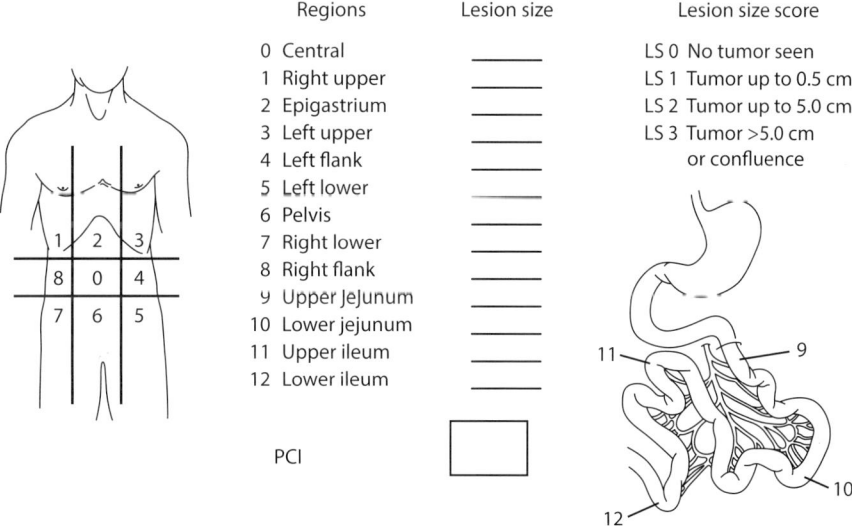

Figure 14.1 The peritoneal cancer index. This index combines a size and a distribution parameter to achieve a numerical score. The lesion size (LS) is used to quantitate the size of peritoneal nodules. LS-0 indicates no tumor seen, LS-1 indicates tumor implants up to 0.5 cm, LS-2 indicates tumor implants between 0.5 and 5 cm, and LS-3 indicates tumor implants larger than 5 cm or a layering of cancer. The distribution of tumor is determined within the 13 abdominopelvic regions. Two transverse planes and two sagittal planes are used to divide the abdomen into nine abdominopelvic regions (AR-0 through AR-8). The upper transverse plane is located at the lowest aspect of the costal margin. The lower transverse plane is placed at the anterior superior iliac spine. The sagittal planes divide the abdomen into three equal sectors. These lines define nine regions that are numbered in a clockwise direction with 0 at the umbilicus and 1 defining the space beneath the right hemidiaphragm. The small bowel is assessed as an additional four abdominopelvic regions designated AR-9 through AR-12 and includes the upper jejunum, lower jejunum, upper ileum, and lower ileum, respectively. The summation of the lesion size score in each of the 13 abdominopelvic regions is the peritoneal cancer index ranging from 0 to 39.

It has been established that CT-PCI significantly underestimated the intraoperative PCI; up until now, preoperative CT in the selection of patients for CRS has been questioned. Rather, CT has been used to establish concerning vs. favorable radiologic features [6,9–11].

Esquivel and colleagues have relied heavily on the CT-PCI to generate prognostic information for the peritoneal surface disease severity score [12,13]. When CT was interpreted in a patient-by-patient analysis rather than abdominopelvic region–by–abdominopelvic region analysis, Esquivel found the true rate of accuracy of the CT scan in the estimation of PCI for the purpose of patient selection for CRS to be 88%. He concluded that CT-PCI does have inherent limitations but can still be useful in patient evaluation for the selection of patient who will have a complete CRS [14].

All groups studying the radiology of PM agree that the there are several "concerning features" that are likely to predict unresectability. These are biliary obstructions or PM intimately associated with the porta hepatis; evidence of retroperitoneal disease especially ureteral obstruction; tumor nodules imaged in small bowel regions 10, 11, or 12; and large-volume disease in abdominopelvic region 2 (epigastric region), suggesting extensive involvement of the lesser curvature of the stomach and right and left gastric arterial arcade. A composite of the concerning radiologic features are used for the selection of patients for CRS and hyperthermic intraperitoneal chemotherapy (HIPEC) with PM from mucinous adenocarcinoma and peritoneal mesothelioma [3,6]. The two most prominent features for mucinous adenocarcinoma were obstruction of bowel segments by tumor volume greater than or equal to 0.5 cm on the small bowel exclusive of terminal ileum [3]. For peritoneal mesothelioma, these two concerning features were tumor greater than 5 cm in the epigastric region combined with class III changes of the small bowel or small bowel mesentery [9]. We agree with Rivard and colleagues that two or more concerning CT imaging features are associated with a higher risk of unresectability [11]. For colorectal cancer, gastric cancer, and ovarian malignancy, the CT-PCI is supported by the literature as an estimate of tumor volume and, with limitations, a part of the selection process for beneficial CRS and HIPEC treatments.

The PCI obtained by visual inspection has been validated in several different abdominal or pelvic cancers. First, Steller and colleagues used it successfully to quantitate IP tumor in a murine peritoneal carcinomatosis model [15]. Gomez and coworkers showed that the PCI could be used to predict long-term survival in patients with peritoneal carcinomatosis from colon cancer undergoing a second cytoreduction [16]. Berthet and coworkers showed that the PCI predicted benefits for treatment of peritoneal sarcomatosis from recurrent visceral or parietal sarcoma [3]. In both of these clinical studies, patients with a favorable prognosis had a score of less than 13. The PCI obtained by visual inspection at the time of the abdominal exploration has been used successfully to select PM patients for treatment in several different diseases including colorectal cancer, gastric cancer, and ovarian cancer.

There are some exceptions to the rules established for the use of the PCI. First, as discussed previously, noninvasive malignancy on peritoneal surfaces may be completely cytoreduced even though the index is very large. Diseases such as pseudomyxoma peritonei, low-nuclear-grade peritoneal mesothelioma, low malignant potential ovarian cancers, and grade 1 sarcoma are in this category. With these minimally invasive tumors, the status of the abdomen and pelvis after cytoreduction may have no relationship to its status at the time of abdominal exploration. In other words, even though the surgeons may find an abdomen with a PCI of 39, it can be converted to an index of 0 by cytoreduction and a high likelihood of long-term benefit. In these diseases, the prognosis is more dependent on the CC score than on the PCI.

A second caveat for the PCI is cancer at crucial anatomic sites. Invasive cancer on the common bile duct, invasion at the base of the bladder, or unresectable disease on a pelvic sidewall may result in residual cancer after cytoreduction and eventuate in a poor prognosis. Perhaps, most common is unresectable cancer on the small bowel. In other words, small foci of invasive cancer at crucial anatomic sites may function as systemic disease in assessing prognosis. In summary, since long-term survival can only occur in patients with a complete cytoreduction, residual disease at anatomically crucial sites may override a favorable score with the PCI.

Completeness of cytoreduction score

The most definitive assessment to be used to assess prognosis with peritoneal surface malignancy is the CC score. This information is of less value to the surgeon in planning treatments than the PCI. The CC score is not available until after the cytoreduction is complete, whereas the PCI is available at the time of abdominal exploration. If during exploration it becomes obvious that cytoreduction will not be complete, the surgeon may decide that a palliative debulking that will provide symptomatic relief is appropriate and discontinue plans for an aggressive CRS. In both noninvasive and invasive peritoneal surface malignancy, the CC score is the major prognostic indicator. It has been shown to function with accuracy in pseudomyxoma peritonei, peritoneal carcinomatosis from colon cancer, gastric cancer, sarcomatosis, peritoneal mesothelioma, and ovarian cancer.

For appendiceal mucinous neoplasms, the CC score has been defined as follows: A CC-0 score indicates that no visible peritoneal seeding exists following the cytoreduction. A CC-1 score indicates that tumor nodules persisting after cytoreduction are less than 2.5 mm. This is a nodule size thought to be penetrable by intracavity chemotherapy and may, therefore, be a complete cytoreduction if surgery and perioperative chemotherapy are used together. A CC-2 score indicates tumor nodules between 2.5 mm and 2.5 cm. A CC-3 score indicates tumor nodules greater than 2.5 cm or a confluence of unresectable tumor nodules at any site within the abdomen or pelvis. CC-2 and CC-3 cytoreductions are considered incomplete (Figure 14.2).

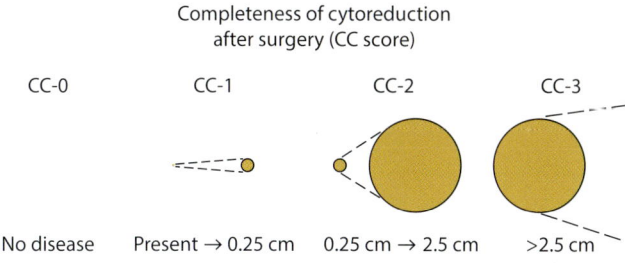

Completeness of cytoreduction
after surgery (CC score)

CC-0   CC-1   CC-2   CC-3

No disease   Present → 0.25 cm   0.25 cm → 2.5 cm   >2.5 cm

Figure 14.2 Completeness of cytoreduction score.

For high-grade nonmucinous neoplasms, more strict criteria for complete cytoreduction are necessary. A complete cytoreduction is restricted to resection to absolutely no visible evidence of disease. Only a CC-0 cytoreduction is scored as a complete cytoreduction.

CYTOREDUCTIVE SURGERY WITH PARIETAL PERITONECTOMY PROCEDURES AND VISCERAL RESECTIONS

Parietal peritonectomy procedures and visceral resections are necessary if one is to successfully treat peritoneal surface malignancies with curative intent [17]. These resections are used in the areas of visible cancer progression in an attempt to leave the patient with only microscopic residual disease. Removal of isolated tumor nodules by scissor dissection or electroevaporation may sometimes be appropriate; however, involvement of the visceral peritoneum usually requires resection of a portion of the stomach, small intestine, or colorectum. Layering of cancer on a parietal peritoneal surface requires peritonectomy.

Locations of peritoneal surface malignancy

PM, especially mucinous tumors, involve the visceral peritoneum in greatest volume at three definite sites [7]. These are sites where the bowel is anchored to the retroperitoneum and peristalsis causes less motion of the visceral peritoneal surface. The rectosigmoid colon, as it emerges from the pelvis, is a nonmobile portion of the bowel. Also, it is located in a dependent site and therefore is frequently layered by PM. Usually, a complete pelvic peritonectomy requires stripping of the pelvic sidewalls, the peritoneum overlying the bladder, the cul-de-sac or rectovesical space, and resection of the rectosigmoid colon. The ileocecal valve region is another area where there is limited mobility and a large peritoneal fluid resorption. Tumor accumulation requires resection of the terminal ileum and a portion of the right colon. A final site often requiring resection is the antrum of the stomach that is fixed to the retroperitoneum at the pylorus. Tumor cells coming in through the foramen of Winslow accumulate in the subpyloric space and may cause intestinal obstruction as a result of gastric outlet obstruction [18]. Large volumes of tumor in the lesser omentum combined with disease in the subpyloric space may cause a confluence of disease that requires a total gastrectomy for complete cytoreduction.

Electroevaporative surgery

In order to adequately perform peritonectomy, the surgeon must use electrosurgery [19]. Peritonectomy performed with high-voltage electrosurgery leaves a margin of heat necrosis that is devoid of viable malignant cells. Not only does electroevaporation of tumor and normal tissue at the margins of resection minimize the likelihood of persistent disease, but also it minimizes blood loss. In the absence of electrosurgery, persistent ooze from stripped peritoneal surfaces may occur.

Peritoneum as a first line of defense in peritoneal metastases

Extensive cancer surgery in the absence of perioperative chemotherapy may actually harm patients in the long run rather than help them. If peritoneal surface malignancy is present, cancer resection without IP chemotherapy will cause tumor cells to become implanted on tissues located beneath the peritoneal layer of the abdomen and pelvis. As cancer progresses, this may contribute to obstruction of vital structures such as the ureter or common bile duct. Also, deep involvement of the pelvic sidewall and tissues along vascular structures will occur. If surgeons attempt to treat peritoneal surface malignancy, they must become thoroughly familiar with the techniques of intraoperative chemotherapy. Complete cytoreduction, aggressive perioperative chemotherapy, and proper patient selection are the three essential requirements of treatment for peritoneal surface malignancy.

Position and incision

The patient is placed in the supine position with the gluteal fold advanced to the end of the operating table to allow full access to the perineum during the surgical procedure.

Abdominal exposure

The abdominal cavity is opened through a midline incision from xiphoid to pubis. The old abdominal incision is widely excised. If laparoscopy port sites are present, the umbilicus is routinely excised; it can be reconstructed if the patient desires. The skin edges are secured at 10 cm intervals by heavy sutures to the self-retaining retractor. Traction on the edges of the abdominal incision elevates the structures of the abdominal wall to facilitate their accurate dissection (Figure 14.3). Strong elevation of abdominal wall helps to avoid damage to bowel loops that are adherent to the anterior parietal peritoneum abdominal wall [20]. Generous abdominal exposure is achieved through the use of a Thompson self-retaining retractor (Thompson Surgical Instruments, Inc., Traverse City, MI). The standard tool used to dissect tumor on peritoneal surfaces from the normal tissues is a 3 mm ball-tipped electrosurgical handpiece (Valleylab, Boulder, CO). The ball-tipped instrument

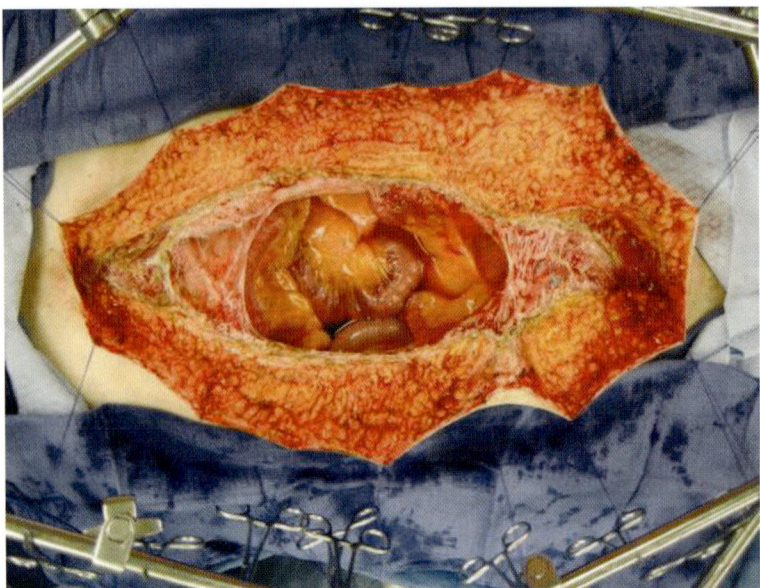

Figure 14.3 Elevation of the edges of the abdominal incision. Skin traction on a self-retaining retractor facilitates dissection of abdominal wall structures and minimizes the likelihood of damage to bowel loops adherent to the abdominal wall. (From Sugarbaker, P.H., An overview of peritonectomy, visceral resections, and perioperative chemotherapy for peritoneal surface malignancy, in: Sugarbaker, P.H., ed., *Cytoreductive Surgery & Perioperative Chemotherapy for Peritoneal Surface Malignancy*, Textbook and Video Atlas, Cine-Med Publishing, Woodbury, CT, 2012, pp. 1–30.)

is placed at the interface of tumor and normal tissues. The focal point for further dissection is placed on strong traction. The electrosurgical generator is used on pure cut at high voltage. Electroevaporative surgery is used cautiously for tumor removal on tubular structures, especially the ureters, small bowel, and colon. Frequent cooling of the dissection site with room temperature saline will prevent excessive heat accumulation. Using ball-tipped electrosurgery on pure cut creates a large volume of plume because of the electroevaporation (carbonization) of tissue. To maintain visualization of the operative field and to preserve a smoke-free atmosphere, a smoke filtration unit is used. The vacuum tip is maintained 2–3 inches from the field of dissection whenever electrosurgery is performed.

Xiphoidectomy

If the preoperative radiologic studies suggest the need for right or left subdiaphragmatic peritonectomy, a xiphoidectomy should be performed [21]. The midline abdominal incision is extended to approximately 4 cm above the xiphoid–sternal junction. The epigastric fat pad is released from the posterior rectus sheath and a self-retaining retractor is used to widely expose the xiphoid bone and its attachments to the sternum.

Using electrosurgical dissection and progressive advancement of the self-retaining retractor, the xiphoid bone is progressively exposed by releasing it from the anterior and posterior rectus sheath. The dissection is performed with electrocoagulation current on high voltage in order to control the numerous arterial bleeding points that are just lateral to the limits of the xiphoid bone.

After the xiphoid is clearly exposed back to its origins on the sternum, a transverse line of high-voltage cutting electrosurgery marks the junction of xiphoid and sternum. The electrosurgical current denatures the protein within the bone at the base of the xiphoid–sternal junction, so the bone is fractured precisely with downward pressure at this line.

The xiphoid is released from the sternum and its base secured with a Kocher clamp. The broad attachments of the diaphragm muscle to the xiphoid are divided as it is peeled away from the underlying tissues. Care is taken to avoid entrance into the left pleural space or the pericardial space.

Total anterior parietal peritonectomy

As the peritoneum is dissected away from the posterior rectus sheath, a single entry into the peritoneal cavity in the upper portion of the incision (peritoneal window) allows the surgeon to assess the requirement for a complete parietal peritonectomy (Figure 14.4). If cancer nodules are palpated on the parietal peritoneum, an anterior parietal peritonectomy is required to achieve a complete cytoreduction. If the parietal peritoneum is not involved by PM, except for the small defect in the peritoneum required for this peritoneal exploration, the remainder of the peritoneum is maintained intact.

The skin traction sutures facilitate the removal of the initial 5-1 of the parietal peritoneum. As this area is cleared of peritoneum, the self-retaining retraction system is steadily advanced along the anterior abdominal wall. This optimizes the broad traction at the point of dissection of the peritoneum from its underlying tissues. Peritoneum is most adherent directly overlying the transversus muscle. In some instances, dissection from inferior to superior aspects of the abdominal

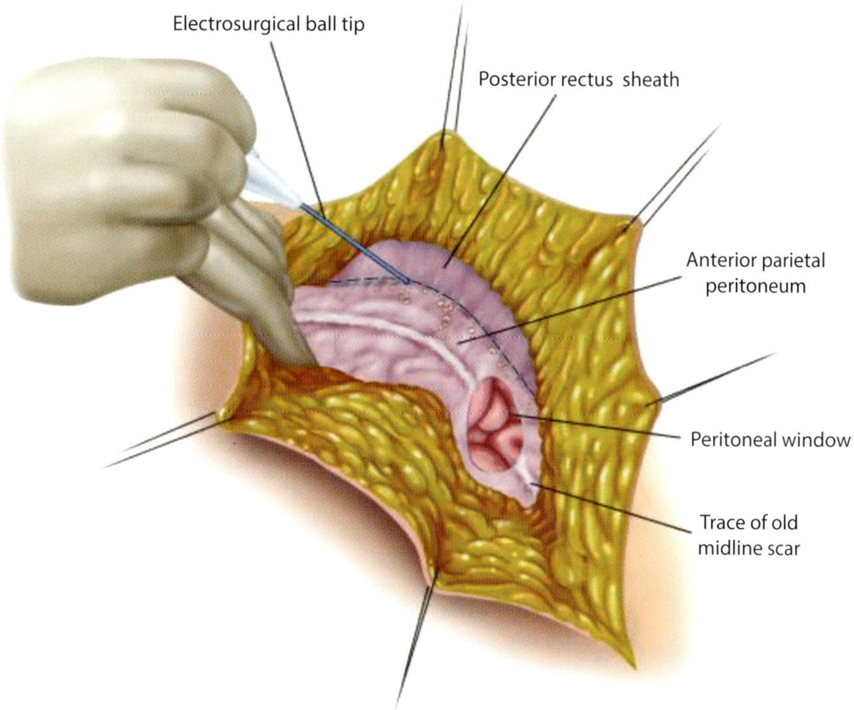

Figure 14.4 Peritoneal window is necessary to assess the need for total anterior parietal peritonectomy. (From Sugarbaker, P.H., An overview of peritonectomy, visceral resections, and perioperative chemotherapy for peritoneal surface malignancy, in: Sugarbaker, P.H., ed., *Cytoreductive Surgery & Perioperative Chemotherapy for Peritoneal Surface Malignancy*, Textbook and Video Atlas, Cine-Med Publishing, Woodbury, CT, 2012, pp. 1–30.)

wall facilitates clearing in this area. The dissection blends in with the right and left subphrenic peritonectomy superiorly and with the complete pelvic peritonectomy inferiorly. As the dissection proceeds to the peritoneum of the paracolic sulcus (line of Toldt), the dissection becomes more rapid with the loose connections of the peritoneum at this anatomic site.

Right subphrenic peritonectomy

Peritoneum is stripped from beneath the right posterior rectus sheath to begin the peritonectomy in the right upper quadrant of the abdomen. Strong traction on the specimen is used to elevate a rolled edge of the hemidiaphragm muscle into the operative field. Again, ball-tipped electrosurgery on pure cut is used to dissect at the interface of tumor and normal tissue. Coagulation current is used to divide the blood vessels between diaphragm and peritoneum as they are encountered and before they bleed.

Stripping of tumor from Glisson's capsule

The stripping of tumor from the right hemidiaphragm continues until the bare area of the liver is encountered. At that point, tumor on the superior surface of the liver is electro-evaporated until the liver surface is cleared (Figure 14.5). With ball-tipped electroevaporation, a thick layer of tumor may be bloodlessly lifted off the liver surface by moving beneath Glisson's capsule (high-voltage pure-cut electrosurgical

dissection). Isolated patches of tumor on the liver surface are electroevaporated with the distal 2 cm of the ball tip bent and stripped of insulation ("hockey-stick" configuration).

Tumor from beneath the right hemidiaphragm and from the surface of the liver forms an envelope as it is removed *en bloc*. The dissection is greatly facilitated if the tumor specimen is maintained intact. The dissection continues laterally on the right to encounter the perirenal fat covering the right kidney. Also, the right adrenal gland is visualized and carefully avoided as tumor is stripped from the right subhepatic space. As the peritoneal reflection onto the undersurface of the liver is divided, care is taken not to traumatize the vena cava or to disrupt the caudate lobe veins that pass between the vena cava and segment 1 of the liver.

Completed right subphrenic peritonectomy

With strong upward traction on the right costal margin by the self-retaining retractor and medial displacement of the right liver, one can visualize the completed right subphrenic peritonectomy. The anterolateral branches of the inferior phrenic artery and vein on the hemidiaphragm are seen and have been preserved. The right hepatic vein and the vena cava have been exposed. The right subhepatic space including the right adrenal gland and perirenal fat covering the right kidney constitutes the base of the dissection.

If the malignancy is invasive, tumor may be densely adherent to the tendinous central portion of the left or right

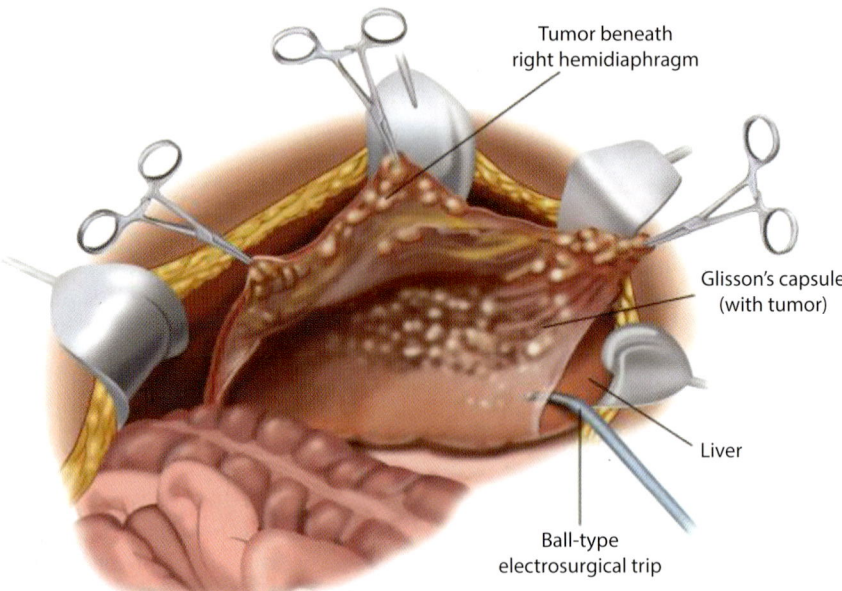

Figure 14.5 Electroevaporation of tumor from the liver surface with resection of Glisson's capsule. (From Sugarbaker, P.H., An overview of peritonectomy, visceral resections, and perioperative chemotherapy for peritoneal surface malignancy, in: Sugarbaker, P.H., ed., *Cytoreductive Surgery & Perioperative Chemotherapy for Peritoneal Surface Malignancy*, Textbook and Video Atlas, Cine-Med Publishing, Woodbury, CT, 2012, pp. 1–30.)

hemidiaphragm. If this occurs, the tissue infiltrated by tumor must be resected. This usually requires an elliptical excision of a portion of the hemidiaphragm on either the right or the left side. The defect in the diaphragm is closed with interrupted sutures. However, the closure occurs after the perioperative chemotherapy of both the chest and abdomen has been completed.

Greater omentectomy and possible splenectomy

To free the midabdomen of a large volume of tumor, the greater omentectomy–splenectomy is performed as the second major resection of the cytoreduction. The greater omentum is elevated and then separated from the transverse colon using electrosurgery. This dissection continues beneath the peritoneum that covers the transverse mesocolon to the lower border of the pancreas. The branches of the gastroepiploic arcade to the greater curvature of the stomach are ligated in continuity and then divided.

If a splenectomy is required, the left subphrenic peritonectomy should be performed first. After the left upper quadrant peritonectomy has been completed, the structures deep beneath the left hemidiaphragm can be elevated. Therefore, under direct vision, the short gastric vessels are litigated and divided. With traction on the spleen, peritoneum on the anterior aspect of the pancreas may be gently stripped from the gland bluntly or by using electrosurgery. If the peritoneum covering the pancreas is free of cancer implants, it remains intact. The splenic artery and vein at the tail of the pancreas are ligated in continuity and proximally suture ligated. Great care is taken not to traumatize the body or tail of the pancreas.

Left subphrenic peritonectomy

The epigastric fat and peritoneum at the edge of the abdominal incision are stripped off the left posterior rectus sheath. Strong traction is exerted on the tumor specimen throughout the left upper quadrant in order to electrosurgically separate tumor from the diaphragmatic muscle, the left adrenal gland, and the perirenal fat. Dissection beneath the hemidiaphragm muscle must be performed with balltipped electrosurgery, not by blunt dissection (Figure 14.6). Numerous blood vessels between the diaphragm muscle and its peritoneal surface must be electrocoagulated before their transection, or unnecessary bleeding will occur as the severed blood vessels retract into the muscle of the diaphragm. However, after the central tendon is visualized, strong traction may effectively separate peritoneum from diaphragm.

Cholecystectomy with stripping of the hepatoduodenal ligament and release of the gastrohepatic ligament

The gallbladder is removed in a routine fashion from its fundus toward the cystic artery and cystic duct. These structures are ligated and divided. The hepatoduodenal ligament is characteristically heavily layered with tumor. After dividing the peritoneal reflection onto the liver, the cancerous tissue that coats the porta hepatis is bluntly stripped using a Russian forceps from the base of the gallbladder bed toward the duodenum. The right gastric artery going to the lesser omental arcade is preserved. Because the triangular ligament of the left lobe of the liver was resected in performing the left subphrenic peritonectomy, the left lateral segment of the liver may be retracted left to right to expose the

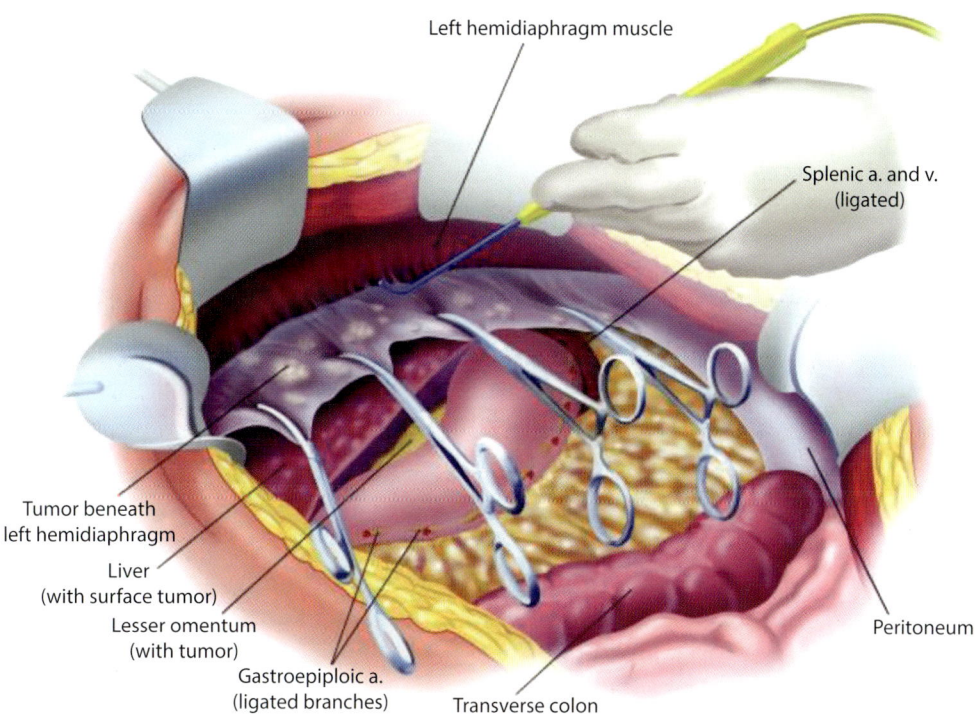

Figure 14.6 Peritoneal stripping of the undersurface of the left diaphragm. (From Sugarbaker, P.H., An overview of perito-nectomy, visceral resections, and perioperative chemotherapy for peritoneal surface malignancy, in: Sugarbaker, P.H., ed., *Cytoreductive Surgery & Perioperative Chemotherapy for Peritoneal Surface Malignancy*, Textbook and Video Atlas, Cine-Med Publishing, Woodbury, CT, 2012, pp. 1–30.)

hepatogastric ligament in its entirety. Under direct vision, the surgeon separates the gastrohepatic ligament from the fissure defined by the ligamentum venosum. Ball-tipped electrosur-gery is used to electroevaporate tumor from the surface of the caudate process. Care is taken not to traumatize the anterior surface of the caudate process, for this can result in excessive and needless blood loss. The segmental blood supply to the cau-date lobe is located on the anterior surface of this segment of the liver, and hemorrhage may occur with only superficial trauma. Also, care must be taken to avoid an accessory left hepatic artery that may arise from the left gastric artery and cross through the hepatogastric ligament. If the artery is embedded in tumor or its preservation occludes clear exposure of the omental bursa, the artery is ligated as it enters the liver parenchyma. It is resected as part of the hepatogastric ligament.

Circumferential resection of the hepatogastric ligament by strong digital dissection

After electrosurgically dividing the peritoneum on the lesser curvature of the stomach, digital dissection with extreme pressure from the surgeon's thumb and index finger sepa-rates the lesser omental fat and tumor from the vascular arcade of the right and left gastric artery along the lesser cur-vature of the stomach (Figure 14.7). As much of the anterior vagus nerve is spared as possible. The tumor and fatty tissue surrounding the right and left gastric arteries are crushed to

isolate the vascular arcade. In this manner, the specimen is centralized over the major branches of the left gastric artery. With strong traction on the specimen, the lesser omentum is released from the left gastric artery and vein.

Stripping of the floor of the omental bursa

A Deaver retractor or the assistant's fingertips beneath the left caudate lobe are positioned to expose the entire floor of the omental bursa. Further electroevaporation of tumor from the caudate process of the left caudate lobe of the liver may be nec-essary to achieve this exposure. Ball-tipped electrosurgery is used to cautiously divide the peritoneal reflection of the liver onto the left side of the subhepatic vena cava. After the perito-neum is divided, Russian forceps assist in a blunt stripping of the peritoneum from the superior recess of the omental bursa, from the crus of the right hemidiaphragm, and from beneath the portal vein. Electroevaporation of tumor from the shelf of liver parenchyma beneath the portal vein that connects the right and left aspects of the caudate lobe may be required. Care is taken while stripping the floor of the omental bursa to stay superficial to the right subphrenic artery.

Clearing the posterior aspect of the hepatoduodenal ligament

In some patients, a large volume of tumor on the posterior aspect of the hepatoduodenal ligament may be difficult to visu-alize. A ½-inch Penrose drain placed around the portal triad

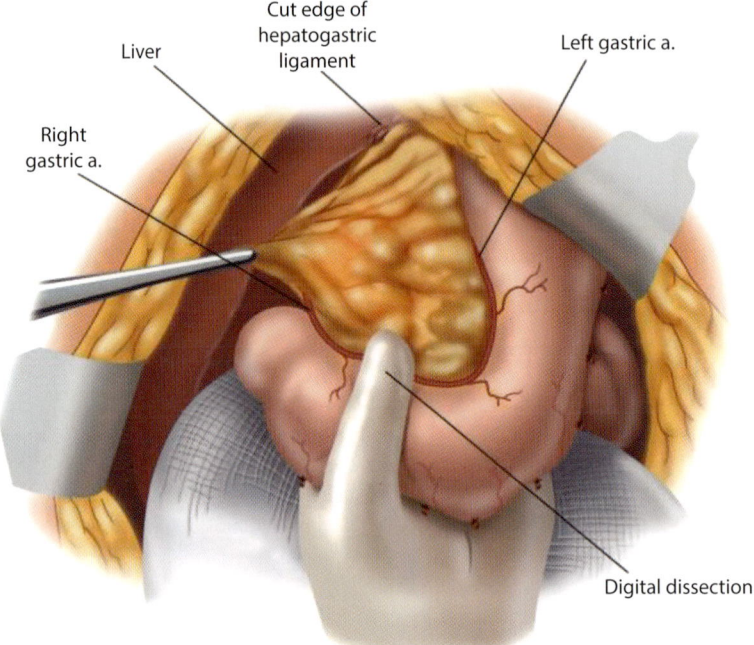

Figure 14.7 Circumferential resection of the hepatogastric ligament and lesser omentum using strong digital dissection to move fat and tumor away from the arcade of the right and left gastric arteries. (From Sugarbaker, P.H., An overview of peritonectomy, visceral resections, and perioperative chemotherapy for peritoneal surface malignancy, in: Sugarbaker, P.H., ed., *Cytoreductive Surgery & Perioperative Chemotherapy for Peritoneal Surface Malignancy*, Textbook and Video Atlas, Cine-Med Publishing, Woodbury, CT, 2012, pp. 1–30.)

may allow improved visualization beneath these structures. Using a Russian forceps tearing away the peritoneum beneath the porta hepatis may be necessary under direct visualization.

Division of the pont hepatique (hepatic bridge) for cytoreduction along the umbilical ligament

The umbilical ligament is a surface structure that defines the separation of the left lateral segment of the liver from liver segment IV. The volume of liver parenchyma that is superficial to the umbilical fissure is extremely variable. Some patients have the umbilical fissure completely open with the umbilical ligament exposed until its entrance into the liver. In other patients, a bridge of liver parenchyma covers the umbilical fissure, the "pont hepatique." The thickness of this bridge of liver parenchyma and the extent to which the umbilical ligament remains visible are extremely variable. The pont hepatique creates a tunnel that surrounds the umbilical ligament. This tunnel is lined by the peritoneum and is at risk for seeding by cancer. In order to inspect the peritoneal surfaces within this tunnel, the liver parenchyma above the umbilical ligament must be divided [22].

Opening the pont hepatique is performed using electrosurgery at high voltage. It can be performed in the absence of any bleeding because no major vascular or ductal structures pass through the pont hepatique. After opening the pont hepatique, the peritoneal lining of the tunnel is carefully inspected and cancer nodules are electroevaporated.

Complete pelvic peritonectomy

The tumor-bearing peritoneum is stripped from the posterior surface of the lower abdominal incision, exposing the rectus muscle. After resection of the peritoneum on the right and left sides of the bladder, the urachus is localized and placed on strong traction using a Babcock clamp. The peritoneum with the underlying fatty tissues is stripped away from the surface of the bladder. Broad traction on the entire anterior parietal peritoneal surface and frequent saline irrigation clears the point for tissue transection that is precisely located between the bladder musculature and its adherent fatty tissue with the peritoneum. The inferior limit of dissection is the cervix in the female or the seminal vesicles in the male.

Hysterectomy

The peritoneal incision around the pelvis is connected to the peritoneal incisions of the right and left paracolic sulci. The round ligaments are divided as they enter the internal inguinal ring. The right and left ureters are identified and preserved. The right and left ovarian veins are ligated at the level of the lower pole of the kidney and divided. Extraperitoneal ligation of the uterine arteries is performed just above the ureter and close to the base of the bladder. The bladder is dissected away from the cervix and the vagina is entered. The vaginal cuff anterior and posterior to the cervix is transected using electrosurgery, and the rectovaginal septum is exposed.

Resection of rectosigmoid colon and cul-de-sacectomy

Electrosurgery is used to dissect pelvic peritoneum from beneath the pararectal fossa toward the rectum at the limits of the mesorectum. The surgeon works in a centripetal fashion. A linear stapler is used to divide the sigmoid colon just above the limits of the pelvic tumor usually at the junction of sigmoid and descending colon. The vascular supply of the distal portion of the bowel is traced back to its origin on the aorta. The inferior mesenteric artery is ligated, suture ligated, and divided. This allows one to pack all the viscera, including the proximal sigmoid colon, in the upper abdomen.

An Allis clamp is placed on the posterior vagina leaving the peritoneum of the cul-de-sac to be included with the intact specimen of the pelvic peritoneum, uterus, and rectum plus the rectosigmoid colon. The perirectal fat is divided on the rectal musculature working from distal to proximal rectum in an attempt to pressure as long a rectal stump as possible. After the rectal musculature is skeletonized using electrosurgery, a stapler is used to close off the rectal stump and free the specimen.

Visceral sparing pelvic peritonectomy

In patients with minimally aggressive PM, such as pseudomyxoma peritonei, the pelvic peritoneum, uterus, ovaries, and tubes can be definitively removed, but the rectum and rectosigmoid colon spared. A layer of fat immediately beneath the rectouterine space in females or the rectovesical space in males can provide a plane of dissection that allows for complete clearing of the pelvic PM but preservation of the rectum. Scissor dissection of noninvasive tumor nodules on the anterior rectum and removal of omental appendages infiltrated by tumor may also be necessary.

Vaginal closure and low colorectal anastomosis

One of the few suture repairs performed prior to the intraoperative chemotherapy is the closure of the vaginal cuff. If one fails to close the vaginal cuff, chemotherapy solution will leak from the vagina. The circular stapled colorectal anastomosis occurs after the intraoperative chemotherapy has been completed. A circular stapling device is passed into the rectum, and the trocar is penetrated to the staple line. A purse-string applicator is used to secure the stapler anvil in the distal descending colon. A monofilament suture is placed through the lateral aspects of the staple line of the rectal stump. As the body of the circular stapler and anvil are mated, these sutures are tied up to include the entire rectal staple line within the circular stapled anastomosis. The stapler is activated to join the colon and rectum. After this, an insufflation into the rectum with a saline filled to the pelvis (bubble test) shows that the circular stapled anastomosis is competent; a second layer of vertical mattress sutures is reinforced to the colorectal staple line circumferentially. If this two-layer anastomosis is technically perfect, no diverting ileostomy is performed.

Left colon mobilization for a tension-free low colorectal anastomosis

An absolute requirement for a complication-free low colorectal anastomosis is the absence of tension on the staple line. Adequate mobilization of the entire left colon is needed, and several steps may be required to accomplish this. The inferior mesenteric artery is ligated on the aorta, and then its individual branches are resected as they arise from this vascular trunk. The Y configuration of the left colic and sigmoidal vessels is converted to a V configuration to keep the intermediate arcade intact. The inferior mesenteric vein is divided as it courses around the duodenum. The mesentery of the transverse colon and splenic flexure are completely elevated away from the perirenal fat surrounding the left kidney. Taking care to avoid the left ureter, the surgeon divides the left colon mesentery from all its retroperitoneal attachments. These maneuvers allow the junction of the sigmoid and descending colon to reach to the low rectum or anus for a tension-free anastomosis. Redundant descending colon should fall into the hollow of the sacrum.

Five types of small bowel involvement by cancer

CRS with perioperative chemotherapy has been most commonly used for the management of mucinous appendiceal neoplasms, but they have been successfully applied to other tumors, especially colon cancer and diffuse malignant peritoneal mesothelioma. The histological features and the depth of invasion of these different tumors into the bowel wall are not uniform. Based on the extent of the invasion, the size of the tumor nodule, and its anatomic location on the bowel wall, small bowel involvement is classified into five types [23]:

Type 1: Noninvasive nodules
Type 2: Small invasive nodules on the antimesenteric portion of the small bowel
Type 3: Moderate-sized invasive nodules on the antimesenteric portion of the small bowel
Type 4: All sizes of invasive nodules at the junction of the small bowel and its mesentery
Type 5: Large invasive nodules

Techniques used in cytoreduction of the small bowel

TYPE 1: NONINVASIVE NODULES

This type of small bowel involvement involves minute nodules of aggressive histology that because of their small size have not invaded past the peritoneum. It would also include large noninvasive nodules of diffuse peritoneal adeno-mucinosis or nuclear grade I peritoneal mesothelioma. The curved Mayo scissors are used to trim these noninvasive nodules from the surface of the small bowel; this results in a localized removal of the peritoneum. Larger nodules are frequently scissor dissected in a piecemeal fashion to avoid damage to the deeper layers of the bowel wall. Considerable skill acquired over time may be needed to avoid damage to the muscularis propria of the bowel. There is usually no need for seromuscular repair.

TYPE 2: SMALL INVASIVE NODULES ON THE ANTIMESENTERIC PORTION OF THE SMALL BOWEL

These invasive nodules do not separate from the muscular layer of the small bowel and a partial thickness resection is required. The seromuscular layer is resected leaving mucosa and submucosa intact. This resection is usually performed with a curved Mayo scissor, but occasionally, it may be performed by pure-cut electrosurgery with frequent irrigation to cool the resection site. Scissor or knife dissection is preferred. The seromuscular layer is repaired by suture plication after the intraoperative chemotherapy is completed.

TYPE 3: MODERATE-SIZED INVASIVE NODULES ON THE ANTIMESENTERIC PORTION OF THE SMALL BOWEL

In contrast to small invasive nodules in this location, larger nodules require a full-thickness elliptical resection of the antimesenteric portion of the bowel wall. The closure is performed in two layers and at two different times. The first layer is a full-thickness closure using absorbable suture. One suture starts at each corner of the defect, and the sutures are then tied at the midportion of the resection. Following the HIPEC, the defect is closed with a second layer of nonabsorbable plication sutures.

TYPE 4: SMALL INVASIVE NODULES AT THE JUNCTION OF SMALL BOWEL AND ITS MESENTERY

These nodules can sometimes be removed by a localized removal with electrosurgery if sufficiently small and if the vascular supply to the segment of bowel is not compromised. A two-layer repair follows this localized resection. More often, these nodules are removed and the incidence of fistula is reduced by a segmental small bowel resection with end-to-end hand-sewn anastomosis (Figure 14.8).

TYPE 5: LARGE INVASIVE NODULES

These lesions require a segmental small bowel resection with generous proximal and distal margins on the bowel wall and on the mesentery. The segment of small bowel and a portion of its mesentery are resected. The bowel is divided and closed using a linear cutter/stapler. The HIPEC is completed prior to a two-layer hand-sewn anastomosis (Figure 14.8).

ADMINISTRATION OF PERIOPERATIVE CHEMOTHERAPY

Hyperthermic intraperitoneal chemotherapy administration

In the operating room, HIPEC is used. Thermal targeting is part of the optimizing process and is used to bring dose

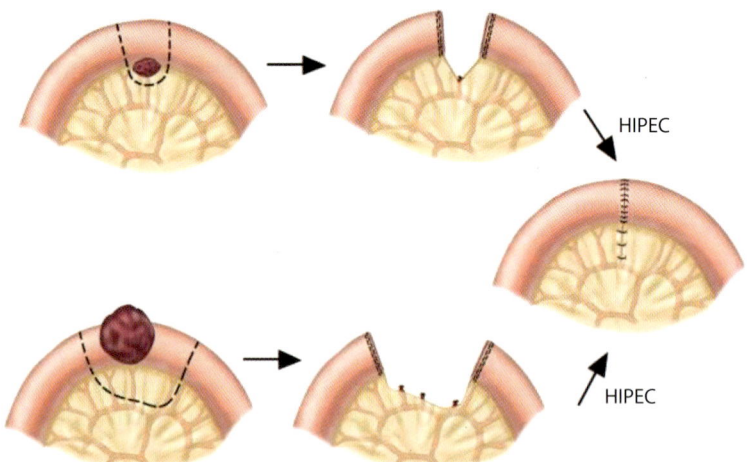

Figure 14.8 Small invasive nodules at the junction of the small bowel and mesentery (type 4) or large invasive nodules (type 5) are resected with generous margins using a linear stapler. After hyperthermic intraperitoneal chemotherapy is complete, a two-layer anastomosis is performed. (From Sugarbaker, P.H., An overview of peritonectomy, visceral resections, and perioperative chemotherapy for peritoneal surface malignancy, in: Sugarbaker, P.H., ed., *Cytoreductive Surgery & Perioperative Chemotherapy for Peritoneal Surface Malignancy*, Textbook and Video Atlas, Cine-Med Publishing, Woodbury, CT, 2012, pp. 1–30.)

intensity to the abdominal and pelvic surfaces. Abdominal and pelvic hyperthermia with IP and IV chemotherapy has several advantages. First, heat by itself has more toxicity for cancerous tissue than for normal tissue. This predominant effect on cancer increases as the vascularity of the malignancy decreases and the duration of the hyperthermia increase. Second, hyperthermia increases the penetration of chemotherapy into tissues. As the lipids in cell walls soften in response to heat, the elevated interstitial pressure of a tumor mass may decrease and allow improved drug penetration. Third, and probably the most important, heat increases the cytotoxicity of selected chemotherapy agents. This synergism occurs only at the interface of heat and body tissue at the peritoneal surface.

After the cancer resection is complete and prior to performing any anastomoses (except for closure of the vaginal cuff), the inflow catheters and outflow drains are placed through the abdominal wall. Temperature probes are secured to the skin edge. Three different methodologies for administering the hyperthermic perioperative chemotherapy are currently utilized. With the closed technique, the skin of the abdomen is closed in a watertight fashion for the duration of the chemotherapy treatments. At most institutions, this temporary closure is then opened for the performance of intestinal anastomoses and then a formal closure of the abdominal wall. At some institutions, the reconstruction is performed, the abdominal wall closed definitively, and then the closed chemohyperthermia treatments administered.

A second technique is the covered technique. After placing the inflow tubes, outflow drains, and temperature probes, a long running monofilament suture is used to elevate the skin edges to a self-retaining retractor. A plastic sheet is incorporated into these sutures to create a covering for the abdominal cavity. A slit in the plastic cover is made to allow the surgeon's double-gloved hand access to the abdomen and pelvis for continuous manipulation during the intraoperative treatments.

A third methodology is the open technique utilizing a vapor barrier. In this technique, the inflow tubes, outflow drains, and temperature probes are placed. The skin edges are elevated on the self-retaining retractor using skin traction sutures. Smoke evacuators are placed at the four corners of the abdominal incision and placed on high flow. These smoke evacuators maintain a vapor barrier above the chemotherapy solution during the hyperthermia treatments. In this technique, the surgeon continuously manipulates all viscera to eliminate adherence of peritoneal surfaces. Also, mesenteric cytoreduction can continue during the 60–120 minutes of the chemohyperthermia treatment (Figure 14.9).

Hyperthermic perioperative chemotherapy treatment regimens

The standardized orders for HIPEC used at the Center for Gastrointestinal Malignancies, MedStar Washington Hospital Center, are given in Table 14.1. Mitomycin C and doxorubicin are used intraoperatively to treat appendiceal, colonic, and gastric cancer. Occasionally, patients with pancreatic cancer or small bowel adenocarcinoma may be appropriate for these drugs. They are appropriate

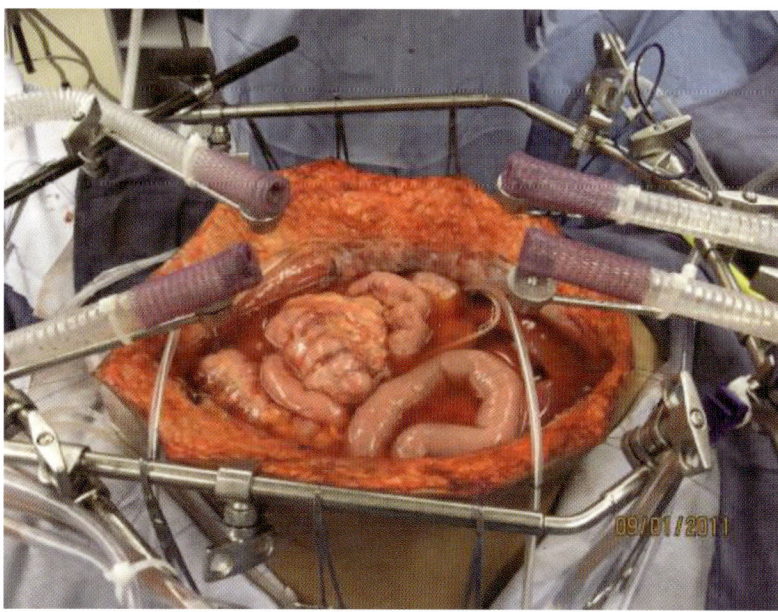

Figure 14.9 Hyperthermic intraperitoneal chemotherapy administered using an open technique. (From Sugarbaker, P.H., An overview of peritonectomy, visceral resections, and perioperative chemotherapy for peritoneal surface malignancy, in: Sugarbaker, P.H., ed., *Cytoreductive Surgery & Perioperative Chemotherapy for Peritoneal Surface Malignancy*, Textbook and Video Atlas, Cine-Med Publishing, Woodbury, CT, 2012, pp. 1–30.)

Table 14.1 Standardized orders for hyperthermic intraperitoneal chemotherapy plus systemic 5-fluorouracil or plus systemic ifosfamide

For pseudomyxoma peritonei and adenocarcinoma from appendiceal and colonic cancer, the following steps apply:
1. Add mitomycin C _____ mg to 2 L of 1.5% peritoneal dialysis solution.
2. Add doxorubicin _____ mg to the same 2 L of 1.5% peritoneal dialysis solution.
3. The dose of mitomycin C and doxorubicin is 15 mg/m^2 for each chemotherapy agent.
4. Add _____ mg 5-fluorouracil (400 mg/m^2) and leucovorin _____ mg (20 mg/m^2) to separate bags of 250 mL normal saline. Begin rapid IV infusion of both drugs simultaneous with IP chemotherapy.

For sarcoma, gastric cancer, ovarian cancer, and peritoneal mesothelioma, the following steps apply:
1. Add cisplatin _____ mg to 2 L of 1.5% peritoneal dialysis solution. The dose of cisplatin is 50 mg/m^2.
2. Add doxorubicin _____ mg to the same 2 L of 1.5% peritoneal dialysis solution. The dose of doxorubicin is 15 mg/m^2.
3. Add ifosfamide (1300 mg/m^2) _____ mg to 1 L 0.9% sodium chloride. Begin continuous IV infusion over 90 minutes simultaneous with IP chemotherapy.
4. Add mesna disulfide (260 mg/m^2) _____ mg in 100 mL 0.9% sodium chloride to be given IV as a bolus 15 minutes prior to ifosfamide infusion.
5. Add mesna disulfide (260 mg/m^2 _____ mg in 100 mL 0.9% sodium chloride to be given IV as a bolus 4 hours after ifosfamide infusion.
6. Add mesna disulfide (260 mg/m^2) _____ mg in 100 mL 0.9% sodium chloride to be given IV as a bolus 8 hours after ifosfamide infusion.

for ovarian cancer patients who have cisplatin neuropathy, hypersensitivity, or drug resistance. Systemic 5-fluorouracil is administered simultaneously with the IP chemotherapy solution.

A combination of doxorubicin and cisplatin is used to treat gastric cancer, ovarian cancer, and peritoneal mesothelioma. Also, papillary serous cancer and primary peritoneal adenocarcinoma are treated with the doxorubicin and cisplatin regimen. Systemic ifosfamide is administered as a continuous infusion over the 90 minutes of IP chemotherapy treatment.

Hyperthermic IP melphalan is often used for patients with recurrence undergoing a second cytoreduction. IP gemcitabine is recommended for patients with resectable pancreatic cancer, ovarian cancer patients who are cisplatin resistant, and peritoneal mesothelioma patients who are cisplatin resistant. Liposomal doxorubicin is used for patients with sarcomatosis or with signet ring adenocarcinoma. The liposomal doxorubicin is often recommended in patients who have an incomplete cytoreduction but a complete exposure of all of the visceral and parietal peritoneal surfaces to the chemotherapy solution.

Early postoperative intraperitoneal chemotherapy with 5-fluorouracil

The standardized orders for early postoperative intraperitoneal chemotherapy (EPIC) with 5-fluorouracil are presented in Table 14.2. After the patient stabilizes postoperatively, the 5-fluorouracil instillation occurs. The patients treated are those with carcinomatosis from adenocarcinoma. In some patients who have extensive small bowel trauma from lysis of adhesions, the early postoperative 5-fluorouracil is withheld for fear of fistula formation. Also, patients who have been treated with multiple cycles of systemic chemotherapy are at risk for severe neutropenia if EPIC with 5-fluorouracil is used.

Table 14.2 Early postoperative intraperitoneal chemotherapy with 5-fluorouracil on postoperative days 1–4

1. 5-Fluorouracil _____ mg (400 mg/m^2 for females and 600 mg/m^2 for males, maximum dose = 1400 mg) and 50 meq sodium bicarbonate in _____ mL 1.5% dextrose peritoneal dialysis solution via Tenckhoff catheter daily for 4 days. Start date _____. Stop date _____.
2. Intraperitoneal fluid volume, 1 L for patients ≤ 2.0 m^2, 1.5 L for > 2.0 m^2.
3. Drain all fluid from the abdominal cavity prior to instillation, and then clamp abdominal drains.
4. Run the chemotherapy solution into the abdominal cavity through Tenckhoff catheter as rapidly as possible. Dwell for 23 hours and drain for 1 hour prior to the next instillation.
5. Use gravity to maximize intraperitoneal distribution of the 5-fluorouracil. Instill the chemotherapy with the patient in a full right lateral position. After ½ hour, direct the patient to turn to the full left lateral position. Change position right to left every ½ hour. Continue turning for the first 6 hours after instillation of chemotherapy solution.
6. Monitor with pulse oximeter during the first 6 hours of intraperitoneal chemotherapy.
7. Continue to drain abdominal cavity after the final dwell until Tenckhoff catheter is removed.

Table 14.3 Early postoperative intraperitoneal chemotherapy with paclitaxel on postoperative days 1–5

1. Paclitaxel _____ mg (20–40 mg/m^2 × _____ m^2) (maximum dose, 80 mg) in 1000 mL 6% Hespan® (B. Braun, Irvine, CA) via Tenckhoff catheter daily.
   Start date _____.   Stop date _____.
2. Instill as rapidly as possible via Tenckhoff catheter. Dwell for 23 hours. Drain using Jackson–Pratt drains for 1 hour prior to next instillation.
3. During the initial 6 hours after chemotherapy infusion, patient's bed should be kept flat. The patient should be on the right side during instillation. Turn at ½-hour postinstillation onto the left side and continue to change sides at ½-hour intervals for 6 hours.
4. Monitor with pulse oximeter during the first 6 hours of intraperitoneal chemotherapy.
5. Continue to drain abdominal cavity by Jackson–Pratt drains after the last dose of intraperitoneal chemotherapy.

Early postoperative intraperitoneal chemotherapy with paclitaxel

The standardized orders for EPIC with paclitaxel are presented in Table 14.3. Patients treated are those with ovarian cancer, papillary serous adenocarcinoma, peritoneal mesothelioma, and gastric cancer.

INDICATIONS FOR HEATED PERIOPERATIVE CHEMOTHERAPY AS AN ONCOLOGIC EMERGENCY

As a primary gastrointestinal cancer is resected, unexpected dissemination of cancer cells on peritoneal surfaces may be documented. Resections of gastrointestinal cancers are performed in which there is a disruption of the cancer specimen resulting in "intraoperative tumor spill." In women, ovarian involvement of a gastrointestinal cancer indicates peritoneal contamination and progressive carcinomatosis. A small volume of localized cancer seeding on the specimen or in the omentum that would be resected as part of the removal of the primary tumor signals generalized peritoneal contamination. Another indication would be a perforated intra-abdominal malignancy when that perforation is through the cancer itself. Positive peritoneal cytology and malignant ascites would also be considered an indication for the oncologic emergency. If HIPEC is available at the time of the primary cancer resection, it should be used as an adjuvant to decrease the likelihood of local–regional relapse in these patients [24].

REFERENCES

1. Ronnett BM, Zahn CM, Kurman RJ, Kass ME, Sugarbaker PH, Shmookler BM. Disseminated peritoneal adenomucinosis and peritoneal mucinous carcinomatosis: A clinicopathologic analysis of 109 cases with emphasis on distinguishing pathologic features, site of origin, prognosis, and relationship to "pseudomyxoma peritonei." *The American Journal of Surgical Pathology*. 1995;19:1390–1408.
2. Cerruto CA, Brun EA, Chang D, Sugarbaker PH. Prognostic significance of histomorphologic parameters in diffuse malignant peritoneal mesothelioma. *Archives of Pathology & Laboratory Medicine*. 2006;130:1654–1661.
3. Berthet B, Sugarbaker TA, Chang D, Sugarbaker PH. Quantitative methodologies for selection of patients with recurrent abdominopelvic sarcoma for treatment. *European Journal of Cancer*. 1999;35:413–419.
4. Sugarbaker PH. Sarcomatosis and imatinib-resistant gistosis: Diagnosis and therapeutic options. In: Sugarbaker PH, ed., *Cytoreductive Surgery & Perioperative Chemotherapy for Peritoneal Surface Malignancy*. Textbook and Video Atlas, Woodbury, CT: Cine-Med Publishing, 2012. pp. 127–136.
5. Jacquet P, Jelinek JS, Steves MA, Sugarbaker PH. Evaluation of computer tomography in patients with peritoneal carcinomatosis. *Cancer*. 1993;72:1631–1636.
6. Jacquet P, Jelinek JS, Chang D, Koslowe P, Sugarbaker PH. Abdominal computed tomographic scan in the selection of patients with mucinous peritoneal carcinomatosis for cytoreductive surgery. *Journal of the American College of Surgeons*. 1995;181:530–538.
7. Carmignani P, Sugarbaker TA, Bromley CM, Sugarbaker PH. Intraperitoneal cancer dissemination: Mechanisms of the patterns of spread. *Cancer and Metastasis Reviews*. 2003;22:465–472.
8. Pestieau SR, Jelinek JS, Chang D, Jacquet P, Sugarbaker PH. CT in the selection of patients with abdominal or pelvic sarcoma for reoperative surgery. *Journal of the American College of Surgeons*. 2000;190:700–710.
9. Yan TD, Haveric N, Carmignani P, Chang D, Sugarbaker PH. Abdominal computed tomography scans in the selection of patients with malignant peritoneal mesothelioma for comprehensive treatment with cytoreductive surgery and perioperative intraperitoneal chemotherapy. *Cancer*. 2005;15:839–849.
10. Koh J-L, Yan TD, Glenn D, Morris DL. Evaluation of preoperative computed tomography in estimating peritoneal cancer index in colorectal peritoneal carcinomatosis. *Annals of Surgical Oncology*. 2009;16:327–333.
11. Rivard JD, Temple WJ, McConnell YJ, Sultan H, Mack LA. Preoperative CT does not predict resectability in peritoneal carcinomatosis. *The American Journal of Surgery*. 2014;207:760–765.

12. Pelz JOW, Stojadinovich A, Nissan A, Hohenberger W, Esquivel J. Evaluation of a peritoneal surface disease severity score in patients with colon cancer with peritoneal carcinomatosis. *Journal of Surgical Oncology.* 2009;99:9–15.

13. Prada-Villaverde A, Esquivel J, Lowy AM, Markman M, Chua T, Pelz J, Baratti D et al. The American Society of Peritoneal Surface Malignancies evaluation of HIPEC with Mitomycin C versus Oxaliplatin in 539 patients with colon cancer undergoing a complete cytoreductive surgery. *Journal of Surgical Oncology.* 2014;110:779–785.

14. Esquivel J, Chua TC. CT versus intraoperative peritoneal cancer index in colorectal cancer peritoneal carcinomatosis: Importance of the difference between statistical significance and clinical relevance. *Annals of Surgical Oncology.* 2009;16:2662–2663.

15. Steller EP. Comparison of four scoring methods for an intraperitoneal immunotherapy model. Enhancement and abrogation: Modifications of host immune influence IL-2 and LAK cell immunotherapy. PhD thesis. Rotterdam, the Netherlands: Erasmus University Rotterdam; November 1988.

16. Gomez Portilla A, Sugarbaker PH, Chang D. Second-look surgery after cytoreductive and intraperitoneal chemotherapy for peritoneal carcinomatosis from colorectal cancer: Analysis of prognostic features. *World Journal of Surgery.* 1999;23:23–29.

17. Sugarbaker PH. Peritonectomy procedures. *Surgical Oncology Clinics of North America.* 2003;12:703–727.

18. Sugarbaker PH. The subpyloric space: An important surgical and radiologic feature in pseudomyxoma peritonei. *European Journal of Surgical Oncology.* 2002;28:443–446.

19. Sugarbaker PH. Dissection by electrocautery with a ball tip. *Journal of Surgical Oncology.* 1994;56:246–248.

20. Sugarbaker PH. Circumferential cutaneous traction for exposure of the layers of the abdominal wall. *Journal of Surgical Oncology.* 2008;98:472–465.

21. De Lima Vazquez V, Sugarbaker PH. Xiphoidectomy. *Gastric Cancer.* 2003;6:127–129.

22. Sugarbaker PH. Pont hepatique (hepatic bridge), an important anatomic structure in cytoreductive surgery. *Journal of Surgical Oncology.* 2010;101:251–252.

23. Bijelic L, Sugarbaker PH. Cytoreduction of the small bowel surfaces. *Journal of Surgical Oncology.* 2008;97:176–179.

24. Glehen O, Yonemura Y, Sugarbaker PH. Prevention and treatment of peritoneal metastases from gastric cancer. In Sugarbaker PH, ed., *Cytoreductive Surgery & Perioperative Chemotherapy for Peritoneal Surface Malignancy.* Textbook and Video Atlas, Woodbury, CT: Cine-Med Publishing, 2012. pp. 79–94.

15

Chemoperfusion techniques and technologies

KIRAN TURAGA

The goal of chemoperfusion is to achieve high tissue concentrations of the cytotoxic drug, with a favorable plasma–peritoneal area under the curve (AUC). Effective delivery of the cytotoxic drug requires a precise balance of numerous components, the most important of which are temperature, flow, volume, and composition of the solution to deliver chemotherapy. In this chapter, we discuss some of the techniques for delivery of intracavitary chemotherapy and the technologies employed with them.

INTRACAVITARY CHEMOPERFUSION

Intracavitary chemoperfusion is generally coupled with a complete cytoreductive surgery in which complete extirpation of the tumor is undertaken before administering chemotherapy. While chemoperfusion has also been employed in the neoadjuvant or palliative setting, the majority of the discussion pertains to the curative paradigm of chemoperfusion [1,2]. The abdominal cavity is the most common site of chemoperfusion for peritoneal surface malignancies occurring from colorectal, appendiceal, ovarian, mesothelial, and other histological primaries. Nevertheless, thoracic cavity perfusions have been employed with success and oncological efficacy for pleural mesotheliomas in conjunction with cytoreductive surgery [3]. Bicavitary chemoperfusion has also been described for patients undergoing chemoperfusion for disease spread to both cavities or for patients undergoing diaphragmectomies for peritoneal disease, thus leading to violation of the thoracic–abdominal

barrier [4,5]. The delivery of the chemoperfusion is usually achieved in one of three ways:

1. *Open chemoperfusion*: This technique of chemoperfusion employs establishing a cavity space with limited to no risk of spillage during manual agitation of the chemoperfusate solution. While this is easily achieved in the thoracic cavity due to the fixed nature of the thoracic wall, to create such a space in the abdomen requires careful planning and preparation by the team. The surgeon incorporates the abdominal wall in sutures that are then suspended by the abdominal wall retractor system such the Thompson or Omni retractors. A plastic barrier is then introduced to avoid aerosol inhalation for the team and a gloved, waterproofed arm is then introduced into the chemoperfusate solution to help circulate the intraperitoneal (IP) chemoperfusate. A smoke evacuator is often placed below the plastic barrier to allow for evacuation of the aerosol created during the perfusion. Catheters are placed in the lateral abdomen to both introduce and drain the IP fluid. Peristaltic pumps (described subsequently) are used to create the perfusion of the solution. This technique allows for adequate delivery of the drug to different regions with adequate spatial diffusion and also facilitates continued cytoreduction during the chemoperfusion period. It can also ensure thermal homogeneity. This has been widely adopted in Europe and some high-volume centers in the United States [6,7]. The disadvantages of the open

chemoperfusion include the potential hazards to the operation room team, the time and expertise needed for the setup, and the need for additional lateral abdominal wall drains in addition to the often used midline incision for cytoreduction.

2. *Closed chemoperfusion*: This technique of chemoperfusion uses the skin of the abdominal wall as an artificial barrier to the chemoperfusate solution as it is being agitated inside the abdominal cavity. After a complete cytoreduction, most frequently, catheters are introduced inside the abdomen through the midline incision and incorporated into a skin closure. After a watertight skin closure is achieved, the abdomen is filled with the perfusate solution. The abdomen is manually agitated in addition to the flow characteristics to obtain adequate distribution of drug. The position of the table is also altered to ensure adequate delivery of the solution. The advantages of this technique alleviate some of the concerns of the operating room personnel and the ease of application. This is used widely in the United States and has been suggested in a recent consensus guidelines paper as a preferred technique for chemoperfusion. The disadvantages of this technique include inadequate delivery of the drug due to altered distribution, inability to continue cytoreduction during this period and greater expertise necessary for troubleshooting as compared to the open technique. It also includes the additional step of opening and closing the skin when creating the barrier for the chemoperfusion. Porcine studies have also indicated altered delivery to the lesser omentum and the right hemidiaphragmatic regions with varied thermal homogeneity, and hence, special attention must be paid to these areas while the inflow cannula are placed [8].

3. *Laparoscopic chemoperfusion*: The technique of laparoscopic chemoperfusion is usually employed in the setting of limited peritoneal disease after a complete cytoreduction or in the setting of palliative evacuation of mucin or palliative perfusion for intractable ascites. In this setting, often 5 and 12 mm ports are used to complete the cytoreduction. The inflow cannulas are bifurcated outside the abdomen and introduced via the port site with purse-string sutures to ensure watertight closure. The outflow cannulas are either single or bifurcated and placed via the port sites and connected to the perfusion pump to create a perfusion. Laparoscopic perfusion is a form of closed perfusion. Alternatively, a single gel port incision for the hand is used to introduce both the inflow and outflow cannulas especially when it is used for cytoreduction as well.

4. *Normothermic IP chemotherapy*: Delivery of IP chemotherapy that occurs via an IP port is not a true chemoperfusion since the flow characteristics of the perfusate are absent. Nevertheless, this technique employs the delivery of drug mixed with a carrier solution warmed to 37°C and introduced when the patient is awake. Hence, the delivery occurs by gravity until the entire perfusate (usually 1 L) is introduced in the abdomen. Authors differ in their practices of either leaving the perfusate in (very common with an IP port) or draining it after a certain time period (commoner in the early postoperative IP chemotherapy, neoadjuvant setting, and those with peritoneal dialysis [Tenckhoff] catheters).

COMPONENTS OF THE CHEMOPERFUSION

The various components of the chemoperfusion that need to be controlled during the chemoperfusion include temperature, flow, volume, perfusate character, perfusion time, drug dosage, and time of delivery.

Temperature

Hyperthermia potentiates the effect of the chemotherapy and is believed to act in numerous ways. It increases the concentration of the drug, improves vascularity to improve delivery, and accentuates cell cycle kinetics to allow more effective cytotoxic effects among others [9]. Hyperthermia during chemoperfusion is delivered by heating the chemoperfusate solution. Unlike other methods of medical hyperthermia, which use radiant heat such as those used for limb sarcomas, chemoperfusion relies on convection to deliver heat. The hyperthermic pump relies on either electromagnetic induction or plate-heated water baths that allow for precise temperature regulation during the delivery of the perfusate. The solution is often heated to 44°C–46°C to allow for radiant heat loss between the roller pump and the patient, although insulation techniques have been tried in some current hyperthermic intraperitoneal chemoperfusion (HIPEC) technologies commercially available. The goal of the chemoperfusion is to maintain the outflow temperature between 40°C and 42°C. Measurement of the peritoneal temperature is performed by placing temperature probes either in the peritoneum or inside the outflow cannulas.

Flow

The impact of the perfusate flow on the oncological aspects of the chemoperfusion is unknown. In animal models, higher flow rates equated with better drug delivery and favorable plasma–peritoneal AUC. A chemoperfusion aims for flow rates of 600–1500 mL/min. While higher flow rates are possible with conventional peristaltic pumps, the effect on the IP viscera might be more unpredictable. Higher flow rates could also lead to more turbulent flow, altering the flow dynamics within the cavity. Increasing the number of inflow cannulas can decrease the individual flow rate unless the overall flow rate is increased by the peristaltic pump. The techniques of chemoperfusion currently use two to four inflow cannulas and 1–8 outflow cannulas.

Volume

The volume of the perfusate used for colorectal peritoneal carcinomatosis has been suggested to be ideal at 3 L in a consensus statement [10]. Regardless, the volume used for open and closed perfusions are different. Open perfusions usually utilize different perfusate volumes (2 L/m²) [6], while most closed perfusions for other histologies utilize 3 (2–4) L of perfusate volume [9]. Addition of the chemotherapy can add additional volume to the perfusate if mixed in additional carrier fluid and needs to be noted carefully. The relationship between volume and pressure has been questioned, and animal models suggest that pressure might be more important for drug delivery than the volume of the perfusate [11,12]. However, due to lack of standardization of the measurement and relevance of pressure, volume is still used as a standardized method for perfusion. Occasionally, due to loss of circuit volume or difficulty in obtaining high flow rates, additional volume can be added to the circuit.

Character

Perfusate solutions could vary from using solutions such as water, 5% dextrose in water, lactated ringers solution, normal saline, and peritoneal dialysate (1.5%) solutions. Choice of the perfusate solution must include the chemotherapy used since platinum products can form adducts with lactated ringers solutions. Hypoosmolar perfusates such as water can cause hyponatremia leading to life-threatening cerebral edema, while normal saline can lead to hyperchloremic acidosis. Although hypotonic solutions have been suggested to have more favorable pharmacokinetic profiles, including the prolonged retention of ascites, studies by some groups revealed high incidence of thrombocytopenia and bleeding [13–16]. The most common perfusate solutions include lactated ringers and 1.5% peritoneal dialysate solution.

Perfusion time

The time for perfusion is usually determined by the plasma–peritoneal AUC and characteristics of the individual drug delivered. The duration of most chemoperfusions with mitomycin C last up to 90 minutes (60–110 minutes) [9] and by consensus were recommended to last 90 minutes [10]. Chemoperfusion with oxaliplatin and irinotecan are usually shorter (30–60 minutes) [6].

Drug dosage and timing

Drugs are usually added at the time point once hyperthermia is achieved using the perfusate solution. Split-dosing regimens have been used for mitomycin, when the drug is added both at time 0 and time 60 minutes [10]. The individual drug dosing regimens are described in detail under the sections dealing with specific histologies. The use of bidirectional chemotherapy has been proposed especially for chemotherapies with synergistic effects with intravenous (IV) chemotherapy. This leads to a bidirectional diffusion gradient between the tissue layers. Bidirectional therapy with IV fluorouracil and IP oxaliplatin/irinotecan or mitomycin C is often used for patients with colorectal or appendiceal primary lesions and with cisplatin and pemetrexed for patients with mesothelioma [13].

PERFUSION TECHNOLOGIES

There are numerous technologies that are currently available in the United States and Europe to deliver hyperthermic IP chemoperfusion. Characteristics of the commercially available perfusion technologies are summarized in Table 15.1 and shown in Figure 15.1.

Table 15.1 Characteristics of commercially available hyperthermia pumps in the United States in 2014

Perfusion characteristics	Belmont hyperthermia pump	Eight medical recirculator 8.0	RanD performer HT	Thermasolutions HT-2000
Heating unit	Electromagnetic induction coil (precision 0.1°C)	Single-use heat exchanger (precision 0.1°C)	High-efficiency plate warmer (precision 0.2°C)	Single-use heat exchanger (heated water bath) (precision 0.1°C)
Maximum perfusion rate (mL/min)	1000	200	2000	2400
Heating system	Integrated (dry)	Integrated (dry)	Integrated (dry)	Integrated (with water tank)
Patient bypass system for troubleshooting		–	+	–
Temperature probes	4	4	8	4
Reservoir volume (L)	4.4–8	8	0.5–9	4–8
Inline pressure monitoring	Yes	Yes	Yes	Yes
Larger size	++	+++	+++	+++
Better touch screen interface with recording ability	+	++	++	++
Higher cost of pump	+	++	++	++
Higher cost of disposables	+	+	+	+

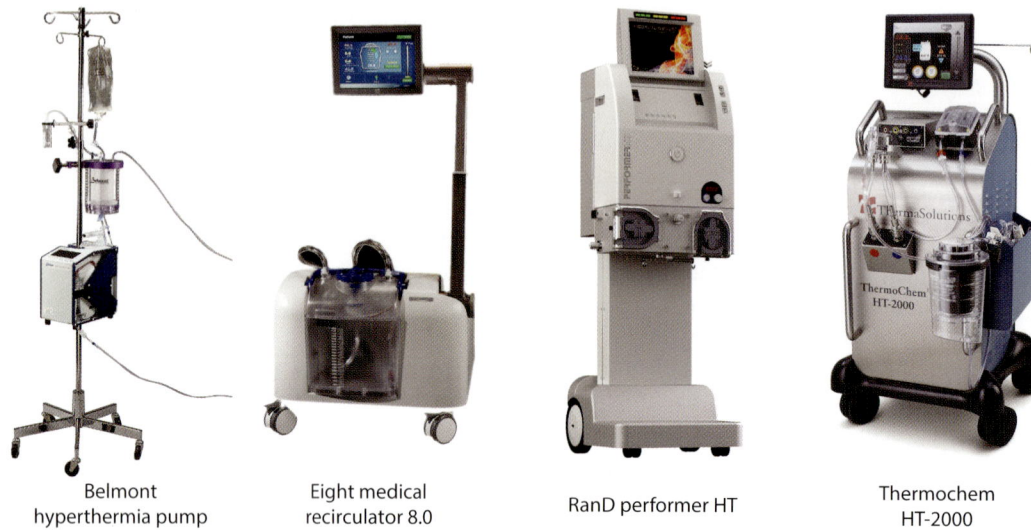

| Belmont hyperthermia pump | Eight medical recirculator 8.0 | RanD performer HT | Thermochem HT-2000 |

Figure 15.1 Commercially available pumps for hyperthermia in the United States.

SPECIAL CONSIDERATIONS

Bicavitary chemoperfusion

In the event that a bicavitary chemoperfusion needs to be performed, the perfusate volume needs to be increased significantly to accommodate the increased cavity space. Often, a 4.5 L perfusate volume is used for bicavitary chemoperfusion, and an additional outflow cannula is placed within the thoracic cavity [4,7]. In bicavitary chemoperfusion, it is imperative to heat and cool slowly given the increased risk of cardiac dysrhythmias with sudden changes in temperature [17]. Troubleshooting a bicavitary circuit is identical to a unicavitary circuit with special attention to loss of reservoir volume that can happen in dependent portions of the chest.

Total gastrectomy/hysterectomy/vaginal cuff resection or total proctectomy with an abdominoperineal resection

After a total gastrectomy, the mediastinal space is often opened to dissect the intra-abdominal and distal thoracic esophagus. Similarly, after a proctectomy requiring an abdominoperineal resection (APR), the perineum is open. These systems lead to loss of IP volume that could impair the ability to chemoperfuse a patient. In such settings, it is advisable to perform the esophagojejunostomy anastomosis for a total gastrectomy prior to performing the chemoperfusion. In patients undergoing APRs, the perineal wound is closed before starting chemoperfusion. Similarly, the vaginal cuff is closed prior to the chemoperfusion after a hysterectomy or a pelvic peritonectomy. This allows for maintenance of the reservoir volume during the HIPEC.

Major abdominal wall resection or resection of previous stoma or port site

Resection of a major portion of the abdominal wall is often performed when there is recurrent disease after a previous cytoreduction. Occasionally, peristomal recurrences requires resection of the stoma site en bloc with the abdominal wall leaving gaping wounds that may not approximate with simple skin sutures. In settings where the skin cannot be closed over the large defect, use of adhesive barriers such as Ioban or Tegaderm has been valuable in maintaining the seal for a closed perfusion. Placing outflow cannulas through the defect might also be considered to allow for smaller space closure with a purse-string suture. The open technique lends itself better to the perfusion of patients with large abdominal wall defects and could be considered if an adequate seal cannot be reached.

Timing of anastomosis

Major series reporting on cytoreductive surgery and HIPEC have reported a median of 0.6–1.2 anastomoses per cytoreductive procedure [18]. There remains considerable ambiguity regarding the optimal timing of the anastomosis during a chemoperfusion procedure. Conventionally, patients have undergone the cytoreductive procedure, followed by the chemoperfusion and then the anastomosis. This allows for resection of perfused staple lines and oncological benefit of limited implantation of disease into the anastomosis. However, this leads to often performing the anastomosis in less than optimal conditions with edematous bowel and toward the end of the procedure when the team may be tired or a new scrub team may be in the room. Some European centers have adopted the technique of performing the anastomosis prior to the chemoperfusion, placing cannulas laterally in the abdominal wall and closing the fascia prior to the chemoperfusion, thus eliminating the step of opening the skin, performing the

Table 15.2 Common troubleshooting techniques during chemoperfusion

Issue	Steps
High inline pressures	Check inflow cannulas that could get kinked during positioning.
	Check the purse-string suture to ensure that it is not occluding the line.
	Reset and reprime the line.
	If perfusion already begun, it is possible that viscera might be occluding the tip. In a closed perfusion, attempt to spin the cannulas gently to allow relief of inline pressure. If persistent, might need to stop perfusion.
Drop in reservoir volume or loss of volume to abdomen	Check the outflow cannula and confirm that it is not kinked or obstructed from the stitch.
	In highly mucinous tumors, mucin can occlude the outflow lines or reservoir. This may need to be flushed.
	If the aforementioned reasons are unlikely then, this error usually occurs when the abdomen is more capacious that the perfusate volume added or if there is a diaphragmatic or perineal opening. This may require interruption of perfusion.
	Adding volume to the perfusate or reducing the flow rate can counter some of the leaks.
Target temperature is not reached	Likely due to malposition of the temperature probes.
	Measure outflow temperature to confirm heated solution is delivered.
	Inflow temperature can be increased, but excessive increases could lead to visceral injury.
Systemic hyperthermia above 39°C	Ensure that bair huggers are placed on ambient rather than off.
	Maximize the cooling blanket temperature. This can be dropped almost to 40°F provided there is a cloth barrier between the patient and cooling blanket.
	Decrease temperature of IV fluids.
	Ice packs can be used near the head.
	Reduce temperature of inflow perfusate.
Flow rates not reached	Check inflow and outflow cannulas as outlined earlier.
	Ensure perfusate volume is adequate, may need to add volume.
	Very viscous perfusions due to mucin may need change of reservoir filter.
	May need to interrupt perfusion and use numerous inflow/outflow cannulas.

anastomosis and then closing the abdomen. Raise patient table or lower reservoir. There is no high-level evidence purporting the benefit of one over the other although the theoretical risk of higher anastomotic leaks in the case of the perfusion performed after the anastomosis is often discussed.

TROUBLESHOOTING THE CHEMOPERFUSION

It is not infrequent to develop interruptions in chemoperfusion given the numerous components involved in achieving a complete perfusion. While simple troubleshooting is possible without much help, more complicated or recurrent issues are best addressed by involving a perfusionist experienced with peritoneal perfusions and a company representative. Table 15.2 outlines some of the common troubleshooting steps that can be undertaken during a chemoperfusion.

REFERENCES

1. Randle RW, Swett KR, Swords DS, Shen P, Stewart JH, Levine EA et al. Efficacy of cytoreductive surgery with hyperthermic intraperitoneal chemotherapy in the management of malignant ascites. *Annals of Surgical Oncology.* 2014;21:1474–1479.

2. Facchiano E, Risio D, Kianmanesh R, Msika S. Laparoscopic hyperthermic intraperitoneal chemotherapy: Indications, aims, and results: A systematic review of the literature. *Annals of Surgical Oncology.* 2012;19:2946–2950

3. Sugarbaker DJ, Gill RR, Yeap BY, Wolf AS, DaSilva MC, Baldini EH et al. Hyperthermic intraoperative pleural cisplatin chemotherapy extends interval to recurrence and survival among low-risk patients with malignant pleural mesothelioma undergoing surgical macroscopic complete resection. *The Journal of Thoracic and Cardiovascular Surgery.* 2013;145:955–963.

4. Senthil M, Harrison LE. Simultaneous bicavitary hyperthermic chemoperfusion in the management of pseudomyxoma peritonei with synchronous pleural extension. *Archives of Surgery.* 2009;144:970–972.

5. Sugarbaker PH, Chang D, Stuart OA. Hyperthermic intraoperative thoracoabdominal chemotherapy. *Gastroenterology Research and Practice.* 2012;2012:623417.

6. Elias D, Goere D, Dumont F, Honoré C, Dartigues P, Stoclin A et al. Role of hyperthermic intraoperative peritoneal chemotherapy in the management of peritoneal metastases. *European Journal of Cancer.* 2014;50:332–340.

7. Sugarbaker P. Management of peritoneal surface malignancy using intraperitoneal therapy and cytoreductive surgery. 2014. Accessed October 5, 2014, at http://www.surgicaloncology.com/.

8. Elias D, Antoun S, Goharin A, Otmany AE, Puizillout JM, Lasser P. Research on the best chemohyperthermia technique of treatment of peritoneal carcinomatosis after complete resection. *International Journal of Surgical Investigation*. 2000;1:431–439.

9. Esquivel J. Technology of hyperthermic intraperitoneal chemotherapy in the United States, Europe, China, Japan, and Korea. *Cancer Journal*. 2009;15:249–254.

10. Turaga K, Levine E, Barone R, Sticca R, Petrelli N, Lambert L et al. Consensus guidelines from The American Society of Peritoneal Surface Malignancies on standardizing the delivery of hyperthermic intraperitoneal chemotherapy (HIPEC) in colorectal cancer patients in the United States. *Annals of Surgical Oncology*. 2014;21:1501–1505.

11. Facy O, Combier C, Poussier M, Magnin G, Ladoire S, Ghiringhelli F et al. High pressure does not counterbalance the advantages of open techniques over closed techniques during heated intraperitoneal chemotherapy with oxaliplatin. *Surgery*. 2015;157(1):72–78.

12. Solass W, Kerb R, Murdter T, Giger-Pabst Urs, Strumberg D, Tempfer C et al. Intraperitoneal chemotherapy of peritoneal carcinomatosis using pressurized aerosol as an alternative to liquid solution: First evidence for efficacy. *Annals of Surgical Oncology*. 2014;21:553–559.

13. Van der Speeten K, Stuart OA, Sugarbaker PH. Pharmacokinetics and pharmacodynamics of perioperative cancer chemotherapy in peritoneal surface malignancy. *Cancer Journal*. 2009;15:216–224.

14. Mohamed F, Marchettini P, Stuart OA, Sugarbaker PH. Pharmacokinetics and tissue distribution of intraperitoneal paclitaxel with different carrier solutions. *Cancer Chemotherapy and Pharmacology*. 2003;52:405–410.

15. Kondo A, Maeta M, Oka A, Tsujitani S, Ikeguchi M, Kaibara N. Hypotonic intraperitoneal cisplatin chemotherapy for peritoneal carcinomatosis in mice. *British Journal of Cancer*. 1996;73:1166–1170.

16. Tsujitani S, Oka A, Kondo A, Katano K, Oka S, Saito H et al. Administration in a hypotonic solution is preferable to dose escalation in intraperitoneal cisplatin chemotherapy for peritoneal carcinomatosis in rats. *Oncology*. 1999;57:77–82.

17. de Bree E, van Ruth S, Schotborgh CE, Baas P, Zoetmulder FA. Limited cardiotoxicity after extensive thoracic surgery and intraoperative hyperthermic intrathoracic chemotherapy with doxorubicin and cisplatin. *Annals of Surgical Oncology*. 2007;14:3019–3026.

18. Chua TC, Yan TD, Saxena A, Morris DL. Should the treatment of peritoneal carcinomatosis by cytoreductive surgery and hyperthermic intraperitoneal chemotherapy still be regarded as a highly morbid procedure?: A systematic review of morbidity and mortality. *Annals of Surgery*. 2009;249:900–907.

16

Port placement for intraperitoneal chemotherapy

LISA M. LANDRUM AND JOAN L. WALKER

INTRODUCTION

In gynecologic oncology, intraperitoneal (IP) chemotherapy has been implemented primarily as front line adjuvant therapy following surgical cytoreduction in patients with advanced epithelial ovarian cancer. This route of delivery gained favor due to the pattern of metastasis for ovarian cancer, which often involves widespread dissemination of tumor implants along peritoneal surfaces of the diaphragm, abdomen, and pelvis but rarely extends outside of the peritoneal cavity. Because advanced endometrial cancer may also present with peritoneal dissemination, there have been a few trials that have evaluated the role of IP delivery of chemotherapy in this patient population [1]. Significant improvement in survival measures have not yet been demonstrated in patients with endometrial cancer, and it is not considered an accepted method for treatment at this time. There have also been a few phase 1 and 2 clinical trials that have used IP chemotherapy in the setting of recurrent ovarian cancer [2–8]. These trials have been met with mixed results and, again, use of IP chemotherapy in this patient population is not evidence based at this time. Conversely, IP chemotherapy has been shown to be superior to intravenous (IV) chemotherapy in treating patients with advanced epithelial ovarian cancer who have small-volume, residual disease following primary cytoreductive surgery in three large, randomized, cooperative-group trials [9–11]. Based on these combined results, the National Cancer Institute (NCI) issued a clinical announcement recommending that women with stage III ovarian cancer who undergo optimal surgical cytoreduction should be considered for IP chemotherapy. To further highlight the relevance of this route of delivery, an ancillary data analysis of the NCI-sponsored, clinical trials published in 2013 revealed patients with advanced ovarian cancer that underwent optimal cytoreductive surgery with only microscopic residual disease and received adjuvant IP chemotherapy had survival measures that exceeded any previously reported with a median progression-free survival (PFS) of 43.2 months (95% CI 32.5–60.4) and median overall survival (OS) of 110 months (95% CI, 60.0–161.3) [12]. Despite these provocative results, there remains reluctance to implement this therapy due to toxicity concerns and a lack of expertise in dealing with the drug delivery device [13,14]. The objectives of this chapter are to review the history of port placement, complications associated with administration of IP chemotherapy, and offer techniques for placement to prevent complications.

HISTORY OF IP CHEMOTHERAPY IN OVARIAN CANCER

The concept of IP chemotherapy first arose in the 1960s, with the initial description of the pharmacokinetics and pharmacodynamic principles provided by Dr. Robert Dedrick and colleagues at the National Institutes of Health [15,16]. The rationale for this novel form of drug delivery was that substantially higher levels of drug concentration could be achieved within the peritoneal cavity than could safely be obtained through IV drug administration. Regional delivery of chemotherapy into the peritoneal cavity provides an advantage by exposing tumor implants to greater concentrations of antineoplastic agents than can be achieved with systemic therapy alone. These initial studies by Dedrick et al. stimulated interest among researchers to begin implementation of this strategy into phase I clinical trials to explore the safety and pharmacologic advantage of treating patients with ovarian cancer. Early studies confirmed that IP chemotherapy could deliver 10–20 times greater concentrations of both carboplatin [17,18] and cisplatin [19–22] than was possible with conventional IV therapy. Likewise, 1000-fold increases in the concentrations of paclitaxel could be obtained with IP delivery compared to systemic delivery [23,24]. Despite the high concentrations that can be achieved, drugs delivered by IP route are only able to penetrate directly into the tumor a few millimeters [25,26]. These data obtained in animal models are further substantiated in phase II trials utilizing cisplatin in second-line treatment of ovarian cancer. Patients with tumor volume greater than 1 cm had minimal objective response rates, with the best activity noted in patients with microscopic or small-volume disease [20,27–30]. As a result of these findings, phase III trials conducted by cooperative groups were restricted to patients that had undergone optimal surgical cytoreduction with minimal amounts of residual tumor. In total, four randomized phase III trials have been completed by cooperative groups, but data have not yet been reported on the most recent trial (Gynecologic Oncology Group [GOG] 252, closed to accrual in November of 2011). The first of three randomized clinical trials was initiated as a collaborative effort by the GOG, the Southwest Oncology Group (SWOG), and the Eastern Cooperative Oncology Group in the mid-1980s [9]. In this study, 546 patients with stage III epithelial ovarian cancer that had previously undergone surgical cytoreduction with residual disease of ≤2 cm were randomized to receive six cycles of IP or IV cisplatin (100 mg/m²) plus IV cyclophosphamide (600 mg/m²). Patients randomized to the IP cisplatin arm experienced a statistically significant improvement in OS (median, 49 v. 41 months; p = 0.02). The hazard ratio for OS was 0.76, indicating a 24% reduction in the risk of death in favor of IP chemotherapy. During this era of patient accrual for SWOG 8501/GOG 104, paclitaxel in combination with IV platinum was just beginning to gain favor a front-line agent in therapy for ovarian cancer, thus the results of the first phase III trial with IP cisplatin were never implemented into standard practice [31]. A second randomized clinical trial was conducted by the GOG (protocol number 114) and compared the "new" standard of care consisting of IV cisplatin (75 mg/m²) and IV paclitaxel (135 mg/m²) with an arm consisting of two cycles of carboplatin (AUC 9) followed by six cycles of IP cisplatin (100 mg/m²) and IV paclitaxel (135 mg/m²) in 532 patients [10]. Eligibility criteria included stage III patients with residual disease of ≤1 cm. Two cycles of single-agent carboplatin were given systemically prior to IP therapy in an effort to further chemically cytoreduce the residual volume of disease; however, the resultant bone marrow suppression

was such that 18% of patients randomized to the experimental arm only received two or fewer cycles of IP chemotherapy. Despite this fact, both PFS (median, 28 v. 22 months; p = 0.05) and OS (median, 63 v. 52 months, p = 0.02) were superior in the IP arm compared to the control group. The hazard ratio was 0.78 for PFS and 0.81 for OS in favor of regional therapy. The next, and most successful, phase III trial (GOG 172) compared IV paclitaxel (135 mg/m² over 24 hours) followed by IP cisplatin (100 mg/m²) on day 2 and IP paclitaxel (60 mg/m²) on day 8 to the control arm consisting of IV paclitaxel (135 mg/m² over 24 hours) followed by IV cisplatin (75 mg/m²) on day 2 [11]. Treatments were given every 21 days for a total of six cycles. Eligible patients had stage III epithelial ovarian or primary peritoneal cancer with residual disease of ≤1 cm after initial surgery. The median PFS was 18.3 and 23.8 months, respectively, for the IV and IP arms. The median survival for the arms was 49.5 and 66.5 months, again favoring the group randomized to IP treatment. The relative risk of death was 0.71 with a 95% confidence interval of 0.54–0.94 for the experimental arm (p = 0.0076). These impressive results were achieved even though only 42% of patients were able to complete six cycles of IP therapy due to toxicity. Grade 3 and 4 hematologic, metabolic, and gastrointestinal toxicities, as well as fatigue, infection, and pain were significantly more common in patients receiving IP chemotherapy (p < 0.001). Walker and colleagues reviewed reasons for failing to complete six cycles of IP chemotherapy in GOG 172 and identified that problems with the drug delivery device resulted in 34% of completion failures [32]. These complications included infection, leaking from the catheter or vagina, and access difficulties.

Since the results of GOG 172 were published, investigators have attempted a number of strategies to improve the tolerability of administration without compromising the survival advantage for patients. This was reflected in the most recent phase III trial (GOG 252) in which the dose of IP cisplatin was reduced from 100 to 75 mg/m² and IP carboplatin was added as an experimental arm of the study. This study has completed accrual and closed in November of 2011, but the data regarding toxicity and survival are not yet available.

CHOOSING A DRUG DELIVERY DEVICE

A venous or peritoneal access device with a large caliber (at least 9.6 French), single lumen, silicone catheter has successfully been used to administer IP chemotherapy [33,34]. Silicone is preferred over polyurethane catheters as these catheters promote fibrin sheath and plug formation and can occlude infusion of chemotherapy agent. There are no clear advantages to using either fenestrated or nonfenestrated catheters as long as silicone catheters are utilized [35]. The size of the access port should be individualized based on the patient's body size and depth of subcutaneous tissue just as one would do with an IV access device. A port should be used that is not too small or sits too deep for chemotherapy nurses to easily access with the Huber needle. Likewise in a thin patient, a correctly positioned port that is too large can cause considerable discomfort overlying the ribs. Port size must be carefully tailored for the individual patient.

TECHNIQUE FOR PLACEMENT

Ideally, the IP port can be placed at the same time as the original ovarian cancer staging and cytoreduction surgery. This enables the surgeon to counsel the patient preoperatively regarding appropriate risks and benefits of IP chemotherapy. Placement of a port at the time of surgery adds minimal time to the procedure, spares the patient an additional visit to the operating room, and if not needed, removal of the port at bedside is always easier than placement. Historically, there has been concern among physicians about placing IP ports at the time of cytoreductive surgery when bowel resections are required [33,36]. Bowel resection is often necessary to achieve optimal cytoreduction, and recent data suggest that ports may safely be placed without increasing risk of intra-abdominal or port site infection [32,37]. In the event of gross bacterial contamination, however, sound clinical judgment should prevail.

Open laparotomy placement

The port pocket is created by making a small horizontal incision (3–4 cm) on the inferior aspect of the thorax overlying a rib at the midclavicular line. The access port should be below the level of the bra to avoid pain and irritation that may come from contact with the port. The incision is then carried down to the underlying fascia, and a pocket just slightly larger than the port is created subcutaneously over the fascia covering the ribs. The catheter is tunneled subcutaneously from the port pocket site for a distance approximately 10 cm and then pulled into the peritoneal cavity well lateral to the midline incision and below the level of the transverse colon to avoid potential entrapment in adhesions (Figure 16.1). The catheter tailored to the proper length at each end is attached to the port, which is then sutured into

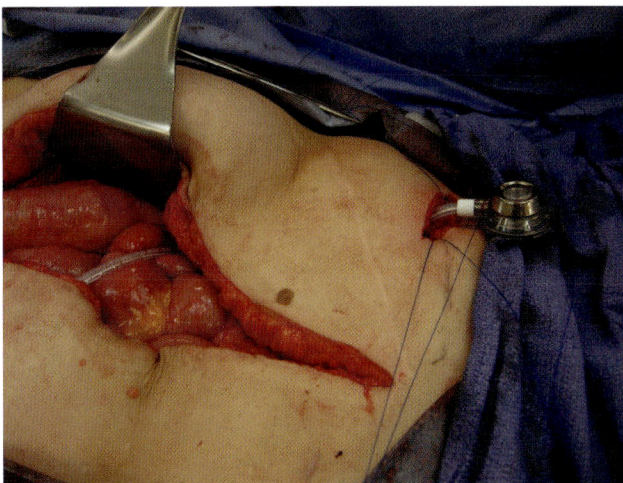

Figure 16.1 Placement of intraperitoneal port at the time of ovarian cancer cytoreduction.

the fascia using 2–0 Prolene at each of the four corners of the device to prevent rotation and subsequent difficulties with access. Once the port is secured in place, the catheter length should be such that approximately 10 cm of length is within the peritoneal cavity to ensure the catheter stays within the abdominal cavity and doesn't retract into the subcutaneous tissue. All perforations in the catheter should be within the peritoneal cavity, and the tip should not reach any bowel anastomosis sites, the bladder or the vagina. A catheter that is too long may create complications such as protrusion through the vaginal cuff, rectum, or bladder. Placement of sodium hyaluronate–carboxymethylcellulose barrier film at the time of port placement may also serve to prevent formation of adhesions that would hinder distribution of IP chemotherapy throughout the abdomen [38–40]. The access port should then be flushed with 10 mL of heparin 100 U/cm^3. The subcutaneous layer of the port pocket and skin are reapproximated with absorbable suture to prevent erosion of the port through the skin.

Delayed port insertion

On occasion, surgeons may not be able to place a port at the time of the original debulking surgery due to an unclear diagnosis, surgical complications, or concerns regarding gross bacterial contamination of the abdominal cavity. Port insertion can be completed at a second surgery by minilaparotomy, laparoscopy, or with assistance from interventional radiology. If the device is placed by minilaparotomy, a 3–4 cm vertical incision is made roughly 6 cm lateral to the umbilicus to avoid adhesions from the transverse colon to the anterior abdominal wall that may be present after an omentectomy. The knowledge of the previous procedures performed will assist its site selection (i.e., rectosigmoid resection vs. ileocecal resection). A port pocket is created at the lower margin of the anterior thorax, and the catheter is tunneled through a small perforation into the peritoneal cavity under direct visualization using a tunneling device or a tonsil under direct visualization to avoid injury to any peritoneal structures. The catheter should not be placed through the abdominal incision, as this incision only serves to provide visualization of catheter placement. A small peritoneal defect around the catheter is preferred rather than a large defect to prevent leaking of ascites and chemotherapy from the abdominal cavity into the port pocket. Finally, all layers of the abdominal incision should be systematically closed to prevent leakage of fluid from the incision.

With port placement in a laparoscopic-assisted fashion, the original abdominal incision can be avoided, and the entire procedure can be completed under direct visualization from a right upper quadrant approach (Figures 16.2 through 16.5) [41,42]. A pneumoperitoneum is established with a Veress needle in the right upper quadrant, after appropriate gastric emptying. A 5 mm trocar is placed for the laparoscope, and the catheter is positioned under direct visualization. The catheter can then be introduced into the peritoneal cavity using a needle, followed by wire, followed

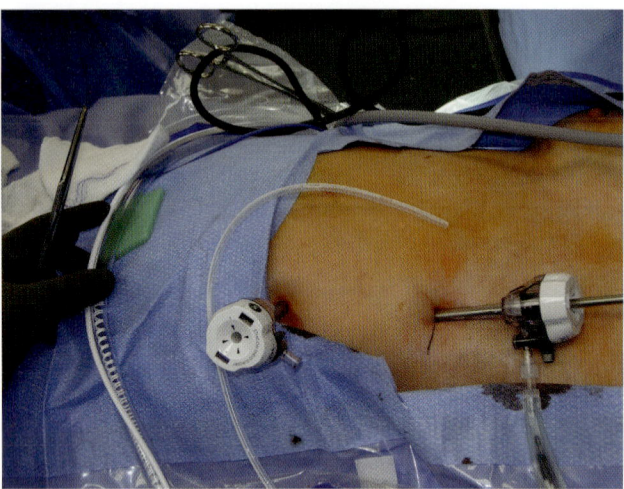

Figure 16.2 Delayed placement of intraperitoneal port by laparoscopy. Abdomen is insufflated, and catheter is placed to appropriate length under direct visualization.

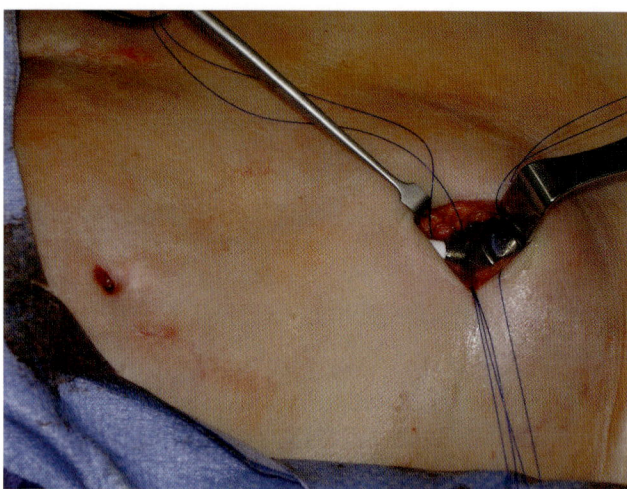

Figure 16.4 Catheter is attached to the port, and the port is secured with permanent suture to the fascia overlying the ribs.

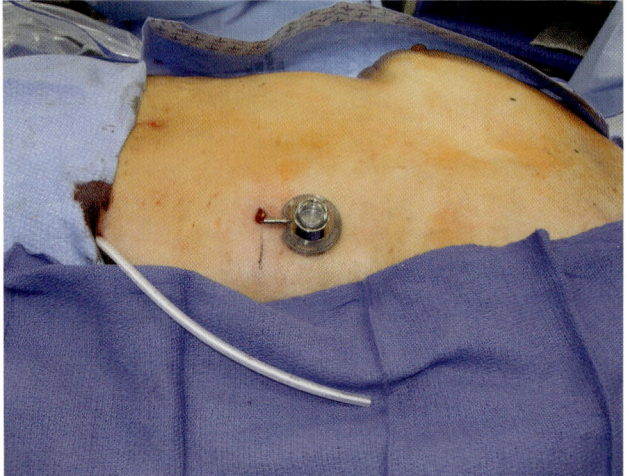

Figure 16.3 Catheter is tunneled to port pocket after placement into the abdominal cavity.

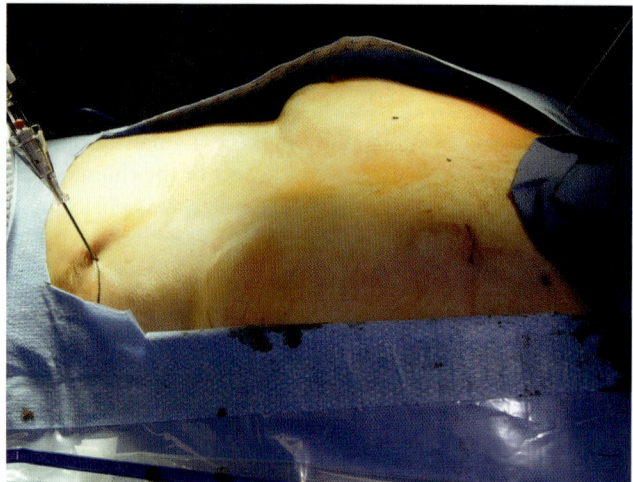

Figure 16.5 The port pocket is closed at time of delayed placement of intraperitoneal port.

by pull away sheath technique. Alternatively, a second 5 mm trocar is placed, and the catheter is passed down the trocar into the peritoneal cavity. The catheter is tunneled through the subcutaneous tissues, using a long tonsil or tunneling device to the site selected on the inferior thorax for the access port. The catheter should have been tailored to the appropriate length at both ends to avoid having any catheter perforations within the abdominal wall, or the catheter too long where it can reach the vagina [43], bladder [44] rectum [45], or any anastomosis sites and result in complications. All port sites should be closed to prevent leakage of fluid, ideally using a Carter–Thompson closure device and 0-vicryl sutures to reapproximate peritoneum and fascia. The interventional radiologist can also place IP catheters under CT or ultrasound guidance. One technique for successful placement by interventional radiology under conscious sedation has been described by Henretta and colleagues in 11 patients with advanced ovarian cancer [46].

All patients had successful placement and had no catheter-related complications in the course of receiving chemotherapy. Greben et al. [47] have also described the percutaneous placement of IP ports in 29 patients with no complications noted at the time of placement. Two patients (6.9%) experienced port-related complications including port site infection, which necessitated removal and obstruction of the port by kinking. The utilization of interventional radiology is an attractive option for delayed port placement because it allows the patient to avoid general anesthesia and have the port placed in a minimally invasive fashion. Admittedly, only small numbers of patients are represented in these case reports, but port placement by interventional radiology appears to be a feasible route. Excellent communication between the gynecologic oncologist and radiologist is strongly encouraged to avoid complications. Review of the individual patient's postoperative anatomy and sites of likely adhesions is helpful.

POSTOPERATIVE CARE AND COMPLICATIONS

Complications are not uncommon during IP chemotherapy. Complications are categorized into port access problems, inflow obstruction, abdominal pain, infections, and leaking into wound, bowel lumen, or out the vagina. The expected complication rate is 10%, and there have been many attempts to reduce these problems. Patients requiring radical surgery, or having a more complicated postoperative course, is expected to have a more difficult time with any chemotherapy given, including IP therapy. Infections have been seen more commonly when there is a midline wound breakdown or a left colon resection. Some centers delay the insertion of the IP catheter after colon resection, others only if an obvious contamination has occurred.

A fever in an IP chemotherapy patient can be evaluated by irrigating and aspirating saline from the port to send to microbiology for evidence of peritoneal or catheter infection. Cellulitis surrounding an IP port is rarely treated with antibiotics alone, the port and catheter are generally removed. Problems with access of the port or inflow obstruction are evaluated by fluoroscopy and a small amount of dilute solution of IV contrast dye. Surgical correction of the device can be considered, but usually the device is removed and IV chemotherapy is given. Successful correction is dependent on the cause being a mechanical problem, rather than a patient specific problem, such as adhesions.

Port malfunction

Difficulties with access can be prevented by securing the port with permanent suture to the fascia overlying the ribs to prevent migration or rotation of the delivery device. The port should also be large enough that it is easily palpated for introduction of the Huber needle and avoidance of needle injuries to the catheter by the nursing staff. Ports can obstruct through a number of different mechanisms including kinking of the catheter, formation of fibrous adhesions, or restriction of circulating chemotherapy by adhesions in neighboring structures, which result in compartmentalization of fluid. The catheter should be of a consistency that is rigid enough that it does not kink but also does not injure peritoneal structures. The caliber should also be large enough that the catheter is not easily obstructed. Distal obstruction prevents inflow of chemotherapy and may result in retrograde flow of ascites or chemotherapy into the subcutaneous tunnel or port pocket. Concern for obstruction should be evaluated by injecting contrast dye into the port and observing by fluoroscopy. Infusion may also be impeded if the catheter retracts from the abdominal cavity into the subcutaneous tissue. The catheter length is a critical factor in preventing retraction out of the peritoneal cavity. The device leaking into the vagina, bladder, or bowel is generally corrected by removal of the device. A laparotomy is not generally needed, unless the patient appears to have peritonitis, free air, or urinoma. Complaints of diarrhea or incontinence of urine with IP chemotherapy administration should be investigated as a potential communication with the catheter.

Abdominal pain

Administration of IP chemotherapy may result in pain due to the stretching and distension of the abdomen that occurs with infusion. Under normal circumstances, the chemotherapy agent is mixed with 1 L of normal saline that has been warmed to 37°C. This is infused through the Huber needle by gravity as rapidly as possible, followed by a second liter of normal saline to facilitate distribution of the drug throughout the peritoneal cavity. When pain is encountered, the initial management should include reducing the rate of infusion. In addition, the second liter saline can be reduced in volume or not given at all [48]. If abdominal pain persists despite alterations in the administration rate or volume, nonopioid analgesics are often adequate to manage the discomfort. There may also be a reaction to the drug, especially paclitaxel, by the peritoneal surface. Assessment of the port site by fluoroscopy may also be helpful to ensure that the catheter tip has not retracted out of the abdominal cavity and into the rectus sheath. This can certainly result in painful infusion for the patient and ultimately ineffective treatment. Some patients will get through therapy with pain pills, and others will refuse further IP administration.

Metabolic issues

Effective antiemetics and careful attention to hydration status is critical in preventing metabolic toxicities when administering IP cisplatin. Pretreatment antiemetics should be given following NCCN guidelines, and include decadron, aprepitant, and ondansetron or an equivalent. The first cycle of chemotherapy is generally given to women within 1–3 weeks following debulking surgery. At this point, many patients are malnourished and often have low serum albumin, ascites, and peripheral edema. Prehydration to expand intravascular volume with 1 L of normal saline should be a minimum requirement before infusion of cisplatin into the peritoneal cavity. Urine output should be documented at 100 cc/min prior to cisplatin administration. Cisplatin, mixed in 1 L of normal saline, should be given next, followed by an additional liter of normal saline to ensure distribution throughout the abdominal cavity. A second liter of IV hydration is performed to maintain urine output post cisplatin infusion. The IP fluid is not a substitute for adequate IV hydration, and to avoid renal toxicity with cisplatin, excellent hydration is mandatory. Patients should go home with strict instructions on home antiemetic use, call parameters, and liberal outpatient hydration. This is crucial in preventing toxicity and patient dissatisfaction. Keeping patients compliant with IP cisplatin requires commitment from the support staff and the patient. The three drug combination of decadron, aprepitant, and ondansetron should make this treatment very tolerable.

REMOVAL OF IP PORT AS OFFICE PROCEDURE

Operative overview

It is unnecessary to remove an IP port in the operating room. They often have to be removed urgently, therefore it is best to have an office set available to make removal quick and easy and timely. It is best to remove these devices as soon as their useful life is over, so a complication will not interfere with overall quality of life.

Preoperative preparation

The patient should not be neutropenic or thrombocytopenic and remember to hold aspirin, plavix, coumadin, lovenox, or other platelet inhibitors. The equipment needed are listed as follows:

1. Sterile field prep and drape
2. Mayo stand and sterile cover
3. Scalpel
4. Mayo scissors
5. Hemostats
6. Needle driver
7. Forceps
8. Retractors
9. Lidocaine
10. 3–0 vicryl SH needle
11. 4–0 vicryl PS-2 needle
12. Electrocautery (optional)

Operative procedure

Sterile skin preparation is first, followed by placement of a sterile drape with a perforation at the site of the port. Next, the area of skin overlying the port as well as the port pocket is infiltrated with 1% lidocaine. Skin incision is made overlying the port through old scar. The adipose tissue is dissected down to the palpable port where the catheter is attached. A dense fibrinous sheath is often found over the port and the catheter, which has to be incised without cutting the catheter itself. The hemostat is used to undermine the catheter and pull it up and out of the abdomen, and this is used for traction. The port is elevated, and the four Prolene sutures are sequentially identified and cut, while cutting through the fibrinous sheath surrounding the port. Be sure to identify and remove all permanent sutures. The port pocket is irrigated with sterile saline, and then the defect is closed in two layers. A prescription for narcotics is often given but nonsteroidal pain medications are generally adequate. Covering the incision for 24 hours is all that is required.

REFERENCES

1. Chambers JT, Chambers SK, Kohorn EI, Carcangiu ML, Schwartz PE. Uterine papillary serous carcinoma treated with intraperitoneal cisplatin and intravenous doxorubicin and cyclophosphamide. *Gynecologic Oncology.* March 1996;60(3):438–442.
2. Feun LG, Blessing JA, Major FJ, DiSaia PJ, Alvarez RD, Berek JS. A phase II study of intraperitoneal cisplatin and thiotepa in residual ovarian carcinoma: A Gynecologic Oncology Group study. *Gynecologic Oncology.* December 1998;71(3):410–415.
3. Skaznik-Wikiel ME, Lesnock JL, McBee WC, Beriwal S, Zorn KK, Richard SD et al. Intraperitoneal chemotherapy for recurrent epithelial ovarian cancer is feasible with high completion rates, low complications, and acceptable patient outcomes. *International Journal of Gynecological Cancer.* February 2012;22(2):232–237.
4. Markman M, Brady M, Hutson A, Berek JS. Survival after second-line intraperitoneal therapy for the treatment of epithelial ovarian cancer: The Gynecologic Oncology Group experience. *International Journal of Gynecological Cancer.* February 2009;19(2):223–239.
5. Armstrong DK, Fleming GF, Markman M, Bailey HH. A phase I trial of intraperitoneal sustained-release paclitaxel microspheres (Paclimer) in recurrent ovarian cancer: A Gynecologic Oncology Group study. *Gynecologic Oncology.* November 2006;103(2):391–396.
6. Alvarez RD, Sill MW, Davidson SA, Muller CY, Bender DP, DeBernardo RL et al. A phase II trial of intraperitoneal EGEN-001, an IL-12 plasmid formulated with PEG-PEI-cholesterol lipopolymer in the treatment of persistent or recurrent epithelial ovarian, fallopian tube or primary peritoneal cancer: A Gynecologic Oncology Group study. *Gynecologic Oncology.* June 2014;133(3):433–438.
7. Barakat RR, Fennelly D, Pizzuto F, Venkatraman ES, Brown C, Curtin JP. Salvage intraperitoneal therapy of advanced epithelial ovarian cancer: Impact of retroperitoneal nodal disease. *European Journal of Gynaecological Oncology.* 1997;18(3):161–163.
8. Markman M. Second-line chemotherapy for refractory cancer: Intraperitoneal chemotherapy. *Seminars in Surgical Oncology.* July 1994;10(4):299–304.
9. Alberts DS, Liu PY, Hannigan EV, O'Toole R, Williams SD, Young JA et al. Intraperitoneal cisplatin plus intravenous cyclophosphamide versus intravenous cisplatin plus intravenous cyclophosphamide for stage III ovarian cancer. *New England Journal of Medicine.* December 26, 1996;335(26):1950–1955.
10. Markman M, Bundy BN, Alberts DS, Fowler JM, Clark-Pearson DL, Carson LF et al. Phase III trial of standard-dose intravenous cisplatin plus paclitaxel versus moderately high-dose carboplatin followed by intravenous paclitaxel and intraperitoneal cisplatin in small-volume stage III ovarian carcinoma: An intergroup study of the Gynecologic

Oncology Group, Southwestern Oncology Group, and Eastern Cooperative Oncology Group. *Journal of Clinical Oncology*. February 15, 2001;19(4):1001–1007.

11. Armstrong DK, Bundy B, Wenzel L, Huang HQ, Baergen R, Lele S et al. Intraperitoneal cisplatin and paclitaxel in ovarian cancer. *New England Journal of Medicine*. January 5, 2006;354(1):34–43.

12. Landrum LM, Java J, Mathews CA, Lanneau GS, Jr., Copeland LJ, Armstrong DK et al. Prognostic factors for stage III epithelial ovarian cancer treated with intraperitoneal chemotherapy: A Gynecologic Oncology Group study. *Gynecologic Oncology*. July 2013;130(1):12–18.

13. Fairfield KM, Murray K, Lachance JA, Wierman HR, Earle CC, Trimble EL et al. Intraperitoneal chemotherapy among women in the Medicare population with epithelial ovarian cancer. *Gynecologic Oncology*. 2014;134(3):473–477.

14. Bowles EJ, Wernli KJ, Gray HJ, Bogart A, Delate T, O'Keeffe-Rosetti M et al. Diffusion of intraperitoneal chemotherapy in women with advanced ovarian cancer in community settings 2003–2008: The effect of the NCI clinical recommendation. *Frontiers in Oncology*. 2014;4:43.

15. Dedrick RL, Myers CE, Bungay PM, DeVita VT, Jr. Pharmacokinetic rationale for peritoneal drug administration in the treatment of ovarian cancer. *Cancer Treatment Reports*. January 1978;62(1):1–11.

16. Dedrick RL, Flessner MF. Pharmacokinetic problems in peritoneal drug administration: Tissue penetration and surface exposure. *Journal of National Cancer Institute*. April 2, 1997;89(7):480–487.

17. DeGregorio MW, Lum BL, Holleran WM, Wilbur BJ, Sikic BI. Preliminary observations of intraperitoneal carboplatin pharmacokinetics during a phase I study of the Northern California Oncology Group. *Cancer Chemotherapy and Pharmacology*. 1986;18(3):235–238.

18. Elferink F, van der Vijgh WJ, Klein I, ten Bokkel Huinink WW, Dubbelman R, McVie JG. Pharmacokinetics of carboplatin after intraperitoneal administration. *Cancer Chemotherapy and Pharmacology*. 1988;21(1):57–60.

19. Casper ES, Kelsen DP, Alcock NW, Lewis JL, Jr. IP cisplatin in patients with malignant ascites: Pharmacokinetic evaluation and comparison with the iv route. *Cancer Treatment Reports*. March 1983;67(3):235–238.

20. Howell SB, Pfeifle CL, Wung WE, Olshen RA, Lucas WE, Yon JL et al. Intraperitoneal cisplatin with systemic thiosulfate protection. *Annals of Internal Medicine*. December 1982;97(6):845–851.

21. Lopez JA, Krikorian JG, Reich SD, Smyth RD, Lee FH, Issell BF. Clinical pharmacology of intraperitoneal cisplatin. *Gynecologic Oncology*. January 1985;20(1):1–9.

22. Pretorius RG, Hacker NF, Berek JS, Ford LC, Hoeschele JD, Butler TA et al. Pharmacokinetics of IP cisplatin in refractory ovarian carcinoma. *Cancer Treatment Reports*. December 1983;67(12):1085–1092.

23. Francis P, Rowinsky E, Schneider J, Hakes T, Hoskins W, Markman M. Phase I feasibility and pharmacologic study of weekly intraperitoneal paclitaxel: A Gynecologic Oncology Group pilot Study. *Journal of Clinical Oncology*. December 1995;13(12):2961–2967.

24. Markman M, Rowinsky E, Hakes T, Reichman B, Jones W, Lewis JL, Jr. et al. Phase I trial of intraperitoneal taxol: A Gynecologic Oncology Group study. *Journal of Clinical Oncology*. September 1992;10(9):1485–1491.

25. Los G, van Vugt MJ, Pinedo HM. Response of peritoneal solid tumours after intraperitoneal chemohyperthermia treatment with cisplatin or carboplatin. *British Journal of Cancer*. February 1994;69(2):235–241.

26. Los G, Mutsaers PH, Lenglet WJ, Baldew GS, McVie JG. Platinum distribution in intraperitoneal tumors after intraperitoneal cisplatin treatment. *Cancer Chemotherapy and Pharmacology*. 1990;25(6):389–394.

27. Markman M, Rothman R, Hakes T, Reichman B, Hoskins W, Rubin S et al. Second-line platinum therapy in patients with ovarian cancer previously treated with cisplatin. *Journal of Clinical Oncology*. March 1991;9(3):389–393.

28. Markman M, Reichman B, Hakes T, Jones W, Lewis JL, Jr., Rubin S et al. Responses to second-line cisplatin-based intraperitoneal therapy in ovarian cancer: Influence of a prior response to intravenous cisplatin. *Journal of Clinical Oncology*. October 1991;9(10):1801–1805.

29. Markman M, Reichman B, Hakes T, Lewis JL, Jr., Jones W, Rubin S et al. Impact on survival of surgically defined favorable responses to salvage intraperitoneal chemotherapy in small-volume residual ovarian cancer. *Journal of Clinical Oncology*. September 1992;10(9):1479–1484.

30. Howell SB, Zimm S, Markman M, Abramson IS, Cleary S, Lucas WE et al. Long-term survival of advanced refractory ovarian carcinoma patients with small-volume disease treated with intraperitoneal chemotherapy. *Journal of Clinical Oncology*. October 1987;5(10):1607–1612.

31. Alberts DS, Markman M, Muggia F, Ozols RF, Eldermire E, Bookman MA et al. Proceedings of a GOG workshop on intraperitoneal therapy for ovarian cancer. *Gynecologic Oncology*. December 2006;103(3):783–792.

32. Walker JL, Armstrong DK, Huang HQ, Fowler J, Webster K, Burger RA et al. Intraperitoneal catheter outcomes in a phase III trial of intravenous

versus intraperitoneal chemotherapy in optimal stage III ovarian and primary peritoneal cancer: A Gynecologic Oncology Group Study. *Gynecologic Oncology.* January 2006;100(1):27–32.

33. Makhija S, Leitao M, Sabbatini P, Bellin N, Almadrones L, Leon L et al. Complications associated with intraperitoneal chemotherapy catheters. *Gynecologic Oncology.* April 2001;81(1):77–81.

34. Landrum LM, Gold MA, Moore KN, Myers TK, McMeekin DS, Walker JL. Intraperitoneal chemotherapy for patients with advanced epithelial ovarian cancer: A review of complications and completion rates. *Gynecologic Oncology.* November 5, 2007.

35. Ivy JJ, Geller M, Pierson SM, Jonson AL, Argenta PA. Outcomes associated with different intraperitoneal chemotherapy delivery systems in advanced ovarian carcinoma: A single institution's experience. *Gynecologic Oncology.* September 2009;114(3):420–423.

36. Davidson SA, Rubin SC, Markman M, Jones WB, Hakes TB, Reichman B et al. Intraperitoneal chemotherapy: Analysis of complications with an implanted subcutaneous port and catheter system. *Gynecologic Oncology.* May 1991;41(2):101–106.

37. Black D, Levine DA, Nicoll L, Chou JF, Iasonos A, Brown CL et al. Low risk of complications associated with the fenestrated peritoneal catheter used for intraperitoneal chemotherapy in ovarian cancer. *Gynecologic Oncology.* April 2008;109(1):39–42.

38. Becker JM, Stucchi AF. Intra-abdominal adhesion prevention: Are we getting any closer? *Annals of Surgery.* August 2004;240(2):202–204.

39. Bristow RE, Montz FJ. Prevention of adhesion formation after radical oophorectomy using a sodium hyaluronate-carboxymethylcellulose (HA-CMC) barrier. *Gynecologic Oncology.* November 2005;99(2):301–308.

40. Leitao MM, Jr., Natenzon A, bu-Rustum NR, Chi DS, Sonoda Y, Levine DA et al. Postoperative intra-abdominal collections using a sodium hyaluronate-carboxymethylcellulose (HA-CMC) barrier at the time of laparotomy for ovarian, fallopian tube, or primary peritoneal cancers. *Gynecologic Oncology.* November 2009;115(2):204–208.

41. Arts HJ, Willemse PH, Tinga DJ, de Vries EG, Van Der Zee AG. Laparoscopic placement of PAP catheters for intraperitoneal chemotherapy in ovarian carcinoma. *Gynecologic Oncology.* April 1998;69(1):32–35.

42. Liou WS, Teng NN, Chan JK. A modified technique for insertion of intraperitoneal port for chemotherapy. *Journal of Surgical Oncology.* June 15, 2005;90(4):247–248.

43. Ghosh K, Geller MA, Twiggs LB. Erosion of an intraperitoneal chemotherapy catheter resulting in an enterovaginal fistula. *Gynecologic Oncology.* May 2000;77(2):327–329.

44. Bryant CS, Shah JP, Triest JA, Schimp VL, Morris RT. Bladder erosion by an intraperitoneal chemotherapy catheter resulting in catheter protrusion through the external urethral meatus. *Gynecologic Oncology.* December 2008;111(3):552–554.

45. Bilsel Y, Balik E, Bugra D, Yamaner S, Akyuz A. A case of protrusion of an intraperitoneal chemotherapy catheter through rectum. *International Journal of Gynecological Cancer.* January 2005;15(1):171–174.

46. Henretta MS, Anderson CL, Angle JF, Duska LR. It's not just for laparoscopy anymore: Use of insufflation under ultrasound and fluoroscopic guidance by Interventional Radiologists for percutaneous placement of intraperitoneal chemotherapy catheters. *Gynecologic Oncology.* November 2011;123(2):342–345.

47. Greben CR, Goldstein GE, Lovecchio J, John V, Putterman D, Caplin D et al. Percutaneous insertion of peritoneal ports. *International Journal of Gynecological Cancer.* February 2012;22(2):328–331.

48. Markman M, Walker JL. Intraperitoneal chemotherapy of ovarian cancer: A review, with a focus on practical aspects of treatment. *Journal of Clinical Oncology.* February 20, 2006;24(6):988–994.

PART 5

Clinical Results of Intraperitoneal Drug Delivery

17

Intraperitoneal chemotherapy for ovarian cancer

ABDULRAHMAN SINNO AND DEBORAH ARMSTRONG

INTRODUCTION

Despite accounting for only 25% of all gynecologic malignancies, ovarian cancer continues to be the leading cause of death in patients with gynecologic cancer. In 2014, it is anticipated that there will be 21,980 newly diagnosed patients with ovarian cancer in the United States, with 14,270 deaths [1]. Primary debulking surgery followed by platinum-based chemotherapy is the standard of care for initial management of ovarian carcinoma, achieving complete remission in 80% of patients. Unfortunately, the majority of patients will recur and eventually succumb to their disease.

Clearly, the recurrence patterns of ovarian carcinoma suggest that residual microscopic disease persists in the peritoneal cavity despite a relatively high rate of optimal cytoreduction and the utilization of adjuvant chemotherapy [2]. Hence, intraperitoneal (IP) chemotherapy has been proposed as a mechanism to achieve higher IP concentrations of cytotoxic agents in an attempt to improve progression-free (PFS) and overall survival (OS).

In this chapter, we will review the rationale behind IP chemotherapy specifically as it pertains to ovarian cancer and the data that support its use. Furthermore, we will discuss limitations to its widespread adoption and future directions aimed at improving tolerability, acceptance, and efficacy of IP chemotherapy in ovarian cancer.

CONSIDERATIONS FOR IP CHEMOTHERAPY SPECIFIC TO OVARIAN CANCER

Surgical considerations

The consistent failure of screening modalities to improve detection of early ovarian cancer [3] results in greater than 60% of ovarian cancer presenting with advanced disease with malignant ascites and diffuse carcinomatosis [2]. Ovarian cancer most often spreads by shedding of tumor cells into the peritoneal cavity with subsequent serosal or peritoneal implantation and varying degrees of invasion and angiogenesis. While hematogenous dissemination and lymphatic spread may occur, this typical pattern of spread indicates that the peritoneal cavity is the major site of disease burden in ovarian carcinoma. This makes the disease amenable to surgical resection, even when widespread dissemination has occurred.

While the goal of surgery is complete cytoreduction of all visible disease, the current definition of optimal cytoreduction is defined by the Gynecologic Oncology Group (GOG) as residual tumor implants <1 cm at the completion of surgery [4]. Achieving this task often requires complex upper abdominal procedures such as diaphragm stripping, liver resection, splenectomies, and urologic and gastrointestinal resections [5]. Aggressive cytoreductive surgery certainly increases short-term perioperative morbidity, but a growing body of evidence over the past three decades has shown a significant survival advantage with this approach [5–8]. In a meta-analysis of 6885 patients with stage III or IV ovarian cancer, Bristow et al. [9] demonstrated a significant association between maximal cytoreductive surgery and survival outcomes. Median survival time of patient cohorts with >75% complete cytoreduction was 50% higher than cohorts with ≤25% maximal cytoreduction (median survival time of 33.9 vs. 22.7 months).

Several hypotheses attempt to explain the biological basis for the role of aggressive upfront cytoreduction. Bulky disease is generally comprised of a poorly oxygenated and perfused core, limiting the effectiveness of chemotherapy. Furthermore, decreasing tumor burden at initial surgery also decreases the burden of intrinsic resistant clones of tumor cells that may otherwise not be sensitive to chemotherapy. Today, optimal cytoreduction can be achieved in 80% of patients with advanced ovarian cancer. This makes any chemotherapeutic option that targets small volume disease located in the peritoneal cavity with higher concentrations of cytotoxic agents an attractive option for this disease. This is the rationale behind the use of IP chemotherapy in ovarian cancer.

Chemotherapeutic considerations

As discussed in previous chapters, the concept of IP chemotherapy is to directly expose residual tumor cells to an antineoplastic agent at a high concentration for a more prolonged period of time. The antineoplastic agent then affects the tumor by (1) direct contact and diffusion into the tumor causing cytotoxic effects superficially (2) diffusion into local leaky capillaries and recirculating into the tumor core and causing cytotoxic effects deep in the tumor (3) causing changes in the tumor microenvironment and (4) being absorbed into the systemic circulation and being delivered hematogenously to both IP and extraperitoneal tumors. The ideal chemotherapeutic agent is one that is able to penetrate the tumor using these mechanisms, highly effective in ovarian cancer, and persists in the peritoneal cavity for prolonged periods but that also results in some degree of systemic exposure.

IP agents active in ovarian cancer

Platinum drugs and taxanes remain the backbone of upfront chemotherapy in ovarian cancer. They exhibit different pharmacokinetic and pharmacodynamic characteristics when given directly into the IP cavity, and understanding these principles is essential to understanding the side effect profile and activity of these drugs when injected IP. Platinum agents are highly water soluble and have a relatively low molecular weight. As such, they rapidly redistribute to systemic circulation after IP injection. Paclitaxel is a large, lipid soluble molecule with minimal diffusion into the systemic circulation. Table 17.1 presents the IP pharmacologic parameters for drugs with known activity in ovarian cancer.

CISPLATIN AND CARBOPLATIN

Following IP administration of cisplatin, peritoneal concentration and area under the curve (AUC) of the active drug are 21- and 12-fold higher in the peritoneal cavity than in the plasma, respectively [10]. However, after IP administration, some cisplatin "leaks" into the plasma so that even those components of tumor supplied only by capillary flow receive exposure to a cytotoxic dose of cisplatin. Pretorius et al. [11] studied the pharmacology of IP cisplatin in canines. While peak serum levels are higher following IV administration, tissue levels are almost identical except in the peritoneum where the peritoneal lining has 2.5–8 times higher levels of drug after IP administration. The amount of drug excreted in the urine was similar regardless of method of administration, with approximately 50% of the injected dose excreted by day 4.

Carboplatin has very low protein binding but is also water soluble. A study by Miyagi et al. [12] showed that similar to cisplatin, the peak plasma concentrations were identical when carboplatin was administered IV or IP, but the 24 hours platinum AUC in the peritoneal cavity was approximately 17 times higher when carboplatin was administered by the IP route. This led the authors to conclude that not only is IP administration of carboplatin feasible but is also a reasonable route for systemic chemotherapy.

Table 17.1 Pharmacologic parameters for intraperitoneal drugs with activity in ovarian cancer

Drug name	Molecular weight	Solubility	Properties	Peritoneal: Plasma peak level	Peritoneal: Plasma AUC
Cisplatin	300.05	Water soluble	High protein binding (>95%) and rapid activation	20	12
Carboplatin	371.25	Water soluble	Low protein binding and slower activation	24	18
Paclitaxel	853.92	Requires lipid/alcohol formulation	High protein binding		1000
Docetaxel	861.94	Water soluble	Very high protein binding		181
Doxorubicin	543.53	Water soluble	Vesicant, high protein binding	474	
Gemcitabine	299.66	Water soluble	Very low protein binding		759
Topotecan	457.91	Water soluble	Moderate protein binding		54

A recent study by Jandial et al. [13] directly compared IP administration of carboplatin to that of cisplatin in a mouse model of ovarian carcinoma. Equimolar and equitoxic doses of carboplatin were injected IP into nude mice with peritoneal carcinomatosis. Tumor nodules were subsequently harvested and analyzed for platinum concentration. While the intratumoral concentration of cisplatin decreased with increasing nodule size, that of carboplatin did not. These results suggest that tumor penetration of carboplatin might even be superior to cisplatin and hence provide support for its use in IP chemotherapy.

PACLITAXEL

The GOG published the results of the first phase 1 trial of IP paclitaxel in 1992 [14]. In this trial, 24 patients with recurrent ovarian cancer and one patient with breast cancer were treated using a standard 3 + 3 design using 21-day cycles. As can be expected from the large molecular weight and the poor water solubility of paclitaxel, there was little absorption of the drug from the peritoneal cavity. Peak levels in the peritoneal cavity were 1000-fold those in the plasma, and the drug persisted for up to 48 hours after instillation. Abdominal pain was the dose-limiting toxicity in this trial and was significant at doses greater than 175 mg/m^2. This led the authors to conclude the administration at that dosage, as required for 21-day cycles, might not be ideal. Interestingly, abdominal pain began 8–24 hours after injection, with little pain prior to that. This suggests that the pain is not a direct function of distention of the abdominal cavity but rather due to the direct effects of paclitaxel on the peritoneal cavity. A subsequent phase 1 trial explored weekly IP paclitaxel and concluded that this treatment schedule resulted in an acceptable toxicity profile and a major pharmacokinetic advantage for cavity exposure [15]. The recommended dose and schedule for weekly IP paclitaxel was 60–65 mg/m^2 weekly.

IP CHEMOTHERAPY AS FIRST-LINE TREATMENT IN OVARIAN CANCER

The first randomized clinical trial comparing IP to IV chemotherapy in ovarian cancer was conducted by the Southwest Oncology Group (SWOG 8501) and the GOG 104 [16]. Patients with less than 2 cm residual disease, the definition of optimal cytoreduction at that time, were randomized to receive six cycles of IV cyclophosphamide (600 mg/m^2) and IV cisplatin (100 mg/m^2) or IV cyclophosphamide and IP cisplatin at the same dose. A total of 654 patients were evaluated of which 546 were eligible for inclusion. The trial was extended to accrue a sufficient number of patients to a subgroup of patients who were cytoreduced to less than 5 mm visible lesions. OS was significantly longer in the IP group (49 months; 95% CI 42–56) compared to the IV group (41 months; 95% CI 34–47). The hazard ratio (HR) for the risk of death was 0.76 (95% CI 0.61–0.96; P = 0.02) in favor of IP therapy. In both the IV and IP groups, 58% of all patients were able to complete all six cycles of cisplatin therapy. Abdominal pain was more common in the IP group, whereas significantly more patients in the intravenous group had grade 2 or 3 neuromuscular toxic effects at the completion of chemotherapy (25%t, vs. 15% in the IP group; P = 0.02). Furthermore, grade 3/4 granulocytopenia and tinnitus, clinical hearing loss were significantly more frequent in the IV group. This was not surprising given the higher peak systemic exposures predicted by the pharmacokinetic and pharmacodynamics of IV cisplatin and the expected side effects when given at a dose of 100 mg/m^2 (Table 17.2).

Table 17.2 Phase III randomized control trials for upfront intraperitoneal chemotherapy

Study name	Number of patients	Eligibility	Control arm regimen	Median OS months	Experimental arm regimen	Median OS months	P value
GOG104 Alberts et al.	546	Stage III <2 cm residual	Cisplatin 100 mg/m^2 IV Cyclophosphamide 600 mg/m^2 IV (q 21 d × 6)	41	Cisplatin 100 mg/m^2 IP Cyclophosphamide 600 mg/m^2 IV (q 21 d × 6)	49	0.02
GOG 114 Markman et al.	462	Stage III <1 cm residual	Paclitaxel 135 mg/m^2 IV (24 hours D1) Cisplatin 75 mg/m^2 IV (D2) (q 21 d × 6)	51	Carboplatin (AUC9) IV (q 28 d x 2) Paclitaxel 135 mg/m^2 IV (24 hours D1) Cisplatin 100 mg/m^2 IP (D2) (q 21 d × 6)	63	0.05
GOG172 Armstrong et al.	459	Stage III <1 cm residual	Paclitaxel 135 mg/m^2 IV (24 hours D1) Cisplatin 75 mg/m^2 IV (D2) (q 21 d 3 × 6)	49	Paclitaxel 135 mg/m^2 IV (24 hours D1) Cisplatin 100 mg/m^2 IP (D2) Paclitaxel 60 mg/m^2 IP (D8) (q 21 d × 6)	67	0.03

This study is interesting for multiple reasons. It provides a direct comparison of cisplatin delivered intravenously to cisplatin delivered intraperitoneally at the same dose. A clear survival benefit was seen in the IP arm. Furthermore, the results of this trial contributed to the evolving surgical paradigm in the definition of optimal debulking among gynecologic oncologists. OS for the subgroup of patients cytoreduced to less than 5 mm of residual disease was 51 months in the IP group (95% CI 44–67) compared to 46 months in the IV group (95% CI 37–57). The HR for this 5-month improvement in the risk of death was 0.80 (95% CI 0.61–0.96; P = 0.10) in favor of IP therapy. Although these differences were not statistically significant, it was notable that the outcomes for both IV and IP therapy were better in this low-volume group compared to the overall group.

Cyclophosphamide in combination with cisplatin was the standard of care at the time that this trial was developed and conducted, and these agents were appropriately used in both arms of the trial. However, in 1996, the same year that the results of GOG 104 were published, McGuire et al. [17] published the results of GOG 111, the landmark trial that demonstrated the superiority of IV cisplatin and paclitaxel over IV cisplatin and cyclophosphamide in ovarian cancer. This minimized the impact of this trial as most practitioners chose to use the new agent, paclitaxel, rather than IP chemotherapy.

The second IP randomized clinical trial to be published was SWOG 9927/GOG114 [18]. Markman et al. randomized 426 patients, with largest residual disease volume less than 1 cm after primary debulking surgery, to receive either paclitaxel at a dose of 135 mg/m² over 24 hours followed by cisplatin 75 mg/m² every 3 weeks for six cycles (control IV arm) or to high-dose IV carboplatin (AUC 9) for two cycles followed by six cycles of IV paclitaxel at a dose of 135 mg/m² and IP cisplatin at 100 mg/m² every 3 weeks for a total of eight cycles of therapy (experimental IP arm). The rationale behind utilizing two cycles of high-dose carboplatin prior to commencing the IP phase of the experimental arm was that IP chemotherapy would work best in the setting of minimal disease volume and that IV carboplatin would chemically cytoreduce residual disease to attain that goal. The experimental IP arm in this trial had a significant PFS and OS advantage (median 28 vs. 22 months; relative risk 0.78; log rank P = 0.01, median 63 vs. 52 months; relative risk 0.81; P = 0.05). Completion of all planned chemotherapy cycles was higher in the control arm (86% vs. 71%), and there was significantly more grade 4 neutropenia, grade 3–4 thrombocytopenia, and grade 3–4 gastrointestinal toxicity in the experimental arm. This trial was heavily criticized for the fact that the experimental arm was clearly more aggressive with an additional two cycles of therapy and a higher total platinum dose given. It was unclear whether the survival advantage was due to the additional cycles of therapy, the increased total platinum administered or due to the IP administration of these drugs.

In January of 2006, the U.S. National Cancer Institute issued a clinical alert strongly encouraging the use of IP chemotherapy in stage III epithelial ovarian cancer patients who were optimally cytoreduced (to <1.0 cm) [19]. This was directly following the publication of the results of GOG 172 [20]. In this landmark trial, 417 patients were randomized to six 21-day cycles of either a control arm of IV paclitaxel (135 mg/m² over 24 hours) and IV cisplatin (75 mg/m²) or to an experimental arm of IV paclitaxel (135 mg/m² over 24 hours) followed by IP cisplatin (100 mg/m²) on day 2, and IP paclitaxel (60 mg/m²) on day 8. Patients in the experimental arm had a significantly improved PFS (median 24 vs. 18 months; relative risk 0.80; log rank P = 0.05) and a significantly improved OS (median 66 vs. 50 months; relative risk 0.75; P = 0.03) in favor of the IV/IP group. Significantly more patients in the IP-therapy group experienced grade 3 or 4 fatigue, pain, or hematologic, gastrointestinal, metabolic, or neurologic toxic effects (P ≤ 0.001).

GOG 172 continues to have the longest reported OS from a phase 3 clinical trial in North America. The survival analyses were based on intent to treat. Thus, the 16-month improvement in OS is potentially more remarkable given that only 42% patients were able to receive all six planned cycles of IP therapy (compared to 90% in the IV group) and that 48% of all patients received less than four cycles of planned IP chemotherapy. It can be concluded that IP chemotherapy offers a survival advantage in ovarian cancer even when less than six cycles are given and that if conditions are optimized to improve tolerance, a greater survival benefit could be achieved. In a meta-analysis of GOG 172 and GOG 114 by Tewari et al. [21], the 5-year survival rate among patients treated with IP therapy increased from 18% with completion of one or two cycles to 33% with three or four cycles, to 59% for patients who completed five or six cycles of treatment. Whether or not the relationship between number of completed cycles and survival is causal as opposed to a reflection of favorable disease characteristics and comorbidities remains to be elucidated.

CONTROVERSIES AND CHALLENGES IN IP CHEMOTHERAPY

Several concerns raised regarding GOG 172 have hindered the widespread adoption of this treatment regimen. In fact, IP utilization at National Comprehensive Cancer Network (NCCN) cancer centers was only 43% during 2009–2012 [22]. At treatment initiation, 43% of patients received modified IP regimens, whereas only 29% received the GOG 172 regimen and 28% received IP chemotherapy as part of a clinical trial.

The control arm of GOG 172, IV cisplatin and 24 hours paclitaxel, reflected the standard of care at the time of the study design. In 2003, Ozols et al. [23] published the results of GOG 158 in which optimally debulked advanced ovarian cancer patients were randomized to receive cisplatin 75 mg/m² plus a 24 hours infusion of paclitaxel 135 mg/m² (control arm) or carboplatin AUC 7.5 plus paclitaxel 175 mg/m² over 3 hours (experimental arm). In this trial, gastrointestinal, renal, and metabolic toxicity, as well as grade 4 leukopenia, were significantly more common in the control arm, without any survival benefit. This led the Gynecologic Cancer Intergroup (GCIG) to adopt IV carboplatin and IV paclitaxel by consensus [24].

A second concern regarding the regimen used in GOG 172 pertains to the addition of day 8 paclitaxel in the experimental arm. Results from Japanese Gynecologic Oncology Group (JGOG 3016) [25], which compared carboplatin AUC 6 and paclitaxel 180 mg/m^2 on day 1 with carboplatin AUC 6 on day 1 and paclitaxel 80 mg/m^2 on days 1, 8, 15 (dose dense therapy), showed a significant 11-month survival benefit to patients receiving dose dense therapy. This questioned whether the survival benefit in GOG172 was due to the IP administration of chemotherapy or due to the addition of day 8 paclitaxel. GOG 252 (see "Substitution of Carboplatin" section) may address this and other questions including the use of IP carboplatin in place of IP cisplatin.

The increased frequency and severity of dose-limiting toxicity seen on the IV/IP arm of GOG 172 resulted in a substantial number of patients being unable to complete the assigned IV/IP therapy. Most toxicities were short term, and there were no differences with regard to treatment-related deaths or quality of life at 1 year [26]. Neurotoxicity, a known side effect of using cisplatin at a dose of 100 mg/m^2, remained higher in the IP group [27]. With the use of contemporary antiemetics and growth factors and hydration, a higher proportion of patients can successfully complete a full regimen of IV/IP chemotherapy, similar to the IV arm of GOG 172 [28].

Catheter-related complications were the most common cause of discontinuation of IP chemotherapy in GOG 172 [29]. The trial protocol allowed both fenestrated and single-lumen catheters to be used. The use of the fenestrated peritoneal dialysis catheters was problematic as the catheter fenestrations in the peritoneal cavity appear to cause a fibrous sheath formation and the resultant causes adhesions. This and the relative novelty of management of IP catheter complications are likely contribution to the high discontinuation rate of IP chemotherapy on GOG 172. The authors concluded that using single-lumen catheters such as venous access devices rather than peritoneal dialysis catheters would improve chances of successful IP administration (Table 17.3).

Another concern with GOG 172 was the increased cost and complexity of the regimen. Cisplatin administered intraperitoneally requires both pre- and posttreatment hydration, which increases chair time. Management of port complications requires increased staff training and time. Furthermore, 24-hour administration of paclitaxel requires inpatient admission, and this accounts for 40% of the cost of this regimen. However, when the survival advantage is taken into account, IV/IP chemotherapy remains cost-effective [30]. Development of an outpatient regimen of IP chemotherapy may improve the cost effectiveness of IP chemotherapy if proven as effective as the current regimen [31]. The complexity of this regimen is reflected by a higher adoption of IP chemotherapy in academic and larger institutions, where expertise is developed as a result of patient and referral volume. This is in line with multiple studies demonstrating a higher proportion of NCCN-adherent care [32] and improved survival outcomes [33] in these tertiary centers. Utilization of IP chemotherapy is significantly less in nonacademic and community centers.

MODIFICATIONS TO STANDARD IP REGIMENS

Schedule and duration of paclitaxel

To offset the cost and complexity of 24-hour infusion of paclitaxel, as used in GOG 114 and 172, many institutions have utilized 3-hour paclitaxel infusion. When given IV followed by IV cisplatin, 3-hour paclitaxel was associated with unacceptable neurologic toxicity [34]. Thus, many will continue to give the subsequent IP cisplatin on day 2, approximately 24 hours after IV paclitaxel. Of note, while absorbed fairly rapidly, the kinetics of IP cisplatin result in a blunted peak plasma concentration with prolongation of systemic exposure [35], and it is likely that the risk of neurologic toxicity of IP cisplatin after same day IV paclitaxel would be significantly less than that seen with same day IV cisplatin after 3 hour IV paclitaxel.

Reduction in cisplatin dosage

As discussed earlier, neurotoxicity secondary to the administration of cisplatin at a dose of 100 mg/m^2 is the major persistent toxicity in the GOG 172 regimen of IP chemotherapy as compared with IV therapy. However, there is no evidence demonstrating an improved survival with increasing the dose or schedule intensity of platinum drugs. The optimal

Table 17.3 Best practices for intraperitoneal port placement

Best practices for IP port placement
May be placed at initial surgery as long as contamination has not occurred.
Avoid peritoneal dialysis catheters and fenestrated catheters.
Preferred catheter caliber is 9.6 Fr; silicone venous access catheter is used to prevent kinking.
The port should be sutured in four quadrants to the fascia to prevent migration.
Wound needs to be closed in layers after implantation to prevent leakage.
When total hysterectomy has been performed, vaginal closure should be water tight to avoid vaginal leakage.
Consider delayed placement when left-sided bowel surgery has been performed.

dose of IP cisplatin is unknown, and there are no randomized trials that directly compare different dose levels of IP cisplatin. Cisplatin at 75 mg/m^2 (IV or IP) has been utilized by many centers to avoid nonhematologic toxicities. Although the effect on survival outcomes is unknown with this modification of the IP cisplatin dose, it has been widely utilized as significantly more patients can complete IP chemotherapy with this modified dose.

Substitution of carboplatin

Alternatively, substitution of cisplatin with carboplatin has been suggested, as carboplatin has been shown to have a more favorable nonhematologic toxicity profile [36]. While early retrospective studies suggested superiority of IP cisplatin is higher than IP carboplatin [37,38], these studies were flawed by using unusually low doses of carboplatin. Similarly, early pharmacologic studies using equimolar doses of the two drugs suggested an inferior outcome with IP carboplatin. However, IP CBDCA has comparable or better drug penetration when compared to DDP given at equitoxic doses, providing support for trials replacing cisplatin with carboplatin in IP treatment of ovarian cancer [13]. Subsequent phase 1 trials established that the optimal dose for carboplatin was with an AUC of 5–6 when given intraperitoneally [39–41].

Two randomized phase III trials of IP versus IV carboplatin are being conducted by GOG (GOG 252) and the Gynecologic Oncology Trial and Investigation Consortium in Japan (GOTIC 001) in collaboration with JGOG 3019. GOG 252, which completed accrual in 2011, randomized patients with epithelial ovarian, fallopian tube, or primary peritoneal carcinoma, stage II, III, or IV with either optimal (=<1 cm residual disease) or suboptimal residual disease into three arms. ARM I: IV carboplatin on day 1 followed weekly dose dense IV paclitaxel (days 1, 8, and 15). ARM II: Carboplatin IP on day 1 followed by weekly dose dense IV paclitaxel. ARM III: Patients receive paclitaxel IV over 3 hours on day 1, cisplatin IP on day 2, and paclitaxel IP on day 8 (control arm). All three arms include bevacizumab on day 1 of cycles 2–6 and as maintenance for 48 weeks after completion of initial therapy. This study will provide a direct and "clean" comparison between IV and IP carboplatin (ARM I vs. ARM II) and between a regimen using IP carboplatin and one using IP cisplatin (ARM II vs. ARM III). This trial also has the potential to address whether the survival advantage in GOG 172 was related to the dose dense paclitaxel (ARM 1 vs. ARM III). Of note, data from a recently reported phase III randomized clinical trial in suboptimal stage III and stage IV ovarian cancer (GOG 262) suggest that the benefit from dose dense weekly administration of paclitaxel might in fact be due to angiogenesis inhibition. In that trial, weekly IV dose dense paclitaxel did not improve outcome compared to every 3-week paclitaxel when bevacizumab was used. However in patients who did not receive bevacizumab, the weekly dose dense paclitaxel therapy resulted in a 4-month prolongation in PFS compared with traditional carboplatin and non-dose dense, every 3-week paclitaxel.

Neoadjuvant chemotherapy

Neoadjuvant chemotherapy in ovarian cancer is often utilized for patients with stage IV disease or those with poor performance status, who cannot tolerate aggressive cytoreductive surgery and when the surgical expertise required to achieve optimal cytoreduction is not available. Patients treated with neoadjuvant chemotherapy generally receive three cycles of chemotherapy followed by interval cytoreductive surgery and a further three to four cycles of chemotherapy after interval surgery. Tiersten et al. published a Phase II trial including women with stage III/IV (pleural effusions only) epithelial ovarian, fallopian tube, or primary peritoneal carcinoma that presented with bulky disease. In this trial, patients received neoadjuvant carboplatin (AUC6) and paclitaxel 175 mg/m^2 administered via IV route every 3 weeks for three cycles followed by interval optimal debulking and adjuvant IP carboplatin (AUC5) and IV paclitaxel 175 mg/m^2 on day 1 and IP paclitaxel 60 mg/m^2 on day 8 for six cycles. Of the 58 eligible patients enrolled, 36 underwent debulking surgery and 26 received postcytoreduction IV/IP chemotherapy. For these 26 patients, the PFS and OS were 29 and 34 months, respectively. Of note, the NCI Canada Clinical Trials Group, in collaboration with the GCIG, is currently conducting a randomized phase II–III trial to evaluate the safety and efficacy of this approach (OV 21/PETROC).

HYPERTHERMIC INTRAPERITONEAL CHEMOTHERAPY

Hyperthermic intraperitoneal chemotherapy (HIPEC) is the instillation of chemotherapy, typically heated to 41°C–43°C, directly into the abdominal cavity at the time of surgery with the aid of a pump that maintains the temperature and circulation of the drug solution. The drugs selected must maintain their effectiveness at the temperatures used and have a high molecular weight and a low water solubility to remain in the IP cavity. Hyperthermia has been shown to be toxic to tumor cells, increase drug penetration, and exhibit synergistic effects when used with conventional cytotoxic chemotherapy [42–44]. Weisberger and Storaasli [45] were first to utilize heated chemotherapy (nitrogen mustard) in seven patients with ovarian cancer with successful palliation of ascites but were associated with minimal survival benefit. Few prospective studies have examined the role of HIPEC in the upfront setting in ovarian carcinoma. Di Giorgio et al. [46] reported on 47 ovarian cancer patients who underwent primary (n = 22) or secondary (n = 25) debulking followed by HIPEC with cisplatin 75 mg/m^2 at a temperature of 42°C–43°C, followed by systemic chemotherapy. Mean OS was 30 months. Major complications were death from pulmonary embolus (n = 2) reoperation (n = 6) and need of interventional radiology procedure n = 3 [46]. Deraco et al. prospectively studied 26 patients in the upfront setting who received cytoreductive surgery followed by HIPEC with cisplatin 40 mg/L and doxorubicin 15 mg/L. Five years OS was 60.7%. Major complications occurred in four patients and postoperative death in one.

There is currently insufficient evidence to recommend HIPEC in the upfront setting for women with ovarian cancer, especially when we take into account the robustness of the evidence and survival benefit with standard IP chemotherapy. Whether or not there is a role for HIPEC in the recurrent setting remains to be elucidated, and prospective randomized clinical trials already underway should help answer that question [47,48].

Future directions

Future studies will continue to evaluate mechanisms to optimize patient outcomes with IP chemotherapy. Variations will most likely explore the use of different chemotherapeutic schedules, agents, and optimal patient selection for this treatment modality.

As previously described, the role of bevacizumab in IP chemotherapy is being explored in GOG 252. One cannot simply extrapolate the data from IV trials into IP chemotherapy due to the effects that IP administration has on the tumor microenvironment and the tumors itself. As such, trials that specifically incorporate novel agents (given IV or IP) in addition to IP chemotherapy are needed. Of these agents, novel tyrosine kinase inhibitors, and PARP inhibitors show promise.

Given the toxicity of IP chemotherapy, are there patients who would not benefit from IP chemotherapy? Lesnock et al. [49] performed an analysis of tumor tissue from patients enrolled in GOG 172. Tumor was stained for BRCA1 protein expression and results were correlated with survival for both the IP and IV arms of the trial. Of the 393 patients in this study who had evaluable tumor blocks, 189 (48%) tumors had aberrant low level and 204 (52%) had normal BRCA1 expression. In patients with aberrant BRCA1 expression, median OS was 84 months in the IP group versus 48 months in the IV group (P = 0.0002). In patients with normal BRCA1 expression, IP chemotherapy provided a nonstatistically significant 8-month OS benefit (P = 0.818). This study suggests that the intensive and prolonged platinum exposure attained with IP cisplatin in GOG 172 is most effective in tumors that have aberrant homologous recombination and are thus less able to repair platinum-induced DNA damage. If these results can be confirmed, they suggest that BRCA1 expression might serve as a biomarker to triage patients into those who would benefit the most from IP chemotherapy.

The role of IP chemotherapy in settings other than upfront chemotherapy for optimally debulked stage IIIC ovarian cancer still requires clarification. Should this modality be used for patients with early stage disease who would otherwise receive routine IV chemotherapy? Will IP chemotherapy have a role in patients who receive neoadjuvant chemotherapy followed by debulking surgery? What is the role of IP chemotherapy in patients with nonepithelial ovarian cancer? Is IP chemotherapy beneficial in patients with recurrent platinum sensitive ovarian cancer who have had optimal debulking?

Many questions remain unanswered regarding IP chemotherapy in ovarian cancer. What is indisputable is the survival benefit this treatment offers patients who have been optimally debulked. Refinement and improvement upon existing regimens will undoubtedly offer strategies to improve acceptability and tolerability of IP chemotherapy, in hopes of improving the lives of patients afflicted with this lethal disease.

REFERENCES

1. Siegel R, Ma J, Zou Z, Jemal A. Cancer statistics, 2014. *CA: A Cancer Journal for Clinicians.* 2014;64(1):9–29.
2. Cannistra SA. Cancer of the ovary. *The New England Journal of Medicine.* 2004;351(24):2519–2529.
3. Moyer VA, Force USPST. Screening for ovarian cancer: U.S. Preventive Services Task Force reaffirmation recommendation statement. *Annals of Internal Medicine.* 2012;157(12):900–904.
4. Whitney CW. Gynecologic Oncology Group surgical procedures manual. Gynecologic Oncology Group, Philadelphia, PA (2010). Available for members at www.gog.org (last accessed July 24, 2015).
5. Eisenhauer EL, Abu-Rustum NR, Sonoda Y, Levine DA, Poynor EA, Aghajanian C et al. The addition of extensive upper abdominal surgery to achiee optimal cytoreduction improves survival in patients with stages IIIC-IV epithelial ovarian cancer. *Gynecologic Oncology.* 2006;103(3):1083–1090.
6. Aletti GD, Dowdy SC, Gostout BS, Jones MB, Stanhope CR, Wilson TO et al. Aggressive surgical effort and improved survival in advanced-stage ovarian cancer. *Obstetrics and Gynecology.* 2006;107(1):77–85.
7. Chang SJ, Bristow RE, Ryu HS. Impact of complete cytoreduction leaving no gross residual disease associated with radical cytoreductive surgical procedures on survival in advanced ovarian cancer. *Annals of Surgical Oncology.* 2012;19(13):4059–4067.
8. Chi DS, Eisenhauer EL, Lang J, Huh J, Haddad L, Abu-Rustum NR et al. What is the optimal goal of primary cytoreductive surgery for bulky stage IIIC epithelial ovarian carcinoma (EOC)? *Gynecologic Oncology.* 2006;103(2):559–564.
9. Bristow RE, Tomacruz RS, Armstrong DK, Trimble EL, Montz FJ. Survival effect of maximal cytoreductive surgery for advanced ovarian carcinoma during the platinum era: A meta-analysis. *Journal of Clinical Oncology.* 2002;20(5):1248–1259.
10. Howell SB, Pfeifle CL, Wung WE, Olshen RA, Lucas WE, Yon JL et al. Intraperitoneal cisplatin with systemic thiosulfate protection. *Annals of Internal Medicine.* 1982;97(6):845–851.

11. Pretorius RG, Petrilli ES, Kean CK, Ford LC, Hoeschele JD, Lagasse LD. Comparison of the iv and ip routes of administration of cisplatin in dogs. *Cancer Treatment Reports.* 1981;65(11–12):1055–1062.

12. Miyagi Y, Fujiwara K, Kigawa J, Itamochi H, Nagao S, Aotani E et al. Intraperitoneal carboplatin infusion may be a pharmacologically more reasonable route than intravenous administration as a systemic chemotherapy. A comparative pharmacokinetic analysis of platinum using a new mathematical model after intraperitoneal vs. intravenous infusion of carboplatin: A Sankai Gynecology Study Group (SGSG) study. *Gynecologic Oncology.* 2005;99(3):591–596.

13. Jandial DD, Messer K, Farshchi-Heydari S, Pu M, Howell SB. Tumor platinum concentration following intraperitoneal administration of cisplatin versus carboplatin in an ovarian cancer model. *Gynecologic Oncology.* 2009;115(3):362–366.

14. Markman M, Rowinsky E, Hakes T, Reichman B, Jones W, Lewis JL, Jr. et al. Phase I trial of intraperitoneal taxol: A Gynecologic Oncology Group study. *Journal of Clinical Oncology.* 1992;10(9):1485–1491.

15. Francis P, Rowinsky E, Schneider J, Hakes T, Hoskins W, Markman M. Phase I feasibility and pharmacologic study of weekly intraperitoneal paclitaxel: A Gynecologic Oncology Group pilot Study. *Journal of Clinical Oncology.* 1995;13(12):2961–2967.

16. Alberts DS, Liu PY, Hannigan EV, O'Toole R, Williams SD, Young JA et al. Intraperitoneal cisplatin plus intravenous cyclophosphamide versus intravenous cisplatin plus intravenous cyclophosphamide for stage III ovarian cancer. *The New England Journal of Medicine.* 1996;335(26):1950–1955.

17. McGuire WP, Hoskins WJ, Brady MF, Kucera PR, Partridge EE, Look KY et al. Cyclophosphamide and cisplatin compared with paclitaxel and cisplatin in patients with stage III and stage IV ovarian cancer. *The New England Journal of Medicine.* 1996;334(1):1–6.

18. Markman M, Bundy BN, Alberts DS, Fowler JM, Clark-Pearson DL, Carson LF et al. Phase III trial of standard-dose intravenous cisplatin plus paclitaxel versus moderately high-dose carboplatin followed by intravenous paclitaxel and intraperitoneal cisplatin in small-volume stage III ovarian carcinoma: An intergroup study of the Gynecologic Oncology Group, Southwestern Oncology Group, and Eastern Cooperative Oncology Group. *Journal of Clinical Oncology: Official Journal of the American Society of Clinical Oncology.* 2001;19(4):1001–1007.

19. Havrilesky LJ, Kulasingam SL, Matchar DB, Myers ER. FDG-PET for management of cervical and ovarian cancer. *Gynecologic Oncology.* 2005;97(1):183–191.

20. Armstrong DK, Bundy B, Wenzel L, Huang HQ, Baergen R, Lele S et al. Intraperitoneal cisplatin and paclitaxel in ovarian cancer. *The New England Journal of Medicine.* 2006;354(1):34–43.

21. Tewari DJJ, Salani R et al. Long-term survival advantage of intraperitoneal chemotherapy treatment in advanced ovarian cancer: An analysis of Gynecologic Oncology Group Ancillary Data Study. Proc SGO. 2013.

22. Wright A, Cronin A, Milne D, Bookman M, Burger R, Cristea M et al. Effect of intraperitoneal chemotherapy on survival for ovarian cancer in clinical practice and frequency of use. *Journal of Clinical Oncology.* 2014;32(Suppl.; abstr 5576):5s.

23. Ozols RF, Bundy BN, Greer BE, Fowler JM, Clarke-Pearson D, Burger RA et al. Phase III trial of carboplatin and paclitaxel compared with cisplatin and paclitaxel in patients with optimally resected stage III ovarian cancer: A Gynecologic Oncology Group study. *Journal of Clinical Oncology: Official Journal of the American Society of Clinical Oncology.* 2003;21(17):3194–3200.

24. du Bois A, Quinn M, Thigpen T, Vermorken J, Avall-Lundqvist E, Bookman M et al. 2004 consensus statements on the management of ovarian cancer: Final document of the 3rd International Gynecologic Cancer Intergroup Ovarian Cancer Consensus Conference (GCIG OCCC 2004). *Annals of Oncology: Official Journal of the European Society for Medical Oncology/ESMO.* 2005;16(Suppl. 8):viii7–viii12.

25. Noriyuki K, Makoto Y, Seiji I, Fumiaki T, Hirofumi M, Eizo K et al. Long-term results of dose-dense paclitaxel and carboplatin versus conventional paclitaxel and carboplatin for treatment of advanced epithelial ovarian, fallopian tube, or primary peritoneal cancer (JGOG 3016): A randomised, controlled, open-label trial. *Lancet Oncology.* 2013;14:1020–1026.

26. Wenzel LB, Huang HQ, Armstrong DK, Walker JL, Cella D, Gynecologic Oncology G. Health-related quality of life during and after intraperitoneal versus intravenous chemotherapy for optimally debulked ovarian cancer: A Gynecologic Oncology Group Study. *Journal of Clinical Oncology: Official Journal of the American Society of Clinical Oncology.* 2007;25(4):437–443.

27. Helm CW. Ports and complications for intraperitoneal chemotherapy delivery. *BJOG: An International Journal of Obstetrics and Gynaecology.* 2012;119(2):150–159.

28. Guile MW, Horne AL, Thompson SD, Gardner GJ, Giuntoli RL, Armstrong DK et al. Intraperitoneal chemotherapy for stage III ovarian cancer using the Gynecologic Oncology Group protocol 172 intraperitoneal regimen: Effect of supportive care using aprepitant and pegfilgrastim on treatment completion rate. *Clinical Ovarian Cancer.* 2008;1 SRC—GoogleScholar:68–71.

29. Walker JL, Armstrong DK, Huang HQ, Fowler J, Webster K, Burger RA et al. Intraperitoneal catheter outcomes in a phase III trial of intravenous versus intraperitoneal chemotherapy in optimal stage III ovarian and primary peritoneal cancer: A Gynecologic Oncology Group Study. *Gynecologic Oncology.* 2006;100(1):27–32.

30. Bristow RE, Santillan A, Salani R, Diaz-Montes TP, Giuntoli RL, 2nd, Meisner BC et al. Intraperitoneal cisplatin and paclitaxel versus intravenous carboplatin and paclitaxel chemotherapy for Stage III ovarian cancer: A cost-effectiveness analysis. *Gynecologic Oncology.* 2007;106(3):476–481.

31. Havrilesky LJ, Secord AA, Darcy KM, Armstrong DK, Kulasingam S, Gynecologic Oncology Group. Cost effectiveness of intraperitoneal compared with intravenous chemotherapy for women with optimally resected stage III ovarian cancer: A Gynecologic Oncology Group study. *Journal of Clinical Oncology.* 2008;26(25):4144–4150.

32. Erickson BK, Martin JY, Shah MM, Straughn JM, Jr., Leath CA, 3rd. Reasons for failure to deliver National Comprehensive Cancer Network (NCCN)-adherent care in the treatment of epithelial ovarian cancer at an NCCN cancer center. *Gynecologic Oncology.* 2014;133(2):142–146.

33. Bristow RE, Zahurak ML, Diaz-Montes TP, Giuntoli RL, Armstrong DK. Impact of surgeon and hospital ovarian cancer surgical case volume on in-hospital mortality and related short-term outcomes. *Gynecologic Oncology.* 2009;115(3):334–338.

34. Piccart MJ, Bertelsen K, James K, Cassidy J, Mangioni C, Simonsen E et al. Randomized intergroup trial of cisplatin-paclitaxel versus cisplatin-cyclophosphamide in women with advanced epithelial ovarian cancer: Three-year results. *Journal of National Cancer Institute.* 2000;92(9):699–708.

35. Howell SB. Pharmacologic principles of intraperitoneal chemotherapy for the treatment of ovarian cancer. *International Journal of Gynecological Cancer.* 2008;18(Suppl. 1):20–25.

36. Jaaback K, Johnson N, Lawrie TA. Intraperitoneal chemotherapy for the initial management of primary epithelial ovarian cancer. *Cochrane Database System Reviews.* 2011;(11):CD005340.

37. Los G, Verdegaal EM, Mutsaers PH, McVie JG. Penetration of carboplatin and cisplatin into rat peritoneal tumor nodules after intraperitoneal chemotherapy. *Cancer Chemotherapy and Pharmacology.* 1991;28(3):159–165.

38. Markman M, Reichman B, Hakes T, Rubin S, Lewis JL, Jr., Jones W et al. Evidence supporting the superiority of intraperitoneal cisplatin compared to intraperitoneal carboplatin for salvage therapy of small-volume residual ovarian cancer. *Gynecologic Oncology.* 1993;50(1):100–104.

39. Gould N, Sill MW, Mannel RS, Thaker PH, DiSilvestro PA, Waggoner SE et al. A phase I study with an expanded cohort to assess feasibility of intravenous docetaxel, intraperitoneal carboplatin and intraperitoneal paclitaxel in patients with previously untreated ovarian, fallopian tube or primary peritoneal carcinoma: A Gynecologic Oncology Group study. *Gynecologic Oncology.* 2012;127(3):506–510.

40. Gould N, Sill MW, Mannel RS, Thaker PH, Disilvestro P, Waggoner S et al. A phase I study with an expanded cohort to assess the feasibility of intravenous paclitaxel, intraperitoneal carboplatin and intraperitoneal paclitaxel in patients with untreated ovarian, fallopian tube or primary peritoneal carcinoma: A Gynecologic Oncology Group study. *Gynecologic Oncology.* 2012;125(1):54–58.

41. Morgan MA, Sill MW, Fujiwara K, Greer B, Rubin SC, Degeest K et al. A phase I study with an expanded cohort to assess the feasibility of intraperitoneal carboplatin and intravenous paclitaxel in untreated ovarian, fallopian tube, and primary peritoneal carcinoma: A Gynecologic Oncology Group study. *Gynecologic Oncology.* 2011;121(2):264–268.

42. Nicoletto MO, Padrini R, Galeotti F, Ferrazzi E, Cartei G, Riddi F et al. Pharmacokinetics of intraperitoneal hyperthermic perfusion with mitoxantrone in ovarian cancer. *Cancer Chemotherapy and Pharmacology.* 2000;45(6):457–462.

43. Ohno S, Siddik ZH, Kido Y, Zwelling LA, Bull JM. Thermal enhancement of drug uptake and DNA adducts as a possible mechanism for the effect of sequencing hyperthermia on cisplatin-induced cytotoxicity in L1210 cells. *Cancer Chemotherapy and Pharmacology.* 1994;34(4):302–306.

44. Vernon C. Hyperthermia in cancer growth regulation. *Biotherapy.* 1992;4(4):307–315.

45. Weisberger AS LB, Storaasli JP. Use of nitrogen mustard in treatment of serous effusions of neoplastic origin. *JAMA.* 1955(159):1704–1707.

46. Di Giorgio A, Naticchioni E, Biacchi D, Sibio S, Accarpio F, Rocco M et al. Cytoreductive surgery (peritonectomy procedures) combined with hyperthermic intraperitoneal chemotherapy (HIPEC) in the treatment of diffuse peritoneal carcinomatosis from ovarian cancer. *Cancer.* 2008;113(2):315–325.

47. Hyperthermic Intra-peritoneal Chemotherapy (HIPEC) in Ovarian Cancer Recurrence (HORSE) ClinicalTrials.gov Identifier: NCT01539785.

48. Hyperthermic Intra-Peritoneal Chemotherapy (HIPEC) in Relapse Ovarian Cancer Treatment (CHIPOR) ClinicalTrials.gov Identifier: NCT01376752.

49. Lesnock JL, Darcy KM, Tian C, Deloia JA, Thrall MM, Zahn C et al. BRCA1 expression and improved survival in ovarian cancer patients treated with intraperitoneal cisplatin and paclitaxel: A Gynecologic Oncology Group Study. *British Journal of Cancer.* 2013;108(6):1231–1237.

18

Cytoreductive surgery and HIPEC in the treatment of advanced epithelial ovarian cancer and serous papillary peritoneal carcinoma

DERACO MARCELLO, KUSAMURA SHIGEKI, AND BARATTI DARIO

INTRODUCTION

Epithelial ovarian cancer (EOC) is the sixth commonest malignancy in women worldwide and has an annual incidence of 200,000 [1]. It is the deadliest of all the gynecological malignancies and the fifth leading cause of cancer death, killing 125,000 lives each year [1,2]. In the United States, it affects more than 22,280 women annually and is responsible for 15,500 deaths [3]. Most patients with EOC present with a specific symptoms of abdominal distension and discomfort at the onset and hence are often diagnosed at an advanced stage, with 60%–70% having stage III or IV disease at the onset [4]. The median 5-year survival is less than 50% [5], and in advanced EOC, this drops to less than 25%. Up to 70% of all patients relapse and eventually succumb to their disease. Moreover, progress in reducing incidence and mortality has been slow [5]. The conventional approach is optimal cytoreductive surgery (CRS) and adjuvant chemotherapy with platinum-based and taxol-based chemotherapy.

CRS AND DEFINITION OF OPTIMAL RESIDUAL DISEASE

The term "optimal cytoreduction" was introduced by the Gynecologic Oncology Group (GOG) in 1986 defined as residual disease (RD) left after surgery <1 cm. The RD is estimated as the largest diameter of remaining tumor after the operation. Although indisputable as crucial point in the treatment, several definitions of optimal RD are retrievable in the literature.

According to a survey conducted by the Society of Gynecologic Oncology, 12.0% think of removing all visible disease as "optimal"; 13.7% use a 0.5 cm cutoff point, 60.8% a 1 cm, 3.6% a 1.5 cm, and 8.7% a 2.0 cm; and 1.3% use other criteria such as the total estimated weight and/or volume of RD [6].

The direct association between survival of patients with advanced EOC and completeness of cytoreduction (CC) has been well established. In 1992 and 1994, Hoskins et al. conducted ancillary data studies on 349 advanced EOC patients with optimal RD (≤1 cm) and 294 patients with suboptimal RD (>1 cm) receiving cisplatin/cyclophosphamide chemotherapy. These data demonstrated that survival of patients improved as the diameter of the largest RD decreased from 2 cm to microscopic. Patients with no gross RD had a 5-year survival rate of 60%, those with 0.1–1 cm or 1–2 cm RD had a 5-year survival rate of 35%, and those with RD > 2 cm had the worst 5-year survival rate of 20%. The maximal diameter of RD was found to be an independent predictor of overall survival after controlling other variables [7,8]. Moreover, in a recent meta-analysis involving 13 relevant studies and 13,327 patients, it was shown by multiple linear regression analysis that each 10% increase in the proportion of patients undergoing complete cytoreduction to no gross RD was associated with a significant and independent 2.3-month increase (95% confidence interval (CI) = 0.6–4.0, p = 0.011) in cohort median survival compared to a 1.8-month increase (95% CI = 0.6–3.0, p = 0.004) in cohort median survival for RD ≤ 1 cm [9].

The different definitions of optimal cytoreduction could be grouped in two schools of thought: the chemotherapy oriented and surgically oriented. The first one stresses the high initial chemosensibility of the disease and adopts the policy of avoiding radical operations to minimize associated surgical morbidity. The chemotherapy-oriented group represents the mainstream of the gynecologic oncology international scenario and states that evidence supporting multivisceral resections and ultraradical surgical maneuvers is insufficient. The ability to obtain an optimal cytoreduction is believed to be mostly dependent on the biological aggressiveness and not on technical dexterity of the surgeon. Therefore, as the likelihood of changing prognosis by surgical effort is severely limited by the biology of the tumor and initial tumor burden, perioperative chemotherapy assumes a major role in the EOC treatment armamentarium [10]. In effect, an exploratory analysis in the context of a large randomized trial (SCOTROC, The Scottish Randomized Trial in Ovarian Cancer) has shown that the significant benefit in terms of progression-free survival obtained with optimal surgery in stage IIIC to IV disease was limited to patients with less disseminated disease [11].

However, there are several data discrediting such a hypothesis. Eisenkop and Spirtos observed that the need to remove an initial large tumor volume correlates with biological aggressiveness and diminished survival, but not significantly enough to preclude long-term survival or justify abbreviation of the surgical effort [6]. The issue of trade-off between tumor biology and actual impact of complete cytoreduction on outcome has been cleared by a study evaluating tumor-infiltrating lymphocytes and/or tumor cell–proliferating activity on 134 stage III/IV EOC patients submitted to primary CRS [12]. Of note, patients with aggressive biology were more likely to benefit from aggressive CRS.

The second school is surgically oriented and tends to push the limits of radicality as far as technically possible. Extensive procedures including multivisceral resections, in order to achieve highest rate of complete cytoreduction, are systematically pursued, despite potential increase in complication rates. Supporters of surgically oriented school represent the minority in the gynecologic oncology scenario. However, interesting data have been published thus far that supports a surgically aggressive policy that is more in line with the kinetics of intraperitoneal (IP) neoplastic dissemination. Once released from the primary tumor, free tumor cells enter the peritoneal fluid circulation that is governed by the respiratory movements, peristaltic activity of the bowel, and force of gravity [13]. Then, they are deposited in the subphrenic area (primarily the right subphrenic space), subhepatic and retrohepatic areas, the lesser omentum, the lesser sac, and the perisplenic area [14].

In 2006, Chi et al. analyzed 465 patients with advanced stage IIIC disease from the Memorial Sloan Kettering Cancer Center [15]. All patients underwent attempted maximal CRS, with extensive upper abdominal surgery (diaphragm stripping/resection, splenectomy, distal pancreatectomy, liver resection, and resection of tumor from *porta hepatis*) in a significant proportion of patients followed by a minimum of six cycles of postoperative platinum-based systemic chemotherapy. The authors demonstrated that patients with no gross RD after primary cytoreduction had median survival of 106 months and proposed that resection of all visible disease significantly improved survival and should be the surgical goal of primary CRS. More recently, the same group of investigators conducted a comparative retrospective analysis between the aggressive surgical policy and the traditional debulking approach. The study groups were well balanced with respect to the distribution of main prognostic factors. They concluded that such aggressive surgical policy resulted in increased optimal cytoreduction rates and significantly survival rates [15].

LOCOREGIONAL APPROACH TO EOC

CRS with hyperthermic intraperitoneal chemotherapy (CRS and HIPEC) was conceived three decades ago as a locoregional intensified combined approach for peritoneal surface malignancies when the peritoneum is the only site of metastasis. This novel strategy has become the standard of care for appendiceal mucinous tumors [16] and mesothelioma [17]. Promising results in terms of overall and progression-free survivals have been reported in the management of colorectal carcinomatosis [18].

EOC represents a perfect clinical circumstance for a locoregional approach as it remains confined to the peritoneal cavity and retroperitoneal lymph nodes for much of its natural history. Mechanisms of death are primarily related to intra-abdominal progression rather than the risk of systemic dissemination.

CRS was based on the technique described by Sugarbaker [19], with some modifications [20]. Briefly, the goal of the cytoreduction is to remove all visible tumor by means of one to six of the following procedures: right diaphragmatic peritonectomy, left diaphragmatic peritonectomy, pelvic peritonectomy, parietal anterior peritonectomy, greater omentectomy, and lesser omentectomy. Small and scattered localizations on visceral surfaces are resected by local excision or electrothermal evaporation. In case of massive involvement, visceral resections are performed. Bowel anastomosis techniques are described previously. Anastomosis could be performed at the completion of the cytoreduction and before or after HIPEC because in both the literature and the experience of the National Cancer Institute (NCI) in Milan, there was no evidence of increased risk for anastomotic complications or isolated disease recurrence on suture lines, which represent the theoretical drawbacks of such time setting for their construction. Protective ostomies are performed only in high-risk patients after HIPEC, to prevent perfusate leak from ostomy tracts through the abdominal wall.

HYPERTHERMIC INTRAPERITONEAL CHEMOTHERAPY

The management of advanced EOC in the last decade has evolved with the introduction of IP chemotherapy. The GOG-172 phase III trial concluded the advantage of the intravenous (IV) plus IP chemotherapy (median overall survival 65.6 months) over IV chemotherapy (median overall survival [OS] 49.7 months) in primary stage III EOC [21]. Successively, a Cochrane meta-analysis of all randomized IP versus IV trials showed a hazard ratio of 0.79 for disease-free survival (DFS) and 0.79 for OS, favoring the IP arms [22,23].

HIPEC was first introduced in the early 1980s for the treatment of peritoneal carcinomatosis. The addition of hyperthermia to the IP chemotherapy has been shown to increase penetration of the chemotherapy into the tumor cells, increasing the intracellular accumulation of the drug [24]. The cytotoxic effect appears to be synergistically enhanced by an impairment of the cells' capacity to repair damaged DNA, exerting a greater antiblastic effect [24,25]. HIPEC is performed intraoperatively under general anesthesia, via a pump that maintains the temperature and circulation of the drug solution. In contrast to the normothermic approach, the HIPEC ensures that the entire peritoneal surface is bathed in the chemotherapeutic agent, prior to the formation of obstructing adhesions that may develop in the postoperative period. HIPEC could be performed using the open or closed techniques and could last from 30 minutes to 2 hours. Most frequent drugs are cisplatin, oxaliplatin, doxorubicin, mitomycin-c, and paclitaxel [26].

CONFLICTING POINTS

The locoregional therapy for EOC is surrounded by various controversies regarding its indications and technical aspects.

Timing of CRS and HIPEC

According to the natural history of EOC, the locoregional therapy can be applied in one of the following time points: upfront, interval debulking, after neoadjuvant chemotherapy (NACT), consolidation (maintenance treatment given following a complete response to frontline treatment), and recurrent disease. Up to date, there are insufficient data clearing the most effective moment for the performance of CRS and HIPEC.

The recent data recommending maximal surgical effort [9] and IP [21] chemotherapy in the primary setting represent indirect evidence that CRS and HIPEC could be tested as upfront treatment in the context of a phase III trial. Deraco et al. conducted a phase II multicentric trial to test CRS and HIPEC with cisplatin and doxorubicin on 26 women with stage III–IV EOC. Patients received adjuvant systemic chemotherapy with carboplatin and paclitaxel for six cycles. Major complications occurred in four patients and postoperative death in one. Five-year overall survival was 60.7% and five-year progression-free survival 15.2% (median 30 months) [27].

The CRS and HIPEC could also be performed following NACT to increase the rates of optimal cytoreduction without the expenses of a high morbidity. Vergote et al. have compared the primary cytoreduction with NACT [28] and reported similar results in terms of progression-free survival (PFS) and OS between the study arms and lower morbidity associated with NACT. These results are in line with a meta-analysis published subsequently [29]. Two prospective trials on locoregional therapy conducted in the interval time point are ongoing (OVHIPEC, NCT00426257; CHORINE, NCT01628380) [30,31].

The CRS and HIPEC have also been applied as consolidation treatment by some investigators [32–34]. The consolidation setting is the time point in which the patient presents complete response to primary treatment. It represents an alluring time point for locoregional approach as the risk of surgical complication is intuitively expected to be low. Gori et al. conducted a multicenter prospective trial on EOC patients with complete response to primary treatment. They compared two nonrandomized groups, one assigned to HIPEC and the other to follow-up. Median overall survival was 64.4 months in the experimental group versus 46.4 months for the control group (p = 0.56) [29]. A group of Korean investigators reported on 18 stage IC–IIIC ovarian cancer patients with a negative second look who were submitted to HIPEC using paclitaxel and observed an 8-year OS of 84%. One criticism to this study was the enrolment of patients with histologies different from epithelial subtype [33]. In contrast, a group of French investigators have not found the same favorable outcomes employing oxaliplatin for HIPEC. Unfortunately, they had to prematurely close the trial due to the emergence of unacceptable rate of side effects associated with HIPEC [34].

CRS and HIPEC could be applied as secondary treatment after partial response or stable disease after primary treatment consisting of upfront incomplete CRS followed by chemotherapy in patients. According to two studies, median OS and DFS for stage III ovarian cancer were 60 months and 26.4–56 months, respectively [35,36]. The 5-year OS and DFS were 53.8%–66.1% and 26.9%, respectively. In these two studies, CRS and HIPEC were compared with CRS alone in a retrospective fashion. DFS and overall survival were significantly better for CRS and HIPEC than CRS alone in stage III ovarian cancer but not in earlier stages. The setting of secondary CRS therefore seems to be a very interesting time point to conduct a randomized trial between CRS and HIPEC and CRS alone in stage III ovarian cancer. Such a trial is ongoing at the Netherlands Cancer Institute (OVHIPEC trial; NCT00426257).

The last time point in which CRS and HIPEC could be employed is as second-line salvage treatment for recurrent disease. Two nonrandomized comparative trials (CRS and HIPEC vs. CRS alone) have been published [37,38]. In the first study on 26 patients, median DFS (48 months) and 5-year OS (67%) were impressive for CRS and HIPEC and significantly better than after CRS alone (24 months and 29%, respectively) [37]. In the second study on 48 patients, median OS was significantly better for CRS and HIPEC (19.4 months) than for CRS alone (11.2 months) [38]. Two prospective randomized trials are ongoing testing CRS and HIPEC versus CRS alone in recurrent disease. The first one is conducted in France (NCT01376752). Four hundred forty-four patients with International Federation of Gynecology and Obstetrics (FIGO) III recurrent EOC will receive six courses of carboplatin–paclitaxel or carboplatin–caelyx. In case of tumor response and if a (near) complete (CC0-1) CRS seems possible, they will be randomized to undergo a second CRS with or without HIPEC. The second in Italy is designed to enroll 158 patients until 2018 (NCT01539785) [39].

Two subsets of patients must be clearly distinguished in the circumstance of a second-line treatment: platinum resistant and platinum sensitive. Although the consensus statement (Milan 2006) considered the platinum-resistant recurrent disease the least favorable time point for the employment of CRS and HIPEC [40], the available literature data are contradictory in this sense. Experimental data sustain that a major synergism between cytotoxicity and heat is achievable in cisplatin-resistant cell lines with respect to platinum-sensitive ones [41]. Based on this favorable in vitro evidence investigators from NCI of Milan launched a phase III trial testing the CRS and HIPEC in platinum-resistant EOC. The few patients that were recruited unfortunately presented high rate of morbidity, and the trial was prematurely closed due to poor patient accrual [42]. Subsequently, two retrospective studies on CRS and HIPEC applied in the recurrent setting, the first conducted in Italy and the second in France, revealed no difference in survival rates between platinum-sensitive and platinum-resistant subsets [43,44].

Time to chemotherapy

One of the criticisms against the locoregional therapy is the potential delay in the beginning of an adjuvant chemotherapy after a major surgical operation. This could impact negatively on outcome. Aletti evaluated retrospectively data from 218 patients with stage IIIC/IV EOC. Mean time to chemotherapy (TTC) interval was 26 days (range, 7–79 days). TTC was not a predictor of OS allowing the conclusions that TTC interval should not be used to justify using a surgically more conservative approach for advanced EOC [45]. In the recent Italian prospective trial, all the patients, except one, underwent systemic chemotherapy at a median of 46 days from combined treatment (range: 29–75), and the TTC did not affect the OS or PFS.

Drugs

Various drug combinations for EOC have been tested by experimental and phase I/II studies on HIPEC. A drug is considered eligible for HIPEC according to its pharmacokinetic profile, tumor chemosensibility, and toxicity. Water solubility and high molecular weight are aspects that ensure a low peritoneal clearance. This, combined with a high systemic clearance, results in pharmacological advantage expressed by the area under the curve (AUC) peritoneal/AUC plasma ratio. HIPEC drug(s) should preferably be cell cycle nonspecific. The optimal choice of the drugs for HIPEC represents another disputed topic in EOC treatment and is still impossible to be done on the basis of the literature data. Agents that have already been employed are cisplatin [46], doxorubicin [47], caelyx [48], mitomycin-c [49], mitoxantrone [50], carboplatin [51], oxaliplatin [39], gemcitabine [52], and paclitaxel [53]. The latter, in particular, although frequently used for HIPEC due to their favorable pharmacokinetic profile with an AUC peritoneal/AUC plasma ratio of 1000, is not an ideal choice for HIPEC. First, there is no evidence of cytotoxicity thermal enhancement. Second, its mechanism of action is prevalently concentrated in the mitotic phase of cell cycle (cycle specific). Such a property in a context of a single-shot therapy like HIPEC represents a disadvantage as not all the neoplastic cell could be killed by the treatment.

MORBIDITY AND MORTALITY

There is no standard classification used to report morbidity. The NCI Common Terminology Criteria for Adverse Events (CTCAE) [54] is available and used by some, and there is increasing use of a surgical classification based on the interventions necessary to address the adverse effect. The absence of homogeneous criteria to classify and grade surgical complications hampers comparisons across series. Postoperative mortality however was not higher after CRS and HIPEC (0.7%) than after CRS only (1.4%). Bristow et al. have recently reported on 32 cases (27 cases of EOC, 3 primary peritoneal cancers, and 2 fallopian tube cancers) treated with CRS and HIPEC in 2 centers. They adopted the NCI CTCAE and observed a combined grade 3/4 morbidity rate of 65.6%. The most frequent morbidities included grade 3 anemia (40.6%), infection (15.6%), and pleural effusion (12.5%). Six patients required readmission (18.8%), and two patients required reoperation (6.2%). There was no postoperative mortality [55].

SEROUS PERITONEAL PAPILLARY CARCINOMA

Serous papillary peritoneal carcinoma (SPPC) was first described by Swerdlow in 1959 [56]. SPPC is histologically similar to advanced stage ovarian carcinoma, and it is clinically defined by predominant peritoneal tumor load, with scant on none ovarian involvement. Historically, SPPC has been variably considered (a) a counterpart of ovarian cancer, arising in the coelomic epithelium of the peritoneum instead of the ovaries, (b) a peritoneal malignancy originating at the coelomic epithelium distinct from ovarian cancer, and (c) a carcinoma of unknown origin [57]. However, the epithelial layer of the ovary and peritoneum has a common embryonic origin from the coelomic epithelium. Conversely, the epithelium of fallopian tubes, endometrium, and endocervix share a common embryological Mullerian origin, and both EOC and SPPC are remarkably similar to Mullerian epithelium. On this basis, SPPC is currently considered as an extraovarian primary carcinoma.

The incidence of SPPC is unclear, but it is estimated to be about 10% of EOC [57]. In cases with massive tumor load in the pelvis, it is often impossible to determine the organ of origin, and SPPC is often misdiagnosed as EOC. Accordingly, both tumors are usually combined in data analysis and there is only scant literature focusing on SPPC [58]. In recent years, the incidence of SPPC has risen in the United States, but it remains unknown whether this trend reflects true increase or better diagnosis. Recently, the GOG developed a set of criteria to diagnose SPPC, thus creating a common standard for pathologic workup and favoring the emergence of homogeneous case series [59] (Table 18.1).

Despite the similarities between SPPC and EOC, a recent systematic review has highlighted a few epidemiological, clinical, and molecular differences [57]. SPPC mostly arises in 55–65-year-old women, that is, an average 3–7 years older than EOC, and it has been exceptionally reported in male. SPPC is more commonly multifocal than EOC and tends to show a more diffuse micronodular pattern of spread in the omentum and peritoneal surfaces. Similar rates of lymph node (20%–70%) and visceral/extraperitoneal spread (<15%) have been reported in SPPC and EOC. Serum CA125 is elevated in 70%–90% of SPPC patients.

As biological features are concerned, SPPC has been demonstrated to harbor similar rates of tumor suppressor gene dysfunction as the ovarian counterparts. However, SPPC showed patterns of loss of heterozygosity at several chromosomal loci different from those of EOC [57]. The reported incidence of germ line BRCA mutations in SPPC is similar to EOC (5%–10%). Of note, women with BRCA1/BRCA2 mutations carry a 5% lifetime risk of developing peritoneal cancer even after prophylactic oophorectomy. On the other side, SPPC showed significantly lower expression of estrogen and progesterone receptors and increased Ki-67 expression than ovarian tumors. Furthermore, a 35%–55% incidence of HER2 overexpression has been reported in SPPC, consistently higher than the 5%–30% rate seen in EOC. HER2 overexpression/amplification is an early tumorigenic event in serous carcinomas of the ovary and endometrium, leading to evasion of apoptosis, angiogenesis, and cellular proliferation and invasion [60]. These data suggested that different molecular events may characterize SPPC, as well as the potential for developing targeted therapeutic approaches. Conversely, no difference in p53 protein overexpression, p53 gene mutations, and abnormal DNA content were seen [57].

TREATMENT

Given the rarity of the disease, the standard treatment of SPPC has not been well established. However, due to the similarities to EOC, SPPC has been often treated by CRS and platinum- and taxane-containing systemic chemotherapy [55]. Most of the available information come from small- to medium-sized retrospective cohort or case-control series, comparing patients with SPPC and EOC. In early series treated by surgical debulking, patient survival was comparable to that of suboptimally cytoreduced EOC. In most recent series, better understanding of the importance of surgical aggressiveness resulted in increasing rate of optimal debulking (residual lesions <1 cm) up to 60%–80% in reference centers. This progress, along with the advent of taxane-/platinum-based chemotherapy, led to median survival of 35–40 months. In comparative studies, however, median survival of SPPC patients is shorter than that of matched EOC patients by 3–6 months, even though no statistical significance is observed. Analogously lower rates of optimal cytoreduction have been sometimes reported in SPPC, although not all the published studies have confirmed this finding [54].

CRS AND HIPEC

The first series of SPPC treated by CRS and HIPEC was reported by Look and Sugarbaker in 2004, retrieving 28 females with either EOC (n = 18) or SPPC (n = 10) from a prospective database [61]. Previously, systemic chemotherapy was given to 16 patients and IP chemotherapy to 2 patients. The patients underwent peritonectomy procedures and (multi)visceral resections with the aim to completely remove the tumor. Optimal cytoreduction was obtained in 16 patients, namely, no visible or ≤2.5 mm RD. HIPEC was performed in 12 patients, EPIC in 13, and no IP intraoperative chemotherapy in 3, due to massive postsurgical tumor load. The authors did not provide separate results for EOC and SPPC patients. In the overall series, median follow-up was 26.9 months and median overall survival 45.8 months. The prognostic indicators of longer

Table 18.1 Gynecologic oncology group criteria to diagnose serous papillary peritoneal carcinoma

1. Both ovaries must be either normal in size or enlarged by a benign process (4.0 cm in largest diameter).
2. The involvement of extraovarian sites must be greater than that on the involved surface of either ovary.
3. Microscopically, the ovarian component must be one of the following:
   a. Nonexistent.
   b. Confined to the ovarian surface epithelium with no evidence of cortical invasion.
   c. Involving the ovarian surface epithelium and underlying cortical stroma, but any given tumor size must be less than 5 × 5 mm.
   d. Tumors less than 5 × 5 mm within the ovarian substance associated with or without surface disease.

survival were the extent of prior surgeries (p < 0.001), CC (p = 0.037), and response to prior chemotherapy (p = 0.012). Patients who had complete cytoreduction had a median survival of 55.9 months, as compared with 8.0 months in those who had incomplete cytoreduction. There were three major postoperative complications (11%) and no mortality.

Bakrin et al. collected 36 patients with SPPC undergoing 39 procedures of CRS with HIPEC in 8 French and 1 Italian centers between 1997 and 2007 [58]. Among them there was one male patient. All patients but one received a previous platinum-based systemic chemotherapy. At the completion of the CRS, RD was not visible in 27 patients and ≤2.5 mm in 5, while 4 patients had grossly incomplete cytoreduction. In the different centers, HIPEC was performed with many variations in exposure techniques (open vs. closed abdomen), duration, IP temperatures, and drugs. Operative mortality occurred in 2/39 procedures (5.6%) and major complication in 7/39 (20.6%). Five-year overall survival was 57.4%, and DFS was 24% (median 16.7 months).

Deraco et al. reported the largest single-center series of SPPC treated by cytoreduction and HIPEC [62]. Eleven females were treated at NCI Milan (Italy) from 2000 to 2012. All the patients had undergone systemic chemotherapy. During the study period, a policy of complete parietal peritonectomy and systematic pelvic and retroperitoneal lymphadenectomy was adopted. This was based on the center's growing experience with this disease and the understanding of SPPC propensity to diffusely involve the peritoneum [54]. Also literature data support the possible multifocal nature of SPPC based on discordant expression of HER2 and p53 in tumors with multiple intrapatient deposits biopsied. All but one patient had macroscopically complete cytoreduction (one had RD ≤ 2.5 mm). Systematic pelvic and retroperitoneal lymphadenectomy was performed in eight patients, with positive nodes found in four. Operative major morbidity occurred in six patients, and operative death in none. Five-year overall survival was 55% (median not reached). Median progression-free survival was 10 months.

CONCLUSION

Data from literature support the evidence that CRS represents one of the most powerful determinants of outcome and the strongest clinician-driven predictor of survival in patients with stage IIIC/IV EOC. Peritonectomy procedures, as a result of a change in surgical paradigm, could overcome limits imposed by the biology of the tumor and improve outcomes, despite disease aggressiveness. The CRS and HIPEC imply higher rates of complications but do not seem to increase surgical mortality, with respect to CRS alone. Eventual delay of systemic chemotherapy following major surgery does not seem to be correlated with worsening of prognosis. The most favorable time point for CRS and HIPEC seems to be persistent disease after incomplete response to first-line therapy and/or platinum-sensitive recurrence.

The results of four randomized ongoing trials are eagerly awaited regarding the effects of CRS and HIPEC in EOC. But anyway, the success in patient accrual of these trials depends on a key element represented by a narrow collaboration between gynecologic oncologist and a surgeon proficient in peritonectomy procedures. Provided that the expertise for peritonectomy procedures is only achievable with a long-lasting training program including at least 140 procedures [63], a shift in the paradigm of EOC treatment would be possible expanding the multidisciplinary environment with the inclusion of a surgeon proficient in the performance of CRS and HIPEC.

SPCC represents another potential clinical setting where CRS and HIPEC could be of benefit. Given that it is rare disease, more data are necessary to confirm the actual efficacy of the locoregional therapy.

REFERENCES

1. Seigal R, Naishadham D, Jemal A. Cancer statistics. *CA: A Cancer Journal for Clinicians*. 2012;62:10–29.
2. Parkin DM, Bray F, Ferlay J, Pisani P. Global cancer statistics, 2002. *CA: A Cancer Journal for Clinicians*. 2005;55(2):74–108.
3. American Cancer Society. *Cancer Facts & Figures 2012*, Atlanta, GA: American Cancer Society, 2012.
4. Coleman RL, Monk BJ, Sood AK, Herzog TJ. Latest research and treatment of advanced-stage epithelial ovarian cancer. *Nature Reviews Clinical Oncology*. 2013;10:211–224.
5. Horner MJ, Ries LA, Krapcho M, Neyman N, Aminou R, Howlader N et al. (eds). SEER cancer statistics review, 1975–2006, Bethesda, MD: National Cancer Institute, 2009. Available at: http://seer.cancer.gov/csr/1975_2006/. Based on November 2008 SEER data submission, posted to the SEER web site, 2009. Accessed August 18, 2012.
6. Eisenkop SM, Spirtos NM. What are the current surgical objectives, strategies, and technical capabilities of gynecologic oncologists treating advanced epithelial EOC? *Gynecologic Oncology*. 2001;82:489–497.
7. Hoskins WJ, McGuire WP, Brady MF, Homesley HD, Creasman WT, Berman M et al. The effect of diameter of largest residual disease on survival after primary cytoreductive surgery in patients with suboptimal residual epithelial ovarian carcinoma. *American Journal of Obstetrics and Gynecology*. 1994;170:974–979, discussion 979–980.
8. Hoskins WJ, Bundy BN, Thigpen JT, Omura GA. The influence of cytoreductive surgery on recurrence-free interval and survival in small-volume stage III epithelial ovarian cancer: A Gynecologic Oncology Group study. *Gynecologic Oncology*. 1992;47:159–166.

9. Chang SJ, Hodeib M, Chang J, Bristow RE. Survival impact of complete cytoreduction to no gross residual disease for advanced-stage ovarian cancer: A meta-analysis. *Gynecologic Oncology.* 2013;130(3):493–498.

10. Pfisterer J, Weber B, Reuss A, Kimmig R, du Bois A, Wagner U et al., AGO-OVAR, GINECO. Randomized phase III trial of topotecan following carboplatin and paclitaxel in first-line treatment of advanced EOC: A gynecologic cancer intergroup trial of the AGO-OVAR and GINECO. *Journal of the National Cancer Institute.* 2006;98:1036–1045.

11. Crawford SC, Vasey PA, Paul J, Hay A, Davis JA, Kaye SB. Does aggressive surgery only benefit patients with less advanced EOC? Results from an international comparison within the SCOTROC-1 Trial. *Journal of Clinical Oncology.* 2005;23:8802–8811. Erratum in: *Journal of Clinical Oncology.* 2006;24:1224.

12. Adams SF, Levine DA, Cadungog MG, Hammond R, Facciabene A, Olvera N et al. Intraepithelial T cells and tumor proliferation: Impact on the benefit from surgical cytoreduction in advanced serous EOC. *Cancer.* 2009;115:2891–2902.

13. Deraco M, Santoro N, Carraro O, Inglese MG, Rebuffoni G, Guadagni S et al. Peritoneal carcinomatosis: Feature of dissemination. A review. *Tumori.* 1999;85(1):1–5.

14. Yonemura Y, Kawamura T, Bandou E et al. In: Gonzalez-Moreno S, ed., *Advances in Peritoneal Surface Oncology.* In: Schlag PM, Senn HJ, eds., *Recent Results in Cancer Research,* New York: Springer, 2007. pp. 11–24.

15. Chi DS, Eisenhauer EL, Zivanovic O, Sonoda Y, Abu-Rustum NR, Levine DA. Improved progression-free and overall survival in advanced EOC as a result of a change in surgical paradigm. *Gynecologic Oncology.* 2009;114:26–31.

16. Chua TC, Moran BJ, Sugarbaker PH, Levine EA, Glehen O, Gilly FN et al. Early- and long-term outcome data of patients with pseudomyxoma peritonei from appendiceal origin treated by a strategy of cytoreductive surgery and hyperthermic intraperitoneal chemotherapy. *Journal of Clinical Oncology.* 2012;30(20):2449–2456.

17. Yan TD, Deraco M, Baratti D, Kusamura S, Elias D, Glehen O et al. Cytoreductive surgery and hyperthermic intraperitoneal chemotherapy for malignant peritoneal mesothelioma: Multi-institutional experience. *Journal of Clinical Oncology.* December 2009;27(36):6237–6242.

18. Esquivel J, Lowy AM, Markman M, Chua T, Pelz J, Baratti D et al. The American Society of Peritoneal Surface Malignancies (ASPSM) Multiinstitution Evaluation of the Peritoneal Surface Disease Severity Score (PSDSS) in 1,013 patients with colorectal cancer with peritoneal carcinomatosis. *Annals of Surgical Oncology.* 2014;21:4195–4201.

19. Sugarbaker Ph. Peritonectomy procedures. *Annals of Surgery.* 1995;221:29–42.

20. Deraco M, Baratti D, Kusamura S, Laterza B, Balestra MR. Surgical technique of parietal and visceral peritonectomy for peritoneal surface malignancies. *Journal of Surgical Oncology.* 2009;100:321–328.

21. Armstrong DK, Bundy B, Wenzel L, Huang HQ, Baergen R, Lele S et al. Intraperitoneal cisplatin and paclitaxel in EOC. *New England Journal of Medicine.* 2006;354:34 43.

22. Jaaback K, Johnson N. Intraperitoneal chemotherapy for the initial management of primary epithelial EOC. *Cochrane Database of Systematic Reviews.* 2006;1:CD005340.

23. Rowan K. Intraperitoneal therapy for EOC: Why has it not become standard? *Journal of the National Cancer Institute.* 2009;101:775–777.

24. Saladino E, Flere F, Irato S, Famulari C, Macri A. The role of cytoreductive surgery and hyperthermic intraperitoneal chemotherapy in the treatment of ovarian cancer relapse. *Updates in Surgery.* 2014;66:109–113.

25. Deraco M, Baratti D, Laterza B, Balestra MR, Mingrone E, Macri A et al. Advanced cytoreduction as surgical standard of care and hyperthermic intraperitoneal chemotherapy as promising treatment in epithelial ovarian cancer. *European Journal of Surgical Oncology.* 2011;37:4–9.

26. Kusamura S, Dominique E, Baratti D, Younan R, Deraco M. Drugs, carrier solutions and temperature in hyperthermic intraperitoneal chemotherapy. *Journal of Surgical Oncology.* September 2008;98(4):247–252.

27. Deraco M, Kusamura S, Virzì S, Puccio F, Macri A, Famulari C et al. Cytoreductive surgery and hyperthermic intraperitoneal chemotherapy as upfront therapy for advanced epithelial ovarian cancer: Multi-institutional phase-II trial. *Gynecologic Oncology.* 2011;122(2):215 220.

28. Vergote I, Tropé CG, Amant F, Kristensen GB, Ehlen T, Johnson N et al., European Organization for Research and Treatment of Cancer-Gynaecological Cancer Group; NCIC Clinical Trials Group. Neoadjuvant chemotherapy or primary surgery in stage IIIC or IV ovarian cancer. *New England Journal of Medicine.* 2010;363(10): 943–953.

29. Kang S, Nam BH. Does neoadjuvant chemotherapy increase optimal cytoreduction rate in advanced ovarian cancer? Meta-analysis of 21 studies. *Annals of Surgical Oncology.* 2009;16:2315–2320.

30. Secondary Debulking Surgery +/- Hyperthermic Intraperitoneal Chemotherapy in Stage III Ovarian Cancer. http://clinicaltrials.gov/show/NCT00426257. Accessed on September 15, 2015.

31. Phase 3 Trial Evaluating Hyperthermic Intraperitoneal Chemotherapy in Upfront Treatment of Stage IIIC Epithelial Ovarian Cancer (CHORINE). http://clinicaltrials.gov/show/NCT01628380. Accessed on September 15, 2015.

32. Gori J, Castaño R, Toziano M, Häbich D, Staringer J, De Quirós DG, Felci N. Intraperitoneal hyperthermic chemotherapy in ovarian cancer. *International Journal of Gynecological Cancer.* 2005;15(2):233–239.

33. Kim JH, Lee JM, Ryu KS, Lee YS, Park HG, Hur SY et al. Consolidation hyperthermic intraperitoneal chemotherapy using paclitaxel in patients with epithelial ovarian cancer. *Journal of Surgical Oncology.* 2010;101:149–155.

34. Pomel C, Ferron G, Lorimier G, Rey A, Lhomme C, Classe JM et al. Hyperthermic intra-peritoneal chemotherapy using oxaliplatin as consolidation therapy for advanced epithelial ovarian carcinoma. Results of a phase II prospective multicentre trial. CHIPOVAC study. *European Journal of Surgical Oncology.* 2010;36:589–593.

35. Bae JH, Lee JM, Ryu KS, Lee YS, Park YG, Hur SY et al. Treatment of ovarian cancer with paclitaxel- or carboplatin-based intraperitoneal hyperthermic chemotherapy during secondary surgery. *Gynecologic Oncology.* 2007;106(1):193–200.

36. Ryu KS, Kim JH, Ko HS, Kim JW, Ahn WS, Park YG et al. Effects of intraperitoneal hyperthermic chemotherapy in ovarian cancer. *Gynecologic Oncology.* 2004;94:325–332.

37. Muñoz-Casares FC, Rufián S, Rubio MJ, Díaz CJ, Diaz R, Casado A et al. The role of hyperthermic intraoperative intraperitoneal chemotherapy (HIPEC) in the treatment of peritoneal carcinomatosis in recurrent ovarian cancer. *Clinical and Translational Oncology.* 2009;11(11):753–759.

38. Spiliotis J, Vaxevanidou A, Sergouniotis F, Lambropoulou E, Datsis A, Christopoulou A. The role of cytoreductive surgery and hyperthermic intraperitoneal chemotherapy in the management of recurrent advanced ovarian cancer: A prospective study. *Journal of Balkan Union of Oncology.* 2011;16(1):74–79.

39. Fagotti A, Costantini B, Vizzielli G, Perelli F, Ercoli A, Gallotta V et al. HIPEC in recurrent ovarian cancer patients: Morbidity-related treatment and long-term analysis of clinical outcome. *Gynecologic Oncology.* 2011;122(2):221–225.

40. Helm CW, Bristow RE, Kusamura S, Baratti D, Deraco M. Hyperthermic intraperitoneal chemotherapy with and without cytoreductive surgery for epithelial ovarian cancer. *Journal of Surgical Oncology.* 2008;98:283–290.

41. Hettinga JV, Lemstra W, Meijer C, Dam WA, Uges DR, Konings AW et al. Mechanism of hyperthermic potentiation of cisplatin action in cisplatin-sensitive and -resistant tumour cells. *British Journal of Cancer.* 1997;75:1735–1743.

42. Deraco M, Raspagliesi F, Kusamura S. Management of peritoneal surface component of ovarian cancer. *Surgical Oncology Clinics of North America.* 2003;12:561–583. Review.

43. Deraco M, Virzì S, Iusco DR, Puccio F, Macrì A, Famulari C, Solazzo M, Bonomi S, Grassi A, Baratti D, Kusamura S. Secondary cytoreductive surgery and hyperthermic intraperitoneal chemotherapy for recurrent epithelial ovarian cancer: A multi-institutional study. *BJOG.* 2012;119(7):800–809.

44. Bakrin N, Cotte E, Golfier F, Gilly FN, Freyer G, Helm W, Glehen O, Bereder JM. Cytoreductive surgery and hyperthermic intraperitoneal chemotherapy (HIPEC) for persistent and recurrent advanced ovarian carcinoma: A multicenter, prospective study of 246 patients. *Annals of Surgical Oncology.* 2012;19(13):4052–4058.

45. Aletti GD, Long HJ, Podratz KC, Cliby WA. Is time to chemotherapy a determinant of prognosis in advanced-stage ovarian cancer? *Gynecologic Oncology.* 2007;104:212–216.

46. Bartlett DL, Buell JF, Libutti SK, Reed E, Lee KB, Figg WD et al. A phase I trial of continuous hyperthermic peritoneal perfusion with tumor necrosis factor and cisplatin in the treatment of peritoneal carcinomatosis. *Cancer.* 1998;83:1251–1261.

47. Rossi CR, Foletto M, Mocellin S, Pilati P, De SM, Deraco M et al. Hyperthermic intraoperative intraperitoneal chemotherapy with cisplatin and doxorubicin in patients who undergo cytoreductive surgery for peritoneal carcinomatosis and sarcomatosis: Phase I study. *Cancer.* 2002;94:492–499.

48. Harrison LE, Bryan M, Pliner L, Saunders T. Phase I trial of pegylated liposomal doxorubicin with hyperthermic intraperitoneal chemotherapy in patients undergoing cytoreduction for advanced intra-abdominal malignancy. *Annals of Surgical Oncology.* 2008;15:1407–1413.

49. Markman M, Brady MF, Spirtos NM, Hanjani P, Rubin SC. Phase II trial of intraperitoneal Paclitaxel in carcinoma of the ovary, tube and peritoneum: A Gynecologic Oncology Group Study. *Journal of Clinical Oncology.* 1998;16:2620–2624.

50. Nicoletto MO, Padrini R, Galeotti F, Ferrazzi E, Cartei G, Riddi F et al. Pharmacokinetics of intraperitoneal hyperthermic perfusion with mitoxantrone in EOC. *Cancer Chemotheraphy and Pharmacology.* 2000;45:457–462.

51. Lentz SS, Miller BE, Kucera GL, Levine EA. Intraperitoneal hyperthermic chemotherapy using carboplatin: A phase I analysis in ovarian carcinoma. *Gynecologic Oncology.* 2007;106:207–210.

52. Morgan RJ Jr, Synold TW, Xi B, Lim D, Shibata S, Margolin K et al. Phase I trial of intraperitoneal gemcitabine in the treatment of advanced malignancies primarily confined to the peritoneal cavity. *Clinical Cancer Research.* 2007;13:1232–1237.

53. de Bree E, Rosing H, Filis D, Romanos J, Melisssourgaki M, Daskalakis M et al. Cytoreductive surgery and intraoperative hyperthermic intraperitoneal chemotherapy with paclitaxel: A clinical and pharmacokinetic study. *Annals of Surgical Oncology.* 2008;15:1183–1192.

54. Younan R, Kusamura S, Baratti D, Cloutier AS, Deraco M. Morbidity, toxicity, and mortality classification systems in the local regional treatment of peritoneal surface malignancy. *Journal of Surgical Oncology.* September 15, 2008;98(4):253–257. Review.

55. Cripe J, Tseng J, Eskander R, Fader AN, Tanner E, Bristow R. Cytoreductive surgery and hyperthermic intraperitoneal chemotherapy for recurrent ovarian carcinoma: Analysis of 30-day morbidity and mortality. *Annals of Surgical Oncology.* 2015;22:655–661.

56. Swerdlow M. Mesothelioma of the pelvic peritoneum resembling papillary cystadenocarcinoma of the ovary. *American Journal of Obstetrics and Gynecology.* 1959;77:197–200.

57. Pentheroudakis G, Pavlidis N. Serous papillary peritoneal carcinoma: Unknown primary tumour, ovarian cancer counterpart or a distinct entity? A systematic review. *Critical Reviews in Oncology/Hematology.* 2010;75:27–42.

58. Bakrin N, Gilly FN, Baratti D, Bereder JM, Quenet F, Lorimier G et al. Primary peritoneal serous carcinoma treated by cytoreductive surgery combined with hyperthermic intraperitoneal chemotherapy. A multi-institutional study of 36 patients. *European Journal of Surgical Oncology.* 2013;39:742–747.

59. Bloss JD, Shu-Yuan L, Buller RE, Manetta A, Berman ML, McMeekin S et al. Extraovarin peritoneal serous papillary carcinoma: A case–control retrospective comparison to papillary adenocarcinoma of the ovary. *Gynecologic Oncology.* 1993;50:347–351.

60. Halperin R, Zehavi S, Hadas E, Habler L, Bukovsky I, Schneider D. Immunohistochemical comparison of primary peritoneal and primary ovarian serous papillary carcinoma. *International Journal of Gynecological Pathology.* 2001;20:341–345.

61. Look M, Chang D, Sugarbaker PH. Long-term results of cytoreductive surgery for advanced and recurrent epithelial ovarian cancers and papillary serous carcinoma of the peritoneum. *International Journal of Gynecological Cancer.* 2004;14:35–41.

62. Deraco M, Baratti D, Kusamura S, Gil Gomez E. Cytoreductive surgery and hyperthermic intraperitoneal chemotherapy for serous peritoneal papillary carcinoma (SPPC). Paper presented at the *Eighth International Symposium on Regional Cancer Therapies*, Palm Springs, CA, February 16–18, 2013.

63. Kusamura S, Baratti D, Deraco M. Multidimensional analysis of the learning curve for cytoreductive surgery and hyperthermic intraperitoneal chemotherapy in peritoneal surface malignancies. *Annals of Surgery.* 2012;255:348–356.

19

Pseudomyxoma peritonei

BETTINA LIESKE AND BRENDAN MORAN

INTRODUCTION

Pseudomyxoma peritonei (PMP) is an uncommon clinical condition characterized by mucinous ascites and predominantly originates from a perforated epithelial neoplasm of the appendix [1,2]. The clinical presentation is variable, often with nonspecific symptoms, and is associated with abdominal distension in advanced cases [1,2]. While traditionally considered benign, it is apparent that there is a spectrum of diseases varying from slowly progressive to aggressively malignant disease such that PMP, at best, should be considered a "borderline" malignancy [2]. Similar clinical, radiological, and pathological features may originate from any abdominal mucinous tumor, in particular the ovary in females or colorectal pathology in males or females. PMP of nonappendiceal origin tends to be at the adverse end of the spectrum. The primary tumor is more likely to be a mucinous adenocarcinoma with a worse prognosis than that in classical PMP of appendiceal origin.

HISTORICAL OVERVIEW

An appendiceal mucocele was first described by Carl Rokitansky, an anatomy professor at the University of Vienna in 1842. The term "pseudomyxoma peritonei" was coined several years later by Werth [3]. Further case reports of the condition were published over the following years, including a remarkable paper by the German obstetrician and gynecologist Robert Michaelis von Olshausen, in which he described his hypothesis that the epithelial cells from the lining of the ruptured appendix cyst were transplanted to the peritoneum, where they took root and continued to secrete gelatinous material [4]. In 1915, Otto Castle published one of the first literature reviews and estimated the occurrence of a mucocele of the appendix at 0.2%, based on autopsy reports [5]. There is some ongoing confusion of the two terms "mucocele" and PMP, but in essence a mucocele, by definition, contains mucus only with no abnormal cells and therefore cannot per se be the source of PMP. PMP requires rupture of an appendix with abnormal mucosal cells that spread and propagate within the peritoneal cavity.

INCIDENCE

There is no substantial information on the true incidence of either appendiceal mucinous tumors or the incidence of PMP. Estimates of an incidence of PMP of one per million per year had been proposed [6], though this was based on a figure with no scientific evidence [2]. An epidemiological analysis by Smeenk et al. in 2008 of a population-based study in the Netherlands [7] reported an incidence of mucinous epithelial neoplasm of the appendix of 0.3% and progression to PMP in 20%. Extrapolations from this paper estimates the incidence of PMP as two per million per year. However, experience in a high-volume centralized treatment center has suggested that the incidence may be higher with three to four operable cases per million per year [8].

PATHOPHYSIOLOGY

PMP is a clinicopathological entity resulting from mucin-producing peritoneal and omental tumor implants secondary to a perforated mucinous neoplasm. This

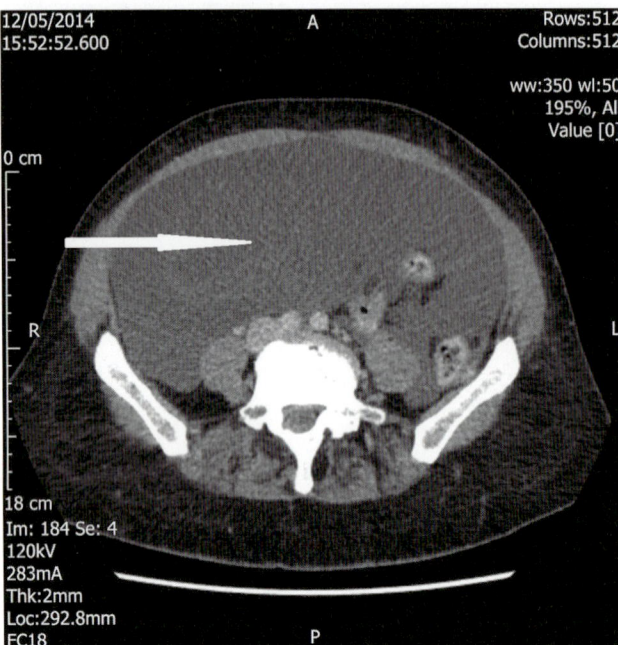

Figure 19.1 CT scan of a "jelly belly." The white arrow is pointing toward the enlarged right ovary surrounded by mucinous ascites.

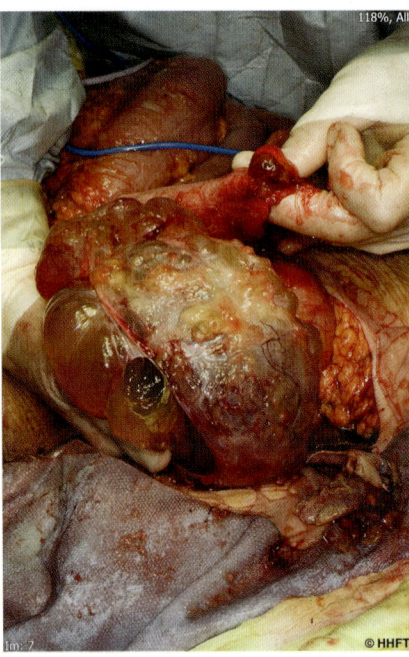

Figure 19.2 Enlarged ovary and appendiceal tumor. Intraoperative picture of the same patient as Figure 19.1 demonstrating the enlarged ovary and the perforated appendix tumor.

phenomenon culminates in the characteristic accumulation of gelatinous mucus in the peritoneal cavity, also commonly referred to as "jelly belly" [9] (Figures 19.1 and 19.2). While the classical PMP appearances originate form an appendiceal tumor, the clinical, radiological, and indeed image-guided biopsy appearances of "jelly belly"

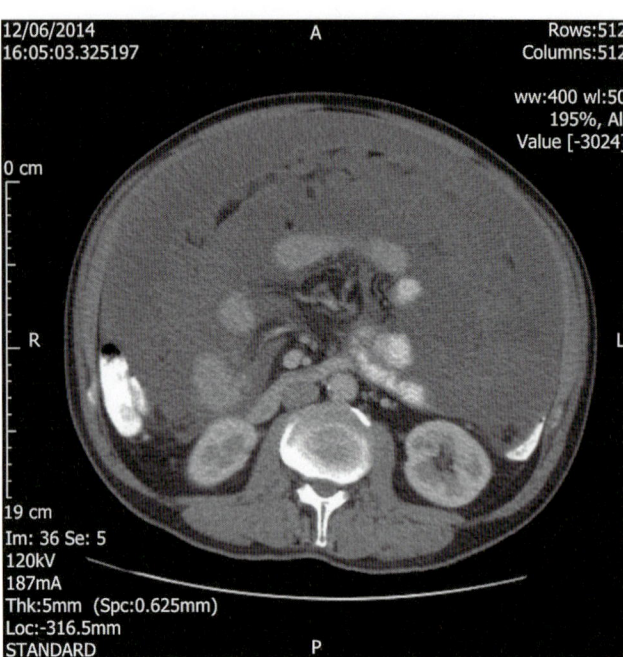

Figure 19.3 CT of omental cake and mucinous ascites. Large omental cake and ascites compressing the contents of the abdominal cavity.

may also originate from a true adenocarcinoma of the appendix, colon, or rectum, primary peritoneal or ovarian malignancies, and there are indeed case reports and a small series of origin of PMP from most intra-abdominal organs, including the stomach, pancreas, liver, gallbladder, urinary bladder, and urachus [2,10].

PMP appears to be more common in females who often present with rapidly progressive abdominal distension as a consequence of ovarian involvement by transcoelomic spread. The long-standing theory of a predominance of ovarian origin of PMP in females has been refuted, and it is now generally accepted that the underlying pathology in most cases is the appendix, with secondary ovarian involvement [2]. Immunohistochemistry and molecular markers have shown that despite advanced ovarian involvement, the disease is predominantly of intestinal origin [11–14].

Presentation of PMP in males at an early stage is less common, unless as an incidental finding in appendicectomy specimens, and many males present with insidious onset advanced disease (Figure 19.3). This presentation of advanced disease in males may represent underinvestigation by cross-sectional imaging in males compared with females and the more rapid and symptomatic progression in females associated with ovarian involvement.

REDISTRIBUTION OF MUCINOUS TUMORS IN THE PERITONEAL CAVITY

The distribution of mucinous tumor implants within the peritoneal cavity is determined by what has been termed "the redistribution phenomenon" [2,15]. Rupture of the

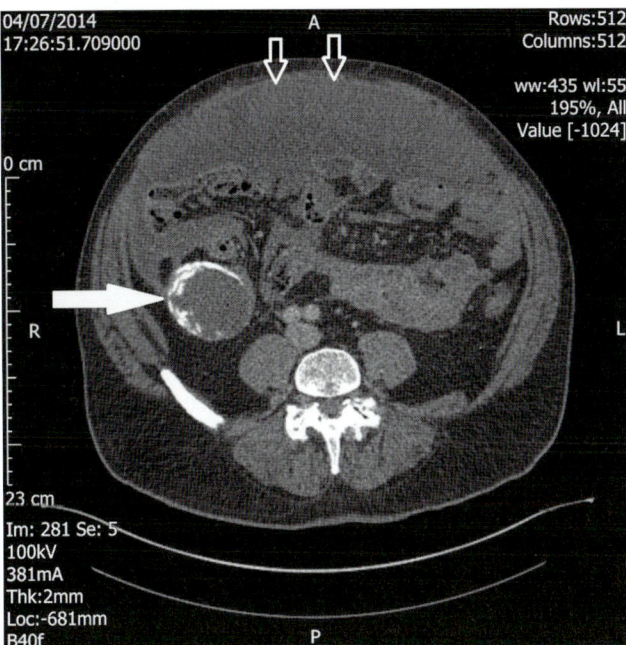

Figure 19.4 CT scan of an appendix tumor and omental cake. The solid white arrow is pointing to the calcified appendix tumor and the arrow outlines are indicating the omental cake.

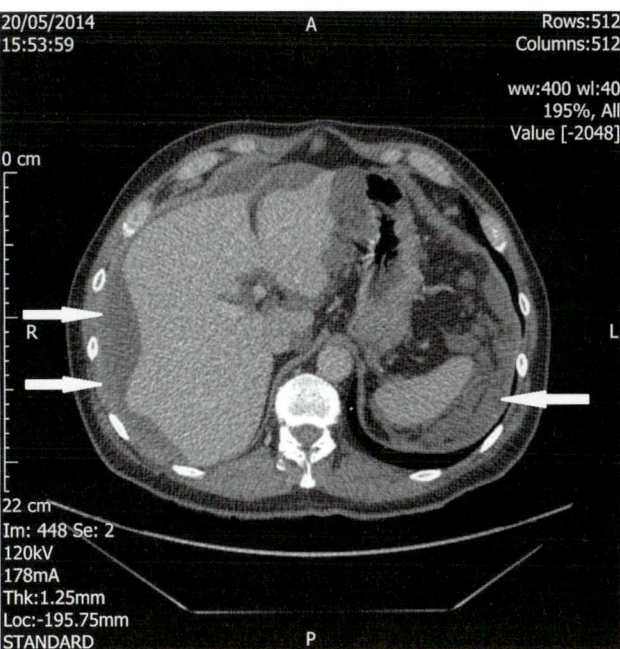

Figure 19.5 CT scan demonstrating subdiaphragmatic disease. The arrows point toward the subdiaphragmatic disease around the liver on the right and the spleen on the left side.

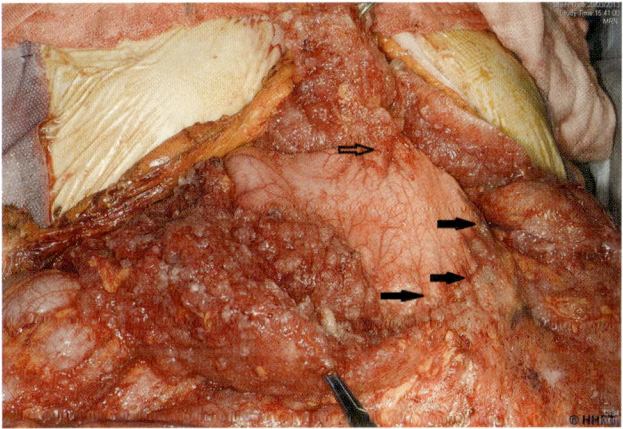

Figure 19.6 Extensive disease in the upper abdomen. Intraoperative picture showing extensive disease in the upper abdomen surrounding the stomach. The solid arrows point toward the greater curve of the stomach, and the arrow outline points toward the lesser curve of the stomach.

primary tumor results in the release of free-floating cells and mucin that disseminate throughout the abdominal cavity. The epithelial tumor cells have either no or low adhesion properties and consequently distribute within and by the peritoneal fluid [15]. Characteristically, cellular deposits accumulate and proliferate in predetermined sites by two main mechanisms, namely, resorption of peritoneal fluid and gravity. The physiology of the peritoneal cavity involves production, circulation, and resorption of peritoneal fluid. The main sites of fluid reabsorption are the greater and lesser omentum (accounting for the classical "omental cake," Figure 19.4) and the undersurface of the diaphragm, particularly the right side, resulting in tumor accumulation in the subdiaphragmatic and suprahepatic regions (Figure 19.5).

The second main mechanism is by gravity with cell accumulation in dependent sites, such as the rectovesical pouch, the right retrohepatic space, and the paracolic gutters [2,15].

Mobile organs such as the small bowel and its mesentery are usually spared, particularly early on in the course of the disease. In contrast, the less mobile, partially retroperitoneal, ascending and sigmoid colon as well as the fixed points of the stomach in its distal portion and the duodenojejunal flexure at the ligament of Treitz can be heavily involved by disease and may warrant bowel resections such as colectomy and distal gastrectomy to remove troublesome deposits (Figures 19.6 and 19.7).

The relative sparing of the motile small bowel and its mesentery allows complete removal of tumor in most patients without the need for substantial small bowel resection.

Extensive small bowel involvement can occur at an early stage in more aggressive tumors and even in less invasive tumors when the disease is at an advanced stage. A further additional factor influencing small bowel involvement is prior attempts at tumor removal, particularly if extensive abdominal surgery has been performed, as tumor proliferates in scar tissue and may involve the small bowel at the sites of adhesions. Extensive small bowel involvement, particularly if the disease involves the serosa or infiltrates at the junction of the small bowel with its mesentery, may prevent a complete tumor removal.

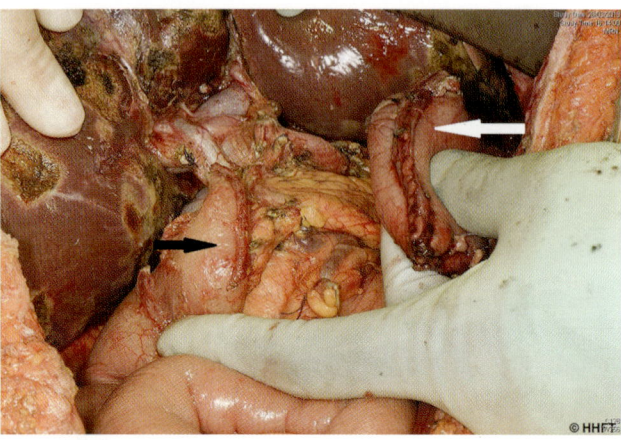

Figure 19.7 Distal gastrectomy. Intraoperative picture of the same patient after distal gastrectomy. The white arrow points toward the proximal stomach remnant and the black arrow toward the duodenum.

CLINICAL SYMPTOMS OF PMP

Patients with classical PMP commonly present with vague abdominal symptoms, and often only when disease burden is marked. Many may even have been investigated by gastroscopy and colonoscopy and been labeled irritable bowel syndrome. The initial lesion in the appendix, though ruptured at initiation of PMP, is commonly asymptomatic, and many patients have no recollection of symptoms such as acute abdominal pain normally associated with appendiceal rupture. The absence of acute symptoms is a consequence of the slowly progressive distension of the appendix and no bacterial contamination of the mucinous rupture as the luminal appendix tumor seals the luminal communication to the cecum.

The increasing mucus accumulation progresses to abdominal distension, abdominal discomfort or pain, and often palpable masses, either ovarian in females or an omental cake in males or females. Eventually, malnutrition, bowel obstruction, and respiratory compromise are apparent and are precursors of a terminal decline.

The presenting features of PMP were outlined in 2000 by Esquivel and Sugarbaker [16], who found that the commonest clinical presentation of a patient with PMP was suspected acute appendicitis (27%), increasing abdominal distension (23%), or a new-onset hernia (14%). Other presentations were ascites, pain, and other vague symptoms, accounting for 17% of cases. In women, the diagnosis was made most commonly during investigation for a suspected ovarian mass (39%). We have recently analyzed the mode of presentation in the modern era in a series of 222 patients undergoing surgery for appendiceal tumors in Basingstoke over a 2-year period from January 2011 to December 2012 [17] and found that overall computed tomography (CT) was the main diagnostic method with 81/222 (36.5%) diagnosed preoperatively with CT alone (with or without image-guided biopsy) and 32/222 (14.4%) following a suspicious CT, which led to operative confirmation. The next most frequent mechanism was during laparoscopy/laparotomy for an acute abdomen or on subsequent

appendix histology in 46/222 (20.7%). Other presentations were new-onset hernia in 5%, diagnostic laparoscopy in 5.4%, and miscellaneous in 3.6%.

It is apparent from both Sugarbaker's [16] and our more recent experience that many patients present with appendicitis or unexpectedly at laparoscopy or laparotomy and increasingly at either cross-sectional imaging for investigation of abdominal symptoms or incidental abnormalities noted on staging or investigational imaging for unrelated pathology [18].

Physical examination in symptomatic patients often reveals a markedly distended soft abdomen, typically not exhibiting shifting dullness, as the mucus is too dense to redistribute during positional changes. Occasionally, an enlarged ovary or omental cake can be felt. Digital rectal examination can reveal disease in the pouch of Douglas in females and rectovesical pouch in males.

INVESTIGATIONS

CT of the chest, abdomen, and pelvis with intravenous and oral contrast is the imaging modality of choice [19,20]. This can reveal the lesion in the appendix, which may be calcified, omental caking and mucinous ascites. The pathognomonic features of "scalloping" of the liver represent liver capsular tumor masses that indent and deform the liver capsule and differentiate peritoneal malignant deposits from ascites (Figure 19.8).

The key feature determining the feasibility of complete tumor resection is not only the involvement of the small bowel in particular but also to a lesser extent gross involvement of the porta hepatis [19,20]. Oral contrast may help to

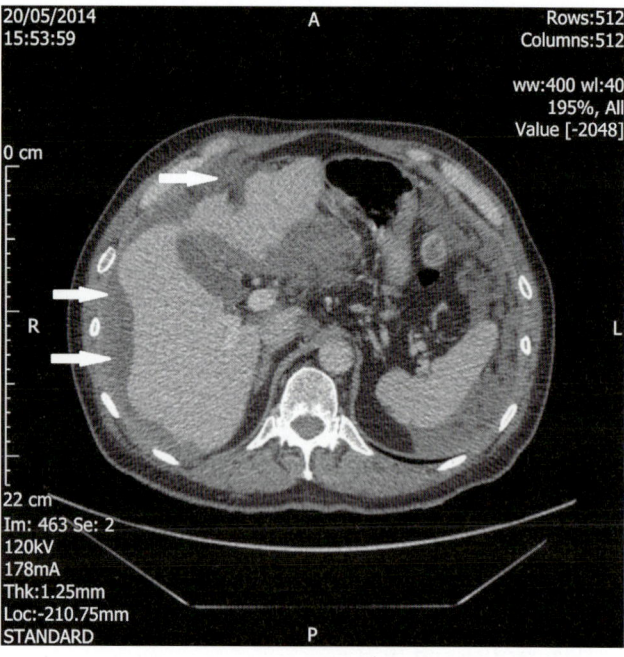

Figure 19.8 CT scan of liver "scalloping." The arrows point toward the disease indenting the surface of the liver.

assess the small bowel and other modalities such as MRI have been proposed by some [21–23]. There is a limited role for functional imaging such as positron emission tomography (PET)–CT in pseudomyxoma, but PET–CT may identify extra-abdominal or intrahepatic metastases in patients with adenocarcinoma [24].

Small bowel involvement in peritoneal malignancy is not accurately determined by any noninvasive modality, and optimal assessment requires direct inspection at laparotomy, though laparoscopy may also be sufficient to detect low-volume extensive disease on the serosa and mesentery of the small bowel in conditions such colorectal peritoneal metastases [25].

Diagnostic laparoscopy is seldom helpful in PMP as the large omental cake and copious mucinous ascites preclude access and visualization of the small bowel.

Percutaneous image-guided biopsy (under CT or US guidance) often is unhelpful, commonly yielding acellular mucin even in patients with mucinous adenocarcinoma.

SERUM TUMOR MARKERS

Tumor marker measurements help to predict the aggressiveness of the tumor and in patients who are secretors can aid detection of recurrence after surgery. Carcinoembryonic antigen (CEA), carbohydrate antigen 125 (CA 125), and carbohydrate antigen 19.9 (CA 19.9) have been found to be of diagnostic and predictive value for the condition, although published studies are small series with short follow-up [26–30].

CEA is expressed in adenocarcinomas of gastrointestinal origin, mainly colorectal cancers. CA 125 is a marker used in ovarian cancers, and CA 19.9 is expressed in diseases and conditions affecting the peritoneum and often raised in peritoneal irritation. All publications to date suggest that patients with elevated tumor markers have an increased risk of recurrence [26–30].

The largest reported series has been by Taflampas et al. [31], who have recently published the results of a study of 519 patients who had complete tumor removal by cytoreductive surgery and hyperthermic intraperitoneal chemotherapy (HIPEC) for perforated appendiceal tumors in Basingstoke. The main finding was that patients with normal tumor markers preoperatively had significantly higher disease-free (DFS) and overall (OS) survival when compared with patients with elevated tumor markers. DFS and OS correlated with the number of elevated markers with a downward shift in the curves by one, two, or all three elevated markers compared with patients who had normal preoperative markers. This finding was independent of underlying histopathological classification into low grade and high grade and seems to suggest that current histopathological grading alone cannot be used as a reliable marker to predict DFS and OS. The paper suggests that tumor markers should be used as an independent prognostic predictor for survival, as their elevation is likely to represent a manifestation of the biology of the disease [31]. The conclusion was that elevated tumor markers might be used to determine consideration for postoperative systemic chemotherapy and both timing and frequency of follow-up.

TREATMENT

The optimal treatment for PMP is complete macroscopic tumor removal, with the aim to remove all visible lesions throughout the entire peritoneal cavity (complete cytoreductive surgery [CCRS]), in combination with intraoperative HIPEC [32–34]. The most important prognostic factor has been consistently reported to be CCRS [35,36].

If complete CCRS is not possible, maximal tumor debulking (MTD), involving a greater omentectomy and either an ileocolic anastomosis or a subtotal colectomy and end ileostomy, can achieve long-term survival and good quality of life when balanced against postoperative morbidity and mortality as recently reported by Dayal et al. [8]. In this study, 205/748 consecutive patients who underwent surgery for PMP had MTD. OS at 3, 5, and 10 years was 47%, 30%, and 22% in the MTD group, compared with 90%, 82%, and 64% in the CCRS group. The median survival in the MTD group was 32.8 months.

CCRS combined with HIPEC is a major intervention with an average procedure time of 9 hours, ranging from 2 to 24 hours [35].

Careful anesthetic assessment and management is required with experienced patient positioning on the operating table, taking into account the need for surgical access to all of the abdomen and the perineum while being aware of the risks of neurological compression and the risks of compartment syndrome.

The abdomen is opened from xiphisternum to symphysis pubis, and the umbilicus and any previous midline scar may need excision if involved by tumor.

Our favored approach is to commence with right parietal peritonectomy and medial mobilization of the cecum to expose the right ureter and gonadals [37]. Peritonectomy is continued cephalad to perform a right diaphragmatic peritonectomy with full mobilization of the liver. A liver capsulectomy is performed if necessary and is generally accomplished by a "roller ball" diathermy at maximal setting. A high-power smoke extraction system is essential to reduce the smoke contamination. Similar steps on the left side begin with left parietal peritonectomy locating the left ureter and gonadals. The left diaphragmatic peritoneum is stripped if necessary.

A radical greater omentectomy (inside the gastroepiploic vessels) is performed and the spleen is carefully assessed, and if involved by disease, the splenic artery and vein are clamped, transfixed, and ligated and a splenectomy performed taking great care to avoid damage to the tail of the pancreas.

The pelvis dissection is commenced by rectal mobilization in the total mesorectal excision plane posteriorly with full mobilization of the rectum, the peritoneal mobilization is carried anteriorly toward the bladder, and the peritoneum is carefully dissected off its posterior surface. Usually the rectum and sigmoid can be preserved, but prior pelvic surgery (especially major gynecological surgery such as hysterectomy and salpingo-oophorectomy) may mean that the tumor has infiltrated the anterior rectal wall, and an anterior resection may be needed.

In females, the ovaries are routinely removed and removal of the uterus may or may not be required.

In many cases, appendicectomy alone may suffice to resect the tumor, but a right hemicolectomy is required if there is extensive peritoneal involvement of the cecum and/ or terminal ileum or if there are suspected involved nodes on the ileocolic chain. Occasionally, a frozen section assessment of an ileocolic node may help in the decision making.

A problematic area on many occasions is the lesser omentum, porta hepatitis, and aortocaval groove on the left side. It is best to commence by removing the lesser omentum from the lesser curve of the stomach (taking care to preserve the left gastric vessels) and continuing to the porta hepatis by lifting the peritoneum with a curved forceps anterior to the portal triad structures (common bile duct, hepatic artery, and portal vein). The gallbladder is removed (often by retrograde cholecystectomy) to facilitate identification of the portal anatomy.

The disease in the aortocaval groove is best approached after full mobilization of the left liver and retraction of the left liver to the right side. The caudate lobe is identified, and the peritoneum extending between the caudate, right crus of the diaphragm, and vena cava is removed (often by traction with an artery forceps).

On occasions, a distal gastrectomy is needed to remove disease surrounding the pylorus (approximately 10% in our series of patients with PMP). The stomach and duodenum are stapled with mechanical staplers, and after HIPEC, the gastric remnant is anastomosed to the duodenum.

Once the peritonectomies and tumor removal are completed, HIPEC is administered by continuous infusion of mitomycin C (10 mg/m^2, with dose adjustments for patients with renal impairment, major obesity, older age, or comorbidities) heated to 42°C for 1 hour.

Any bowel anastomosis is performed after the HIPEC, and if the rectum has been resected, a stapled colorectal anastomosis is performed and generally protected by a defunctioning ileostomy.

It is our practice to insert a chest drain if a diaphragm has been stripped of its peritoneum. Thus many patients will have two chest drains and may require overnight ventilation in an intensive care unit.

Some centers combine HIPEC with early postoperative intraperitoneal chemotherapy using 5-fluorouracil. Our policy is to selectively use 5-fluorouracil at 15 mg/kg for 4 days postoperatively via a Tenckhoff catheter inserted at operation.

HISTOLOGY

There are several histological classifications and ongoing confusion partly attributable to the different terminology in these classification systems. However, the general trend has been toward the consensus that PMP is a malignant process with varying degrees of malignant potential.

One of the first internationally recognized histopathological classification systems was reported by Ronnett et al. in 1995 [38], in which PMP is described as a heterogeneous group of pathological lesions that may have in common only the presence of abundant extracellular mucin and may or may not contain epithelial cells. Ronnett's classification divides PMP into three categories: disseminated peritoneal adenomucinosis (DPAM), peritoneal mucinous carcinomatosis (PMCA), and an intermediate category in tumors with inconsistent or discordant features (PMCA-I/D). In this classification system, cases of DPAM are characterized by peritoneal lesions composed of abundant extracellular mucin containing scant simple to focally proliferative mucinous epithelium with little cytological atypia or mitotic activity, with or without an associated appendiceal mucinous adenoma. Cases of PMCA are characterized by peritoneal lesions composed of more abundant mucinous epithelium with the architectural and cytologic features of carcinoma, with or without an associated primary mucinous adenocarcinoma. While this system is widely used, it is important to note that this categorization was on patients who had undergone cytoreductive surgery and was retrospective. In addition, the term DPAM suggests a "benign" entity and is not in keeping with the behavior of PMP, even some of those at the lower end of the histological spectrum.

Bradley et al. attempted a reclassification in their study in 2006 [39], using the same pathological criteria as described by Ronnett et al. [38]. After reviewing patient outcomes, they proposed the classification into two distinct categories: mucinous carcinoma peritonei low grade (MCP-L) and mucinous carcinoma peritonei high grade (MCP-H). MCP-L incorporated Ronnett's cases with DPAM and those categorized by Ronnett et al. as PMCA-I. Cases that are moderately to poorly differentiated are classified as MCP-H, including cases with signet ring cells.

In 2010, WHO published a classification that divides PMP into low and high grades [40].

Carr et al. [41] subsequently reviewed the histology of over 270 cases and correlated their findings with clinical information and survival data. They found that the categorization as either low grade or high grade by WHO criteria correlates with prognosis. The group also correlated the grade of PMP with the grade of the primary tumor and found that the grade of the PMP is generally consistent with the grade of the primary appendiceal neoplasm.

Work is ongoing to achieve consensus of the leading pathologists on appendiceal tumors using a Delphi process being conducted by Carr on behalf of Peritoneal Surface Oncology Group International with plans for conclusion over the next year.

OUTCOMES

DFS and OS after surgical procedures for PMP have improved over time with the appreciation of the need for CCRS and the added benefit of HIPEC [42,43]. Two publications from the Mayo Clinic in the early 1990s reported a

10-year survival rate of 32% for low-grade PMP and a 5-year survival rate of 6% for adenocarcinoma originating from the appendix [44,45].

Subsequent publications incorporating the concepts of CCRS and HIPEC have reported much better outcomes, with operative mortality rates ranging between 1.6% and 4.4% and morbidity rates between 7% and 49%. Disease- or progression-free survival at 1, 5, and 10 years were reported as 75%, 56%–70%, and 67%. The overall 5-year survival rate was 69%–75% and overall 10-year survival rate was 57% [26,34,36,46,47].

An expert consensus concluded in 2006 that there was a survival benefit with this approach comparing results to historical controls [32]; however, due to the rarity of the disease, long-term outcome data for larger series were not available until a pooled analysis was published by Chua et al. in 2012 [35]. This review included 2298 patients from 16 centers with a strategy of CCRS, if feasible, combined with HIPEC. In this multicenter study, the overall 3-, 5-, 10-, and 15-year survival rates were 80%, 74%, 63%, and 59%, respectively. Postoperative mortality was 2% and major complication rate was 24%.

The review emphasized the completeness of cytoreduction (CCR) as a major predictor for outcome, independent of histological grade.

Residual disease following CRS was scored according to the CCR score [48]. CCR0 indicates no macroscopic residual cancer; CCR1 indicates no residual nodule larger than 2.5 mm in diameter; CCR2 indicates residual nodules between 2.5 mm and 2.5 cm in diameter; and CCR3 implies residual disease greater than 2.5 cm in diameter. Overall CC0 and CC1 equate to a complete cytoreduction with optimal outcomes and significantly better than patients who have CCR2 or CCR3 cytoreduction.

For patients with an incomplete cytoreduction (analogous to debulking surgery), the 5 year survival rate was 24% (in patients with CCR2 or CCR3) compared with 85% in patients who had CCR0 and 80% in those who had CCR1 [35]. This difference remained significant when stratified by histopathological subtype on multivariate analysis. This supports complete cytoreduction as optimal treatment.

However, CCR depends on a number of factors, including the histological grade and extent of the disease. Previous surgery, especially attempts at major debulking, diminishes the chances of CCRS due to tumor deposition and entrapment at scar tissue and adhesions [49].

FOLLOW-UP AFTER CYTOREDUCTIVE SURGERY

With increasing experience in management of PMP, a follow-up strategy is needed to detect and treat recurrence. Current follow-up strategies include CT scanning and serum tumor markers at regular intervals. Our standard practice for PMP is CT and tumor markers at 1 year after surgery and annually thereafter for 10 years.

Earlier imaging may be warranted if symptoms manifest or disease recurrence is suspected.

Once disease progression is detected by imaging or suspected by elevated tumor markers, further management is problematic with no consensus. Repeat laparotomy and HIPEC is advocated by some with others suggesting that systemic chemotherapy and/or sequential monitoring with intervention only for treatable symptoms.

CONCLUSION

PMP is an uncommon and heterogeneous clinicopathological entity generally originating from a perforated mucinous appendiceal neoplasm. It is, at best, a borderline malignancy, and optimal management is by complete cytoreductive surgery, combined with hyperthermic intraperitoneal chemotherapy. The surgery is complex, with major complications and a significant mortality risk and is best performed in experienced centers.

Experience with PMP has been extrapolated to the management of other peritoneal malignancies, particularly mesothelioma, ovarian tumors, and colorectal peritoneal metastases.

Experience gained and lessons learned with PMP have advanced knowledge on all aspects of diagnosis, management, and outcome improvements for a selection of the vast numbers of patients who present with primary and secondary synchronous and metachronous peritoneal malignancies.

REFERENCES

1. Sugarbaker PH. Pseudomyxoma peritonei. *Cancer Treatment Research.* 1996;81:105–119.
2. Moran BJ, Cecil TD. The etiology, clinical presentation, and management of pseudomyxoma peritonei. *Surgical Oncology Clinics of North America.* 2003;12:585–603.
3. Werth R. Klinische und Anatomische Untersuchungen zur Lehre von den Bauchgeschwuelsten und der Laparotomie. *Archives of Gynaecology and Obstetrics.* 1884;24:100–118.
4. Weaver CH. Mucocele of appendix with pseudomucinous degeneration. *The American Journal of Surgery.* 1937;36(2):523–526.
5. Castle OL. Cystic dilatation of the vermiform appendix. *Annals of Surgery.* 1915;61:582–588.
6. National Institute for Health and Clinical Excellence. Complete cytoreduction for pseudomyxoma peritonei (Sugarbaker technique). NICE interventional procedure guidance 56, 2004. http://www.nice.org.uk/guidance/IPG56. Accessed June 16, 2015.
7. Smeenk RM, van Velthuysen ML, Verwaal VJ, Zoetmulder FA. Appendiceal neoplasms and pseudomyxoma peritonei: A population based study. *European Journal of Surgical Oncology.* 2008;34:196–201.

8. Dayal S, Taflampas P, Riss S, Chandrakumaran K, Cecil TD, Mohamed F, Moran BJ. Complete cytoreduction for pseudomyxoma peritonei is optimal but maximal tumor debulking may be beneficial in patients in whom complete tumor removal cannot be achieved. *Diseases of the Colon and Rectum.* 2013;56(12):1366–1372.

9. Behling H. Mucocele of the appendix and jelly-belly. *Minnesota Medicine.* July 1967;50(7):1109–1112.

10. Smeenk RM, Bex A, Verwaal VJ, Horenblas S, Zoetmulder FA. Pseudomyxoma peritonei and the urinary tract: Involvement and treatment related complications. *Journal of Surgical Oncology.* 2006;93:20–23.

11. Ronnett BM, Shmookler BM, Diener-West M, Sugarbaker PH, Kurman RJ. Immunohistochemical evidence supporting the appendiceal origin of pseudomyxoma peritonei in women. *International Journal of Gynecological Pathology.* 1997;16:1–9.

12. Szych C, Staebler A, Connolly DC, Wu R, Cho KR, Ronnett BM. Molecular genetic evidence supporting the clonality and appendiceal origin of pseudomyxoma peritonei in women. *American Journal of Pathology.* 1999;154:1849–1855.

13. Chuaqui RF, Zhuang Z, Emmert-Buck MR, Bryant BR, Nogales F, Tavassoli FA, Merino MJ. Genetic analysis of synchronous mucinous tumors of the ovary and appendix. *Human Pathology.* 1996;27:165–171.

14. Guerrieri C, Frånlund B, Fristedt S, Gillooley JF, Boeryd B. Mucinous tumors of the vermiform appendix and ovary, and pseudomyxoma peritonei: Histogenetic implications of cytokeratin 7 expression. *Human Pathology.* 1997;28:1039–1045.

15. Sugarbaker PH. Pseudomyxoma peritonei. A cancer whose biology is characterized by a redistribution phenomenon. *Annals of Surgery.* 1994;219:109–111.

16. Esquivel J, Sugarbaker PH. Clinical presentation of the pseudomyxoma peritonei syndrome. *British Journal of Surgery.* 2000;87:1414–1418.

17. Glaysher M, Gordon-Dixon A, Chandrakumaran K, Cecil TD, Moran BJ. Pseudomyxoma peritonei of appendiceal origin: Mode of presentation in the modern era. *Colorectal Disease.* 2014;16(Suppl. 2):53.

18. Murphy EM, Farquharson SM, Moran BJ. Management of an unexpected appendiceal neoplasm. *British Journal of Surgery.* 2006;93:783–792.

19. Jacquet P, Jelinek JS, Chang D, Koslowe P, Sugarbaker PH. Abdominal computed tomographic scan in the selection of patients with mucinous peritoneal carcinomatosis for cytoreductive surgery. *Journal of the American College of Surgeons.* 1995;181:530–538.

20. Sulkin TV, O'Neill H, Amin AI, Moran B. CT in pseudomyxoma peritonei: A review of 17 cases. *Clinical Radiology.* 2002;57(7):608–613.

21. Cotton F, Pellet O, Gilly FN, Granier A, Sournac L, Glehen O. MRI evaluation of bulky tumor masses in the mesentery and bladder involvement in peritoneal carcinomatosis. *European Journal of Surgical Oncology.* December 2006;32(10):1212–1216.

22. Tirumani SH, Fraser-Hill M, Auer R, Shabana W, Walsh C, Lee F, Ryan JG. Mucinous neoplasms of the appendix: A current comprehensive clinicopathologic and imaging review. *Cancer Imaging.* February 2013;13:14–25.

23. Low RN, Low RN, Barone RM, Gurney JM, Muller WD. Mucinous appendiceal neoplasms: Preoperative MR staging and classification compared with surgical and histopathologic findings. *American Journal of Roentgenology.* 2008;190:656–665.

24. Passot G, Glehen O, Pellet O, Isaac S, Tychyj C, Mohamed F, Giammarile F, Gilly FN, Cotte E. Pseudomyxoma peritonei: Role of 18F-FDG PET in preoperative evaluation of pathological grade and potential for complete cytoreduction. *European Journal of Surgical Oncology.* 2010;36(3):315–323.

25. Moran BJ, Cecil TD. Treatment of surgically resectable colorectal peritoneal metastases. *British Journal of Surgery.* January 2014;101(2):5–7.

26. Chua TC, Yan TD, Smigielski ME, Zhu KJ, Ng KM, Zhao J et al. Long-term survival in patients with pseudomyxoma peritonei treated with cytoreductive surgery and perioperative intraperitoneal chemotherapy: 10 years of experience from a single institution. *Annals of Surgical Oncology.* 2009;16:1903–1911.

27. Baratti D, Kusamura S, Martinetti A, Seregni E, Laterza B, Oliva DG et al. Prognostic value of circulating tumor markers in patients with pseudomyxoma peritonei treated with cytoreductive surgery and hyperthermic intraperitoneal chemotherapy. *Annals of Surgical Oncology.* 2007;14:2300–2308.

28. Carmignani CP, Hampton R, Sugarbaker CE, Chang D, Sugarbaker PH. Utility of CEA and CA 19.9 tumor markers in diagnosis and prognostic assessment of mucinous epithelial cancers of the appendix. *Journal of Surgical Oncology.* 2004;87:162–166.

29. Van Ruth S, Hart AA, Bonfrer JM, Verwaal VJ, Zoetmulder FA. Prognostic value of baseline and serial carcinoembryonic antigen and carbohydrate antigen 19.9 measurements in patients with pseudomyxoma peritonei treated with cytoreduction and hyperthermic intraperitoneal chemotherapy. *Annals of Surgical Oncology.* 2002;9:961–967.

30. Alexander-Sefre F, Chandrakumaran K, Banerjee S, Sexton R, Thomas JM, Moran B. Elevated tumour markers prior to complete tumour removal in patients with pseudomyxoma peritonei predict early recurrence. *Colorectal Disease.* 2005;7:382–386.

31. Taflampas P, Dayal S, Chandrakumaran K, Mohamed F, Cecil TD, Moran BJ. Pre-operative tumour marker status predicts recurrence and survival after complete cytoreduction and hyperthermic intraperitoneal

chemotherapy for appendiceal pseudomyxoma peritonei: Analysis of 519 patients. *European Journal of Surgical Oncology.* May 2014;40(5):515–520.

32. Moran B, Baralli D, Yan TD, Kusamura S, Deraco M. Consensus statement on the loco-regional treatment of appendiceal mucinous neoplasms with peritoneal dissemination (pseudomyxoma peritonei). *Journal of Surgical Oncology.* September 2008;98(4):277–282.

33. Sugarbaker PH, Chang D. Results of treatment of 385 patients with peritoneal surface spread of appendiceal malignancy. *Annals of Surgical Oncology.* 1999;6(8):727–731.

34. Youssef H, Newman C, Chandrakumaran K, Mohamed F, Cecil TD, Moran BJ. Operative findings, early complications, and long-term survival in 456 patients with pseudomyxoma peritonei syndrome of appendiceal origin. *Diseases of the Colon and Rectum.* March 2011;54(3):293–299.

35. Chua TC, Moran BJ, Sugarbaker PH, Levine EA, Glehen O, Gilly FN et al. Early- and long-term outcome data of patients with pseudomyxoma peritonei from appendiceal origin treated by a strategy of cytoreductive surgery and hyperthermic intraperitoneal chemotherapy. *Journal of Clinical Oncology.* July 2012;30(20):2449–2456.

36. Yan TD, Bijelic L, Sugarbaker PH. Critical analysis of treatment failure after complete cytoreductive surgery and perioperative intraperitoneal chemotherapy for peritoneal dissemination from appendiceal mucinous neoplasms. *Annals of Surgical Oncology.* 2007;14:2289–2299.

37. Taflampas P, Moran BJ. Extraperitoneal resection of the right colon for locally advanced colon cancer. *Colorectal Disease.* January 2013;15(1):e56–e59.

38. Ronnett BM, Zahn CM, Kurman RJ, Kass ME, Sugarbaker PH, Shmookler BM et al. Disseminated peritoneal adenomucinosis and peritoneal mucinous carcinomatosis. A clinicopathologic analysis of 109 cases with emphasis on distinguishing pathologic features, site of origin, prognosis and relationship to "pseudomyxoma peritonei". *American Journal of Surgical Pathology.* 1995;19:1390–1408.

39. Bradley RF, Stewart JH, Russell GB, Levine EA, Geisinger KR. Pseudomyxoma peritonei of appendiceal origin. *American Journal of Surgical Pathology.* 2006;30:551–559.

40. Carr NJ, Sobin LH. Adenocarcinoma of the appendix. In: Bosman FT, Carneiro F, Hruban RH et al., eds., *WHO Classification of Tumors of the Digestive System*, IARC: Lyon, France, 2010. pp. 122–125.

41. Carr NJ, Finch J, Ilesley IC, Chandrakumaran K, Mohamed F, Mirnezami A, Cecil T, Moran B. Pathology and prognosis in pseudomyxoma peritonei: A review of 274 cases. *Journal of Clinical Pathology.* October 2012;65(10):919–923.

42. Sugarbaker PH. Surgical treatment of peritoneal carcinomatosis: 1988 Du Pont lecture. *Canadian Journal of Surgery.* 1989;32:164–170.

43. Sugarbaker PH. Peritonectomy procedures. *Annals of Surgery.* 1995;221:29–42.

44. Gough DB, Donohue JH, Schutt AJ, Gonchoroff N, Goellner JR, Wilson TO et al. Pseudomyxoma peritonei: Long-term patient survival with an aggressive regional approach. *Annals of Surgery.* 1994;219:112–119.

45. Nitecki SS, Wolff BG, Schlinkert R, Sarr MG. The natural history of surgically treated primary adenocarcinoma of the appendix. *Annals of Surgery.* 1994;219:51–57.

46. Elias D, Gilly F, Quenet F, Bereder JM, Sidéris L, Mansvelt B et al. Pseudomyxoma peritonei: A French multicentric study of 301 patients treated with cytoreductive surgery and intraperitoneal chemotherapy. *European Journal of Surgical Oncology.* 2010;36:456–462.

47. Omohwo C, Nieroda CA, Studeman KD, Thieme H, Kostuik P, Ross AS et al. Complete cytoreduction offers long term survival in patients with peritoneal carcinomatosis from appendiceal tumors of unfavorable histology. *Journal of the American College of Surgeons.* 2009;209:308–312.

48. Jacquet P, Sugarbaker PH. Current methodologies for clinical assessment of patients with peritoneal carcinomatosis. *Journal of Experimental & Clinical Cancer Research.* 1996;15:49–58.

49. Spiliotis J, Efstathiou E, Halkia E, Vaxevanidou A, Datsis A, Sugarbaker P. The influence of tumor cell entrapment phenomenon on the natural history of pseudomyxoma peritonei syndrome. *Hepatogastroenterology.* May 2012;59(115):705–708.

Cytoreductive surgery and hyperthermic intraperitoneal chemotherapy for metastatic colorectal cancer with peritoneal surface disease

EDWARD A. LEVINE AND CHUKWUEMEKA OBIORA

Over the past 20 years, the treatment of metastatic colorectal cancer has undergone major changes. New chemotherapeutic and biologic agents have improved the median overall survival (OS) for some stage IV patients to 20+ months and beyond [1]. However, when patients present with isolated colorectal hepatic metastases (HMs) or pulmonary metastases, surgical resection has been shown in multiple large retrospective series to provide 5-year survival rates of 25%–40% with a median OS of 30–40 months [2–10]. In fact, a recent study from Memorial Sloan Kettering Cancer Center [8] reported on 10-year survivors after resection of liver metastases from colorectal cancer and found 17%–25% appeared to be cured of their disease. Based on these data and the improved safety of hepatic resection using modern operative techniques and better critical care support, a surgical approach to isolated metastatic disease to the liver has become the standard of care accepted by oncologists of all disciplines [11]. Resection of isolated pulmonary metastases has similar long-term outcomes. However, the resection and therapy of isolated peritoneal metastases has been more controversial.

At initial diagnosis, the peritoneal surface is involved by tumor in 10%–15% of patients with colorectal cancer [12–14]. Next to the liver, the peritoneal surface is the most common site for recurrence after purported curative primary tumor resections, occurring in as many as 50% of patients [12,15,16]. In 10%–35% of all patients with recurrent disease, the peritoneal surface is the only site of cancer [12–14]. Though patients with isolated peritoneal surface disease (PSD) from colorectal carcinoma have traditionally been treated with systemic therapy, there are few prospective studies documenting the natural history of this subset of patients. Systemic chemotherapy for metastatic colorectal cancer has clearly improved significantly since the turn of the century [17,18]. The availability of newer agents such as oxaliplatin and irinotecan and biologic agents such as cetuximab and bevacizumab has more than doubled the survival with systemic therapy alone [18,19]. There are no randomized trials of modern systemic therapy limited to patients with PSD. However, a retrospective study of the North Central Cancer Treatment Group 9741 and 9841 trials of systemic therapy for metastatic colon cancer stratified response by site of metastases [19]. That study clearly showed inferior outcomes with "modern" systemic therapy for patients with peritoneal metastases compared with metastases to other sites (12.7 vs. 17.6 months OS p < 0.001 and 5.8 vs. 7.2 months progression-free survival, p < 0.001). Despite this poorer outcome, it is noteworthy that with "modern" chemotherapy, there were a few 5-year survivors (4.1% with peritoneal metastases and 6% without peritoneal metastases), which represents a clear change from the era before newer agents for metastatic colorectal cancer became available [17,19].

The use of cytoreductive surgery (CS) and hyperthermic intraperitoneal chemotherapy (HIPEC) for PSD from colorectal cancer is a more recent development in oncologic surgery. Although originally described by Spratt at the University of Louisville in 1980, the concept of aggressive cytoreduction and HIPEC was initially investigated by a handful of centers [17,20,21] (see Figure 20.1). The rationale for CS for PSD is based on the idea of the peritoneum representing another organ site (such as the liver or lung) that can be completely resected and HIPEC being used as an "adjuvant" to treat microscopic residual disease. The literature supporting such an approach is not as extensive as it is for hepatic resection; it mainly consists of many single institutional series [17,22–29], one international multicenter retrospective review [12], and notably only a single prospective randomized trial [30]. Yet the reported outcomes are remarkably consistent, demonstrating 5-year OS rates of approximately 25%–40% for patients undergoing a complete cytoreduction. These studies, as well as recent reports of improved outcomes of intraperitoneal chemotherapy for advanced ovarian cancer [31], have fueled increasing interest in the use of CS and HIPEC for metastatic colorectal cancer over the past decade. However, despite the publication of consensus statements on the role of CS and HIPEC for PSD from colorectal cancer [32], the controversy continues regarding its efficacy, safety, and application in these patients. In contrast to hepatic resection, which is performed at virtually all major cancer centers throughout the world, only a handful of high-volume institutions have significant experience in this procedure. Due to the nature of this disease presentation, the surgical procedures required for complete cytoreduction of PSD have been associated with significant (but improving [29]) postoperative morbidity and mortality, which stresses patients, health-care resources, and personnel. Finally, attempts to conduct prospective randomized clinical trials to further define the efficacy of this approach have proven to be extremely difficult to conduct.

This chapter reviews our experience using CS–HIPEC to treat PSD from colorectal cancer and examine demographics, clinical outcomes, and prognostic factors for OS.

PATIENT SELECTION

It is imperative that appropriate candidates be selected for CS–HIPEC for peritoneal dissemination from any site, but particularly for colorectal cancer patients. Although distal rectal cancer arises in a retroperitoneal position, proximal rectal primary tumors can also be considered for HIPEC [33]. Preoperative evaluation includes complete history, physical examination, pathologic review, contrast-enhanced computed tomography (CT) or MRI, and laboratory examination including blood counts, CEA level, and renal and liver function panel. The requisite thorough preoperative evaluation may include endoscopy (if not done within the last 2 years); diagnostic laparoscopy has also been employed to determine the resectability of PSD prior to CS–HIPEC [34,35].

Previously published selection criteria for our group include the following:

1. The patient is sufficiently medically fit to undergo CS–HIPEC.
2. There is no extra-abdominal disease.
3. Peritoneal disease burden is potentially resectable (with residual lesions <5 mm).
4. No or limited and completely resectable parenchymal HM.
5. There is no bulky retroperitoneal disease or biliary obstruction [26,29].

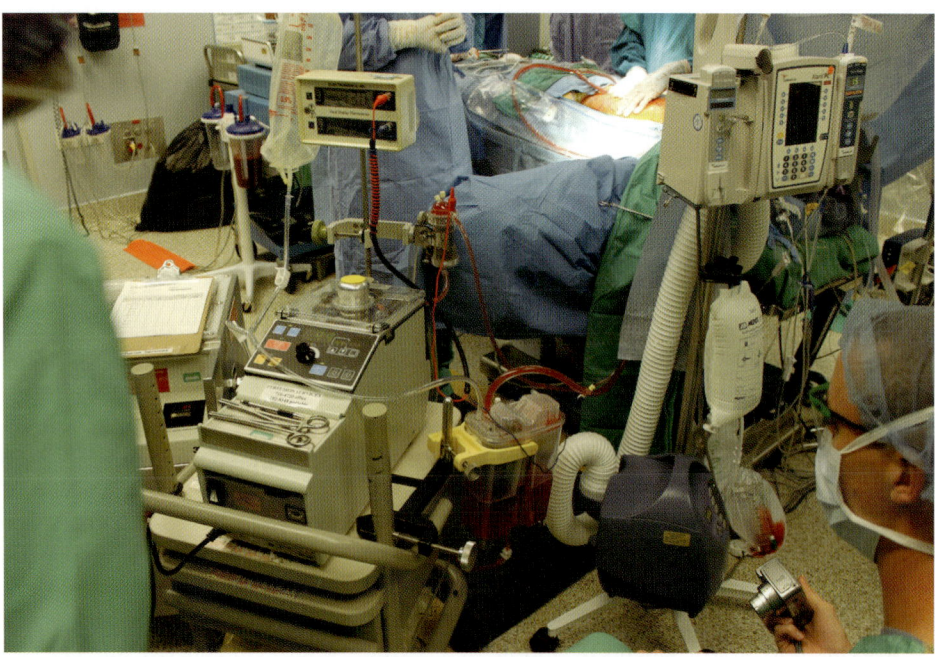

Figure 20.1 HIPEC perfusion (closed technique).

Although not an absolute contraindication, poor performance status and depression have been worse outcomes after CS–HIPEC. Patients with Eastern Cooperative Oncology Group performance status scores >2 are no longer candidates for the procedure in our clinics [29,36] Age [37] and obesity [38] are risk factors for any major oncologic resection; however, HIPEC can be performed in such patients and is not an absolute contraindication.

Other clinical factors we consider in selecting patients include the presence of a bowel obstruction (unless unifocal), malnutrition (albumin <3 g/dL), progression of disease on the best chemotherapy, and malignant ascites (which is a strong predictor of incomplete resection and as such also predicts worse survival) [39]. Scoring systems have been suggested as an aid to select patients most likely to be able to undergo complete cytoreductions [17,40]. However, such scoring systems (such as the PSD scoring system) have long-term survivors even in this highest-risk groups; therefore, it is difficult to deny a patient a HIPEC based upon a score alone [17].

CS–HIPEC FOR SYNCHRONOUS PERITONEAL AND LIVER METASTASIS

The role of CS–HIPEC in the setting of synchronous liver and peritoneal metastasis has long been debated. Glehen and coworkers [41] suggested that synchronous resection of liver metastasis at the time of CS–HIPEC for peritoneal carcinomatosis from colorectal cancer have negative prognostic value. However, results from Kianmanesh et al. [42] and Carmignani et al. [43] showed no difference in outcome with synchronous CS and liver resection. Our group [44] reported, respectively, OS of 23 months versus 15.8 months (p = 0.39) in patients undergoing CS–HIPEC with and without synchronous liver metastasis. However, most patients had a single small (median size 3 cm) liver lesion that was treated with minor hepatic resection. Hence, our practice has been to perform liver resection as part of CS for small lesion(s). Our most recent data, however, show that hepatic resection in the setting of an R0/R1 resection is associated with significantly worse median OS (21.2 vs. 33.6 months; p = 0.03) [45]. Currently, we consider patients for concomitant liver resections only if all disease can be resected/ablated, and the hepatic resection can be accomplished without the need for lobectomy.

GOAL OF CS–HIPEC

Complete cytoreduction of all gross disease is the primary objective for CS prior to HIPEC. It is quite clear that complete cytoreduction is a strong predictor of improved survival [12,25,26,29,30,46–48]. While long-term disease-free survival or cure can be achieved in a minority of cases, it is important to realize that essentially all long-term survivors have undergone a complete cytoreduction. Despite this, since most patients will recur even with a complete resection, attempts must be made to reduce as much of the tumor

burden as possible without compromising the safety (and future quality of life [QOL]) of the patient for cases in which complete cytoreduction is not feasible [29,46]. This is the crux of the learning curve for surgeons performing HIPEC, and substantial experience is therefore required with these challenging patients [17,29,49,50].

POSTOPERATIVE MORBIDITY AND MORTALITY

Given the magnitude of the surgical resections required to achieve adequate cytoreduction, it should not be surprising that the morbidity in these cases is significant. Overall major morbidity following CS–HIPEC ranges from 12% to 68% though comparison between studies is difficult due to the lack of a universally accepted grading system [29,46,50,51]. Complications are frequently divided into two groups based on whether they are believed to have arisen from the operation itself or represent toxicity from the chemotherapeutic agent. Operative mortality has been reported as high as 11% following CS–HIPEC, but is generally about 4% [12,17,29,52,53]. Common causes of death are bowel perforation, respiratory failure, bone marrow suppression, thromboembolic events, and various infections. Preoperatively, the presence of ascites, bowel obstruction, and poor performance status predicts mortality [17,29,50]. It is clear that morbidity and mortality rates are decreasing in recent years at larger centers, as surgeon/center experience and patient selection criteria continue to improve.

CLINICAL FOLLOW-UP

The clinical follow-up at our institution is typically scheduled at 1 month postprocedure and at least every 3–6 months thereafter for up to 5 years. The follow-up is coordinated with medical oncologists. After 5 years from their date of surgery, follow-up was annual. Chest x-ray or chest CT and abdominal/pelvic CT scans with oral and IV contrast were obtained along with a CEA (if elevated prior to resection) at each follow-up visit and when clinically indicated. Patients were typically followed up jointly with medical oncologists and received "adjuvant" systemic chemotherapy at their discretion on a case-by-case basis. Further, some patients who had undergone complete cytoreduction initially may become candidates for repeat procedures. With most recurrences being intraperitoneal, surveillance for such candidates is mandatory [54].

The experience with CS–HIPEC for colorectal cancer is predominantly retrospective (see Table 20.1). However, there is a single prospective randomized trial [30] and an international multicenter registry review [12]. In the one prospective randomized study, 105 patients with PSD from colorectal cancer were assigned to systemic chemotherapy consisting of 5-fluorouracil/leucovorin with or without palliative surgery or CS–HIPEC with mitomycin C followed by systemic chemotherapy. The initial publication reported a 9.7-month survival advantage in the experimental arm

Table 20.1 Outcomes following CRS–HIPEC for colorectal cancer

Author	Year	n	Drug	Median follow-up (months)	Median overall survival (months)	5-Year survival (%)	Major morbidity (%)	Mortality (%)
Shen et al. [26]	2004	77	MMC	15	16	17	30	12
Glehen et al. [12]	2004	506	Oxaliplatin or CDDP or 5-FU or LCV	53	19	19	22.9	4
Chua et al. [67]	2009	55	MMC HIPEC + 5-FU EPIC	19	36	60[a]	30.9	0
Elias et al. [68]	2010	523	Multiple regimens	45	30.1	27	31	3.3
Verwaal et al. [55]	2008	105	MMC	96	22.2	20	NR	NR
Elias et al. [28]	2009	48	Oxaliplatin	63	62.7	51	NR	NR
Franko et al. [69]	2010	67	MMC	NR	34.7	25	NR	NR
Levine et al. [29]	2014	232	MMC	54.1	16.4	18	31.3	2.6

NR, not reported; MMC, mitomycin C; CDDP, cisplatin; 5-FU, 5-fluorouracil; LCV, leucovorin.
[a] Three-year survival.

(p = 0.032). An update of this study with a median follow-up of 94 months reported a disease-specific survival of 12.6 months in the control arm and 22.2 months in the HIPEC arm (p = 0.028) [55]. Though randomized, the study was only from a single institution, and the systemic therapy regimen used is now outdated and so does not represent the standard of care at this time. The study has also been criticized because 17% of patients had appendiceal cancer with a better outcome (although the distribution of appendiceal cases favored the standard arm). In addition, the mortality rate for the experimental group was 8%, which is higher than reported in most other series.

The large multi-institutional study from Glehen et al. [12] included 506 patients from 28 institutions with a median follow-up of 53 months. The morbidity and mortality rates were 22.9% and 4%, respectively. Patients who underwent a complete cytoreduction had a median survival of 32.4 months. Positive independent prognostic factors for OS were complete cytoreduction, treatment by a second procedure, limited extent of peritoneal disease, age less than 65 years, and use of adjuvant chemotherapy. The survival outcomes from this study are consistent with smaller series from single institutions including the current series [17,26,28,40,56].

A multicenter retrospective report from Elias et al. examined the outcomes of 48 patients undergoing HIPEC with oxaliplatin compared to a group of 48 patients with limited PSD who were treated with systemic chemotherapy [28]. The control group in this manuscript was comprised of patients who were at centers that did not offer HIPEC and could not be referred to the reference center because of its limited capacity. The 5-year OS rates for the HIPEC and systemic therapy–only group were 51% and 13%, respectively. Median survival was 62.7 months in the HIPEC group versus 23.9 months in the systemic chemotherapy group (p < 0.05). Both groups received systemic therapy with a median of 2.3 regimens per patient. This report was the first to provide a comparison of patients with limited PSD from colorectal cancer treated

with modern systemic chemotherapy alone versus the addition of CS–HIPEC. Though the results with systemic therapy alone, with a median of 24 months, represent a substantial improvement over the 12.8-month median survival of similar patients in the randomized trail from Verwaal et al. [55], the addition of CS–HIPEC improved the median survival to 63 months. This trial supports the utility of CS and HIPEC even though retrospective and nonrandomized.

QUALITY OF LIFE AFTER CS–HIPEC

Unfortunately, most patients who undergo CS–HIPEC for colorectal cancer are not cured. The procedure can be a life-changing experience for some patients, and consideration of QOL after the procedure is a crucial part of preoperative and intraoperative decision making. Besides the considerable morbidity, some patients may have to deal with permanent ostomies as well as changes in bowel habits due to extensive removal of the small bowel and/or colon. All these factors play a role in affecting their postoperative QOL. Despite initial impairment in the QOL, several studies have shown improvement of the QOL in long-term survivors [57,58]. Passot et al. [59] prospectively followed 216 patients undergoing CS–HIPEC and found that the QOL significantly decreased for the first 6 months but subsequently returned to baseline at 12 months. Our group has published extensively comparing the QOL before and after HIPEC [36,58,60–63]. Data from these reports [60] indicate that patients initially have decreased physical and functional well-being scores, but these increase relative to baseline at 3, 6, and 12 months. However, depression symptoms may persist even 12 months after surgery. This highlights the importance of psychosocial support services to help patients deal with survivorship issues. Further, baseline QOL assessments can predict outcomes [36]. We have found that poor performance status, depressive symptoms, and poor baseline QOL predict poor outcomes; thus they should be considered in initial patient evaluations. Understanding the implications of the procedure on QOL is crucial for preoperative discussions with the patients and for selecting appropriate candidates.

CONSENSUS STATEMENTS

In an effort to promote cooperation among surgical oncologists who perform CS–HIPEC, consensus statements have been published, outlining a proposed algorithmic approach to the management of patients with PSD from colorectal cancer [32,64]. They stated that patients with resectable PSD without evidence of extra-abdominal disease should be referred to a peritoneal surface malignancy center to undergo evaluation for CS–HIPEC. This was a promising start toward standardization and increasing awareness of the role of CS–HIPEC for patients with carcinomatosis from colorectal cancer. However, simply printing guidelines does little to increase the acceptance of this procedure among medical oncologists, who are the primary referral physicians.

The results of these studies suggest that the peritoneum can be a target for a combined approach of aggressive resection and HIPEC when metastatic disease is confined to its surface. The oncologic principle is similar to that found in patients undergoing resection of colorectal HMs, resulting in a subset of patients achieving long-term survival. In fact, the OS in our study cohort was similar to patients undergoing hepatic resection for colorectal liver metastases at our institution. Further, resection (or ablation) of synchronous HMs (if complete) yields encouraging survival rates [45].

Patients with PSD from colorectal cancer should be referred to a peritoneal surface malignancy center to be evaluated for CS–HIPEC. A multidisciplinary strategy should then be formulated with the express goal of achieving a complete (R0/R1 or CC0) cytoreduction followed by HIPEC. The use of preoperative or adjuvant systemic therapy would be planned as well. It is time to reconsider our perception of peritoneal metastases from colorectal cancer with regard to potential for long term survival. Not all patients with PSD will succumb to the disease and approaching this with nihilism is no longer justified.

CURRENT CLINICAL TRIALS

The current level of evidence [32,64], however, may be insufficient to produce enough consensus among medical oncologists to change current practice for colorectal cancer with peritoneal metastases. Another phase III multicenter randomized trial is needed to validate and confirm the efficacy of this intervention. Additionally, this would accomplish other secondary objectives such as helping to define patient selection criteria and major prognostic factors prospectively. Preoperative imaging, surgical approaches, HIPEC techniques, and the optimal chemotherapeutic agents for the perfusion could also be evaluated and standardized. Despite substantial sustained efforts, randomized surgical trials have proven difficult to perform in the United States.

The single prospective trial that was opened supported by the Walter Reed Army Medical Center in collaboration with the NCI in August 2010 (NCT 1167725). Unfortunately, this trial accrued but a single patient (from Wake Forest), and so was closed. Further, cooperative group trials are not currently on the horizon in North America.

Despite difficulties conducting trials for PSD from colorectal cancer, several centers have persevered, with European centers making significant progress. There is an ongoing French trial called "Prodige 7," which randomizes patients with peritoneal dissemination from colon cancer after complete cytoreduction to observation or HIPEC (with oxaliplatin 460 mg/m^2 for 30 minutes at 42°C). This trial of 280 patients is nearing completion of accrual and should give insights into the contribution of HIPEC to cytoreduction. The investigators have suggested that OS is better than anticipated in both arms of the trial [65]. However, the applicability of this study, if negative, will be debated since both the high dose of oxaliplatin and short-duration HIPEC, are not commonly utilized outside of France. Another interesting trial from the French Prodige group is the Prodige 15 study. This trial planned for 130 patients is evaluating "high-risk" colorectal patients (those with perforation, ovarian metastasis, or a few peritoneal lesions completely resected with the primary lesion) and randomizing them, after 6 months of adjuvant systemic therapy to surveillance or second-look surgery with HIPEC [66].

CONCLUSIONS

Outcomes for patients with PSD from colorectal cancer optimally treated with CS–HIPEC result in approximately a quarter of patients achieving long-term survival. Further, the quality of life of long-term survivors is good, although returning to preoperative levels may take 1–6 months [62,63]. More work with preoperative imaging and definitions of resectability need to be done to improve the R0/R1 resection rate. Further study is required to determine the role of new intraperitoneal chemotherapy agents and neoadjuvant/adjuvant therapies. Systemic chemotherapy has clearly improved substantially over the past decade for colorectal cancer and remains the mainstay for treatment of stage IV disease. Patients with PSD do not fare as well as metastatic disease to other sites; however, CS–HIPEC should be considered in addition to systemic chemotherapy, not in lieu of it.

Patients with isolated PSD should be referred to a peritoneal surface malignancy center for a multidisciplinary evaluation. All too often, patients not treated in a multimodality environment face disease progression and referral (if at all) to a center only after the peritoneal carcinomatosis index (PCI) is too high to consider CS–HIPEC, and only palliative procedures remain an option. While systemic therapy should be part of treatment for essentially all patients with PSD from colorectal cancer, the optimal timing (preoperative, postoperative, or both) remains unclear at present. We currently favor a single course (four to six cycles) of chemotherapy prior to cytoreductive surgery and HIPEC for PSD from colorectal cancer. However, we hope that late referral of overtly symptomatic patients only after all conceivable chemotherapy options are exhausted be relegated to oncologic history. It is clear that intervention with CS–HIPEC has better outcomes when performed on patients with lower disease burden (PCI) and performance status not excessively degraded by extensive systemic therapy prior to intervention. Timely referral of patients (such as now commonplace for patients with hepatic metastasis) for CS–HIPEC is associated with better outcomes than found with systemic therapy alone. No longer do all patients with PSD rapidly succumb to the disease, and approaching this with nihilism is no longer justified.

REFERENCES

1. Kelly H, Goldberg RM. Systemic therapy for metastatic colorectal cancer: Current options, current evidence. *Journal of Clinical Oncology.* 2005;23:4553–4560.

2. Hughes KS, Rosenstein RB, Songhorabodi S, Adson MA, Ilstrup DM, Fortner JG et al. Resection of the liver for colorectal carcinoma metastases. A multi-institutional study of long-term survivors. *Diseases of the Colon and Rectum.* 1988;31:1–4.

3. Scheele J, Stang R, Altendorf-Hofmann A, Paul M. Resection of colorectal liver metastases. *World Journal of Surgery.* 1995;19:59–71.

4. Rosen CB, Nagorney DM, Taswell HF, Helgeson SL, Ilstrup DM, van Heerden JA, Adson MA. Perioperative blood transfusion and determinants of survival after liver resection for metastatic colorectal carcinoma. *Annals of Surgery.* 1992;216:493–504.

5. Gayowski TJ, Iwatsuki S, Madariaga JR, Selby R, Todo S, Irish W, Starzl TE. Experience in hepatic resection for metastatic colorectal cancer: Analysis of clinical and pathologic risk factors. *Surgery.* 1994;116:703–710.

6. Nordlinger B, Guiguet M, Vaillant JC, Balladur P, Boudjema K, Bachellier P, Jaeck D. Surgical resection of colorectal carcinoma metastases to the liver. A prognostic scoring system to improve case selection, based on 1568 patients. Association Française de Chirurgie. *Cancer.* 1996;77:1254–1262.

7. Jamison RL, Donohue JH, Nagorney DM, Rosen CB, Harmsen WS, Ilstrup DM. Hepatic resection for metastatic colorectal cancer results in cure for some patients. *Archives of Surgery.* 1997;132:505–510.

8. Fong Y, Fortner J, Sun RL, Brennan MF, Blumgart LH. Clinical score for predicting recurrence after hepatic resection for metastatic colorectal cancer: Analysis of 1001 consecutive cases. *Annals of Surgery.* 1999;230:309–318.

9. Choti MA, Sitzmann JV, Tiburi MF, Sumetchotimetha W, Rangsin R, Schulick RD et al. Trends in long-term survival following liver resection for hepatic colorectal metastases. *Annals of Surgery.* 2002;235:759–766.

10. Rees M, Tekkis PP, Welsh FK, O'Rourke T, John TG. Evaluation of long-term survival after hepatic resection for metastatic colorectal cancer: A multifactorial model of 929 patients. *Annals of Surgery.* 2008;247:125–135.

11. Adam R, Delvart V, Pascal G, Valeanu A, Castaing D, Azoulay D et al. Rescue surgery for unresectable colorectal liver metastases downstaged by chemotherapy: A model to predict long-term survival. *Annals of Surgery.* 2004;240:644–658.

12. Glehen O, Kwiatkowski F, Sugarbaker PH, Elias D, Levine EA, De Simone M et al. Cytoreductive surgery combined with perioperative intraperitoneal chemotherapy for the management of peritoneal carcinomatosis from colorectal cancer: A multi-institutional study. *Journal of Clinical Oncology.* 2004;22:3284–3292.

13. Dawson LE, Russell AH, Tong D, Wisbeck WM. Adenocarcinoma of the sigmoid colon: Sites of initial dissemination and clinical patterns of recurrence following surgery alone. *Journal of Surgical Oncology.* 1983;22:95–99.

14. Chu DZ, Lang NP, Thompson C, Osteen PK, Westbrook KC. Peritoneal carcinomatosis in non-gynecologic malignancy. A prospective study of prognostic factors. *Cancer.* 1989;63:364–367.

15. Knorr C, Reingruber B, Meyer T, Hohenberger W, Stremmel C. Peritoneal carcinomatosis of colorectal cancer: Incidence, prognosis, and treatment modalities. *International Journal of Colorectal Disease.* 2004;19:181–187.

16. Improved survival with preoperative radiotherapy in resectable rectal cancer. Swedish Rectal Cancer Trial. *The New England Journal of Medicine.* 1997;336:980–987.

17. Lambert LA. Recent advances in understanding and treating peritoneal carcinomatosis. *CA: A Cancer Journal for Clinicians.* July 2015;65(4):283–298.

18. Cersosimo RJ. Management of advance colorectal cancer, Part 1. *American Journal of Health-System Pharmacy.* 2013;70:395–406.

19. Franko J, Shi Q, Goldman CD, Pockaj BA, Nelson GD, Goldberg RM et al. Treatment of colorectal peritoneal carcinomatosis with systemic chemotherapy: A pooled analysis of North Central Cancer Treatment Group phase III trials N9741 and 9841. *Journal of Clinical Oncology.* 2012;30:263–267.

20. Spratt JS, Adcock RA, Muskovin M, Sherrill W, McKeown J. Clinical delivery system for intraperitoneal hyperthermic chemotherapy. *Cancer Research.* 1980;40(2):260.

21. Speyer JL, Collins JM, Dedrick RL, Brennan MF, Buckpitt AR, Londer H et al. Phase I and pharmacological studies of 5-flourouracil administered intraperitoneally. *Cancer Research*. 1980;40:567–572.

22. Sugarbaker PH, Jablonski KA. Prognostic features of 51 colorectal and 130 appendiceal cancer patients with peritoneal carcinomatosis treated by cytoreductive surgery and intraperitoneal chemotherapy. *Annals of Surgery*. 1995;221:124–132.

23. Loggie BW, Fleming RA, McQuellon RP, Russell GB, Geisinger KR. Cytoreductive surgery with intraperitoneal hyperthermic chemotherapy for disseminated peritoneal cancer of gastrointestinal origin. *The American Surgeon*. 2000;66:561–568.

24. Pestieau SR, Sugarbaker PH. Treatment of primary colon cancer with peritoneal carcinomatosis: Comparison of concomitant vs. delayed management. *Diseases of the Colon and Rectum*. 2000;43:1341–1348.

25. Elias D, Blot F, El Otmany A, Antoun S, Lasser P, Boige V et al. Curative treatment of peritoneal carcinomatosis arising from colorectal cancer by complete resection and intraperitoneal chemotherapy. *Cancer*. 2001;92:71–76.

26. Shen P, Hawksworth J, Lovato J, Loggie BW, Geisinger KR, Fleming RA, Levine EA. Cytoreductive surgery and intraperitoneal hyperthermic chemotherapy with mitomycin C for peritoneal carcinomatosis from nonappendiceal colorectal carcinoma. *Annals of Surgical Oncology*. 2004;11:178–186.

27. Barratti D, Kusamura S, Lusco D, Bonomi S, Grassi A, Virzi S et al. Postoperative complications after cytoreductive surgery and hyperthermic intraperitoneal chemotherapy affect long-term outcome of patients with peritoneal metastases from colorectal cancer: A two-center study of 101 patients. *Diseases of the Colon and Rectum*. 2014;57(7):858–868.

28. Elias D, Lefevre JH, Chevalier J, Brouquet A, Marchal F, Classe JM et al. Complete cytoreductive surgery plus intraperitoneal chemohyperthermia with oxaliplatin for peritoneal carcinomatosis of colorectal origin. *Journal of Clinical Oncology*. 2009;27:681–685.

29. Levine EA, Stewart JH, Shen P, Russell GB, Loggie BL, Votanopoulos KI. Cytoreductive surgery and intraperitoneal hyperthermic chemotherapy for peritoneal surface malignancy: Experience with 1,000 patients. *Journal of the American College of Surgeons*. 2014;518:573–587.

30. Verwaal VJ, van Ruth S, de Bree E, van Slooten GW, van Tinteren H, Boot H, Zoetmulder FA. Randomized trial of cytoreduction and hyperthermic intraperitoneal chemotherapy versus systemic chemotherapy and palliative surgery in patients with peritoneal carcinomatosis of colorectal cancer. *Journal of Clinical Oncology*. 2003;21:3737–3743.

31. Armstrong DK, Bundy B, Wenzel L, Huang HQ, Baergen R, Lele S et al. Intraperitoneal cisplatin and paclitaxel in ovarian cancer. *The New England Journal of Medicine*. 2006;354:34–43.

32. Esquivel J, Sticca R, Sugarbaker P, Levine E, Yan TD, Alexander R et al. Cytoreductive surgery and hyperthermic intraperitoneal chemotherapy in the management of peritoneal surface malignancies of colonic origin: A consensus statement. *Annals of Surgical Oncology*. 2007;14:128–133.

33. Votanopoulos KI, Aaron Blackham A, Ihemelandu C, Shen P, Stewart JH, Swett K, Levine EA. Cytoreductive surgery with hyperthermic intraperitoneal chemotherapy in peritoneal carcinomatosis from rectal cancer. *Annals of Surgical Oncology*. 2013;20:1088–1092.

34. Garofalo A, Valle M. Staging videolaparoscopy of peritoneal carcinomatosis. *Tumori*. July 2003;89(4 Suppl.):70–77.

35. Pomel C, Appleyard TL, Gouy S, Rouzier R, Elias D. The role of laparoscopy to evaluate candidates for complete cytoreduction of peritoneal carcinomatosis and hyperthermic intraperitoneal chemotherapy. *European Journal of Surgical Oncology*. June 2005;31(5):540–543.

36. Ihemelandu CU, McQuellon R, Shen P, Stewart JH, Votanopolos KI, Levine EA. Predicting postoperative morbidity following cytoreductive surgery with hyperthermic intraperitoneal chemotherapy (CS + HIPEC) with preoperative FACT - C (Functional Assessment of Cancer Therapy) and patient rated performance status. *Annals of Surgical Oncology*. 2013;20:3519–3526.

37. Votanopoulos KI, Newman NA, Russell G, Ihemelandu C, Shen P, Stewart JH, Levine EA. Outcomes of cytoreductive surgery (CRS) with hyperthermic intraperitoneal chemotherapy (HIPEC) in patients older than 70 years; survival benefit at considerable morbidity and mortality. *Annals of Surgical Oncology*. 2013;20:3497–3503.

38. Votanopoulos KI, Swords DS, Swett KR, Randle RW, Shen P, Stewart JH, Levine EA. Obesity and peritoneal surface disease; outcomes following cytoreductive surgery (CRS) with hyperthermic intraperitoneal chemotherapy (HIPEC) for appendiceal and colon primaries. *Annals of Surgical Oncology*. 2013;20:3899–3904.

39. Randle RR, Swett KR, Swords DS, Shen P, Stewart JH, Levine EA, Votanopoulos KI. Efficacy of cytoreductive surgery with hyperthermic intraperitoneal chemotherapy in the management of malignant ascites. *Annals of Surgical Oncology*. 2014;21(5):1474–1479.

40. Pelz JO, Stojandinovic A, Nissan A, Hohenberger W, Esquivel J. Evaluation of a peritoneal surface disease severity score in patients with colon cancer with peritoneal carcinomatosis. *Journal of Surgical Oncology*. 2009;99:9–15.

41. Cotte E, Passot G, Gilly FN, Glehen O. Selection of patients and staging of peritoneal surface malignancies. *World Journal of Gastrointestinal Oncology.* 2010;2:31–35.

42. Kianmanesh R, Scaringi S, Sabate JM, Castel B, Pons-Kerjean N, Coffin B, Hay JM, Flamant Y, Msika S. Iterative cytoreductive surgery associated with hyperthermic intraperitoneal chemotherapy for treatment of peritoneal carcinomatosis of colorectal origin with or without liver metastases. *Annals of Surgery.* April 2007;245(4):597–603.

43. Carmignani CP, Ortega-Perez G, Sugarbaker PH. The management of synchronous peritoneal carcinomatosis and hematogenous metastasis from colorectal cancer. *European Journal of Surgical Oncology.* May 2004;30(4):391–398.

44. Varban O, Levine EA, Stewart JH, McCoy TP, Shen P. Outcomes associated with cytoreductive surgery and intraperitoneal hyperthermic chemotherapy in colorectal cancer patients with peritoneal surface disease and hepatic metastases. *Cancer.* August 2009;115(15):3427–3436.

45. Blackham AU, Russell GB, Stewart JH, Votanopoulos K, Levine EA, Shen P. Metastatic colorectal cancer: Survival comparison of hepatic resection versus cytoreductive surgery and hyperthermic chemotherapy. *Annals of Surgical Oncology.* 2014;21:2667–2674.

46. Levine EA, Stewart JH, Russell GB, Geisinger KR, Loggie BL, Shen P. Cytoreductive surgery and intraperitoneal hyperthermic chemotherapy for peritoneal surface malignancy: Experience with 501 procedures. *Journal of the American College of Surgeons.* May 2007;204(5):943–953.

47. Gonzalez-Moreno S. Peritoneal surface oncology: A progress report. *European Journal of Surgical Oncology.* August 2006;32(6):593–596.

48. Glockzin G, Schlitt HJ, Piso P. Peritoneal carcinomatosis: Patients selection, perioperative complications and quality of life related to cytoreductive surgery and hyperthermic intraperitoneal chemotherapy. *World Journal of Surgical Oncology.* 2009;7:5.

49. Kusamura S, Baratti D, Deraco M. Multidimensional analysis of the learning curve for cytoreductive surgery and hyperthermic intraperitoneal chemotherapy in peritoneal surface malignancies. *Annals of Surgery.* February 2012;255(2):348–356.

50. Mohamed F, Moran BJ. Morbidity and mortality with cytoreductive surgery and intraperitoneal chemotherapy: The importance of a learning curve. *Cancer Journal.* May 2009;15(3):196–199.

51. Dindo D, Demartines N, Clavien PA. Classification of surgical complications: A new proposal with evaluation in a cohort of 6336 patients and results of a survey. *Annals of Surgery.* 2004;240:205–213.

52. Sugarbaker, PH. Cytoreductive surgery plus hyperthermic perioperative chemotherapy for selected patients with peritoneal metastases from colorectal cancer: A new standard of care or an experimental approach. *Gastroenterology Research and Practice.* 2012;2012:309417.

53. Jafari MD, Halabi WJ, Stamos MJ, Nguyen VQ, Carmichael JC, Mills SD, Pigazzi A. Surgical outcomes of hyperthermic intraperitoneal chemotherapy analysis of American College of Surgeons National Surgical Quality Improvement Program. *JAMA Surgery.* 2014;149(2):170–175.

54. Votanopoulos KI, Ihemelandu C, Shen P, Stewart JH 4th, Russell GB, Levine EA. Outcomes of repeat cytoreductive surgery with hyperthermic intraperitoneal chemotherapy for the treatment of peritoneal surface malignancy. *Journal of the American College of Surgeons.* September 2012;215(3):412–417.

55. Verwaal VJ, Bruin S, Boot H, van Slooten G, van Tinteren H. 8-Year follow-up of randomized trial: Cytoreduction and hyperthermic intraperitoneal chemotherapy versus systemic chemotherapy in patients with peritoneal carcinomatosis of colorectal cancer. *Annals of Surgical Oncology.* 2008;15:2426–2432.

56. Yan TD, Morris DL. Cytoreductive surgery and perioperative intraperitoneal chemotherapy for isolated colorectal peritoneal carcinomatosis: Experimental therapy of standard of care? *Annals of Surgery.* 2008;248:829–835.

57. Schmidt U, Dahlke MH, Klempnauer J, Schlitt HJ, Piso P. Perioperative morbidity and quality of life in long-term survivors following cytoreductive surgery and hyperthermic intraperitoneal chemotherapy. *European Journal of Surgical Oncology.* February 2005;31(1):53–58.

58. McQuellon RP, Loggie BW, Lehman AB, Russell GB, Fleming RA, Shen P, Levine EA. Long-term survivorship and quality of life after cytoreductive surgery plus intraperitoneal hyperthermic chemotherapy for peritoneal carcinomatosis. *Annals of Surgical Oncology.* March 2003;10(2):155–162.

59. Passot G, Bakrin N, Roux AS, Vaudoyer D, Gilly FN, Glehen O, Cotte E. Quality of life after cytoreductive surgery plus hyperthermic intraperitoneal chemotherapy: A prospective study of 216 patients. *European Journal of Surgical Oncology.* May 2014;40(5):529–535.

60. McQuellon RP, Loggie BW, Fleming RA, Russell GB, Lehman AB, Rambo TD. Quality of life after intraperitoneal hyperthermic chemotherapy (IPHC) for peritoneal carcinomatosis. *European Journal of Surgical Oncology.* February 2001;27(1):65–73.

61. McQuellon RP, Danhauer SC, Russell GB, Shen P, Fenstermaker J, Stewart JH, Levine EA. Monitoring health outcomes following cytoreductive surgery plus intraperitoneal hyperthermic chemotherapy for peritoneal carcinomatosis. *Annals of Surgical Oncology.* March 2007;14(3):1105–1113.

62. Duckworth KE, McQuellon RP, Russell GB, Cashwell CS, Shen P, Stewart JH, Levine EA. Patient reported outcomes and survivorship following cytoreductive surgery plus hyperthermic intraperitoneal chemotherapy (CS+HIPEC). *Journal of Surgical Oncology.* September 2012;106(4):376–380.

63. Hill AR, McQuellon RP, Russell GB, Shen P, Stewart JH, Levine EA. Survival and quality of life following cytoreductive surgery plus hyperthermic intraperitoneal chemotherapy for peritoneal carcinomatosis of colonic origin. *Annals of Surgical Oncology.* December 2011;18(13):3673–3679.

64. Turaga K, Levine E, Barone R, Sticca R, Petrelli N, Lambert L et al. Consensus guidelines from The American Society of Peritoneal Surface Malignancies on standardizing the delivery of hyperthermic intraperitoneal chemotherapy (HIPEC) in colorectal cancer patients in the United States. *Annals of Surgical Oncology.* 2014;21(5):1501–1505.

65. Elias D, Goere D, Dumont F, Honoré C, Dartigues P, Stoclin A et al. Role of hyperthermic intraoperative chemotherapy in the management of peritoneal metastases. *European Journal of Cancer.* 2014;50:332.

66. Elias D, Quenet F, Goere D. Current status and future directions in the treatment of peritoneal dissemination from colorectal carcinoma. *Surgical Oncology Clinics of North America.* 2012;21:611–623.

67. Chua TC, Yan TD, Zhao J, Morris DL. Peritoneal carcinomatosis and liver metastasis from colorectal cancer treated with cytoreductive surgery perioperative intraperitoneal chemotherapy and liver resection. *European Journal of Surgical Oncology.* December 2009;35(12):1299–1302.

68. Elias D, Gilly F, Boutitie F, Quenet F, Bereder JM, Mansvelt B, Lorimier G, Dube P, Glehen O. Peritoneal colorectal carcinomatosis treated with surgery and perioperative intraperitoneal chemotherapy: Retrospective analysis of 523 patients from a multicentric French study. *Journal of Clinical Oncology.* January 2010;28(1):63–68.

69. Franko J, Ibrahim Z, Gusani NJ, Holtzman MP, Bartlett DL, Zeh HJ 3rd. Cytoreductive surgery and hyperthermic intraperitoneal chemoperfusion versus systemic chemotherapy alone or colorectal peritoneal carcinomatosis. *Cancer.* August 2010;116(16):3756–3762.

21

Diffuse malignant peritoneal mesothelioma: Current concepts in evaluation and management

KELI M. TURNER AND H. RICHARD ALEXANDER, JR.

INTRODUCTION

In 1908, Drs. James Miller and William Wynn, both pathologists working in Birmingham, England, published a case report of a 32-year-old male miller who presented with weight loss and ascites. Over the course of 7 months, he underwent repeated paracenteses that drained large amounts of viscous fluid. He was eventually explored via a small infraumbilical incision, at which time a copious amount of mucinous ascites was evacuated. The visualized peritoneum was noted to be studded with innumerable soft, friable tissue nodules that varied in size. The patient was deemed inoperable and subsequently died. Autopsy revealed the diffuse nature of this process as tissue growths were noted covering the liver, spleen, and intestines; however, on microscopic analysis, the tumor cells appeared to infiltrate these organs rather than arise from them. Of particular interest was the absence of tumor cells in the lymphatics as well as lung or brain metastases indicating this process, even at an advanced stage, remained localized to the abdominal cavity. This published report is believed to be the first to describe malignant peritoneal mesothelioma. Although published over 100 years ago, the description of disease progression almost invariably within the abdominal cavity has become well established and serves as the basis for the development of cytoreductive surgery (CRS) with concomitant intraperitoneal chemotherapy [1].

Diffuse malignant peritoneal mesothelioma or DMPM is a rare cancer arising from the peritoneal lining of the abdominal cavity. There are approximately 250–500 cases of peritoneal mesothelioma in the United States each year with an equal incidence in males and females [2,3]. Several factors have been implicated in the development of mesothelioma including exposure to the mineral erionite [4], infection with simian virus 40 [5], and abdominal radiation [6]; however, the strongest association for the development of DMPM lies with asbestos exposure [7].

PRESENTATION, DIAGNOSIS, AND STAGING

DMPM has a heterogeneous tumor biology with some patients surviving years and others succumbing within months of diagnosis (Figure 21.1). The outcome of a cohort of 35 patients with DMPM has been reported recently and provides important insights into the natural history of this disease and factors associated with survival [8]. The report originated from Turkey where most patients are diagnosed late and only palliative or supportive care options are usually offered. The median survival time from diagnosis was 16 months; on multivariate analysis, factors associated with shortened survival were age greater than 60 years, poor Eastern Cooperative Oncology Group (ECOG) performance status (ECOG 3 vs. 0–2), and a long exposure to asbestos.

The initial presentation of patients with DMPM is typically nonspecific. The most common age range at initial presentation is between 40 and 65 years [9]. Patients most commonly present with abdominal pain and increasing abdominal girth, usually caused by ascites in over 60% of

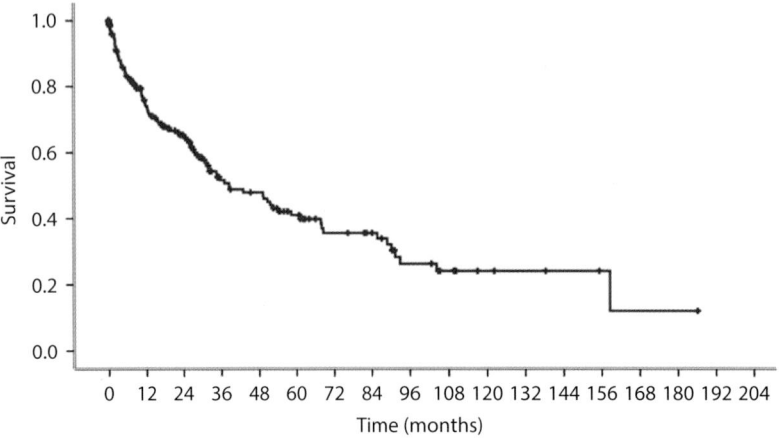

Figure 21.1 Long-term overall survival of a cohort of patients with peritoneal mesothelioma treated with cytoreductive surgery and hyperthermic intraperitoneal chemotherapy.

patients (Figure 21.2). Weight loss can also be noted, even in the presence of ascites. Occasionally, a palpable mass may be felt on abdominal examination [10–12]. The disease tends to remain confined to the abdominal cavity, although in late stages, spread to the lungs may occur via direct extension into the diaphragm or through transdiaphragmatic lymphatics. The condition is uniformly fatal with death being secondary

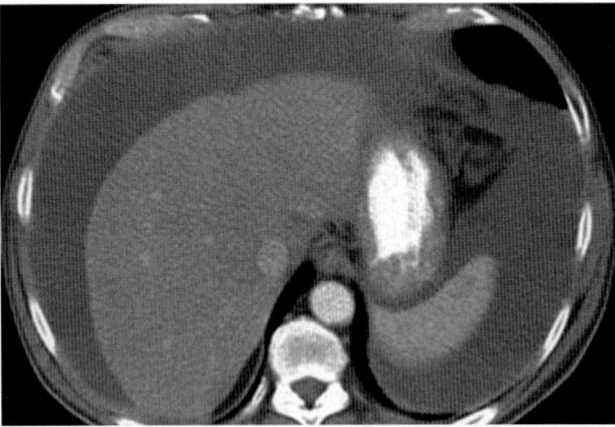

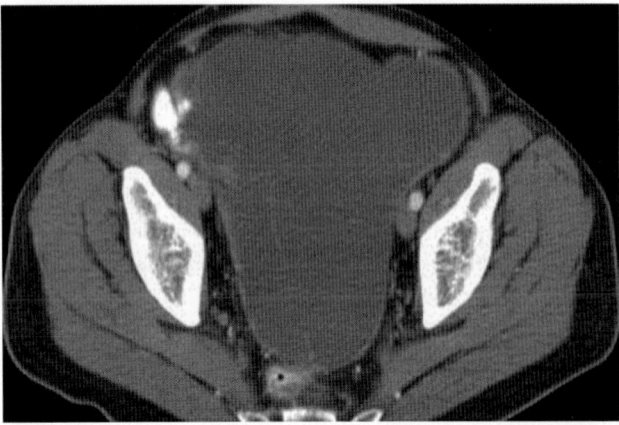

Figure 21.2 Computed tomographic images of a patient with diffuse malignant peritoneal mesothelioma manifested by ascites throughout the abdominal cavity.

to the consequences of intra-abdominal disease progression, namely, small bowel obstruction and cachexia [13]. Hematogenous and nodal metastases are rare occurrences.

The diagnosis of a patient with DMPM begins with a thorough history and physical examination that may demonstrate a protuberant abdomen with a fluid wave or palpable masses as mentioned earlier. Laboratory investigation may reveal an elevated CA-125; however, this value is not specific for diagnosis and is best used for patients with DMPM to monitor for disease recurrence or progression [14]. The imaging modality most commonly employed for diagnosis is contrast-enhanced computed tomography (CT) as it is the most useful at detecting many of the subtle findings characteristic of DMPM. The findings on abdominal CT concerning for peritoneal mesothelioma include peritoneal thickening, masses arising from the omentum or peritoneum, omental caking, and scalloping of solid abdominal organs that is reflective of tumor infiltration [15] (Figure 21.3). Assessment of the small bowel mesentery is critical as it provides information related to the feasibility of surgical resection in patients with DMPM [16]. As tumor infiltrates the mesentery of the small bowel, it may take on a pleated appearance while the mesenteric vessels develop an uncharacteristically straightened course [17]. The small bowel thickens as tumor invades its serosal surface. At the extreme of disease progression, the mesenteric vessels are obscured as the mesenteric fat is replaced by solid tumor, and bowel obstruction may be evident. These latter findings are associated with a suboptimal surgical resection and worse outcome [16]. Recent data suggest that diffusion-weighted and dynamic contrast-enhanced MRI may have an important role in assessing the extent of disease or peritoneal cancer index (PCI) in patients with peritoneal metastases who are being considered for CRS. In 33 patients undergoing CRS (only one had DMPM), the PCI was correctly predicted in 29 (88%) [18].

It is important to note that peritoneal metastases are most commonly secondary to dissemination from another organ such as the ovary or colon. Thus, patients who present

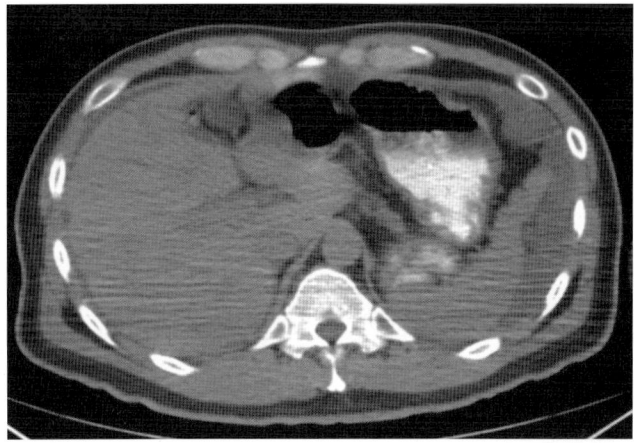

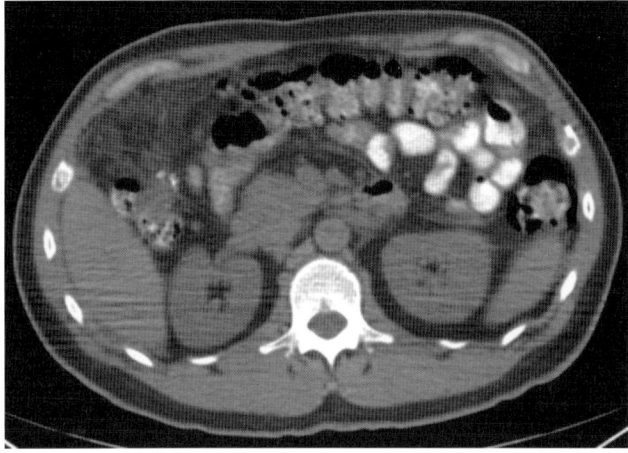

Figure 21.3 Computed tomographic images of a patient with diffuse malignant peritoneal mesothelioma demonstrating extensive peritoneal thickening and intra-abdominal soft tissue mass (top panel) along with omental thickening (bottom panel).

with evidence of a neoplastic process involving the peritoneum should also be evaluated for a primary malignancy elsewhere. For women, the malignancy that most commonly disseminates to the peritoneum is of epithelial ovarian origin, while a colorectal tumor is the most common malignancy leading to carcinomatosis in males. Additional neoplasms that spread to the peritoneum are stomach and pancreas. Upper and lower endoscopy should be included in the workup of any patient with peritoneal dissemination in whom the diagnosis of DMPM is questionable.

To definitively diagnose DMPM, tissue sampling is required. This may be performed by CT-guided core biopsy or diagnostic laparoscopy. Diagnostic laparoscopy allows for the assessment of tumor burden and thus the feasibility of successful operative intervention [19]. This is particularly advantageous as CT scan often underestimates the volume of disease. Patients with ascites often undergo diagnostic paracentesis, but this usually does not provide enough cellular material to establish a diagnosis of malignant mesothelioma [12]. When diagnostic paracentesis is suggestive of malignant mesothelioma, a pathologic specimen is still

required for immunohistochemical staining that definitively establishes the diagnosis. Antibodies that stain positive in DMPM are cytokeratin 5/6, calretinin, and vimentin. DMPM also stains positive for epithelial membrane antigen and Wilms tumor 1. Negative staining for CEA, Ber-EP4, TTF-1, and PAX-2 supports the diagnosis of DMPM [20].

If immunohistochemical staining is equivocal, electron microscopy can be utilized to identify DMPM. Electron microscopy is most beneficial for well- to moderately differentiated epithelioid tumors that show features typical of mesothelial cells such as long, thin microvilli and the presence of a basal lamina [21]. There are three well-established histopathological subtypes of DMPM: epithelioid, sarcomatous, and mixed/biphasic type. The epithelioid type is the most common and is associated with the best prognosis, while sarcomatoid features confer a poor prognosis [22,23] (Figure 21.4).

A modified "TNM" staging system has been proposed that stratifies the extent of disease in the peritoneum for the epithelial subtype of DMPM [24]. In this staging system, the PCI denotes the "T" stage, intra-abdominal nodal disease the "N" stage, and extra-abdominal disease the "M" stage. T1 represents a PCI less than or equal to 10, T2 a PCI between 11 and 20, T3 a PCI between 21 and 30, and T4 greater than 30. Based on this staging system, overall survival by stage has been reported as shown in the Table 21.1.

SYSTEMIC THERAPY

Without treatment, malignant peritoneal mesothelioma is uniformly fatal with an estimated survival of 6–16 months from the time of diagnosis [8,11,25]. Systemic therapy for peritoneal mesothelioma has been difficult to evaluate due to the rarity of the disease. One of the earliest trials that demonstrated the efficacy of systemic chemotherapy in the treatment of patients with DMPM was published in 1983. In this study, 14 chemotherapy naïve patients with peritoneal mesothelioma and measurable disease were evaluated for response after being treated with a doxorubicin-containing regimen. Six of the 14 patients (43%) had a response. The median survival of these patients was 22 months versus 5 months for the remaining eight patients with stable or progressive disease [10].

The largest study to evaluate the activity of systemic chemotherapy in patients with DMPM was published by Jänne and colleagues in 2005 [26]. This study was a nonrandomized trial that enrolled 98 patients with surgically unresectable peritoneal mesothelioma as part of an expanded access program prior to the approval of pemetrexed for the treatment of patients with pleural mesothelioma. Seventy-three patients were ultimately evaluated for tumor response by the RECIST criteria; 43 of those patients had been previously treated with chemotherapy. Patients received pemetrexed either alone or in combination with cisplatin. The median survival for patients who received the pemetrexed/cisplatin combination was longer than for patients who received pemetrexed alone (13.1 vs. 8.7 months). Moreover,

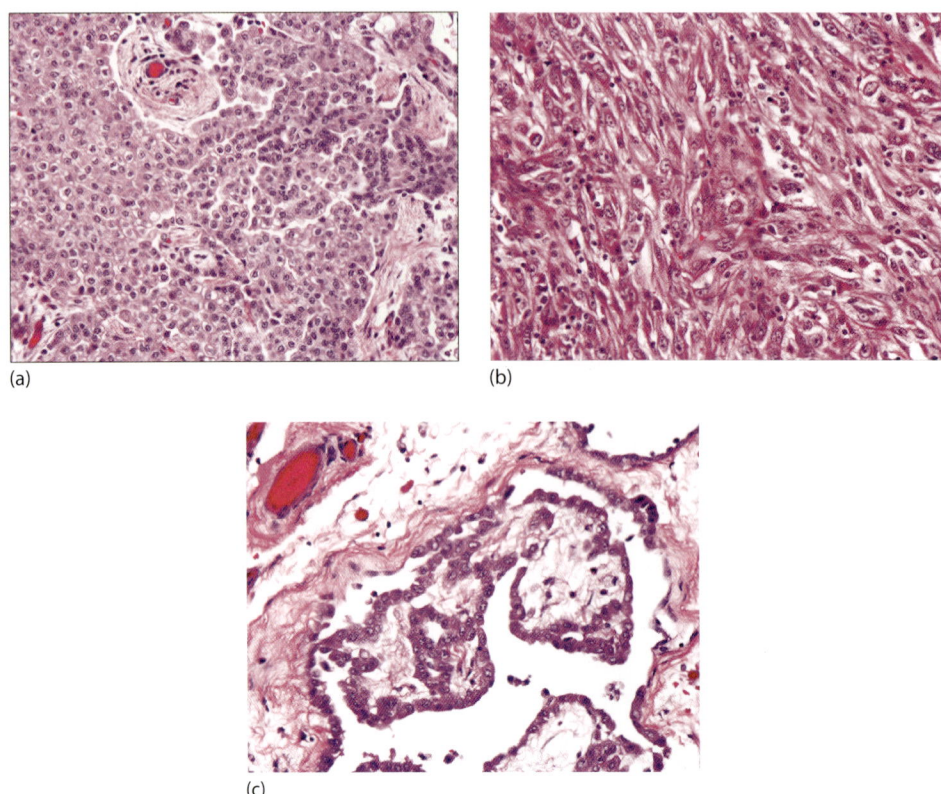

Figure 21.4 Light micrographs depicting the three main histological types of malignant peritoneal mesothelioma (a, epithelioid; b, sarcomatous; c, tubulopapillary).

Table 21.1 Staging system and survival data for 294 patients with diffuse malignant peritoneal mesothelioma

Stage	TNM	Median overall survival	5-year overall survival (%)
I	T1 N0 M0	Not reached	87
II	T2–3 N0 M0	67	53
III	T4 N0–1 M0–1	26	29
	T1–4 N1 M0–1		
	T1–4 N0–1 M1		

Source: Adapted from Yan, T.D. et al., *Cancer*, 117, 1855, 2010.

the response rate for patients who received the combination regimen was greater than for patients who received pemetrexed alone (30% for pemetrexed/cisplatin combination vs. 19% for pemetrexed). Of note, all of the complete responders in this study received the combination regimen. The results from this study established pemetrexed in combination with a platinum agent as first-line chemotherapy for patients with DMPM.

Immunotherapeutic approaches are now being tested as systemic treatment in patients with DMPM. Recently, the anti-CTLA-4 agent tremelimumab was administered to 29 patients with DMPM who had progressed after receiving a platinum-containing regimen. There were no complete responders, two partial responders, and seven patients with stable disease accounting for a disease control rate of 31%. The median overall survival (mos) was 10.7 months and the

median progression-free survival was 6.2 months. The most common side effects were dermatologic and gastrointestinal, which resolved with steroids when administered [27]. This phase II study is the first to evaluate the role of an immunologic agent in patients with DMPM. While the disease control rate and median overall survival were noteworthy, further study is warranted to determine the value of this agent in the treatment of patients with peritoneal mesothelioma.

OPERATIVE CYTOREDUCTION AND REGIONAL CHEMOTHERAPY

DMPM typically remains localized in the abdomen, with morbidity and mortality as consequences of disease progression there. Clinically, significant systemic metastases are very rare. Based on this natural history, operative strategies designed to control disease progression within the abdominal cavity have been developed. Currently, CRS with hyperthermic intraperitoneal chemotherapy (HIPEC) usually with mitomycin C or cisplatin has been established as standard of care for patients with DMPM.

The purpose of CRS and HIPEC is to eradicate disease within the abdominal cavity. CRS involves the systematic resection or ablation of tumors within the abdomen and pelvis combined with removal of the peritoneum underneath the diaphragm, along the abdominal wall, and within the pelvis [28]. Tumor implants on the small bowel mesentery and solid organ surfaces are treated with electrofulguration. Once gross disease is removed, heated chemotherapy is circulated into the abdomen via a perfusion circuit to eradicate small tumor deposits and microscopic disease. The technique of HIPEC has been described elsewhere [29]; in brief, large bore catheters are placed into the abdominal cavity and connected to an extracorporeal perfusion circuit consisting of a reservoir, heat exchanger, and roller pump. Temperature probes are placed in the abdominal wall or within the inflow and outflow cannulas to monitor the degree of hyperthermia. A 4–6 L perfusion is recirculated through the abdomen at a rate of about 1.5 L/min to provide a target tissue hyperthermia of approximately 40°C–41°C. During the perfusion, the abdomen is gently manipulated so that there is uniform distribution of the perfusate to all the serosal surfaces. The agents that are typically used for DMPM are mitomycin C and cisplatin. At the completion of the procedure, the perfusate is drained and the abdomen is closed.

There are two scoring systems utilized in CRS and HIPEC to codify tumor burden prior to and after CRS. PCI is an assessment of the size and distribution of cancer implants within the abdomen and pelvis calculated before surgery. The lowest score is zero (no disease burden) while the highest score is 39. The completeness of cytoreduction (CCR) score is calculated after operative resection to describe disease remaining after CRS and HIPEC. A score of 0 is assigned if no gross disease remains, while a score of 1 is given if tumor nodules remain that are ≤2.5 mm in diameter. Both of these scores are considered as evidence of a therapeutic cytoreduction. Residual disease that is greater than 2.5 mm in diameter is assigned a CCR of 3 or 4 depending on the size and extent of the tumor left behind. A decreased tumor burden after surgery as defined by a CCR of 0 or 1 has been shown to be independently associated with improved survival in several studies [30–32].

The morbidity of CRS and HIPEC in patients with DMPM can be quite significant (up to 31% in selected studies); thus, patient selection is critical to reduce morbidity and optimize patient outcome (Table 21.2) [22,30,32]. Only patients with a good performance status and who have disease that appears amenable to complete gross cytoreduction should be considered for this treatment approach. Yan and colleagues evaluated radiographic findings that signify the likelihood of a suboptimal cytoreduction and noted that patients with a tumor mass >5 cm in the epigastric region or those with grossly abnormal architecture of the small bowel such as nodular thickening and lack of mesenteric vessel clarity had a greater risk of suboptimal cytoreduction [16]. Relative contraindications to CRS and HIPEC are evidence of disease outside the peritoneal cavity, poor performance status, and severe cardiac, pulmonary, hepatic, or renal dysfunction. Morbidity from the procedure is usually secondary to intra-abdominal complications including fistula and abscess [30,32,33] (Table 21.2). The mortality rate following CRS and HIPEC is between 0% and 7% [22,30–32].

There are two large multicenter retrospective reviews and a number of single institutional retrospective reports detailing outcomes of patients undergoing CRS and HIPEC for DMPM (Table 21.3). Based on the long-term survival associated with CRS and HIPEC, this approach has been established as standard of care for selected patients with DMPM based on single-institution studies that consistently show an increased survival from this approach compared to survival data from treatment with systemic chemotherapy alone or in conjunction with palliative surgery. The overall median survival for patients treated with CRS and HIPEC ranges from 34.2 to 92 months in these studies [22,30–32,34,35].

Table 21.2 Complications after cytoreductive surgery and hyperthermic intraperitoneal chemotherapy in 211 diffuse malignant peritoneal mesothelioma patients

Patients returned to OR	9.4%
Operative mortality	2.3%
Length of hospital stay (median in days and range)	11 (2–64)
Types of Complications:	
Intra-abdominal (fistula, perforation, dehiscence, infection)	9.6%
Surgical site infection	4.4%
Noninfectious cardiopulmonary (pulmonary embolism, pleural effusion, atrial fibrillation)	12%
Gastrointestinal (ileus, vomiting, obstruction)	5.2%
Vascular (thrombosis, arterial injury)	3%
Hematologic	3.7%

Source: Adapted from *Surgery*, 153, Alexander, H.R., Jr., Bartlett, D.L., Pingpank, J.F., Libutti, S.K., Royal, R., Hughes, M.S., Holtzman, M. et al., Treatment factors associated with long-term survival after cytoreductive surgery and regional chemotherapy for patients with malignant peritoneal mesothelioma, 779–786, Copyright 2013, with permission from Elsevier.

Table 21.3 Results of two large multicenter reviews, a meta-analysis and a population study in diffuse malignant peritoneal mesothelioma

Center	N	Overall survival	Major findings of the study
Multicenter, United States, 2013 [32]	211	38 m (median) 5-year OS: 41% 10-year OS: 26%	CCR 0–1, age <60 years associated with better OS. HIPEC with cisplatin better OS than mitomycin C. Trend toward female gender and improved OS. CCR 0–1: 50%.
Multicenter, International, 2009 [30]	405	53 m (median) 3-year OS: 60% 5-year OS: 47%	Mean PCI: 20. CCR 0–1: 46%. Absence of LN mets better OS. CCR 0–1 better OS.
Meta-analysis, 2014 [43]	1047	5-year OS: 42%	Mean age at diagnosis: 51 years. Female gender: 59%. Median PCI: 19. CCR 0–1 achieved in 67%.
SEER database 2014 [44]	1591	9 m (median) In patients undergoing operation: 15 m (median) (1991–1995) 38 m (median) (2006–2010)	Includes all U.S. patients diagnosed in 1973–2010. Factors associated with shortened outcome were advancing age, male gender, biphasic histology, advanced tumor burden. Patients treated with operation had better OS.

A multi-institutional registry combining retrospective data on patients with DMPM treated with CRS and HIPEC at 29 clinical centers worldwide was published in 2009 [30]. This registry included 405 patients with DMPM; a variety of intraperitoneal chemotherapeutic agents was utilized during HIPEC including cisplatin, mitomycin C, and doxorubicin. The median actuarial overall survival was 53 months with 1-, 3-, and 5-year survival rates of 81%, 60%, and 47%, respectively. Prognostic factors that were shown to be independently associated with improved survival on multivariate analysis were epithelioid subtype, the absence of lymph node metastasis, CCR 0 or CCR 1, and the use of HIPEC. A second multicenter retrospective analysis of 211 patients treated with CRS and HIPEC at 3 centers in the Unites States has recently been reported [32]. All patients underwent CRS with HIPEC using either mitomycin C or cisplatin; the median overall survival was 38 months and the 5- and 10-year actuarial survival rates were 41% and 26%, respectively. Prognostic factors in this study that were associated with prolonged survival included age less than 60 years, complete or near-complete resection (CCR 0 or 1), low versus high histologic grade, and the use of cisplatin versus mitomycin C (Figure 21.5). The observation that the outcome was statistically better in patients treated with cisplatin than with mitomycin C was provocative; the salutary effect was seen only in the subgroup who had a complete or near-complete cytoreduction that strongly suggests a therapeutic effect of HIPEC with cisplatin.

The results of single-center studies provide additional insights into the use of CRS and HIPEC in the treatment of patients with DMPM. For example, investigators at Wake Forest University published an analysis of outcomes in patients with DMPM and showed that the use of cisplatin was associated with a better, but not statistically improved, survival compared to patients treated with mitomycin C. This is consistent with the findings in the multicenter study from the United States but in a separate patient cohort [36]. An older single-center study from the NCI on 49 patients with DMPM was reported in 2003. In this study, the 49 patients with DMPM underwent CRS and HIPEC with cisplatin [22]. Thirty-five patients were also treated with a single intraperitoneal dose of fluorouracil and paclitaxel on postoperative day 7–10. The median progression-free survival was 17 months, and the median actuarial overall survival was 92 months. The clinical or treatment parameters that were independent factors associated with prolonged survival were age 60 or younger and complete or near-complete cytoreduction. The pathological parameter associated with favorable outcome was the absence of deep tissue invasion and patients who had a history of a previous cytoreduction procedure. These latter two factors most likely represent surrogates for favorable tumor biology. More recently, a study from the University of Maryland also demonstrated the independent prognostic significance of tissue invasion on microscopic evaluation [20]. Tumor specimens from 73 patients with DMPM were codified with respect to the degree of tissue invasion as absent (0), into stroma (I), into fat (II), or into adjacent structures (III). Incomplete cytoreduction and degree of tissue invasion were independently associated with shortened survival. Conceptually, the two parameters are likely related and reflect aggressive tumor biology.

Several centers have reported results using various additional chemotherapy regimens based around a cytoreduction procedure. At New York-Presbyterian Hospital, a multimodal two-stage operative approach has been employed [37,38]. Between an initial operative exploration

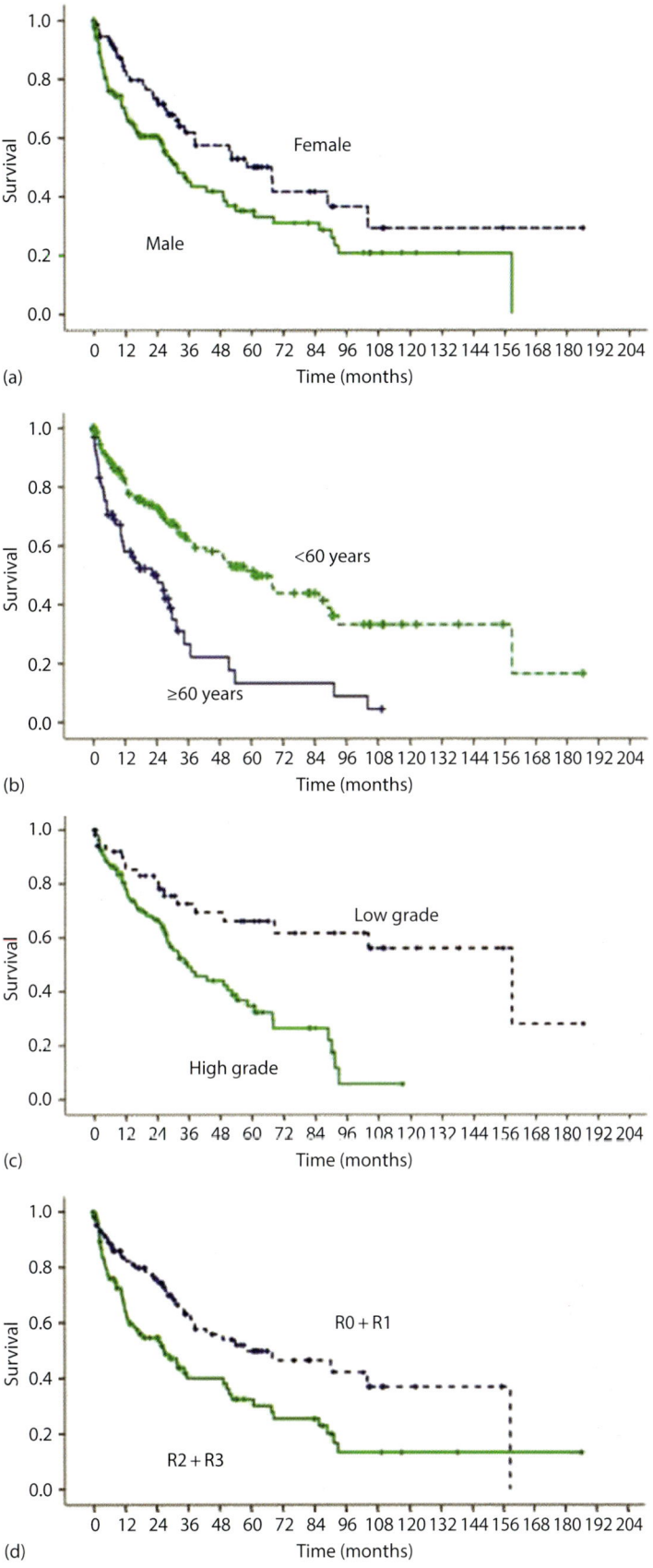

Figure 21.5 Overall survival of 211 patients with diffuse malignant peritoneal mesothelioma treated with cytoreductive surgery and hyperthermic intraperitoneal chemotherapy stratified by **(b)** age, **(a)** gender, **(c)** tumor grade, and **(d)** extent of cytoreduction.

and partial cytoreduction, patients receive intraperitoneal cisplatin, doxorubicin, and gamma interferon. Whole abdominal radiation has been eliminated from the regimen due to toxicity; the median overall survival was 70 months. The Washington Hospital Center has reported results of early postoperative intraperitoneal pemetrexed and intravenous cisplatin and CRS and HIPEC. The authors showed a favorable pharmacokinetic advantage to intraperitoneal pemetrexed [39]. Investigators from the NCI of Milan reported results in 116 patients with DMPM. In this study, some patients received pre- and/or postoperative systemic chemotherapy. Interestingly, there was no association between the use of preoperative chemotherapy and CCR or operative morbidity. Chemotherapy given pre- or postoperatively was not associated with an improvement in survival compared to those that did not receive chemotherapy [40].

Other important observations that have been reported are that CRS and HIPEC results in palliation of malignant ascites in this patient population in over 90% of patients [41]. Moreover, the use of a repeat CRS and HIPEC is associated with long-term survival in selected patients [22,42].

Two population-based studies have been reported regarding the use of CRS and HIPEC in DMPM patients. A meta-analysis of 1047 patients with DMPM undergoing CRS and HIPEC derived from 20 publications reported an estimated 5-year actuarial survival of 42% [43]. Complete or near-complete CRS was achieved in 42%. An analysis of 1591 patients diagnosed with DMPM between 1973 and 2010 were identified in the Surveillance, Epidemiology, and End Results database [44]. Factors identified with shortened survival include advancing age, male gender, biphasic versus epithelioid histology, and advanced burden of disease.

FUTURE DIRECTIONS

Recent studies have established a possible role of phosphatidylinositol-3 kinase and mammalian target of rapamycin (PI3K/mTOR) signaling pathways and mutations in the epidermal growth factor receptor in DMPM [45]. In the first study, a gene expression analysis on 41 tumor samples was performed to identify potentially important genes and pathways in DMPM. Investigators showed that patients with poor survival had tumors with significantly higher expression of the genes of PI3K/mTOR signaling. Moreover, inhibiting the PI3K/mTOR pathway in mesothelioma cell lines led to inhibition in DMPM cell proliferation.

CONCLUSIONS

Diffuse malignant peritoneal mesothelioma (DMPM) is a rare malignancy that affects the peritoneal surfaces of the abdominal cavity. Considerable progress has been made toward a cure for this condition since Miller and Wynn's sentinel paper over 100 years ago. In recent decades, treatment with systemic chemotherapy has resulted in prolonged survival for this disease when compared to historical controls. However, the combined approach of cytoreductive surgery (CRS) and hyperthermic intraperitoneal chemotherapy (HIPEC) has become the standard of care for patients with DMPM as it has been shown to consistently result in durable long-term survival. This treatment strategy continues to be refined as data emerge regarding the optimal intraperitoneal chemotherapeutic agent and the efficacy of CRS and HIPEC performed in a repeated fashion. Moreover, adjunctive therapies utilizing systemic chemotherapy, immunotherapy, and targeted molecular therapy are increasingly being utilized to augment this surgical strategy in order to create a multimodal approach to the treatment of this condition.

REFERENCES

1. Miller JA, Wynn WH. Malignant tumor arising from endothelium of peritoneum, and producing mucoid ascitic fluid. *The Journal of Pathology and Bacteriology.* 1908;12:267–278.
2. Price B, Ware A. Mesothelioma trends in the United States: An update based on Surveillance, Epidemiology, and End Results Program data for 1973 through 2003. *American Journal of Epidemiology.* 2004;159:107–112.
3. Moolgavkar SH, Meza R, Turim J. Pleural and peritoneal mesotheliomas in SEER: Age effects and temporal trends, 1973–2005. *Cancer Causes and Control.* 2009;20:935–944.
4. Carbone M, Emri S, Dogan AU, Steele I, Tuncer M, Pass HI et al. A mesothelioma epidemic in Cappadocia: Scientific developments and unexpected social outcomes. *Nature Reviews. Cancer.* 2007;7:147–154.
5. Rivera Z, Strianese O, Bertino P, Yang H, Pass H, Carbone M. The relationship between simian virus 40 and mesothelioma. *Current Opinion in Pulmonary Medicine.* 2008;14:316–321.
6. Gilks B, Hegedus C, Freeman H, Fratkin L, Churg A. Malignant peritoneal mesothelioma after remote abdominal radiation. *Cancer.* 1988;61:2019–2021.
7. Selikoff IJ, Churg J, Hammond EC. Relation between exposure to asbestos and mesothelioma. *The New England Journal of Medicine.* 1965;272:560–565.
8. Kaya H, Sezgi C, Tanrikulu AC, Taylan M, Abakay O, Sen HS et al. Prognostic factors influencing survival in 35 patients with malignant peritoneal mesothelioma. *Neoplasma.* 2014;61:433–438.
9. Alexander HR, Hanna N, Pingpank JF. Clinical results of cytoreduction and HIPEC for malignant peritoneal mesothelioma. *Cancer Treatment and Research.* 2007;134:343–355.
10. Antman K, Pomfret F, Aisner J, MacIntyre J, Osteen RT, Greenberger JS. Peritoneal mesothelioma: Natural history and response to chemotherapy. *Journal of Clinical Oncology.* 1983;1:386.
11. Moertel C. Peritoneal mesothelioma. *Gastroenterology.* 1972;63:346–350.

12. Sugarbaker PH, Welch LS, Mohamed F, Glehen O. A review of peritoneal mesothelioma at the Washington Cancer Institute. *Surgical Oncology Clinics of North America.* 2003;12:605–621, xi.

13. Antman KH, Blum RH, Greenberger JS, Flowerdew G, Skarin AT, Canellos GP. Multimodality therapy for malignant mesothelioma based on a study of natural history. *American Journal of Medicine.* 1980;68:356–362.

14. Baratti D, Kusamura S, Martinetti A, Seregni E, Laterza B, Oliva DG et al. Prognostic value of circulating tumor markers in patients with pseudomyxoma peritonei treated with cytoreductive surgery and hyperthermic intraperitoneal chemotherapy. *Annals of Surgical Oncology.* 2007;14:2300–2308.

15. Park JY, Kim KW, Kwon HJ, Park MS, Kwon GY, Jun SY et al. Peritoneal mesotheliomas: Clinicopathologic features, CT findings, and differential diagnosis. *AJR American Journal of Roentgenology.* 2008;191:814–825.

16. Yan TD, Haveric N, Carmignani CP, Chang D, Sugarbaker PH. Abdominal computed tomography scans in the selection of patients with malignant peritoneal mesothelioma for comprehensive treatment with cytoreductive surgery and perioperative intraperitoneal chemotherapy. *Cancer.* 2005;103:839–849.

17. Levy AD, Arnaiz J, Shaw JC, Sobin LH. From the archives of the AFIP: Primary peritoneal tumors: Imaging features with pathologic correlation. *Radiographics.* 2008;28:583–607.

18. Low RN, Barone RM. Combined diffusion-weighted and gadolinium-enhanced MRI can accurately predict the peritoneal cancer index preoperatively in patients being considered for cytoreductive surgical procedures. *Annals of Surgical Oncology.* 2012;19:1394–1401.

19. Deraco M, Bartlett D, Kusmaura S, Baratti D. Consensus statement on peritoneal mesothelioma. *Journal of Surgical Oncology.* 2008;98:268–272.

20. Lee M, Alexander HR, Burke A. Diffuse mesothelioma of the peritoneum: A pathological study of 64 tumours treated with cytoreductive therapy. *Pathology.* 2013;45:464–473.

21. Husain AN, Colby TV, Ordonez NG, Krausz T, Borczuk A, Cagle PT et al. Guidelines for pathologic diagnosis of malignant mesothelioma: A consensus statement from the International Mesothelioma Interest Group. *Archives of Pathology & Laboratory Medicine.* 2009;133:1317–1331.

22. Feldman AL, Libutti SK, Pingpank JF, Bartlett DL, Beresnev TH, Mavroukakis SM et al. Analysis of factors associated with outcome in patients with malignant peritoneal mesothelioma undergoing surgical debulking and intraperitoneal chemotherapy. *Journal of Clinical Oncology.* 2003;21:4560–4567.

23. Cerruto CA, Brun EA, Chang D, Sugarbaker PH. Prognostic significance of histomorphologic parameters in diffuse malignant peritoneal mesothelioma. *Archives of Pathology & Laboratory Medicine.* 2006;130:1654–1661.

24. Yan TD, Deraco M, Elias D, Glehen O, Levine EA, Moran BJ et al. A novel tumor-node-metastasis (TNM) staging system of diffuse malignant peritoneal mesothelioma using outcome analysis of a multi-institutional database. *Cancer.* 2010;117:1855–1863.

25. Eltabbakh GH, Piver MS, Hempling RE, Recio FO, Intengen ME. Clinical picture, response to therapy, and survival of women with diffuse malignant peritoneal mesothelioma. *Journal of Surgical Oncology.* 1999;70:6–12.

26. Jänne PA, Wozniak AJ, Belani CP, Keohan ML, Ross HJ, Polikoff JA et al. Open-label study of pemetrexed alone or in combination with cisplatin for the treatment of patients with peritoneal mesothelioma: Outcomes of an expanded access program. *Clinical Lung Cancer.* 2005;7:40–46.

27. Calabro L, Morra A, Fonsatti E, Cutaia O, Amato G, Giannarelli D et al. Tremelimumab for patients with chemotherapy-resistant advanced malignant mesothelioma: An open-label, single-arm, phase 2 trial. *The Lancet Oncology.* 2013;14:1104–1111.

28. Sugarbaker PH. Peritonectomy procedures. *Annals of Surgery.* 1995;221:29–42.

29. Turner KM, Hanna NN, Zhu Y, Jain A, Kesmodel SB, Switzer RA et al. Assessment of neoadjuvant chemotherapy on operative parameters and outcome in patients with peritoneal dissemination from high-grade appendiceal cancer. *Annals of Surgical Oncology.* 2013;20:1068–1073.

30. Yan TD, Deraco M, Baratti D, Kusamura S, Elias D, Glehen O et al. Cytoreductive surgery and hyperthermic intraperitoneal chemotherapy for malignant peritoneal mesothelioma: Multi-institutional experience. *Journal of Clinical Oncology.* 2009;27:6237–6242.

31. Sugarbaker PH, Yan TD, Stuart OA, Yoo D. Comprehensive management of diffuse malignant peritoneal mesothelioma. *European Journal of Surgical Oncology.* 2006;32:686–691.

32. Alexander HR Jr., Bartlett DL, Pingpank JF, Libutti SK, Royal R, Hughes MS et al. Treatment factors associated with long-term survival after cytoreductive surgery and regional chemotherapy for patients with malignant peritoneal mesothelioma. *Surgery.* 2013;153:779–786.

33. Deraco M, Casali P, Inglese MG, Baratti D, Pennacchioli E, Bertulli R et al. Peritoneal mesothelioma treated by induction chemotherapy, cytoreductive surgery, and intraperitoneal hyperthermic perfusion. *Journal of Surgical Oncology.* 2003;83:147–153.

34. Brigand C, Monneuse O, Mohamed F, Sayag-Beaujard AC, Issac S, Gilly FN et al. Peritoneal mesothelioma treated by cytoreductive surgery and intraperitoneal hyperthermic chemotherapy: Results of a prospective study. *Annals of Surgical Oncology.* 2006;13:405–412.

35. Loggie BW, Fleming RA, McQuellon RP, Russell GB, Geisinger KR, Levine EA. Prospective trial for the treatment of malignant peritoneal mesothelioma. *The American Surgeon.* 2001;67:999–1003.

36. Blackham AU, Shen P, Stewart JH, Russell GB, Levine EA. Cytoreductive surgery with intraperitoneal hyperthermic chemotherapy for malignant peritoneal mesothelioma: Mitomycin versus cisplatin. *Annals of Surgical Oncology.* 2010;17:2720–2727.

37. Hesdorffer ME, Chabot JA, Keohan ML, Fountain K, Talbot S, Gabay M et al. Combined resection, intraperitoneal chemotherapy, and whole abdominal radiation for the treatment of malignant peritoneal mesothelioma. *American Journal of Clinical Oncology.* 2008;31:49–54.

38. Hassan R, Alexander R, Antman K, Boffetta P, Churg A, Coit D et al. Current treatment options and biology of peritoneal mesothelioma: Meeting summary of the first NIH peritoneal mesothelioma conference. *Annals of Oncology.* 2006;17:1615–1619.

39. Bijelic L, Stuart OA, Sugarbaker P. Adjuvant bidirectional chemotherapy with intraperitoneal pemetrexed combined with intravenous cisplatin for diffuse malignant peritoneal mesothelioma. *Gastroenterology Research and Practice.* 2012;2012:Article ID:890450.

40. Deraco M, Baratti D, Hutanu I, Bertuli R, Kusamura S. The role of perioperative systemic chemotherapy in diffuse malignant peritoneal mesothelioma patients treated with cytoreductive surgery and hyperthermic intraperitoneal chemotherapy. *Annals of Surgical Oncology.* 2013;20:1093–1100.

41. Randle RW, Swett KR, Swords DS, Shen P, Stewart JH, Levine EA et al. Efficacy of cytoreductive surgery with hyperthermic intraperitoneal chemotherapy in the management of malignant ascites. *Annals of Surgical Oncology.* 2014;21:1474–1479.

42. Ihemelandu C, Bijelic L, Sugarbaker PH. Iterative cytoreductive surgery and hyperthermic intraperitoneal chemotherapy for recurrent or progressive diffuse malignant peritoneal mesothelioma: Clinicopathologic characteristics and survival outcome. *Annals of Surgical Oncology.* 2015;22:1680–1685.

43. Helm JH, Miura JT, Glenn JA, Marcus RK, Larrieux G, Jayakrishnan TT et al. Cytoreductive surgery and hyperthermic intraperitoneal chemotherapy for malignant peritoneal mesothelioma: A systematic review and meta-analysis. *Annals of Surgical Oncology.* 2015;22:1686–1693.

44. Miura JT, Johnston FM, Gamblin TC, Turaga KK. Current trends in the management of malignant peritoneal mesothelioma. *Annals of Surgical Oncology.* 2014;21:3947–3953.

45. Varghese S, Chen Z, Bartlett DL, Pingpank JF, Libutti SK, Steinberg SM et al. Activation of the phosphoinositide-3-kinase and mammalian target of rapamycin signaling pathways are associated with shortened survival in patients with malignant peritoneal mesothelioma. *Cancer.* 2011;117:361–371.

22

Gastric cancer and intraperitoneal chemotherapy

VALERIE FRANCESCUTTI, JOHN M. KANE III, AND JOSEPH J. SKITZKI

EPIDEMIOLOGY

Gastric cancer is a worldwide health problem and is second to lung cancer as the leading cause of cancer-related mortality [1]. It remains the fourth most common cancer globally, and incidence over the last several decades has been steadily falling [2]. The incidence remains the highest in the Asian countries including China and Japan and also in South America [3].

In the United States, gastric cancer rarely occurs before the age of 40, with the peak of incidence in the seventh decade. It is also at least twice as common in men as in women and more common in African, Hispanic, and Native Americans compared with Caucasians [4].

HISTOLOGY AND ANATOMY

Over 90% of gastric cancers are adenocarcinomas, with the remaining 10% consisting of lymphomas, neuroendocrine tumors, and gastrointestinal stromal tumors [3]. Considering all gastric adenocarcinomas, the incidence of adenocarcinoma of the distal stomach is falling, whereas the incidence of proximal adenocarcinomas, mainly of the gastric cardia, is rising [5]. The most widely accepted histologic classification system for gastric adenocarcinoma is that proposed by Lauren; the intestinal-type adenocarcinomas are generally located in the distal stomach and are usually well differentiated, whereas the diffuse-type adenocarcinomas present with a linitis plastica type of picture have signet-ring features and are generally more aggressive with a worse prognosis [6].

DIAGNOSIS AND STAGING

One of the main difficulties in treating gastric adenocarcinoma is the fact that diagnosis generally occurs at a late stage, especially in North American countries, related to low disease prevalence and lack of screening programs that exist in Asian countries. Diagnostic esophagogastroduodenoscopy is generally the first test used to obtain a tissue diagnosis, in particular when symptoms of ongoing dyspepsia, weight loss, hematemesis, melena, or anemia occur [7].

The AJCC TNM staging system used for gastric cancer includes the T stage, which is depth of invasion into the gastric wall; N stage, which includes regional lymph node metastases; and M stage, which includes distant metastatic disease (Table 22.1) [8]. In general, computed tomography (CT) scan is the main modality used to evaluate for M stage, in particular liver and lung metastases. However, CT has not been found to be particularly helpful in evaluating nodal metastases or peritoneal metastases.

An adjunct to the staging process has included endoscopic ultrasound (EUS) to assist in evaluating T stage, with a cited accuracy of approximately 80%–90%, compared with 20%–30% for CT scan. For N stage, EUS has had an accuracy of 70%–80%, compared with 30%–40% with CT [9]. For M stage, EUS has been able

Table 22.1 TNM staging system for gastric cancer

Tumor (T)

TX	Primary tumor cannot be assessed.
T0	No evidence of primary tumor.
Tis	Carcinoma in situ, intraepithelial tumor without invasion of the lamina propria.
T1	Tumor invades lamina propria, muscularis mucosae, or submucosa.
T1a	Tumor invades lamina propria or muscularis mucosae.
T1b	Tumor invades submucosa.
T2	Tumor invades muscularis propria.
T3	Tumor penetrates subserosal connective tissue without invasion of visceral peritoneum or adjacent structures.
T4	Tumor invades serosa or adjacent structures.
T4a	Tumor invades serosa.
T4b	Tumor invades adjacent structures.

Lymph nodes (N)

NX	Regional lymph node(s) cannot be assessed.
N0	No regional lymph node metastasis.
N1	Metastases in 1–2 regional lymph nodes.
N2	Metastases in 3–6 regional lymph nodes.
N3	Metastases in ≥7 regional lymph nodes.
N3a	Metastases in 7–15 regional lymph nodes.
N3b	Metastases in ≥16 regional lymph nodes.

Distant metastasis (M)

M0	No distant metastasis.
M1	Distant metastasis.

Source: Adapted from Edge, S.B. et al., *Ann. Surg. Oncol.*, 17(6), 1471, 2010.

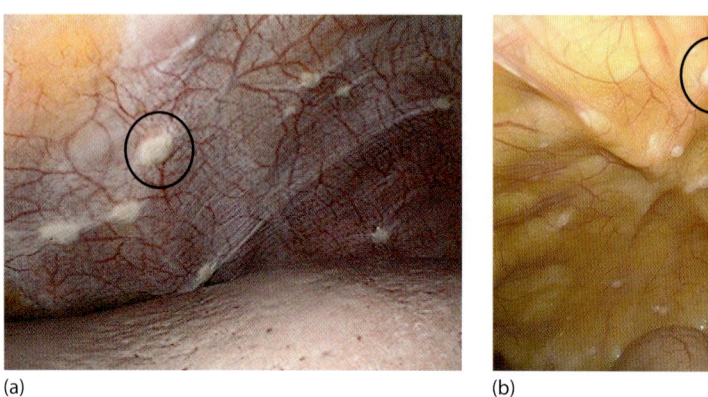

(a)   (b)

Figure 22.1 Intraoperative video screen capture during diagnostic laparoscopy shows **(a)** scattered gastric cancer peritoneal nodules on the surface of the left hemidiaphragm and **(b)** peritoneal nodules on the anterior abdominal wall looking into the pelvis.

to demonstrate low-volume ascites or small left-sided liver metastases not seen on CT. This modality can also be used to obtain fine-needle aspiration samples of suspicious appearing lymph nodes, ascites fluid, or liver masses for staging [10].

In the past, peritoneal metastases were typically discovered at the time of attempted curative gastric resection, given poor detection on preoperative staging CT scans. The introduction of laparoscopy permitted a more minimally invasive manner in which to evaluate the peritoneal cavity for metastases prior to embarking on resection. Direct visualization of suspicious peritoneal deposits, cytological evaluation of small volume ascites, and the addition of laparoscopic ultrasound have been found to further enhance staging [11,12] (Figure 22.1). In the absence of visible peritoneal metastases or ascites, the use of peritoneal lavage for cytology to evaluate for free intraperitoneal (IP) tumor cells has been shown to be efficacious, and a positive result is now defined as M1 disease [13,14]. In general, positive peritoneal cytology is associated with T3 or T4 primary gastric tumors and is considered an important addition to standard staging procedures [15].

TREATMENT OF GASTRIC CANCER BASED ON STAGE

In general, the treatment of gastric cancer is multimodal, as surgical, medical, and radiation treatments in isolation have not been found to be efficacious.

Surgery

Gastric resection has received considerable debate, regarding the extent of resection and perioperative morbidity and mortality. In patients with cancers in the distal half of the stomach, comparable survival for subtotal gastrectomy versus total gastrectomy was found in a French multicenter randomized trial and Italian Gastrointestinal Tumor Study Group trial [16,17]. However, at 1 year postoperatively, quality of life was found to be significantly better in patients with subtotal gastrectomy [18]. In general, for gastric cancers of the cardia or proximal stomach, transabdominal total gastrectomy is the preferred surgery, with more extensive esophagectomy not found to improve survival [19]. Overall, an R0 resection is desired, including at least 4 cm margins for T1b-T3 tumors and en bloc resection of other involved organs for T4 tumors [20].

More controversial has been the extent of lymphadenectomy for gastric resections. The lymphatic drainage of the stomach is variable related to several different blood vessels providing perfusion, thus making lymph node involvement unpredictable with the potential for skip metastases [21]. The concept of first-level (perigastric, or D1) and second-level (regional, or D2) lymphadenectomy has been debated, related to the aggressiveness of gastric cancer and possible benefit derived [22]. D2 lymphadenectomy includes the hepatic, left gastric, celiac, splenic artery, and splenic hilum nodes, in its more aggressive form including the tail of the pancreas and spleen [23]. Several prospective and retrospective trials have compared D1 to D2 lymphadenectomy, attempting to address many preexisting opinions that have affected adoption of the more aggressive approach, including advanced stages of disease presentation in North American/European patients, balance of benefit of approach versus operative morbidity and mortality, and the learning curve required to complete a thorough D2 lymphadenectomy [24].

There are several large randomized controlled trials comparing aggressive D2 lymphadenectomy to limited D1 lymphadenectomy. The Dutch Gastric Cancer Trial and the British Medical Research Council (MRC) Gastric Cancer Surgical Trial showed high overall mortality rates (4%–13%), with high postoperative morbidity (25%–46%) and a nonsignificant difference in a 5-year survival between groups [23,25–27]. Despite these results, further stage stratification within the Dutch trial showed that the patients most likely to benefit from D2 lymphadenectomy were those with midstage (II, IIIA) gastric cancer [28]. A more recent randomized controlled trial evaluating D1 versus D2 pancreas and spleen-preserving lymphadenectomy showed a lower (16%) morbidity rate with no mortality [29]. Since

D1 lymphadenectomies generally do not provide sufficient (15 or greater) lymph nodes for evaluation and appropriate staging according to current AJCC staging, pancreas and spleen-preserving D2 lymphadenectomies are standardly recommended for patients where a gastrectomy is being performed with curative intent.

Systemic therapy

Adjuvant chemotherapy has been prescribed given the aggressiveness of gastric adenocarcinoma, supported by several studies published over the last three to four decades, represented in seven systematic review and meta-analysis studies [30–32]. Chemotherapy regimens represented in these studies are 5-FU-based regimens, including anthracyclines, mitomycin C, or capecitabine. Comparing results of pooled analyses, an apparent survival benefit was noted for patients administered chemotherapy after curative tumor resection versus surgery alone with observation. Benefit was observed for patients having nonmetastatic tumors with the exception of those that were Tis and T1. However, these studies include both Western and Asian patients; when Asian patients are removed from these analyses, the beneficial effect of the systemic therapy are lost, which may be reflective of more advanced disease state in Western patients [31].

Perioperative or neoadjuvant chemotherapy

The NCCN Guidelines for gastric cancer recommend that for any patient with M0 gastric cancer that is T2 or greater with any demonstrated nodal disease, neoadjuvant chemotherapy be considered prior to curative resection. The British MRC MAGIC trial evaluated the use of perioperative chemotherapy for resectable gastroesophageal cancers (74% of patients had gastric cancers). The majority of patients had T2 or greater cancers, and more than two-thirds had node-positive cancer. Despite reported issues with methodology, the use of pre- and postoperative ECF (epirubicin, cisplatin, 5-FU) chemotherapy was found to improve overall survival and progression-free survival; 5-year survival was 36% in the chemotherapy group, 23% in the surgery alone group [33].

Radiation therapy

Radiation therapy (RT) has been used in the treatment of gastric cancer in a pre- or postoperative setting, alone and in conjunction with chemotherapy. In pilot studies of chemoradiation therapy in gastric cancer using external beam RT and infusional 5-FU, pathologic response rates of 63% with complete response rates of 11% were seen [20].

IP CHEMOTHERAPY FOR GASTRIC CANCER

Peritoneal spread is particularly problematic for the successful treatment of gastric cancer. With approximately 700,000 people worldwide dying annually of gastric cancer, 60% of deaths are associated with peritoneal carcinomatosis (PC) [34]. PC from gastric cancer can be found either at presentation or at the time of disease recurrence. Alarmingly, 5%–20% of patients who are deemed to have "localized" disease and potentially curative gastric resection are found to have PC [35]. Furthermore, following an R0 gastric resection, the recurrence rate for PC is estimated to be 30%. Despite improvements in combination systemic chemotherapies for gastric cancer as previously mentioned, the peritoneum may represent a sanctuary site due to poor penetration of the plasma–peritoneal interface [36]. Accordingly, the inability of systemic chemotherapy to treat PC from gastric cancer is exemplified by much lower response rates compared to other sites of metastases such as liver or lymph nodes.

A basic knowledge of the structure and function of the peritoneal lining is necessary to understand the unique circumstances associated with the treatment of gastric PC. The peritoneal surface is quite extensive and likely functions to reduce friction between intra-abdominal structures by production of a serous lubricant. Additionally, lymphoid aggregates are dispersed throughout the peritoneum and are potentially associated with both innate and adaptive immune responses to IP infections [36]. In combination, the surface features including a glycocalyx and lubricant along with growth factors associated with the lymphoid aggregates may support tumor cell implantation and growth. Additionally, the anatomic structure of the peritoneum limits transportation of molecules including systemically delivered chemotherapeutic agents. The total thickness of the peritoneal lining is approximately 90 μm and is composed of an inner layer of mesothelial cells, a basement membrane, and several layers of connective tissue. Submesothelial capillaries are the major interface for the peritoneum with the systemic circulation and interestingly remain a barrier to drug distribution even when the overlying mesothelium is removed during cytoreduction procedures [36]. When evaluating the distribution of intravenously administered 5-FU, it has been noted that there is a peak concentration of drug in the plasma–peritoneal barrier at 15 minutes with near complete elimination over 90 minutes. However, the concentration of drug within the peritoneal cavity is minimal due to the slow release across the plasma–peritoneal barrier and does not reach tumoricidal levels [34]. While the particular features of the plasma–peritoneal barrier limit the utility of systemic chemotherapy agents for gastric PC, these same characteristics may be taken advantage of during the delivery of IP chemotherapeutics. The rationale for IP chemotherapy delivery is that tumoricidal doses can be achieved within the peritoneum with limited absorption across the plasma–peritoneal barrier, thus limiting systemic toxicities.

The degree of tissue penetration for IP chemotherapy agents is dependent upon many factors, but a 2 mm depth is likely maximum [36]. Combined with standard oncologic gastric resections, cytoreduction of any visible tumor deposits within the peritoneum is postulated to enhance the tumoricidal effects of IP chemotherapy on any remaining microscopic deposits, particularly those less than 2 mm in size. As absorbed IP chemotherapy has been demonstrated to enter the portal system, there may be a theoretical benefit for microscopic liver metastasis as well; however, this is only a secondary consideration [37].

The methods of delivering IP chemotherapy for gastric cancer have varied and include normothermic IP chemotherapy and hyperthermic IP chemotherapy (HIPEC) at the time of resection and early postoperative IP chemotherapy (EPIC) and delayed postoperative IP chemotherapy in the postoperative period [38]. Data regarding these approaches for gastric cancer PC have been accumulating since the 1980s with the majority of reports originating from clinical trials in Asia.

CLINICAL DATA FOR IP CHEMOTHERAPY IN GASTRIC CANCER

While data regarding IP chemotherapy for gastric PC are plagued by the variability in patient selection; treatment or prophylactic intent; surgical technique; chemotherapies utilized; method of delivery, HIPEC (open vs. closed technique, temperature, and time) or EPIC; the duration of treatment; and confounding variables associated with systemic chemotherapy, trends in morbidity and mortality are clearly evident. In a large meta-analysis of randomized clinical trials (RCTs) for gastric cancer PC treated with IP chemotherapy, 20 distinct trials were identified including translation of Chinese and Japanese literature [35]. Of the 20 RCTs, 15% were considered to be of high quality, 75% fair quality, and the remaining 10% low quality. A total of 2145 patients were analyzed with 54% randomized to radical resection and IP chemotherapy compared to 46% randomized to radical resection alone. Interestingly, the overall 1-, 2-, and 3-year mortality rates were significantly favorable for the surgery and IP chemotherapy arm (OR = 0.31, 0.27, and 0.29, respectively). The overall 5-year mortality did not demonstrate any statistically significant difference between groups (OR = 0.99). When examining the mortality of patients specifically with and without PC (treatment or prophylactic intent), a similar pattern was noted with significantly improved 1-, 2-, and 3-year mortality rates in patients treated with surgery and IP chemotherapy compared to surgery alone. The 5-year mortality rate in these patients, however, failed to show any statistical difference between treatment arms. Overall recurrence rates were significantly favorable for the surgery and IP chemotherapy groups compared to surgery alone. Specifically, peritoneal recurrence was statistically less likely in the surgery and IP chemotherapy group (OR = 0.50), but concerning lymph node recurrence, there was no statistical difference between treatment arms (OR = 0.94). Hematogenous recurrence was also noted to be significantly lower in the surgery and IP chemotherapy–treated patients (OR = 0.63). Regarding the 1- and 2-year mortality in patients with serosal involvement, the surgery and IP chemotherapy group was significantly better than surgery alone (OR = 0.33, 0.27, respectively). However, when considering morbidity, the surgery alone group was more favorable compared to the surgery and IP chemotherapy groups (OR = 1.82).

Viewed collectively, the findings of this meta-analysis suggest an early survival benefit in the first 3 years following surgery and IP chemotherapy but a lack of durability at the 5-year mark. The mortality data for patients with and without gastric PC would also imply an early benefit for both a treatment and prophylactic IP chemotherapy approach during the first 3 years, but not maintained at 5 years. Consistent with the high correlation between gastric serosal involvement and PC, IP chemotherapy also demonstrated an improved survival at early time points in these patients. Not surprisingly, morbidity was higher in the surgery and IP chemotherapy–treated groups compared to surgery alone, although detailed analysis of the degree of morbidity was not performed.

Limited morbidity data may be gleaned from an analysis of prospective and retrospective case series examining cytoreduction and HIPEC for gastric cancer. Unlike the prior meta-analysis, the majority of centers were either European or American (70%) compared to Asian, and HIPEC was the method of delivery, which may further limit any generalizations [39]. However, an overall mortality rate of 4.8% was reported out of a total of 467 patients treated with cytoreduction and HIPEC. The overall morbidity was 21.5% and commonly included abscesses, fistulas, hematologic toxicities, and anastomotic leaks. In general, these mortality and morbidity rates are within accepted parameters for other major oncological procedures.

A detailed analysis of the most recent Phase III clinical trial may offer insight regarding the application of cytoreduction and HIPEC for established gastric PC in contemporary settings [40]. In the study by Yang et al. published in 2011, 68 patients with PC from gastric cancer were randomized to receive cytoreduction alone or cytoreduction/HIPEC. The cytoreduction included the standard gastric resections to clear margins and the associated lymph node basins, any involved surrounding tissue, and selective peritonectomy of involved surfaces. The HIPEC procedure was performed in a closed fashion with 120 mg of cisplatin and 30 mg of mitomycin C with flows of 500 mL/min, temperature held at 43°C for 60–90 minutes. The extent of cytoreduction was recorded as CC-0 (no residual disease), CC-1 (less than 2.5 mm residual disease), CC-2 (2.5 mm to 2.5 cm residual disease), or CC-3 (greater than 2.5 cm residual disease). There were no significant differences in baseline patient characteristics between the two groups making this a fair comparison of two different treatments. The median follow-up was 32 months, and disease-specific death was 97.1% in the cytoreduction alone group versus 85.3% in the cytoreduction/HIPEC-treated patients. Overall survival for the cytoreduction alone group was 6.5 months and 11.0 months for cytoreduction/HIPEC. An early benefit within the first year was noted for patients receiving cytoreduction/HIPEC

with 1-, 2-, and 3-year survival rates (41.2%, 14.7%, and 5.9%, respectively) as compared to the cytoreduction alone group (29.4%, 5.9%, and 0%, respectively). These data are similar to the large meta-analysis with an early survival benefit but a lack of durability in response over time. Similar to other tumor types, the completeness of cytoreduction was directly related to better survival. Interestingly, in patients with an incomplete cytoreduction, the addition of HIPEC offered statistically improved overall survival (8.2 vs. 4.0 months). Morbidity was equal between the two groups but, when present, negatively impacted survival. In the vast majority of patients, recurrence or progression of peritoneal disease was the cause of death in both groups. When evaluating this study, an overall survival advantage of 4.5 months may seem meager; however, current chemotherapeutic agents are approved with far less benefit. The real question regarding this short improvement is whether this prolonged survival has a reasonable quality of life. Based upon the reported morbidity of 14.7% in the HIPEC-treated patients, it can be inferred that most patients enjoyed a reasonable quality of life; however, specific quality of life analysis was not conducted during this study.

The data for the addition of IP chemotherapy appear to support a role for regional therapy for gastric cancer; however, the demonstration of prolonged benefits has been lacking. As the most common site of failure for gastric cancer is the peritoneum, it can be postulated that the types of chemotherapy agents used have some transient effect but are not generally curative. A variety of chemotherapeutics have been employed for IP delivery to treat gastric PC, including mitomycin C, cisplatin, and 5-FU. As there is no definitive evidence of superiority for any of these agents, standard recommendations are lacking. Additionally, the optimal method of IP chemotherapy delivery, the duration of treatment, and the use of the so-called bidirectional chemotherapy remain unknown.

CONSIDERATIONS FOR IP CHEMOTHERAPY OF GASTRIC CANCER

Stratifying gastric cancer patients with PC may be useful for prognostication and for comparison of clinical trials. Current strategies for classifying the extent of gastric PC include the Japanese classification, Lyon or Gilly classification, and peritoneal cancer index (PCI) (Table 22.2) [41]. In the *Japanese General Rules for Gastric Cancer Study*, three categories of peritoneal spread are identified: P1 is the peritoneal dissemination in upper abdomen above the transverse colon, P2 is few to several peritoneal nodules in the distant peritoneum, and P3 is the numerous nodules in the distant peritoneum. The Lyon or Gilly classification is described in stages: stage 0 is positive peritoneal cytology, stage I is tumor nodules <5 mm localized, stage II is tumor nodules <5 mm diffuse, stage III is tumor nodules 5 mm to 2 cm, and stage IV is large >2 cm tumor implants. The PCI score, dividing the abdomen into nine areas and four additional sections of small bowel, is more complex but

Table 22.2 Comparison of three classification systems for extent and location of peritoneal metastases in gastric cancer

Japanese classification	Lyon (Gilly) classification	Peritoneal cancer index
P1, dissemination in upper abdomen (above the transverse colon)	Stage 0, positive peritoneal cytology	Lesion size
	Stage I, localized nodules <5 mm	0, no tumor
	Stage II, diffuse nodules <5 mm	1, up to 0.5 cm
P2, few to several nodules in distant peritoneum	Stage III, nodules 5 mm to 2 cm	2, up to 5.0 cm
	Stage IV, >2 cm tumor implants	3, >5.0 cm or confluence
P3, numerous nodules in distant peritoneum		

offers an accurate description of the distribution of gastric PC. Japanese P1 and P2 correspond to Lyon stages I and II and a PCI < 13. A Japanese P3 compares to Lyon stages III and IV and a PCI > 13. Each of these classification systems offers good prognostic data with a worse prognosis directly proportional to the extent of gastric PC. Additional prognostic information can be obtained after a cytoreduction procedure by scoring the completeness of cytoreduction. Evaluation of disease extent at the time of resection as well as the presence of any residual disease may help identify patients who are most likely to benefit from cytoreduction and IP chemotherapy or, alternatively, those who will not receive clinical benefit.

Although definitive patient selection criteria have yet to be established, there are general considerations that should be taken into account when considering cytoreduction and IP chemotherapy for treating gastric PC based upon current data. For example, patients deemed to have extensive PC that would preclude the potential for a complete or near complete cytoreduction are unlikely to improve from an extensive procedure and risk significant morbidity. Patients with significant ascites or omental cake are likely to have diffuse and potentially extensive disease (Figure 22.2). Patients who manifest any evidence of hematogenous metastasis are also unlikely to receive benefit from cytoreduction and IP chemotherapy. Accordingly, poor performance status in patients who cannot tolerate a major surgery is prohibitive. Also, significant progression of disease while receiving systemic chemotherapy is often a harbinger of poor survival and outcomes.

Even though it is debatable in terms of morbidity and risk/benefit profiles, surgery and IP chemotherapy can be considered for both treatment and/or prophylactic intent in high-risk gastric cancer patients. When PC is noted on preoperative imaging or during diagnostic laparoscopy, the use of cytoreduction and IP chemotherapy can be considered to have treatment intent. When cytoreduction and IP chemotherapy are performed for gastric cancer with no obvious evidence of PC, such as T3 or T4 tumors, serosal involvement prior to neoadjuvant chemotherapy, or cytology that was positive, but rendered negative with neoadjuvant chemotherapy, then these cases are considered to have prophylactic intent. As previously mentioned, meta-analysis has shown survival improvement for cytoreduction and IP chemotherapy for both treatment and prophylactic intent. For a direct comparison, a study from France compared variables and outcomes associated with treatment and prophylactic approaches [42]. A total of 37 patients (11 prophylactics, 26 treatments) who underwent cytoreduction and HIPEC (mitomycin C and cisplatin for 60–90 minutes at 41°C–43°C) were evaluated. The 2-year recurrence rates were 36% for the prophylactic group and 50% for the treatment group. The median survival favored the prophylactic group as compared to the treatment group (23.4 vs. 6.6 months, respectively). Importantly, there were three deaths associated with the prophylactic treated group and morbidity was significant in all patients. While this study demonstrated a survival benefit, it remains unclear if prophylactic HIPEC generates a lead-time bias that may artificially inflate survival with potential for significant morbidity and mortality. A true comparison would include similarly matched patients without evidence of gastric PC treated by surgery alone versus surgery and HIPEC.

Currently, a large prospective RCT, called GASTRICHIP, is being undertaken in France [43]. The GASTRICHIP study intends to randomize 306 patients intraoperatively, at the end of curative surgery, to either receive or not receive HIPEC. The primary endpoint is overall survival at 5 years and secondary

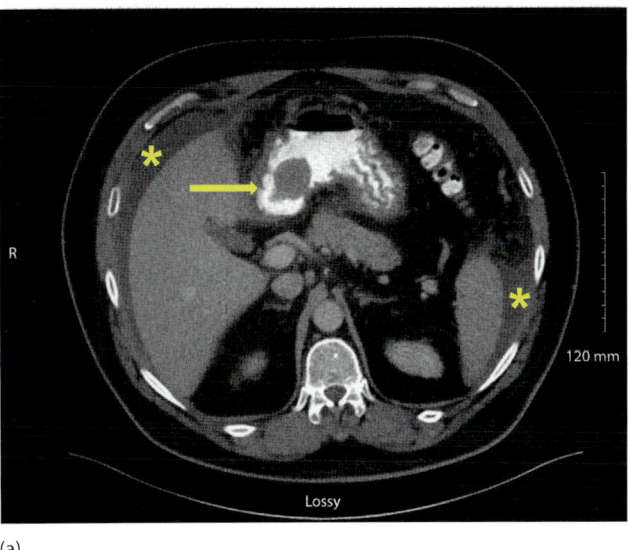
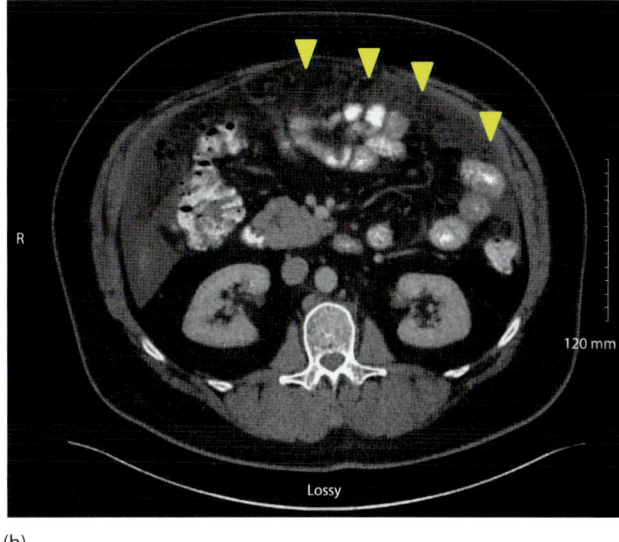

(a)   (b)

Figure 22.2 CT scan of abdomen with oral and i.v. contrast demonstrating (a) large primary tumor in the lumen of the stomach and associated ascites around the liver and spleen and (b) omental cake adjacent to the anterior abdominal wall.

endpoints will be 3- and 5-year recurrence-free survival. Additionally, the sites of recurrence, procedure morbidity, and quality of life will be examined. The HIPEC will consist of intravenous 5-FU and leucovorin combined with oxaliplatin (250 mg/m^2) given IP (30 minutes at 42°C–43°C, open or closed technique). The results of GASTRICHIP should be able to address the utility of treatment and prophylactic approaches and gather much needed quality of life data. Ancillary investigations in these patients will include cytology taken before and after curative resection in both groups to determine any influence on survival and outcomes.

Technical considerations

If an IP chemotherapy approach is being considered, several technical details can assist in the best care of gastric PC patients. Knowing that a complete cytoreduction typically entails the excision of any scars that may harbor tumor cells, this can alter the approach for staging or diagnostic laparoscopy. For example, as most cytoreduction/HIPEC procedures are performed through a generous midline incision, keeping the camera port and any other associated working ports in the midline may be awkward at the time but will facilitate an easy reexcision in the future. Also, when percutaneous biopsy is being performed (e.g., omental cake or peritoneal nodule), the biopsy approach should also take this into consideration if possible.

Operative considerations

At the time of cytoreduction/HIPEC, patients should have at a minimum two large bore intravenous lines and an arterial line for blood pressure monitoring. Patients with comorbidities may require more intense monitoring including a central line for central venous pressure measurements or even transesophageal echocardiogram if necessary. Patients typically should not routinely receive mechanical bowel preparation as it is not only unnecessary but may cause volume depletion that may lead to hypotension during the systemic vasodilation associated with HIPEC. A mechanical retractor system is almost mandatory for complete exposure and access to the peritoneum, particularly the upper abdomen. Therefore, the arms are usually abducted to allow for the post of the retractor system to attach to the operating room table. The position of the arms also gives ready access to the anesthesia team for the placement of lines as the case begins. A nasogastric tube and Foley catheter are placed for use during the operation and also for the postoperative care of the patient. If regional anesthesia is available, such as an epidural catheter, it should be placed at this time for use in the postoperative setting. Depending on the extent of PC, the patient should be situated on the operating room table in a way that would allow for lithotomy position if extensive pelvic work is necessary. The entire abdomen is prepped and a generous midline incision from the xiphoid process to the pubic symphysis is employed. The initial incision may start in the upper midline, and after a cursory inspection to ensure that the disease is resectable and that no liver metastases are present, the incision is continued to its full extent. Care should be taken to excise any prior scars that may have been seeded with tumor cells. The umbilicus and its associated lymphatic tissue are also typically taken to treat or prevent Sister Mary Joseph nodules. The falciform ligament and its continuation as the ligamentum teres of the liver is also taken as it often harbors occult or visible tumor nodules. The recess of the liver in which the ligamentum teres enters is particularly prone to have tumor deposits and should be inspected, cleared, or ablated completely. The gastric resection including the associated lymph node basins is performed in a standard fashion depending upon the location of the tumor in the stomach as mentioned previously. As the greater omentum is prone to tumor cell implantation, it is taken completely regardless if the disease is evident or occult. As the gastric resection and greater omentectomy are completed, a close inspection of the lesser sac should be performed and any involved peritoneal surfaces removed or ablated. A splenectomy may be necessary if the spleen is involved with PC. The left, and eventually right, lobes of the liver should be fully mobilized and the diaphragmatic peritoneal surfaces inspected. Any involved peritoneum should be removed or ablated; uninvolved peritoneum is usually not disturbed. Attention should be turned to Morrison's pouch and the area surrounding the ligament of Treitz as these areas may have PC involvement and should be treated in a similar manner. The paracolic gutters and pelvic peritoneum should be inspected with particular attention to the perirectal space as this is often a site of drop metastases. The small bowel and colon are inspected in their entirety with care to examine both surfaces of the mesentery. Any nodularity should be excised or ablated as necessary. Limited small bowel involvement or colonic involvement may require a segmental resection, but this carries the risk of postoperative leak and is often a marker for extensive disease that may limit the benefits of cytoreduction/HIPEC. Once all visible disease is removed, a HIPEC is performed according to the preferences of the particular institute (e.g., choice of technique [open vs. closed], chemotherapy, hyperthermia, and duration of perfusion). All anastomoses are created after the HIPEC procedure for two reasons. Theoretically, performing the anastomosis first may entrap tumor cells and limit their exposure to the HIPEC. Also, the tissue swelling associate following HIPEC may create problems with any anastomoses and predispose to leak. All areas of the abdomen are inspected for hemostasis and this may require hemostatic agents such as Surgicel® (Ethicon, Somerville, NJ) over areas of raw muscle (particularly the right hemidiaphragm where the smooth Glisson's capsule of the liver does not offer a matrix to form clot). If EPIC is to be performed, catheters should be placed at this time and positioned into the areas to be targeted. If the preference is to place a feeding jejunostomy, it should be performed at this time and kept away from the midline closure. The nasogastric tube should be placed according to preference and secured by anesthesia so as not to migrate postoperatively. Seprafilm® (Sanofi-Aventis, Bridgewater, NJ) to prevent adhesions may also be placed at this time and the abdominal wall fascia reapproximated. If an epidural catheter was not placed or is not preferred, small diameter pain catheters for the controlled delivery of local anesthetic can be placed at the level of the fascia and the midline subcutaneous tissue for excellent postoperative pain control. A JP drain (or similar closed drain system) is placed in the subcutaneous space as delayed fat necrosis associated with chemotherapy exposure is common. The skin is closed with staples. The majority of patients should be able to be extubated immediately and close monitoring for the first 24 hours is typical.

Postoperatively, fluid resuscitation is key and patients are usually started on 1.5 intravenous maintenance rates of isotonic fluids to avoid problems. Most issues in hemodynamics will typically respond with the delivery of intravenous fluids and adequate resuscitation. During the postoperative recovery phase, any sudden or unexplained tachycardia may represent the first sign of an anastomotic leak and should be aggressively investigated.

FUTURE DIRECTIONS

The literature clearly supports the fact that the lower the overall PC disease burden, the better the overall response to HIPEC and overall prognosis from gastric cancer. For those patients with no obvious gross PC, diagnostic laparoscopy with peritoneal washings is undertaken as part of staging. Currently, standard cytology techniques and immunohistochemistry and microscopy are used to evaluate peritoneal washings used for staging in gastric cancer. It has been proposed that the use of other molecular techniques, such as PCR, can assist in detecting PC earlier allowing for earlier treatment decisions including HIPEC [44].

In addition, the use of new targeted drugs in place of standard IP chemotherapy may have a role in improving outcomes for patients with gastric cancer PC. Current chemotherapy drugs have well-defined toxicity profiles, but newer targeted drugs may lessen these side effects allowing for increased dosing and fewer complications.

Finally, although the literature is rich with reports of outcomes including overall survival, studies including quality of life information following cytoreduction/HIPEC for gastric cancer are lacking. The previously mentioned GASTRICHIP study has proposed the use of several quality of life scoring systems to evaluate this issue, and results will assist in having a more comprehensive understanding of the effect on quality of life, as well as the suitability of such scales for this measurement in cytoreduction/HIPEC.

REFERENCES

1. WHO. Global health observatory (GHO), cancer mortality and morbidity. 2014. Available from: www.who.int/gho/ncd/mortalitymorbidity/cancertext/en. Retrieved July 1, 2014.
2. Bertuccio P, Chatenoud L, Levi F, Praud D, Ferlay J, Negri E et al. Recent patterns in gastric cancer: A global overview. International Journal of Cancer Journal International du Cancer. 2009;125(3):666–673.
3. Fuchs CS, Mayer RJ. Gastric carcinoma. The New England Journal of Medicine. 1995;333(1):32–41.
4. Howlander N, Noone A, Kraphcho M, Garshell J, Miller D, Altekruse S et al. SEER cancer statistics review, 1975–2011, National Cancer Institute. 2014. Available from: http://seer.cancer.gov/csr/1975 2011/sections.html. Retrieved July 1, 2014.

5. Kubo A, Corley DA. Marked regional variation in adenocarcinomas of the esophagus and the gastric cardia in the United States. *Cancer.* 2002;95(10):2096–2102.

6. Bamba M, Sugihara H, Kushima R, Okada K, Tsukashita S, Horinouchi M et al. Time-dependent expression of intestinal phenotype in signet ring cell carcinomas of the human stomach. *Virchows Archiv: An International Journal of Pathology.* 2001;438(1):49–56.

7. Gupta JP, Jain AK, Agrawal BK, Gupta S. Gastroscopic cytology and biopsies in diagnosis of gastric malignancies. *Journal of Surgical Oncology.* 1983;22(1):62–64.

8. Edge SB, Compton CC. The American Joint Committee on Cancer: The 7th edition of the AJCC cancer staging manual and the future of TNM. *Annals of Surgical Oncology.* 2010;17(6):1471–1474.

9. Pollack BJ, Chak A, Sivak MV Jr. Endoscopic ultrasonography. *Seminars in Oncology.* 1996;23(3):336–346.

10. Chang KJ, Katz KD, Durbin TE, Erickson RA, Butler JA, Lin F et al. Endoscopic ultrasound-guided fine-needle aspiration. *Gastrointestinal Endoscopy.* 1994;40(6):694–699.

11. Conlon KC, Karpeh MS Jr. Laparoscopy and laparoscopic ultrasound in the staging of gastric cancer. *Seminars in Oncology.* 1996;23(3):347–351.

12. Stell DA, Carter CR, Stewart I, Anderson JR. Prospective comparison of laparoscopy, ultrasonography and computed tomography in the staging of gastric cancer. *The British Journal of Surgery.* 1996;83(9):1260–1262.

13. Bryan RT, Cruickshank NR, Needham SJ, Moffitt DD, Young JA, Hallissey MT et al. Laparoscopic peritoneal lavage in staging gastric and oesophageal cancer. *European Journal of Surgical Oncology: The Journal of the European Society of Surgical Oncology and the British Association of Surgical Oncology.* 2001;27(3):291–297.

14. Ribeiro U Jr., Gama-Rodrigues JJ, Safatle-Ribeiro AV, Bitelman B, Ibrahim RE, Ferreira MB et al. Prognostic significance of intraperitoneal free cancer cells obtained by laparoscopic peritoneal lavage in patients with gastric cancer. *Journal of Gastrointestinal Surgery: Official Journal of the Society for Surgery of the Alimentary Tract.* 1998;2(3):244–249.

15. Bentrem D, Wilton A, Mazumdar M, Brennan M, Coit D. The value of peritoneal cytology as a preoperative predictor in patients with gastric carcinoma undergoing a curative resection. *Annals of Surgical Oncology.* 2005;12(5):347–353.

16. Bozzetti F, Marubini E, Bonfanti G, Miceli R, Piano C, Gennari L. Subtotal versus total gastrectomy for gastric cancer: Five-year survival rates in a multicenter randomized Italian trial. Italian Gastrointestinal Tumor Study Group. *Annals of Surgery.* 1999;230(2):170–178.

17. Gouzi JL, Huguier M, Fagniez PL, Launois B, Flamant Y, Lacaine F et al. Total versus subtotal gastrectomy for adenocarcinoma of the gastric antrum. A French prospective controlled study. *Annals of Surgery.* 1989;209(2):162–166.

18. Davies J, Johnston D, Sue-Ling H, Young S, May J, Griffith J et al. Total or subtotal gastrectomy for gastric carcinoma? A study of quality of life. *World Journal of Surgery.* 1998;22(10):1048–1055.

19. Siewert JR, Stein HJ, Sendler A, Fink U. Surgical resection for cancer of the cardia. *Seminars in Surgical Oncology.* 1999;17(2):125–131.

20. National Comprehensive Cancer Network N. Gastric cancer clinical practice guidelines. 2014. Available from: www.nccn.org. Retrieved July 1, 2014.

21. Kitagawa Y, Fujii H, Kumai K, Kubota T, Otani Y, Saikawa Y et al. Recent advances in sentinel node navigation for gastric cancer: A paradigm shift of surgical management. *Journal of Surgical Oncology.* 2005;90(3):147–151; discussion 51–52.

22. Hartgrink HH, van de Velde CJ, Putter H, Bonenkamp JJ, Klein Kranenbarg E, Songun I et al. Extended lymph node dissection for gastric cancer: Who may benefit? Final results of the randomized Dutch gastric cancer group trial. *Journal of Clinical Oncology: Official Journal of the American Society of Clinical Oncology.* 2004;22(11):2069–2077.

23. Bonenkamp JJ, Hermans J, Sasako M, van de Velde CJ, Welvaart K, Songun I et al. Extended lymph-node dissection for gastric cancer. *The New England Journal of Medicine.* 1999;340(12):908–914.

24. Stabile BS, B. Cancer of the stomach: Surgical management. In: Silberman HSA, ed., *Principles and Practice of Surgical Oncology*, 1st edn., Philadelphia, PA: Lippincott Williams & Wilkins, 2010. p. 639.

25. Bonenkamp JJ, Songun I, Hermans J, Sasako M, Welvaart K, Plukker JT et al. Randomised comparison of morbidity after D1 and D2 dissection for gastric cancer in 996 Dutch patients. *Lancet.* 1995;345(8952):745–748.

26. Cuschieri A, Fayers P, Fielding J, Craven J, Bancewicz J, Joypaul V et al. Postoperative morbidity and mortality after D1 and D2 resections for gastric cancer: Preliminary results of the MRC randomised controlled surgical trial. The Surgical Cooperative Group. *Lancet.* 1996;347(9007):995–999.

27. Cuschieri A, Weeden S, Fielding J, Bancewicz J, Craven J, Joypaul V et al. Patient survival after D1 and D2 resections for gastric cancer: Long-term results of the MRC randomized surgical trial. Surgical Co-operative Group. *British Journal of Cancer.* 1999;79(9–10):1522–1530.

28. Siewert JR, Bottcher K, Stein HJ, Roder JD. Relevant prognostic factors in gastric cancer: Ten-year results of the German Gastric Cancer Study. *Annals of Surgery.* 1998;228(4):449–461.

29. Degiuli M, Sasako M, Calgaro M, Garino M, Rebecchi F, Mineccia M et al. Morbidity and mortality after D1 and D2 gastrectomy for cancer: Interim analysis of the Italian Gastric Cancer Study Group (IGCSG) randomised surgical trial. *European Journal of Surgical Oncology: The Journal of the European Society of Surgical Oncology and the British Association of Surgical Oncology.* 2004;30(3):303–308.

30. Earle CC, Maroun JA. Adjuvant chemotherapy after curative resection for gastric cancer in non-Asian patients: Revisiting a meta-analysis of randomised trials. *European Journal of Cancer.* 1999;35(7):1059–1064.

31. Hu JK, Chen ZX, Zhou ZG, Zhang B, Tian J, Chen JP et al. Intravenous chemotherapy for resected gastric cancer: Meta-analysis of randomized controlled trials. *World Journal of Gastroenterology: WJG.* 2002;8(6):1023–1028.

32. Panzini I, Gianni L, Fattori PP, Tassinari D, Imola M, Fabbri P et al. Adjuvant chemotherapy in gastric cancer: A meta-analysis of randomized trials and a comparison with previous meta-analyses. *Tumori.* 2002;88(1):21–27.

33. Cunningham D, Allum WH, Stenning SP, Thompson JN, Van de Velde CJ, Nicolson M et al. Perioperative chemotherapy versus surgery alone for resectable gastroesophageal cancer. *The New England Journal of Medicine.* 2006;355(1):11–20.

34. Yonemura Y, Endou Y, Sasaki T, Hirano M, Mizumoto A, Matsuda T et al. Surgical treatment for peritoneal carcinomatosis from gastric cancer. *European Journal of Surgical Oncology: The Journal of the European Society of Surgical Oncology and the British Association of Surgical Oncology.* 2010;36(12):1131–1138.

35. Coccolini F, Cotte E, Glehen O, Lotti M, Poiasina E, Catena F et al. Intraperitoneal chemotherapy in advanced gastric cancer. Meta-analysis of randomized trials. *European Journal of Surgical Oncology: The Journal of the European Society of Surgical Oncology and the British Association of Surgical Oncology.* 2014;40(1):12–26.

36. Van der Speeten K, Stuart OA, Sugarbaker PH. Using pharmacologic data to plan clinical treatments for patients with peritoneal surface malignancy. *Current Drug Discovery Technologies.* 2009;6(1):72–81.

37. Speyer JL. The rationale behind intraperitoneal chemotherapy in gastrointestinal malignancies. *Seminars in Oncology.* 1985;12(3 Suppl. 4):23–28.

38. Roviello F, Caruso S, Neri A, Marrelli D. Treatment and prevention of peritoneal carcinomatosis from gastric cancer by cytoreductive surgery and hyperthermic intraperitoneal chemotherapy: Overview and rationale. *European Journal of Surgical Oncology: The Journal of the European Society of Surgical Oncology and the British Association of Surgical Oncology.* 2013;39(12):1309–1316.

39. Gill RS, Al-Adra DP, Nagendran J, Campbell S, Shi X, Haase E et al. Treatment of gastric cancer with peritoneal carcinomatosis by cytoreductive surgery and HIPEC: A systematic review of survival, mortality, and morbidity. *Journal of Surgical Oncology.* 2011;104(6):692–698.

40. Yang XJ, Huang CQ, Suo T, Mei LJ, Yang GL, Cheng FL et al. Cytoreductive surgery and hyperthermic intraperitoneal chemotherapy improves survival of patients with peritoneal carcinomatosis from gastric cancer: Final results of a phase III randomized clinical trial. *Annals of Surgical Oncology.* 2011;18(6):1575–1581.

41. Yonemura Y, Bandou E, Kawamura T, Endou Y, Sasaki T. Quantitative prognostic indicators of peritoneal dissemination of gastric cancer. *European Journal of Surgical Oncology: The Journal of the European Society of Surgical Oncology and the British Association of Surgical Oncology.* 2006;32(6):602–606.

42. Scaringi S, Kianmanesh R, Sabate JM, Facchiano E, Jouet P, Coffin B et al. Advanced gastric cancer with or without peritoneal carcinomatosis treated with hyperthermic intraperitoneal chemotherapy: A single western center experience. *European Journal of Surgical Oncology: The Journal of the European Society of Surgical Oncology and the British Association of Surgical Oncology.* 2008;34(11):1246–1252.

43. Glehen O, Passot G, Villeneuve L, Vaudoyer D, Bin-Dorel S, Boschetti G et al. GASTRICHIP: D2 resection and hyperthermic intraperitoneal chemotherapy in locally advanced gastric carcinoma: A randomized and multicenter phase III study. *BMC Cancer.* 2014;14:183.

44. Fujiwara Y, Doki Y, Taniguchi H, Sohma I, Takiguchi S, Miyata H et al. Genetic detection of free cancer cells in the peritoneal cavity of the patient with gastric cancer: Present status and future perspectives. *Gastric Cancer: Official Journal of the International Gastric Cancer Association and the Japanese Gastric Cancer Association.* 2007;10(4):197–204.

Cytoreductive surgery and hyperthermic intraperitoneal chemotherapy for peritoneal carcinomatosis from small bowel adenocarcinoma

EDWARD A. LEVINE

INTRODUCTION

Despite the variety of malignant tumors of the small bowel, such lesions are rare, representing only 1%–3% of all gastrointestinal malignancies [1–4]. Small bowel tumors are difficult to identify at an early stage by most endoscopic or imaging modalities. Further, its vague presentation and low index of suspicion by physicians contribute to its diagnostic challenges [4,8]. There are several types of small bowel malignancy, but of these different types, small bowel adenocarcinoma (SBA) is the most common histologic variant [4–6]. It is estimated that approximately 2–5000 patients are diagnosed with SBA each year in the United States [4]. SBA is most commonly seen in the duodenum and least commonly in the ileum. SBA has historically been known for its poor prognosis, with a median overall survival ranging from 12 to 20 months [1–4]. With current treatment, survival for patients with SBA has remained relatively unchanged over the last 20 years [7].

At the time a definitive diagnosis is made, more than a quarter of SBA cases have regional lymph node and/or peritoneal dissemination [1]. These late presentations are associated with a median overall survival of only 10–20 months and a dismal 5-year survival rate [1–3]. Peritoneal carcinomatosis (PC) has also been found to be the most common site of disease progression for SBA [1]. The late presentation, along with a lack of consensus on standard treatment, makes the prognosis grim. PC has limited response to systemic chemotherapy, and radiation plays a very limited role [8].

Due to the poor results of traditional treatment, aggressive therapies, including cytoreductive surgery (CS), and hyperthermic intraperitoneal chemotherapy (HIPEC), have become more attractive options that have been gaining momentum in the last few decades [9–14]. Extrapolating from experience with HIPEC data of appendiceal and colorectal origins [13,14], there have been efforts to employ this modality for SBA. The data on HIPEC for peritoneal dissemination from non-SBA small bowel malignancy are extremely limited [12,15]. We at Wake Forest have recently published the largest series to date, which examines our experience with 17 consecutive patients diagnosed with PC secondary to SBA who were treated with HIPEC at our institution.

WAKE FOREST UNIVERSITY EXPERIENCE

From November 1995 to June 2011, 17 patients from Wake Forest University Baptist Hospital, who underwent HIPEC at least once for PC due to primary SBA, were identified from a prospective database. Patients were selected for the HIPEC operation based on our standard criteria, which included but was not limited to medical fitness, resectable (or previously resected) primary lesion, and absence of extra-abdominal metastasis. We also did not consider patients with a duodenal primary lesion. Preoperative images, including CT, MRI, and PET scans, were routinely used to rule out any extra-abdominal disease and determine the resectability of PC. Our techniques for HIPEC have been described elsewhere and are briefly described below [13–15]. All patients

Table 23.1 Demographic, histologic, and survival data of 17 patients with variables in perioperative and postoperative outcome

Patient	Age at HIPEC	Gender	Primary site	Interval between primary diagnosis and HIPEC (months)	Survival after primary diagnosis (months)	Survival after HIPEC (months)	Number of visceral resection	Duration of HIPEC (hours)	Length of ICU stay (days)	Length of hospital stay (days)	Clavien–Dindo classification (grade) [20]
1	35	F	Jejunum	6	36	30	2	11	1	11	—
2	37	M	Ileum	10	55	45	3	8	0	6	—
3	61	F	Jejunum	12	64	52	5	7.5	1	13	—
4	47	F	Jejunum	20	51	31	3	7.5	2	11	—
5	53	F	Jejunum	46	57	11	3	6.5	0	6	IIIa
6	54	F	Jejunum	16	21	5	3	8.3	2	20	—
7	60	M	Ileum	23	28	5	4	7	1	13	—
8	59	M	Ileum	12	15	3	3	9	2	24	—
9	55	M	Duodenum	21	40	19	2	7	1	7	—
10	64	F	Jejunum	6	33	27	3	8.2	0	6	—
11	32	M	Ileum	7	12	5	6	5.5	0	15	—
12	58	M	Ileum	2	47	45	3	8.2	2	7	IIIa
13	40	F	Ileum	7	21	14	3	5.5	0	7	—
14	65	M	Jejunum	33	35	2	3	6.5	0	6	—
15	63	F	Ileum	7	31 (alive)	24	1	10	1	6	—
16	44	F	Jejunum	35	42	7	3	7.35	1	9	—
17	60	F	Jejunum	6	14 (alive)	8	4	5.3	0	7	—
Mean	52.2			17.1	37.1	18.4	3.2	7.55	0.82	10.2	

Source: Sun, Y. et al., Am. Surg., 79, 644, 2013.

underwent surgical resection based on their symptoms and extent of disease on imaging modalities; additional therapies varied among the 17 patients. CS consisted of the resection of the primary tumor (if still present), as well as the resection of all gross tumor feasible. Peritonectomy procedures were performed for gross disease only; not on a routine basis. Complete lysis of adhesions was also routinely performed if necessary to improve chemotherapy flow at the time of HIPEC.

During CS, patients were passively cooled to a core temperature of 34°C–35°C prior to HIPEC. Inflow and outflow catheters for peritoneal perfusion were placed into the abdominal cavity, and the abdominal skin incision was temporarily closed, with a running cutaneous suture. A perfusion circuit with a 3 L crystalloid solution prime utilized to initiate perfusion, at a flow rate of approximately 1 L/min, by a roller pump managed by a perfusionist. The circuit was run through the roller pump and a heat exchanger, and perfusate temperature was strictly monitored by temperature probes on the inflow and outflow catheters. Once outflow temperatures exceeded 39°C, 30 mg of mitomycin C was added to the perfusate. After 60 minutes, an additional 10 mg was added, and the total perfusion time was 120 minutes. The abdomen was gently massaged throughout the perfusion to optimize drug distribution. After completion of the perfusion, the peritoneum was washed with several liters of crystalloid solution; the abdomen was opened and requisite anastomoses and stomas created prior to final closure if needed.

All patients in this series were diagnosed with a primary SBA and had peritoneal dissemination at the time of HIPEC. Ten of the 17 patients were female. Three of the 17 patients had a repeat HIPEC (11, 21, and 20 months after the initial HIPEC procedure). The mean age at the time of HIPEC was 52.2 years (range, 32–65 years). Primary locations of SBA differed among 17 patients; 1 was in the duodenum (early in the experience), 9 in the jejunum, and 7 in the ileum. Demographic, histologic, and survival data along with perioperative and postoperative variables are shown in Table 23.1. Most patients (13/17) received chemotherapy prior to their HIPEC; 5 of the 17 patients received chemotherapy after their HIPEC; 3 of whom did not have chemotherapy prior to surgery. Fifteen of 17 patients underwent omentectomy (2 had prior omentectomy); 13 had a colectomy; 12 had small bowel resection; 4 had splenectomy; 3 appendectomy, cholecystectomy, and liver resection; 2 distal pancreatectomy; 1 nephrectomy; 1 hysterectomy; and 1 oophorectomy. Fourteen patients had either R0 or R1 resections, while the remainder of the patients had R2 resections.

The median survival after HIPEC procedure was 20.1 months excluding the two patients who are still alive (at the time of writing this chapter). The 1-year survival was 52%, with a 3-year survival of 23%. Overall survival of the 17 patients after the HIPEC operation is shown in Figure 23.1 Two patients are still alive, one of whom has no evidence of disease; however, 15 have died of progressive

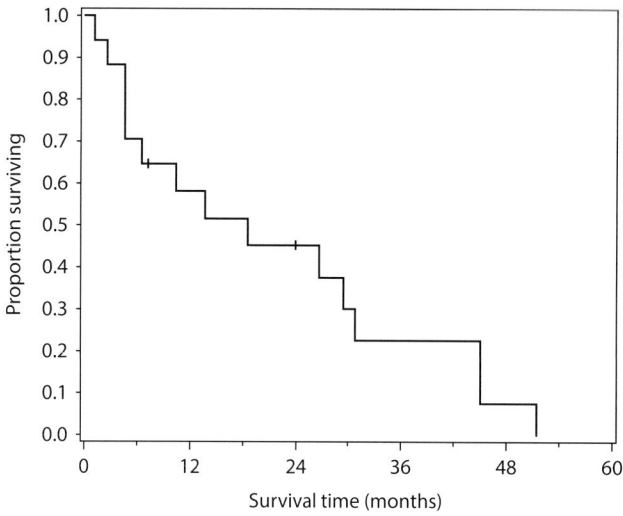

Figure 23.1 Kaplan–Meier analysis of postoperative survival in 17 patients with peritoneal carcinomatosis originating from small bowel adenocarcinoma. Two patients, 15 and 17, are still alive at 24 and 7 months, respectively. (From Sun, Y. et al., *Am. Surg.*, 79, 644, 2013.)

intra-abdominal disease. A mean overall survival *after diagnosis* of 37.1 months was achieved in the study, with a 1-, 2-, 3-, and 5-year overall survival of 93.3%, 73.3%, 53.3%, and 6.7%, respectively.

The extent of disease, the magnitude of cytoreduction, the duration of the operation, and health status of the patients all made morbidity and mortality significant. The mean duration of the HIPEC procedure was 7.5 hours (range, 6.5–11), and total length of hospital stay was 10 days (range, 6–24). There was no HIPEC-related mortality. Six patients were readmitted to the hospital within 30 days of discharge. A total of 47% experienced a postoperative complication.

REVIEW OF LITERATURE AND DISCUSSION

PC from SBA continues to be a diagnostic and treatment challenge to physicians, due to its rarity and poor prognosis when compared with PC originating from other gastrointestinal sources [17–19]. Several studies have reported the natural history of PC derived from gastrointestinal malignancies, which have found a median survival of only 3–7 months in patients not being aggressively treated with HIPEC [8]. Treatment for PC from SBA with systemic chemotherapy and "conventional surgery" has been attempted in the past, with limited efficacy. Systemic chemotherapy regimens are typically utilized as an extrapolation of the experience with colon cancer. In a study from 2011, an overall survival of 11.8 months was achieved in patients with advanced SBA who received chemotherapy alone [20]. However, the use of chemotherapy with newer platinum containing regimens could potentially add to survival benefits [3]. Although the utility of using systemic chemotherapy (despite its limitations) in combination with HIPEC remains unproven,

Table 23.2 Published series of cytoreductive surgery and hyperthermic intraperitoneal chemotherapy for peritoneal carcinomatosis originating from small bowel adenocarcinoma

Source	Patients (n)	Mean age (years)	Institution[b]	Survival s/p HIPEC (months)
Jacks et al.	6	47.7	WFU	30.1
Marchettini	6	45.7	WHC	27.0
Chua et al.	7	44.7	UNSW	21.2
Sun et al.[a]	17	52.2	WFU	18.4
Total	30	49.1		22.2

Source: Sun, Y. et al., Am. Surg., 79, 644, 2013.
[a] Current series includes the six patients published in our group's original series [18].
[b] WFU, Wake Forest University; WHC, Washington Hospital Center; UNSW, University of New South Wales.

we routinely recommend it. Further, similar to HIPEC procedures for other primary sites, the HIPEC is best utilized with systemic therapy, not in lieu of it.

The rarity of small bowel carcinoma makes experience with PC from this site extremely limited. A literature search identified three published studies on the outcome of HIPEC in patients with PC originating from SBA [12,16,18], all of which showed similar outcomes. In the first of these studies, we had previously published a series of six patients treated with HIPEC [18]. Marchettini and Sugarbaker [12] and Chua et al. [16] each showed similar results with their data and from the meta-analysis of all three series published at the time. In this series, we have expanded our patient population from the initial six patients published in our first series, to include all SBA patients who underwent HIPEC in the past 15 years. At 17 patients, this is the largest cohort that has been reported. Our patients had an overall postoperative survival of 27.6 months after HIPEC, if they had the operation within 12 months of initial diagnosis. The same survival benefit dropped to 11.4 months if they underwent the procedure longer than 1 year after diagnosis, suggesting earlier intervention is likely more beneficial than waiting until after extensive chemotherapy (Table 23.2).

Whether a repeat HIPEC would improve outcome in patients with primary SBA is unclear. However, the three patients in this series who underwent a repeat HIPEC, and other studies published on PC arising from other gastrointestinal malignancies, support such a possibility. Additional prospective studies, via multi-institutional registry data, should be investigated in this patient population. The rarity of the diagnosis makes prospective trials unfeasible.

It seems that treating PC originating from SBA with HIPEC is a reasonable surgical option for selected patients. In comparison, after HIPEC in patients with advanced disease who had already undergone chemotherapy (with an average survival of 12 months [3,18,19]), the average post-HIPEC survival of 22 months had been achieved at all three centers reporting results, nearly doubling the survival time accomplished by medical therapy alone. HIPEC appears to have lengthened their survival, and likely the quality of life, by an average of more than 18 months. Ideally, this finding would be confirmed by a randomized trial; however, the rarity of this disease makes such a study implausible. Even though HIPEC has not been a curative treatment for advanced SBA, results from the largest published experience, as well as multiple centers, point to HIPEC with systemic therapy being the most effective option for this population.

REFERENCES

1. Dabaja BS, Suki D, Pro B et al. Adenocarcinoma of the small bowel: Presentation, prognostic factors, and outcome of 217 patients. Cancer. 2004;101:518–526.
2. Locher C, Malka D, Boige V et al. Combination chemotherapy in advanced small bowel adenocarcinoma. Oncology. 2005;69:290–294.
3. Overman MJ, Kopetz S, Wen S et al. Chemotherapy with 5-fluorouracil and a platinum compound improves outcomes in metastatic small bowel adenocarcinoma. Cancer. 2008;113:2038–2045.
4. Talamonti MS, Goetz LH, Rao S et al. Primary cancers of the small bowel: Analysis of prognostic factors and results of surgical management. Archives of Surgery. 2002;137:564–570.
5. North JH, Pack MS. Malignant tumors of the small intestine: A review of 144 cases. The American Surgeon. 2000;66:46–51.
6. Frost DB, Mercado PD, Tyrell JS. Small bowel cancer: A 30-year review. Annals of Surgical Oncology. 1994;1:290–295.
7. Bilimoria KY, Bentrem DJ, Wayne JD et al. Small bowel cancer in the United States. Changes in epidemiology, treatment and survival over the last 20 years. Annals of Surgery. 2009;249:63–71.
8. Sadeghi B, Arvieux C, Glehen O et al. Peritoneal carcinomatosis from non-gynecologic malignancies: Results of the EVOCAPE 1 multicentric prospective study. Cancer. 2000;88:358–363.
9. Tsushima T, Taquri M, Honma Y et al. Multicenter retrospective study of 132 patients with unresectable small bowel adenocarcinoma treated with chemotherapy. Oncologist. May 2012.
10. Witkamp AJ, de Bree E, Kaag MM et al. Extensive cytoreductive surgery followed by intra-operative hyperthermic intraperitoneal chemotherapy with

mitomycin-C in patients with peritoneal carcinomatosis of colorectal origin. *European Journal of Cancer.* 2001;37:979–984.

11. Sugarbaker PH. Cytoreductive surgery and perioperative intraperitoneal chemotherapy as a curative approach to pseudomyxoma peritonei syndrome. *European Journal of Surgical Oncology.* 2001;27:239–243.

12. Marchettini P, Sugarbaker PH. Mucinous adenocarcinoma of the small bowel with peritoneal seeding. *European Journal of Surgical Oncology.* 2002;28:19–23.

13. Shen P, Levine EA, Hall J et al. Factors predicting survival after intraperitoneal hyperthermic chemotherapy with mitomycin C after cytoreductive surgery for patients with peritoneal carcinomatosis. *Archives of Surgery.* 2003;138:26–33.

14. McQuellon RP, Loggie BW, Lehman AB et al. A long-term survivorship and quality of life after cytoreductive surgery plus intraperitoneal hyperthermic chemotherapy for peritoneal carcinomatosis. *Annals of Surgical Oncology.* 2003;10:155–162.

15. Levine EA, Stewart JH, Shen P, Russell GB, Loggie BL, Votanopoulos KI. Cytoreductive surgery and intraperitoneal hyperthermic chemotherapy for peritoneal surface malignancy: Experience with 1,000 patients. *Journal of the American College of Surgeons.* 2014;518:573–587.

16. Chua TC, Koh JL, Yan TD et al. Cytoreductive surgery and perioperative intraperitoneal chemotherapy for peritoneal carcinomatosis from small bowel adenocarcinoma. *Journal of Surgical Oncology.* 2009;100:139–143.

17. Jemal A, Siegel R, Ward E et al. Cancer statistics, 2008. *CA: A Cancer Journal for Clinicians.* 2008;58:71–96.

18. Jacks SP, Hundley JC, Shen P et al. Cytoreductive surgery and intraperitoneal hyperthermic chemotherapy for peritoneal carcinomatosis from small bowel adenocarcinoma. *Journal of Surgical Oncology.* 2005;91:112–117.

19. Sun Y, Shen P, Stewart JH, Russell GB, Levine EA. Cytoreductive surgery and hyperthermic intraperitoneal chemotherapy for peritoneal carcinomatosis from small bowel adenocarcinoma. *The American Surgeon.* 2013;79:644–648.

20. Koo DH, Yun SC, Hong YS et al. Systemic chemotherapy for treatment of advanced small bowel adenocarcinoma with prognostic factor analysis: Retrospective study. *BMC Cancer.* 2011;11:205.

24

Peritoneal surface malignancy from neuroendocrine tumors

MLADJAN PROTIĆ, ITZHAK AVITAL, AND ALEXANDER STOJADINOVIC

INTRODUCTION

According to the definition by the National Cancer Institute, neuroendocrine tumors (NETs) arise from cells that release hormones into the blood stream in response to signals originating from the nervous system [1]. NETs are a very heterogeneous group of tumors, and in this group of neoplasms, there are carcinoid (serotonin or prostaglandin secreting) tumors, gastroenteropancreatic NETs (GEP-NETs) (e.g., insulinoma, gastrinoma, vasoactive intestinal peptideoma, medullary tumors of the thyroid gland, catecholamine secreting tumors [e.g., pheochromocytoma, paraganglioma, neuroblastoma, ganglioneuroblastoma, ganglioneuroma, and sympathoblastoma]), NETs of the skin (Merkel cell cancer), small-cell lung tumors, large-cell neuroendocrine carcinoma (a rare type of lung cancer), and pituitary tumors [1,2]. These tumors may be either benign or malignant. These tumors can also secrete various types of hormones in enormous quantities with resultant symptoms and clinical picture determined by the type of hormone secreted.

Peritoneal surface malignancy (PSM) of NET origin is known to extend from primary NETs of the digestive tract or pancreas (GEP-NETs). These tumors originate from the mucosa of the stomach, the jejunum, ileum, colon, rectum, and islets of Langerhans in the pancreas. The incidence of these tumors is on the rise and has increased fivefold over the past 30 years [3]. It is estimated that the annual incidence of GEP-NETs is 5.25/100,000 people and the prevalence 35/100,000 people. The GEP-NETs can occur at any age, with highest incidence after the fifth decade of life. Carcinoid of the small intestine typically occurs around 40 years of age. Incidence rates are somewhat higher in men than in women. Patients with multiple endocrine neoplasia type 1 and von Hippel-Lindau's disease typically manifest clinical manifestations of the disease 15–20 years earlier than sporadic NET [4].

PSM of NET origin has as its primary tumor site the pancreas or the gastrointestinal tract. In small series of patients undergoing surgical treatment of well-differentiated digestive endocrine carcinomas, the prevalence of peritoneal carcinomatosis (PC) has been reported in the range of 10%–33% [5,6]. According to the data collected prospectively, the French National Registry of 508 patients with GEP-NETS estimated the prevalence of related PSM to be 17.5% [7]. In 603 consecutively treated patients with tumors of the small intestine in Uppsala, the prevalence of PSM was 17% [8]. According to the U.S. National Cancer Institute Surveillance, Epidemiology, and End Results (SEER) report in 2003 on 13,715 cases, the prevalence of PSM of NET intestinal origin was 13.6%. It is more common for GEP-NETs to metastasize only to regional lymph nodes (89.8%) and liver

(44.1%) rather than the peritoneal surface [3]. The association between the presence of regional lymph node and liver metastases and PSM has been reported in the range of 30%–80%. The most common site of primary tumor in the case of PSM of NET origin is the small intestine. According to Elias et al., 20 of 37 patients (54%) with PSM of NET origin had a midgut primary tumor source [5]. Vasseur et al. in the same clinical situation found midgut NET spread to the peritoneal surface in 8 of 11 patients (73%) [6].

The clinical significance of PSM in the case of NET remains a matter of debate. Some authors have argued that the presence of PSM in NETs has no effect on survival; therefore, the treatment of PSM of NET origin is not considered useful [6,9]. However, Mayo et al. examined the surgical treatment of hepatic metastases of NET origin in 339 patients and found that the presence of extrahepatic metastasis was a negative predictor of survival in these patients. Median survival among patients who, at time of surgery of the liver for NET metastases, also had extrahepatic disease was 85.1 months, while those who had only hepatic NET metastases had a median survival of 148.1 months (p < 0.001). Elias et al. investigated 111 cases with well-differentiated NET with PSM and found that untreated PC was directly responsible for 40% of deaths and recommended cytoreductive surgery (CRS) with intraperitoneal chemotherapy to improve clinical outcome as well as palliate-related symptoms [5].

SYMPTOMATOLOGY

There are no specific symptoms related to PSM of NET origin, for they are similar to other types of tumors involving the peritoneal surface. Sometimes, the clinical picture is dominated by symptoms of the primary tumor. Almost half of patients are asymptomatic or have nonspecific symptoms such as abdominal pain or discomfort at time of diagnosis of peritoneal disease. Peritoneal disease is typically detected incidentally during clinical examination or diagnostic testing or during surgical exploration. Symptoms related to PSM of NET origin most commonly mimic symptoms of incomplete intestinal obstruction and resemble the symptoms often seen in inflammatory bowel disease [10,11]. Patients with advanced disease may have weight loss or even an increase in body weight in the case of ascites [5,12]. The clinical picture of these patients may be affected by excess circulating hormones produced by these tumors, as an example, carcinoid syndrome [13–15].

DIAGNOSIS, GRADING, AND STAGING OF NET

All GEP-NETs are confirmed histopathologically by primary tumor samples obtained with endoscopic and/or surgical biopsy, targeted biopsies of the involved liver and/or cytological examination of ascites fluid. Detailed description of macroscopic, microscopic, and immunohistochemical features are central to accurate diagnosis of NET, its classification, staging, and grading [16]. Although NETs are a very heterogeneous group of tumors, they all share a common phenotype in the form of immunohistochemical reactivity of the so-called pan-neuroendocrine markers including chromogranin A and synaptophysin. Neuron-specific enolase and CD56 are often present in GEP-NETs but are not specific to these tumor types. Determination of Ki-67 (MIB-1) is required to determine the grade of the tumor according to the new classification of the World Health Organization (WHO), Table 24.1 [17,18]. For the purpose of disease classification and staging, both the WHO classification and the TNM classification systems are utilized, Table 24.2 [19].

Table 24.1 WHO 2010 grading classes, rules of application, and projected malignancy

WHO class	Definition	Grade	Ki67%[a,b] Range	Ki67%[a,b] Rules of application	Mitotic index[a,b] Range	Mitotic index[a,b] Rules of application	Malignancy[c] (expected)
1	NET	G1	≤2	Assessed on 500–2000 cells, hot spots[d]	<2	Assessed per 10 HPF,[e] hot spots,[d] 50 fields as recommended	+
2	NET	G2	3–20		2–20		++
3	NEC	G3	>20		>20		+++
4	MANEC[f]	mr	mr	mr	mr	mr	Variable
5	Hyperplasia/dysplasia	na	na	na	na	na	na

Source: Rindi, G. et al., Endocr. Pathol., 25(2), 186, June 2014, Available from: http://www.ncbi.nlm.nih.gov/pubmed/24699927, retrieved on September 28, 2014.

NET, neuroendocrine tumor; NEC, neuroendocrine carcinoma; MANEC, mixed adenoneuroendocrine carcinoma; mr, missing recommendation from current WHO 2010; na, not applicable.

a Round up to a lower value when 0.1–0.4 and to a higher value when 0.5–0.9 (proposed but not present in WHO 2010 [10]).
b In case of grade discrepancy as defined by Ki67% and mitosis is recommended to apply the higher value observed.
c Expected malignancy as estimated from reported literature (see text and references).
d Areas of highest nuclear labeling (Ki67)/density (mitosis)—the latter one not present in WHO 2010 [10] but defined so by ENETS [14,15].
e High-power fields = 2 mm².
f 30% of either component required.

Table 24.2 Tumor, node, and metastases classification and disease staging for neuroendocrine tumor of the duodenum/ampulla/proximal jejunum

Tumor, node, and metastases				
T—Primary tumor				
TX	Primary tumor cannot be assessed.			
T0	No evidence of primary tumor.			
T1	Tumor invades lamina propria or submucosa and size ≤1 cm.[a]			
T2	Tumor invades muscularis propria or size >1 cm.			
T3	Tumor invades pancreas or retroperitoneum.			
T4	Tumor invades peritoneum or other organs. For any T, add (m) for multiple tumors.			
N—Regional lymph nodes				
NX	Regional lymph nodes cannot be assessed.			
N0	No regional lymph node metastasis.			
N1	Regional lymph node metastasis.			
M—Distant metastases				
MX	Distant metastasis cannot be assessed.			
M0	No distant metastases.			
M1[b]	Distant metastasis.			
Stage				
Disease stages				
Stage	I	T1	N0	M0
Stage	II	T2	N0	M0
	IIb	T3	N0	M0
Stage	IIIa	T4	N0	M0
	IIIb	Any T	N1	M0
Stage	IV	Any T	Any N	MI

Source: Rindi, G. et al., Virchows Arch., 451(4), 757, October 2007, Available from: http://www.ncbi.nlm.nih.gov/pubmed/17674042, retrieved on September 25, 2014.

[a] Tumor limited to ampulla of Vater for ampullary gangliocytic paraganglioma.

[b] M1-specific sites defined according to the TNM staging system.

DIAGNOSIS OF PSM OF NET ORIGIN

The diagnosis of PSM of NET origin is primarily based on morphology and diagnostic imaging such as computed tomography (CT) scan, magnetic resonance imaging (MRI), and somatostatin receptor scintigraphy. These techniques can visualize tumor nodules ≥1 cm in diameter. Minor disease-related anatomical changes are usually not evident on these diagnostic procedures so that the number and extent of lesions detected intraoperatively usually exceed that seen using imaging procedures. According to the European Neuroendocrine Tumor Society (ENETS), extra level of detection of extrahepatic disease within the abdomen by CT examination is approximately 81%, while the sensitivity of the method is 75% (63%–90%) and specificity 99% (98%–100%). The corresponding diagnostic accuracy, sensitivity, and specificity of MRI are 68%, 89%, and 100%, respectively [20]. CT enterography and MRI enterography may be of use in the diagnosis of the primary tumor of the small intestine and/or luminal narrowing or obstruction of the small intestine caused by a primary lesion or secondary lesions (e.g., carcinomatosis) as well as the eventual presence of the retraction of the mesentery often seen with NETs of

small bowel origin [20–22]. PET-CT can significantly influence surgical decision making in the assessment of the extent of PSM and determination of resectability and thereby prevent unnecessary surgical exploration with tumor burden and extent making complete cytoreduction unlikely [23,24].

In the case of ascites, peritoneal fluid cytological examination can confirm the presence of malignancy. However, it is important to note that negative cytological findings do not exclude the presence of PSM of NET origin [6].

Surgical exploration certainly provides the most accurate and certainly the best assessment of the nature, extent, and quantifiable tumor burden, hence the staging of PSM of NET origin. Surgical exploration may be performed laparoscopically (minimally invasive) or by way of open exploration (laparotomy).

Laparoscopy lends itself in most cases to complete peritoneal cavity exploration, to confirm the diagnosis and determine the precise stage of the disease, and to select patients who are suitable for CRS [25,26]. Laparotomy can be performed for even more detailed exploration, for securing tissue samples for pathological examination, conducting intraoperative ultrasonography (e.g., of liver and pancreas), and accurately determining the extent peritoneal involvement

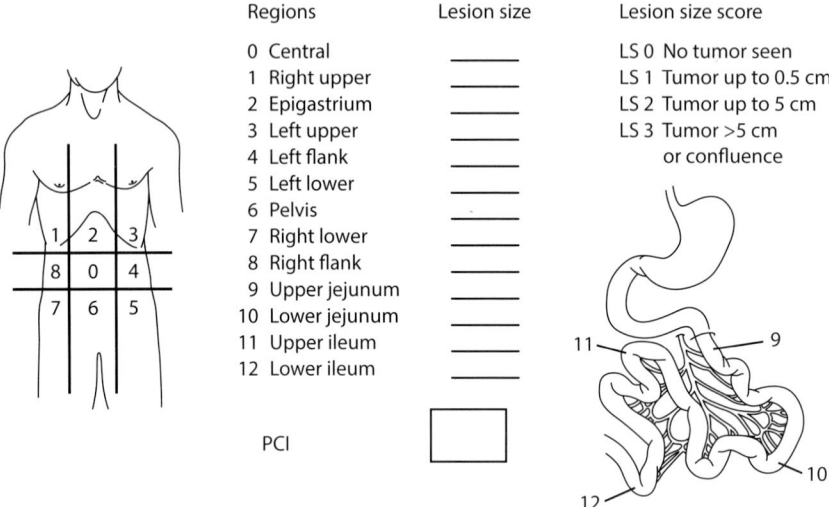

Figure 24.1 Peritoneal cancer index classification. (From Kianmanesh, R. et al., *Neuroendocrinology*, 91(4), 333, January 2010.)

and stage of disease. Surgical exploration must include careful assessment of both subdiaphragmatic spaces; lesser and greater omentum; lesser omental bursa; the lateral abdominal regions adjacent to the right, left, and sigmoid colon; mesenteric blood vessels; and the pelvis (pouch of Douglas) [12].

CLASSIFICATION OF PERITONEAL SURFACE MALIGNANCY

Classification systems are used to assess the severity and quantifiable extent of PSM and inform determination of resectability, treatment approach, and estimate prognosis. Most of the classification systems for PSM were developed for other histological types of primary tumors, primarily adenocarcinoma (e.g., appendix or colon). In practice, both preoperative and intraoperative assessment is utilized for assessing extent of PSM of NET origin and arriving at individualized treatment approaches. It is important to note that the classification systems used to assess the quantifiable extent of PSM are not solely reliable to assess surgical resectability of PSM of NET origin [12].

In practice, the most commonly used classification systems are the peritoneal cancer index (PCI) and Gilly's classification.

Peritoneal cancer index

The PCI quantifies pre- and intraoperative spread of peritoneal surface disease in each region of the abdomen and pelvis and then summed and expressed as a numerical score that ranges from 0 to 39 for the entire peritoneal cavity. It is based on the anatomical site and size of tumor nodule(s) in each region. The abdomen and pelvis are divided into nine regions (0–8). The small intestine is divided into 4 regions, so that regions 9 and 10 define the upper and lower part of the jejunum and regions 11 and 12 define the upper and lower part of the ileum. Lesion size (LS), that is, the largest size of the lesion, is recorded for each region of the abdomen. LS is expressed in four categories: LS-0, no visible lesions; LS-1,

lesion(s) up to 0.5 cm; LS-2, ranges from >0.5 to 5 cm; and LS-3, lesion greater than 5 cm (Figure 24.1).

When the PCI score exceeds 20, the disease is typically regarded as in its advanced stages, and it is considered "unresectable" for "curative" intent [27]. PCI is a comprehensive classification system and is most effectively applied in specialized medical centers.

PCI CLASSIFICATION

The abdomen and the pelvic regions are divided by lines into nine regions (0–8). The small bowel is then divided into four regions. Regions 9 and 10 define the upper and lower portions of the jejunum; regions 11 and 12 define the upper and lower portions of the ileum. The LS (i.e., the largest implant size) is scored in each abdominal region. Implants are scored as LS-0 to LS-3. LS-0 means no implants are seen throughout the region; this measurement is made after complete adhesiolysis and complete inspection of all parietal and visceral peritoneal surfaces. LS-1 refers to implants that are visible up to 0.5 cm in greatest diameter. LS-2 identifies nodules greater than 0.5 cm and up to 5 cm. LS-3 refers to implants 5 cm or greater in diameter.

Gilly's classification

Gilly's classification system for PSM is based on nodule size and is a simpler system for estimating peritoneal surface involvement by tumor than the PCI. There are five stages in the Gilly's classification system ranging from 0 to 4. Stage 0 represents no macroscopic disease. Stage 1 is defined by lesions <5 mm in one part of the abdominal cavity. Stage 2 lesions are also <5 mm in diameter but are diffusely distributed throughout the abdominal cavity. Stage 3 lesions range in size from 5 to 20 mm and are localized or diffuse in anatomical distribution. Stage 4 disease is characterized by localized or diffuse lesions larger than 2 cm in diameter (Table 24.3).

This classification is simple and easy to use. However, although Gilly's Stage 3 and 4 are considered advanced stages

Table 24.3 Gilly classification is based on nodule size and simplified extent of intraperitoneal involvement (localized or diffuse)

Stage 0	No macroscopic disease
Stage 1	Malignant granulations less than 5 mm in diameter localized in one part of the abdomen
Stage 2	Malignant granulations less than 5 mm in diameter diffuse to the whole abdomen
Stage 3	Localized or diffuse malignant granulations 5–20 mm in diameter
Stage 4	Localized or diffuse large malignant masses (more than 2 cm in diameter)

Source: Kianmanesh, R. et al., Neuroendocrinology, 91(4), 333, January 2010, Available from: http://www.ncbi.nlm.nih.gov/pubmed/20424420, retrieved on January 24, 2014.

Note: Scores vary from 0 to 4. Patients with Gilly Stage 3 or 4 have macroscopic advanced disease, which is often associated with a worse prognosis.

Table 24.4 European Neuroendocrine Tumor Society proposal of a gravity peritoneal carcinomatosis score grading system based on the association of peritoneal carcinomatosis with lymph node and liver metastases

	0 Point	1 Point	2 Points	3 Points
Lymph node metastases	Local[a]	Regional[b]	Distant abdominal (retroperitoneal, hepatic pedicle)	Extra-abdominal
Liver metastases	No macroscopic nodule	One lobe less than 5 nodules	Both lobes 5–10 nodules	Both lobes more than 10 nodules
PC	No macroscopic nodule	Gilly I–II resectable	Gilly III–IV resectable	Gilly I–II–III–IV unresectable

Source: Kianmanesh, R. et al., Neuroendocrinology, 91(4), 333, January 2010, Available from: http://www.ncbi.nlm.nih.gov/pubmed/20424420, retrieved on January 24, 2014.

Note: GPS grade A, 0–3 points; GPS grade E, 4–6 points; GPS grade C, 7–9 points. To avoid including patients with nonmalignant ascites, patients with positive malignant cells obtained by peritoneal biopsies and/or positive cytology of the peritoneal fluid are considered as having proven PC.

[a] Local: first (adjacent) to the primary tumor territory relay.
[b] Regional: secondary tumor drainage territory relay.

of disease, generally associated with poor prognosis, Gilly's classification system is relatively imprecise in that regard.

ENETS classification

Apart from the extent of peritoneal surface score values, it is important to note the presence of lymph node and hepatic metastases, as well as the presence or absence of retraction of the mesentery. The type of PSM should also be characterized: nodular, infiltrative, or both. It is also very important to determine the nature and extent of peritoneal infiltration in relation to the primary tumor, which may be in continuity, at a distance or consist of both of these types [12]. As PSM of NET origin is often associated with metastases to lymph nodes or the liver, it is clear that the usual scoring systems that take into account only peritoneal surface or small bowel involvement are not sufficient to adequately define the extent of this disease. Therefore, the group of experts at ENETS proposed a scoring system in its consensus guidelines for PC of GEP-NET origin, which includes the presence of metastases in the lymph nodes and/or the liver, the so-called abdominal gravity PC score (GPS) (Table 24.4). Total scores can range from 0 to 9 patients with 3 or fewer points representing a GPS grade of A, considered to have a low risk of intra-abdominal spread. A GPS grade of B is defined by 4–6 points and is associated with a moderate risk, while those having 7–9 points

are classified as grade C and at high risk [12]. This system has yet to be critically evaluated and validated in clinical practice.

TREATMENT OF PERITONEAL CARCINOMATOSIS OF NET ORIGIN

The presence of PC of GEP-NET origin is not rare, as it occurs in about 17% of GEP-NET cases [7,8]. Despite this, treatment recommendations for this particular disease presentation (PSM of GEP-NET origin) remain to be precisely defined, validated, and broadly implemented. The meta-analysis by Gurusamy et al. that was published in 2009 represents an important critical review of palliative CRS versus other palliative interventions for unresectable hepatic metastases of GEP-NET origin [28]. As part of that meta-analysis, an extensive database search (including The Cochrane Hepato-Biliary Group Controlled Trials Register, the Cochrane Central Register of Controlled Trials in The Cochrane Library, MEDLINE, EMBASE, Science Citation Index Expanded, and LILACS) failed to identify a single randomized controlled trial of CRS for unresectable hepatic metastases of GEP-NET origin [28]. Recognizing the modest-to-poor quality of published evidence for this particular clinical presentation, the ENETS consensus conference proposed resection or CRS for PC of NET origin in carefully selected patients within specialized centers [12].

SURGICAL TREATMENT

As with other metastatic disease, surgical treatment of PSM of GEP-NET origin can be with either curative or palliative intent depending on the nature and extent of disease and careful assessment of patient operability and disease resectability. Surgical resection may be indicated for PSM of GEP-NET origin

1. To prevent intraluminal visceral obstruction
2. To prevent consequences (e.g., visceral ischemia) associated with a desmoplastic mesenteric reaction causing fibrosis and critical narrowing of mesenteric vascular structures
3. To prevent visceral obstruction in patients with macronodular disease in the pouch of Douglas
4. To treat gastrointestinal hemorrhage
5. To relive segmental portal venous hypertension [12]

According to ESMO Clinical Practice Guidelines for diagnosis, treatment, and follow-up of PSM of GEP-NET origin, CRS may be justified if more than 70% of the tumor mass can be safely resected, which could improve quality of life (QOL) by reducing endocrine and local symptoms due to tumor, and enhance the efficacy of systemic therapy by way of cytoreduction to minimal residual tumor burden [16].

As with CRS for PSM of other tumor origin, this form of surgery for PSM of NET origin must carefully take into account risk/benefit ratio, on a case-by-case basis [27,29]. It was once thought that the mere presence of PC was associated with adverse oncological outcome (poor overall survival [OS]). As a result of this philosophy, some authors recommended against an aggressive surgical approach to patients with PSM of NET origin [6,9,30]. Vasseur et al. [6] observed, unlike NET liver metastases, no significant difference in 5-year actuarial survival of 64% and 84% in patients with and without PC, respectively. However, Elias et al. [31] compared 20 patients with unresectable PC with 17 patients that underwent resection of PC and intraperitoneal chemotherapy (65% of patients in this group having resection of synchronous liver metastases) and found that the PC was the direct cause of death in 40% of unresectable or untreated patients (mortality due to liver failure or bowel obstruction). Five-year survival was significantly longer in the treated versus untreated group (66% vs. 41%, P = 0.007). Norlén et al. [8] in their series of 608 patients with small intestinal NETs identified the following independent prognostic factors for survival by multivariate analysis: mesenteric nodal metastases, distant nodal metastases, extra-abdominal metastases, PC, liver tumor load, Ki-67 index (WHO grade), and locoregional (cytoreductive) surgery. These findings suggest that surgical treatment of PC might benefit patients with locoregionally advanced NETs.

MORBIDITY AND MORTALITY

Treatment of PC consists of aggressive surgical cytoreduction and hyperthermic intraperitoneal chemotherapy (HIPEC). Tumor-bearing peritonectomy or cytoreduction is a demanding surgical procedure, and for it to be reasonably applied in the setting of PSM of NET origin, one must have an experienced team with demonstrated acceptable perioperative morbidity and low operative mortality. Chambers et al. [32] in their series of 66 patients undergoing aggressive treatment of hepatic metastases and PSM of NET origin reported postoperative morbidity of 22% and 0% operative mortality. Elias et al. recently reported corresponding morbidity and mortality of 56% and 2% (1 out of 41), respectively. Boudreaux et al. [33] reported a 3% intraoperative morbidity, 49% postoperative morbidity, and that 39% of these were minor complications. Postoperative 30-day mortality was 3% (5 of 189). Overall operative morbidity in the published literature ranges from 10% to 60%, and operative mortality ranges from 0% to 10% [12,34]. These rates are acceptable when considering the risk/benefit ratio of CRS, which must take into consideration operative selection criteria: operable patients with good performance status, normal renal function, and adequate nutritional status, among other selection criteria. Aggressive CRS and regional heated intraperitoneal chemotherapy should be considered in the context of multidisciplinary case review, deliberation, and consensus treatment recommendations for each particular case [12].

SHORT-TERM RESULTS

An aggressive surgical approach seems to provide good short-term outcomes, as it significantly relieves QOL-limiting symptoms of the disease. Chambers et al. [32] determined the palliative benefit of an aggressive surgical approach in 24 patients with small bowel obstruction due to advanced NETs and 56 patients with carcinoid syndrome; clinical improvement was identified in 75% of these cases. The authors concluded that aggressive surgery represents an effective palliative treatment approach in carefully selected patients with both hepatic and mesenteric metastases from NETs. Boudreaux et al. [35], in their series of 82 patients with advanced carcinoid tumors (one-third had intestinal obstruction, and nearly half of these patients had mesenteric vascular encasement and ischemia) treated with aggressive surgery, reported a significant improvement in Karnofsky performance scores from 65 to 85 (P < 0.0001). Four-year survival for patients with no or unilateral hepatic metastases was 89%, and for patients with bilateral hepatic metastasis, 4-year survival was 52%, leading the authors to recommend multimodal surgical therapy for advanced-stage carcinoid tumors and to advocate for primary tumor resection even in the presence of distant disease spread.

LONG-TERM RESULTS

In addition to satisfying the short-term outcome measures of CRS (reduction in tumor burden, improvement of tumor-related symptoms, and QOL), there are publications showing an associated benefit in survival. Chambers et al. [32] reported a 5-year survival rate of 74% for aggressive surgical intervention for both hepatic and mesenteric metastases of NET origin. Boudreaux et al. [33] in their series of 189 consecutive patients with well-differentiated NETs underwent a total of 229 CRS procedures. Mean OS from time of diagnosis of NET was ~20 months. 5-, 10-, and 20-year survival rates were 87%, 77%, and 41%, respectively, in that single institutional experience. Elias et al. [31] in a comparative study analyzed 37 patients with PSM of well-differentiated GEP-NET origin. Twenty patients could not undergo complete resection of peritoneal surface tumor, while 17 patients had complete CRS and immediate intraperitoneal chemotherapy. Five-year survival was 40.9% and 60.2% (P = 0.007) for the group with incomplete and complete cytoreduction, respectively. The same group of authors published a paper in 2014 describing the results of 41 patients treated with CRS for PSM of NET origin; 28 patients undergoing CRS + HIPEC and 13 undergoing CRS alone. Liver metastases were treated at time of CRS in 66% of patients. Overall, 5- and 10-year survival rates were 69% and 52%, respectively. Five years after CRS, peritoneal and liver metastases were observed in 47% and 66% of cases, respectively. OS was not statistically significant between patients undergoing CRS with or without HIPEC; however, disease-free interval was greater in the HIPEC group (P = 0.018), primarily due to lower incidence of bone and lung metastases in the CRS + HIPEC group [36].

SYSTEMIC THERAPY

Chemotherapy

There are a small number of prospective randomized trials for NET representing Level I evidence basis for the treatment of this disease with systemic therapy [37]. Systemic chemotherapy agents utilized in the treatment of NET include 5-fluorouracil (5-FU), dacarbazine, doxorubicin, and streptozocin. When used as single agents, these chemotherapeutics have shown little benefit in terms of shrinkage of tumor or disease control. For these reasons, studies have been carried out utilizing a combination of these drugs; however, no combination of cytotoxic chemotherapy agents has produced a response rate higher than 15% in small intestinal NETs when tumor diameter reduction <50% is taken as a response criterion [38].

For NETs of pancreatic islet, the cell origin response rate to treatment with cytotoxic chemotherapy regimens has ranged from 6% to 69%. A retrospective analysis of 84 patients with locally advanced or metastatic pancreatic neuroendocrine carcinoma treated with 5-FU, doxorubicin, and streptozocin identified a 39% response rate [39]. Two-year progression-free survival (PFS) was 41%, and 2-year OS was 74% in that study. Both PFS and OS correlated with extent of hepatic metastatic disease; >75% replacement of liver by tumor was associated with significantly worse PFS and OS.

Sun et al. in a Phase II/III randomized trial of 249 patients with advanced NET showed a significantly longer mean survival of 24.3 months in the group that received streptozocin plus 5-FU compared to 15.6 months for doxorubicin plus 5-FU. There was no significant difference observed in terms of response rate or PFS between the two randomized study groups [40].

Meyer et al. randomized 86 patients with advanced GEP-NETs to receive either capecitabine and streptozocin with cisplatin or capecitabine and streptozocin without cisplatin; treatment response rate was similar between groups, 16% and 12%, respectively. Median PFS was 9.7 and 10.2 months for the three- and two-drug regimen, respectively. OS was similar between the two groups, 27.5 and 26.7 months for capecitabine/streptozocin/cisplatin and capecitabine/streptozocin, respectively. The two-drug regimen was better tolerated than the three-drug regimen with 44% and 68% of patients experiencing Grade 3 or higher adverse events, respectively [41].

Somatostatin analogues

NET-secreting cells have on their surface various types of somatostatin receptors. Specifically, there are five types of somatostatin receptors (sstr1–5). Binding to these receptors, somatostatin inhibits secretion of various hormones, including serotonin, insulin, gastrin, and glucagon, among others [42]. Each type of NET cell can have more than one subtype of somatostatin receptor. Activation of subtypes sstr2 and sstr5 causes antisecretory effect of somatostatin and somatostatin analogs and thereby inhibits the secretion of hormones in functional NETs. On the other hand, there is evidence that subtypes sstr1, sstr2, sstr4, and sstr5 have an antitumor effect through inhibition of tumor cell growth and induction of apoptosis [43].

Octreotide (Sandostatin) was the first commercially available somatostatin analogue noted for its prolonged half-life of 2 hours. Octreotide has great affinity for sstr2 and moderate affinity for sstr3 and sstr5. Octreotide is administered on a daily basis; a longer acting form (octreotide long-acting repeatable [LAR]) is administered on a monthly basis. Octreotide was initially shown to improve symptoms of carcinoid syndrome, which was associated with a reduced level of excretion of 5-HIAA in the urine [44,45]. Several studies have confirmed the efficacy of octreotide LAR for both symptomatic and biochemical control of disease in patients with NET. It was also observed that octreotide contributed to stabilization of disease and control of NET growth in 50%–75% of cases, even in the presence of metastatic disease [46–49].

It was also noted that the use of somatostatin analogs prolongs survival in these patients [50]. Indeed, data from the SEER have shown dramatic improvement in survival for patients who were treated from 1988 to 2004 compared to those treated earlier, and this improvement coincided with a period when the somatostatin analogues were introduced into daily clinical practice. Historically (prior to the routine use of somatostatin analogs), 5-year survival was 18%, but, in the last 20 years, has reached 67% in patients who received somatostatin analogs [4]. Although about two-thirds of patients treated with these drugs have stable disease for more than 5 years, only 5% of patients had an objective tumor response to therapy [46,48,50,51]. Rinke et al. [51] conducted the first major double-blind, placebo-controlled Phase III trial in patients with well-differentiated metastatic NET (Placebo-controlled prospective Randomized study on the antiproliferative efficacy of Octreotide LAR in patients with metastatic neuroendocrine MIDgut tumors [PROMID]). Patients received either placebo or octreotide LAR (30 mg intramuscularly in monthly intervals until disease progression or death). The primary end point was time to tumor progression and secondary end points were survival and tumor response. The study group treated with octreotide LAR had a twofold increase in PFS (14.3 months) as compared to the placebo study arm (6 months; P < 0.001). After 6 months of on study treatment, stable disease was achieved in 67% of patients in the octreotide LAR arm, versus 37% in the placebo group. Actively secreting NETs responded equally to therapy as nonfunctioning NETs. The best treatment results were achieved in a group of patients with low-volume hepatic disease and resected primary tumors [51]. The hazard ratio for OS was 0.81 (95% CI, 0.30–2.18).

The effect of Sandostatin analogues on PC of NET origin was specifically examined. The PROMID study indicates that extrahepatic metastases do not belong to the favorable predictors of response to octreotide [51]. Panzuto et al. [50] concluded that the presence of extrahepatic metastases is the main predictor of poor treatment response for metastatic, well-differentiated GEP-NET. The authors also concluded that the absence of response after 6 months of therapy means a poor prognosis and that one should consider other therapeutic options.

Somatostatin analogs are commonly used for the treatment of postoperative complications. However, there are very few studies that examine the perioperative use of these analogs in patients with NET. Massimino et al. [52] retrospectively analyzed perioperative use of octreotide LAR and octreotide bolus and correlated the use of these agents with occurrence of intraoperative complications in patients with carcinoid tumors undergoing abdominal operations. They found that the intraoperative complications often occur (24%) in the patients having liver resection due to metastases, regardless of the presence of the carcinoid syndrome and perioperative application of octreotide (octreotide LAR or single prophylactic dose of octreotide). Postoperative complications were associated with the occurrence of intraoperative complications (60% versus 31% postoperative morbidity in patients with or without intraoperative morbidity). The authors concluded the necessity of further studies to determine whether the benefits of perioperative application of octreotide are clinically meaningful.

Other somatostatin analogs have been applied clinically—lanreotide and pasireotide. Lanreotide pharmacological effects are similar to Sandostatin. Pasireotide modulates four of five somatostatin receptors (sstr1, sstr2, sstr3, and sstr5) and shows a stronger affinity for more potent functional activity of sstr5 than octreotide. Therefore, one can utilize this drug when a clinical response to octreotide or lanreotide is lacking [38]. Kvols et al. found pasireotide effective in 27% of nonresponders to octreotide LAR [53].

Interferon-alpha

Patients with functioning NETs of the jejunum and ileum and low Ki-67 proliferation index may be treated with interferon-alpha therapy as a second-line approach [54]. A pooled analysis of trials investigating interferon-alpha in patients with NETs showed that about 40% of patients had biochemical responses (comparable with responses observed with octreotide and lanreotide), and about 10% had objective tumor responses [38]. A few studies evaluating a strategy of combination therapy with interferon-alpha and octreotide to control symptom and tumor progression simultaneously did not show significant improvement in survival compared with octreotide monotherapy in patients with NETs [46,55].

Targeted therapy

Gaining new knowledge about the biology of the tumor has led to the development of targeted therapy on specific processes or molecular biological pathways within the tumor, which may prevent tumor growth and progression.

Everolimus

A potential target for NETs is mammalian target of rapamycin (mTOR), a central protein in the synthesis of proteins, which in tumors is active in promoting cell growth, cell proliferation, angiogenesis, and cellular metabolism. Everolimus or RAD001 (afinitor) inhibits the mTOR pathway by binding to an intracellular receptor, FKBP-12 [38,56]. Everolimus can be used alone or in combination with somatostatin or cytotoxic drugs.

Randomized, double-blind, placebo-controlled Phase III RADIANT-2 trial has demonstrated the benefits of everolimus (10 mg/day) in combination with octreotide LAR (30 mg/month) for patients with advanced NET [57]. The authors have shown that these patients have a 23% lower risk of disease progression compared to a group that received placebo plus octreotide LAR. They showed a significant improvement in survival of 5.1 months (16.4 vs. 11.3, respectively) with combination therapy [57]. The RADIANT-3 study has demonstrated a clinically meaningful benefit of PFS (11.0 vs. 4.6 months) in patients treated with everolimus versus placebo, in 410 patients with low or intermediate grade, advanced NET [58].

Tyrosine kinase inhibitors

The best known representatives of this group of targeted therapeutics are sunitinib and pazopanib. They inhibit cell growth and neo-angiogenesis. Raymond et al. conducted a randomized, double-blinded, placebo-controlled international trial in patients with advanced pancreatic NET

[59]. One hundred seventy-one patients were randomized to receive either sunitinib (37.5 mg/day) or best supportive care. The trial was ended earlier than planned due to the significantly increased incidence of adverse events in the placebo group [59]. PFS was significantly longer (11.4 months) in the sunitinib group than (5.5 months) in the placebo group [59].

Radionuclide therapy

Systemic peptide receptor-targeted radiotherapy is a treatment option available for symptomatic patients with nonresectable somatostatin receptor-positive tumor metastases who have evidence of uptake of MIBG 123I- or 111In-octreotide at all known tumor sites during diagnostic imaging [60]. This therapy may be considered for functional and nonfunctional tumors that have positive somatostatin receptors unrelated to the origin of the primary tumor [16]. Based on Phase II clinical trials, more than 1000 patients in total have been treated with radionuclide therapy in Europe with objective response rates ranging from 20% to 40% (III, A). Response rates are higher in pancreatic compared with small intestinal NETs (III, A) [61].

REFERENCES

1. NCI. Dictionary of Cancer Terms—National Cancer Institute. Retrieved on September 23, 2014. Available from: http://www.cancer.gov/dictionary?cdrid=44904.
2. Barakat MT, Meeran K, Bloom SR. Neuroendocrine tumors. *Endocrine-Related Cancer*. Retrieved on January 23, 2014. March 2004;11(1):1–18. Available from: http://www.ncbi.nlm.nih.gov/pubmed/15027882.
3. Modlin IM, Lye KD, Kidd M. A 5-decade analysis of 13,715 carcinoid tumors. *Cancer*. Retrieved on January 15, 2014. February 15, 2003;97(1):934–959. Available from: http://www.ncbi.nlm.nih.gov/pubmed/12569593.
4. Yao JC, Hassan M, Phan A, Dagohoy C, Leary C, Mares JE et al. One hundred years after "carcinoid": Epidemiology of and prognostic factors for neuroendocrine tumors in 35,825 cases in the United States. *Journal of Clinical Oncology*. Retrieved on January 13, 2014. June 20, 2008;26(18):3063–3072. Available from: http://jco.ascopubs.org/content/26/18/3063.abstract.
5. Elias D, Sideris L, Liberals G, Ducreux M, Malka D, Lasser P et al. Surgical treatment of peritoneal carcinomatosis from well-differentiated digestive endocrine carcinomas. *Surgery*. Retrieved on January 27, 2014. April 2005; 137(4):411–416. Available from: http://www.ncbi.nlm.nih.gov/pubmed/15800487.
6. Vasseur B, Cadiot G, Zins M, Fléjou JF, Belghiti J, Marmuse JP et al. Peritoneal carcinomatosis in patients with digestive endocrine tumors. *Cancer*. Retrieved on January 27, 2014. October 15, 1996;78(8):1686–1692. Available from: http://www.ncbi.nlm.nih.gov/pubmed/8859181.
7. Mitry E, O'Toole D, Louvet C, Bouché O, Lecomte T, Seitz JF et al. Résultats préliminaires de l'enquête nationale FFCD-ANGH-GERCOR sur les tumeurs endocrines à localisation digestive. *Gastroentérologie clinique et biologique*. 2003;27:A135.
8. Norlén O, Stalberg P, Öberg K, Eriksson S, Hedberg J, Hessman A et al. Long-term results of surgery for small intestinal neuroendocrine tumors at a tertiary referral center. *World Journal of Surgery*. Retrieved on September 10, 2014. June 2012;36(6):1419–1431. Available from: http://www.ncbi.nlm.nih.gov/pubmed/21984144.
9. Landry CS, Brock G, Scoggins CR, McMasters KM, Martin RM. A proposed staging system for small bowel carcinoid tumors based on an analysis of 6,380 patients. *American Journal of Surgery*. Retrieved on January 28, 2014. December 2008;196(6):896–903; discussion 903 Available from: http://www.ncbi.nlm.nih.gov/pubmed/19095106.
10. Koppe MJ, Boerman OC, Oyen WJG, Bleichrodt RP. Peritoneal carcinomatosis of colorectal origin: Incidence and current treatment strategies. *Annals of Surgery*. Retrieved on September 5, 2014. February 2006;243(2):212–222. Available from: http://www.pubmedcentral.nih.gov/articlerender.fcgi?artid=1448921&tool=pmcentrez&rendertype=abstract.
11. Lifante JC, Glehen O, Cotte E, Beaujard AC, Gilly FN. Natural history of peritoneal carcinomatosis from digestive origin. *Cancer Treatment and Research*. Retrieved on January 28, 2014. January 2007;134:119–129. Available from: http://www.ncbi.nlm.nih.gov/pubmed/17633050.
12. Kianmanesh R, Ruszniewski P, Rindi G, Kwekkeboom D, Pape UF, Kulke M et al. ENets consensus guidelines for the management of peritoneal carcinomatosis from neuroendocrine tumors. *Neuroendocrinology*. Retrieved on January 24, 2014. January 2010;91(4):333–340. Available from: http://www.ncbi.nlm.nih.gov/pubmed/20424420.
13. Askew JW, Connolly HM. Carcinoid valve disease. *Current Treatment Options in Cardiovascular Medicine*. Retrieved on January 28, 2014. October 2013;15(5):544–555. Available from: http://www.ncbi.nlm.nih.gov/pubmed/23955119.
14. Salyers WJ, Vega KJ, Munoz JC, Trotman BW, Tanev SS. Neuroendocrine tumors of the gastrointestinal tract: Case reports and literature review. *World Journal of Gastrointestinal Oncology*. Retrieved on January 28, 2014. August 15, 2014;6(8):301–310. Available from: http://www.pubmedcentral.nih.gov/articlerender.fcgi?artid=4133797&tool=pmcentrez&rendertype=abstract.
15. Vani BR, Thejaswini MU, Kumar BD, Murthy VS, Geethamala K. Carcinoid tumor of appendix in a child: A rare case at an uncommon site.

African Journal of Paediatric Surgery. Retrieved on September 28, 2014. 2014;11(1):71–73. Available from: http://www.ncbi.nlm.nih.gov/pubmed/24647300.

16. Öberg K, Knigge U, Kwekkeboom D, Perren A. neuroendocrine gastro-entero-pancreatic tumors: ESMO Clinical Practice Guidelines for diagnosis, treatment and follow-up. *Annals of Oncology.* Retrieved on August 4, 2014. October 2012;23(Suppl. 7):vii124–vii130. Available from: http://www.ncbi.nlm.nih.gov/pubmed/22997445.

17. Rindi G, Petrone G, Inzani F. The 2010 WHO classification of digestive neuroendocrine neoplasms: A critical appraisal four years after its introduction. *Endocrine Pathology.* Retrieved on September 28, 2014. June 2014;25(2):186–192. Available from: http://www.ncbi.nlm.nih.gov/pubmed/24699927.

18. Klöppel G, Couvelard A, Perren A, Komminoth P, McNicol A-M, Nilsson O et al. ENETS Consensus Guidelines for the Standards of Care in Neuroendocrine Tumors: Towards a standardized approach to the diagnosis of gastroenteropancreatic neuroendocrine tumors and their prognostic stratification. *Neuroendocrinology.* Retrieved on September 28, 2014. January 2009;90(2):162–166. Available from: http://www.ncbi.nlm.nih.gov/pubmed/19060454.

19. Rindi G, Klöppel G, Couvelard A, Komminoth P, Körner M, Lopes JM et al. TNM staging of midgut and hindgut (neuro) endocrine tumors: A consensus proposal including a grading system. *Virchows Archiv.* Retrieved on September 25, 2014. October 2007;451(4):757–762. Available from: http://www.ncbi.nlm.nih.gov/pubmed/17674042.

20. Sundin A, Vullierme M-P, Kaltsas G, Plöckinger U. ENETS Consensus Guidelines for the Standards of Care in Neuroendocrine Tumors: Radiological examinations. *Neuroendocrinology.* Retrieved on September 28, 2014. January 2009;90(2):167–183. Available from: http://www.ncbi.nlm.nih.gov/pubmed/19077417.

21. Schmid-Tannwald C, Zech CJ, Panteleon A, Sommer WH, Auernhammer C, Herrmann KA. Characteristic imaging features of carcinoid tumors of the small bowel in MR enteroclysis. *Radiologe.* Retrieved on September 28, 2014. March 2009;49(3):242–245, 248–251. Available from: http://www.ncbi.nlm.nih.gov/pubmed/19198795.

22. Woodbridge LR, Murtagh BM, Yu DFQC, Planche KL. Midgut neuroendocrine tumors: Imaging assessment for surgical resection. *Radiographics.* Retrieved on September 28, 2014. 34(2):413–426. Available from: http://www.ncbi.nlm.nih.gov/pubmed/24617688.

23. Königsrainer I, Aschoff P, Zieker D, Beckert S, Glatzle J, Pfannenberg C et al. Selection criteria for peritonectomy with hyperthermic intraoperative chemotherapy (HIPEC) in peritoneal carcinomatosis. *Zentralblatt für Chirurgie.* Retrieved on September 28, 2014. September 2008;133(5):468–472. Available from: http://www.ncbi.nlm.nih.gov/pubmed/18924046.

24. Berthelot C, Morel O, Girault S, Verrièle V, Poirier A-L, Moroch J et al. Use of FDG-PET/CT for peritoneal carcinomatosis before hyperthermic intraperitoneal chemotherapy. *Nuclear Medicine Communications.* Retrieved on September 28, 2014. January 2011;32(1):23–29. Available from: http://www.ncbi.nlm.nih.gov/pubmed/21042225.

25. Jayakrishnan TT, Zacharias AJ, Sharma A, Pappas SG, Gamblin TC, Turaga KK. Role of laparoscopy in patients with peritoneal metastases considered for cytoreductive surgery and hyperthermic intraperitoneal chemotherapy (HIPEC). *World Journal of Surgical Oncology.* Retrieved on September 29, 2014. January 2014;12:270. Available from: http://www.pubmedcentral.nih.gov/articlerender.fcgi?artid=4153918&tool=pmcentrez&rendertype=abstract.

26. D'Angelica M, Fong Y, Weber S, Gonen M, DeMatteo RP, Conlon K et al. The role of staging laparoscopy in hepatobiliary malignancy: Prospective analysis of 401 cases. *Annals of Surgical Oncology.* Retrieved on September 29, 2014. March 2003;10(2):183–189. Available from: http://www.ncbi.nlm.nih.gov/pubmed/12620915.

27. Sugarbaker PH. A curative approach to peritoneal carcinomatosis from colorectal cancer. *Seminars in Oncology.* Retrieved on September 30, 2014. December 2005;32(6 Suppl. 9):S68–S73. Available from: http://www.ncbi.nlm.nih.gov/pubmed/16399436.

28. Gurusamy KS, Pamecha V, Sharma D, Davidson BR. Palliative cytoreductive surgery versus other palliative treatments in patients with unresectable liver metastases from gastro-entero-pancreatic neuroendocrine tumours. *Cochrane Database of Systematic Reviews.* Retrieved on September 30, 2014. January 2009;(1):CD007118. Available from: http://www.ncbi.nlm.nih.gov/pubmed/19160322.

29. Sugarbaker PH, Stuart OA, Yoo D. Strategies for management of the peritoneal surface component of cancer: Cytoreductive surgery plus perioperative intraperitoneal chemotherapy. *Journal of Oncology Pharmacy Practice.* Retrieved on September 30, 2014. September 2005;11(3):111–119. Available from: http://www.ncbi.nlm.nih.gov/pubmed/16390599.

30. Mayo SC, de Jong MC, Pulitano C, Clary BM, Reddy SK, Gamblin TC et al. Surgical management of hepatic neuroendocrine tumor metastasis: Results from an international multi-institutional analysis. *Annals of Surgical Oncology.* Retrieved on

September 28, 2014. December 2010;17(12):3129–3136. Available from: http://www.ncbi.nlm.nih.gov/pubmed/20585879.

31. Elias D, Sideris L, Liberale G, Ducreux M, Malka D, Lasser P et al. Surgical treatment of peritoneal carcinomatosis from well-differentiated digestive endocrine carcinomas. *Surgery*. Elsevier; Retrieved on September 27, 2014. April 4, 2005;137(4):411–416. Available from: http://www.surgjournal.com/article/S0039606004007147/fulltext.

32. Chambers AJ, Pasieka JL, Dixon E, Rorstad O. The palliative benefit of aggressive surgical intervention for both hepatic and mesenteric metastases from neuroendocrine tumors. *Surgery*. Retrieved on October 1, 2014. October 2008;144(4):645–651; discussion 651–653. Available from: http://www.ncbi.nlm.nih.gov/pubmed/18847650.

33. Boudreaux JP, Wang Y-Z, Diebold AE, Frey DJ, Anthony L, Uhlhorn AP et al. A single institution's experience with surgical cytoreduction of stage IV, well-differentiated, small bowel neuroendocrine tumors. *Journal of the American College of Surgeons*. Retrieved on September 24, 2014. April 2014;218(4):837–844. Available from: http://www.ncbi.nlm.nih.gov/pubmed/24655881.

34. Au JT, Levine J, Aytaman A, Weber T, Serafini F. Management of peritoneal metastasis from neuroendocrine tumors. *Journal of Surgical Oncology*. Retrieved on September 7, 2014. November 2013;108(6):385–386. Available from: http://www.ncbi.nlm.nih.gov/pubmed/24142576.

35. Boudreaux JP, Putty B, Frey DJ, Woltering E, Anthony L, Daly I et al. Surgical treatment of advanced-stage carcinoid tumors: Lessons learned. *Annals of Surgery*. Retrieved on September 30, 2014. June 2005;241(6):839–845; discussion 845–846. Available from: http://www.pubmedcentral.nih.gov/articlerender.fcgi?artid=1357164&tool=pmcentrez&rendertype=abstract.

36. Elias D, David A, Sourrouille I, Honoré C, Goéré D, Dumont F et al. Neuroendocrine carcinomas: Optimal surgery of peritoneal metastases (and associated intra-abdominal metastases). *Surgery*. Retrieved on September 18, 2014. January 2014;155(1):5–12. Available from: http://www.ncbi.nlm.nih.gov/pubmed/24084595.

37. Valle JW, Eatock M, Clueit B, Gabriel Z, Ferdinand R, Mitchell S. A systematic review of non-surgical treatments for pancreatic neuroendocrine tumours. *Cancer Treatment Reviews*. Retrieved on October 9, 2014. April 2014;40(3):376–389. Available from: http://www.ncbi.nlm.nih.gov/pubmed/24296109.

38. Oberg KE. The management of neuroendocrine tumours: Current and future medical therapy options. *Clinical Oncology (Royal College of Radiology)*. Retrieved on October 6, 2014. May 2012;24(4):282–293. Available from: http://www.ncbi.nlm.nih.gov/pubmed/21907552.

39. Kouvaraki MA, Ajani JA, Hoff P, Wolff R, Evans DB, Lozano R et al. Fluorouracil, doxorubicin, and streptozocin in the treatment of patients with locally advanced and metastatic pancreatic endocrine carcinomas. *Journal of Clinical Oncology*. Retrieved on October 9, 2014. December 1, 2004;22(23):4762–4771. Available from: http://jco.ascopubs.org/content/22/23/4762.abstract.

40. Sun W, Lipsitz S, Catalano P, Mailliard JA, Haller DG. Phase II/III study of doxorubicin with fluorouracil compared with streptozocin with fluorouracil or dacarbazine in the treatment of advanced carcinoid tumors: Eastern Cooperative Oncology Group Study E1281. *Journal of Clinical Oncology*. Retrieved on October 9, 2014. August 1, 2005;23(22):4897–4904. Available from: http://jco.ascopubs.org/content/23/22/4897.abstract.

41. Meyer T, Qian W, Caplin ME, Armstrong G, Lao-Sirieix S-H, Hardy R et al. Capecitabine and streptozocin ± cisplatin in advanced gastroenteropancreatic neuroendocrine tumours. *European Journal of Cancer*. Retrieved on November 23, 2014. March 2014;50(5):902–911. Available from: http://www.ncbi.nlm.nih.gov/pubmed/24445147.

42. Møller LN, Stidsen CE, Hartmann B, Holst JJ. Somatostatin receptors. *Biochimica et Biophysica Acta*. Retrieved on October 9, 2014. September 22, 2003;1616(1):1–84. Available from: http://www.ncbi.nlm.nih.gov/pubmed/14507421.

43. Susini C, Buscail L. Rationale for the use of somatostatin analogs as antitumor agents. *Annals of Oncology*. Retrieved on October 9, 2014. December 2006;17(12):1733–1742. Available from: http://www.ncbi.nlm.nih.gov/pubmed/16801334.

44. Kvols LK, Buck M, Moertel CG, Schutt AJ, Rubin J, O'Connell MJ et al. Treatment of metastatic islet cell carcinoma with a somatostatin analogue (SMS 201–995). *Annals of Internal Medicine*. Retrieved on October 10, 2014. August 1987;107(2):162–168. Available from: http://www.ncbi.nlm.nih.gov/pubmed/2886085.

45. Kvols LK, Moertel CG, O'Connell MJ, Schutt AJ, Rubin J, Hahn RG. Treatment of the malignant carcinoid syndrome. Evaluation of a long-acting somatostatin analogue. *New England Journal of Medicine*. Retrieved on October 10, 2014. September 11, 1986;315(11):663–666. Available from: http://www.ncbi.nlm.nih.gov/pubmed/2427948.

46. Arnold R, Trautmann ME, Creutzfeldt W, Benning R, Benning M, Neuhaus C et al. Somatostatin analogue octreotide and inhibition of tumour growth in metastatic endocrine gastroenteropancreatic tumours.

Gut. Retrieved on October 10, 2014. March 1, 1996;38(3):430–438. Available from: http://gut.bmj.com/content/38/3/430.abstract.

47. Welin SV, Janson ET, Sundin A, Stridsberg M, Lavenius E, Granberg D et al. High-dose treatment with a long-acting somatostatin analogue in patients with advanced midgut carcinoid tumours. *European Journal of Endocrinology.* Retrieved on October 10, 2014. July 2004;151(1):107–112. Available from: http://www.ncbi.nlm.nih.gov/pubmed/15248829.

48. Shojamanesh H, Gibril F, Louie A, Ojeaburu JV, Bashir S, Abou-Saif A et al. Prospective study of the antitumor efficacy of long-term octreotide treatment in patients with progressive metastatic gastrinoma. *Cancer.* Retrieved on October 10, 2014. January 15, 2002;94(2):331–343. Available from: http://www.ncbi.nlm.nih.gov/pubmed/11900219.

49. Angeletti S, Corleto VD, Schillaci O, Moretti A, Panzuto F, Annibale B et al. Single dose of octreotide stabilize metastatic gastro-entero-pancreatic endocrine tumours. *Italian Journal of Gastroenterology and Hepatology.* Retrieved on October 10, 2014. 31(1):23–27. Available from: http://www.ncbi.nlm.nih.gov/pubmed/10091100.

50. Panzuto F, Di Fonzo M, Iannicelli E, Sciuto R, Maini CL, Capurso G et al. Long-term clinical outcome of somatostatin analogues for treatment of progressive, metastatic, well-differentiated entero-pancreatic endocrine carcinoma. *Annals of Oncology.* Retrieved on September 29, 2014. March 2006;17(3):461–466. Available from: http://www.ncbi.nlm.nih.gov/pubmed/16364959.

51. Rinke A, Müller H-H, Schade-Brittinger C, Klose K-J, Barth P, Wied M et al. Placebo-controlled, double-blind, prospective, randomized study on the effect of octreotide LAR in the control of tumor growth in patients with metastatic neuroendocrine midgut tumors: A report from the PROMID Study Group. *Journal of Clinical Oncology.* Retrieved on September 12, 2014. October 1, 2009;27(28):4656–4663. Available from: http://www.ncbi.nlm.nih.gov/pubmed/19704057.

52. Massimino K, Harrskog O, Pommier S, Pommier R. Octreotide LAR and bolus octreotide are insufficient for preventing intraoperative complications in carcinoid patients. *Journal of Surgical Oncology.* Retrieved on October 11, 2014. June 2013;107(8):842–846. Available from: http://www.ncbi.nlm.nih.gov/pubmed/23592524.

53. Kvols LK, Oberg KE, O'Dorisio TM, Mohideen P, de Herder WW, Arnold R et al. Pasireotide (SOM230) shows efficacy and tolerability in the treatment of patients with advanced neuroendocrine tumors refractory or resistant to octreotide LAR: Results from a phase II study. *Endocrine-Related Cancer.* Retrieved on October 6, 2014. October 2012;19(5):657–666. Available from: http://www.ncbi.nlm.nih.gov/pubmed/22807497.

54. Eriksson B, Klöppel G, Krenning E, Ahlman H, Plöckinger U, Wiedenmann B et al. Consensus guidelines for the management of patients with digestive neuroendocrine tumors—Well-differentiated jejunal-ileal tumor/carcinoma. *Neuroendocrinology.* Retrieved on October 5, 2014. January 2008;87(1):8–19. Available from: http://www.ncbi.nlm.nih.gov/pubmed/18097129.

55. Kölby L, Persson G, Franzén S, Ahrén B. Randomized clinical trial of the effect of interferon alpha on survival in patients with disseminated midgut carcinoid tumours. *British Journal of Surgery.* Retrieved on October 12, 2014. June 2003;90(6):687–693. Available from: http://www.ncbi.nlm.nih.gov/pubmed/12808615.

56. Ortolani S, Ciccarese C, Cingarlini S, Tortora G, Massari F. Suppression of mTOR pathway in solid tumors: Lessons learned from clinical experience in renal cell carcinoma and neuroendocrine tumors and new perspectives. *Future Oncology.* 2015;11(12):1809–1828.

57. Pavel ME, Hainsworth JD, Baudin E, Peeters M, Hörsch D, Winkler RE et al. Everolimus plus octreotide long-acting repeatable for the treatment of advanced neuroendocrine tumours associated with carcinoid syndrome (RADIANT-2): A randomised, placebo-controlled, phase 3 study. *Lancet.* Retrieved on October 12, 2014. December 10, 2011;378(9808):2005–2012. Available from: http://www.ncbi.nlm.nih.gov/pubmed/22119496.

58. Yao JC, Shah MH, Ito T, Bohas CL, Wolin EM, Van Cutsem E et al. Everolimus for advanced pancreatic neuroendocrine tumors. *New England Journal of Medicine.* Retrieved on October 10, 2014. February 10, 2011;364(6):514–523. Available from: http://www.ncbi.nlm.nih.gov/pubmed/21306238.

59. Raymond E, Dahan L, Raoul J-L, Bang Y-J, Borbath I, Lombard-Bohas C et al. Sunitinib malate for the treatment of pancreatic neuroendocrine tumors. *New England Journal of Medicine.* Retrieved on October 7, 2014. February 10, 2011;364(6):501–513. Available from: http://www.ncbi.nlm.nih.gov/pubmed/21306237.

60. Ramage JK, Davies AHG, Ardill J, Bax N, Caplin M, Grossman A et al. Guidelines for the management of gastroenteropancreatic neuroendocrine (including carcinoid) tumours. *Gut.* Retrieved on October 6, 2014. June 2005;54(Suppl. 4):iv1–iv16. Available from: http://www.pubmedcentral.nih.gov/articlerender.fcgi?artid=1867801&tool=pmcentrez&rendertype=abstract.

61. Kwekkeboom DJ, de Herder WW, Kam BL, van Eijck CH, van Essen M, Kooij PP et al. Treatment with the radiolabeled somatostatin analog [177 Lu-DOTA 0,Tyr3] octreotate: Toxicity, efficacy, and survival. *Journal of Clinical Oncology.* Retrieved on October 9, 2014. May 1, 2008;26(13):2124–2130. Available from: http://jco.ascopubs.org/content/26/13/2124.abstract.

25

Treatment considerations for high-grade appendiceal adenocarcinoma

SEAN P. DINEEN, MELISSA TAGGART, RICHARD E. ROYAL, PAUL MANSFIELD, AND KEITH F. FOURNIER

INTRODUCTION

Appendiceal neoplasms are relatively rare tumors, originally thought to occur in about 0.12 cases per 1,000,000 persons per year [1,2]. More recent data suggest that the incidence has been rising since the early 1970s to the current high of 0.5–6 cases per 1,000,000. Although the exact cause for this observed increase is uncertain, it is likely secondary to an increased availability of high-quality imaging studies and the liberal use of laparoscopy [3]. The diagnosis of an appendiceal tumor is made preoperatively in less than 25% of cases; they are most commonly found incidentally in appendectomy specimens [1]. Thus, most treatment decisions are made only after the appendix has been resected and a formal pathologic diagnosis rendered.

The varied presentations of appendiceal cancer, the relative rarity of the disease, and the general lack of understanding of the molecular mechanisms underlying the disease have led to several classification schemes. The lack of one, uniform classification system has contributed to confusion regarding proper terminology and probably has led to an underappreciation of the malignant nature of the disease. One of the unfortunate results of this confusion is that some patients may not receive the aggressive and potentially curative treatments that have been developed over the past 30 years. Additionally, these differences in terminology make

comparison of results across clinical studies challenging. Despite all of this, it is very clear that high-grade tumors have a distinctly different natural history than their low-grade counterparts. The often quoted aphorism from Dr. Blake Cady "tumor biology is king, selection is queen and technical endeavors are the prince/princess of the realm. Occasionally the prince and princess try to usurp the throne; they almost always fail to overcome the powerful forces of the king and queen." This is undeniably true with regard to appendiceal neoplasms in that low-grade and high-grade tumors have distinctly different biologic behaviors and outcomes; in many ways, they vary different disease processes. The decision to proceed with definitive therapies such as cytoreductive surgery (CRS) and hyperthermic intraperitoneal chemotherapy (HIPEC) requires careful consideration and thoughtful patient selection due to the high morbidity of the procedure and the significant early, negative impact on the patients' quality of life. This chapter will focus on the treatment of high-grade appendiceal neoplasms with specific emphasis on how treatment differs from that of low-grade tumors.

PATHOLOGY

Appendiceal neoplasms can be broadly separated into epithelial and nonepithelial tumors. Nonepithelial tumors include lymphoma and other soft-tissue neoplasms including sarcoma and gastrointestinal (GI) stromal tumors. Epithelial tumors broadly include adenomas, adenocarcinomas, neuroendocrine tumors (carcinoid tumor) and carcinomas, and other unique tumors such as the goblet cell carcinoid tumor. Surveillance, Epidemiology, and End Results (SEER) data suggest that adenocarcinoma of the appendix accounts for approximately two-thirds of appendiceal cancers, with neuroendocrine tumors being the second most common tumor [1,3,4].

The definitive management of an adenoma is typically an appendectomy. However, it should be recalled that as many as 20% of patients will have associated primary malignancies in other locations within the GI tract, so a thorough workup should be performed, particularly a complete colonoscopy [5,6]. Appendiceal adenomas are common in patients with familial adenomatous polyposis syndrome and in patients with ulcerative colitis [7]. One lesion that remains controversial is the mucinous cystic neoplasm, which was previously designated as mucinous cystadenoma (or sometimes erroneously as mucoceles). These neoplastic lesions are mucin producing and typically present with appendicitis. The majority shows simplified epithelium with banal cytologic features. A minor subset may result in extra-appendiceal proliferation and mucin production, which, when severe, may result in pseudomyxoma peritonei (discussed in the succeeding text). Unfortunately, definitive criteria predicting which lesions will be cured with appendectomy and which may progress as pseudomyxoma peritonei are lacking. Therefore, we and others have used the term low-grade appendiceal mucinous neoplasm (LAMN) for these lesions [8].

As previously noted, adenocarcinomas are the most common type of appendiceal neoplasm. The best known risk factors for the development of an adenocarcinoma are an underlying history of inflammatory bowel disease, familial adenomatous polyposis syndromes, and patients who have defects in MMR genes [7]. The major histologic subtypes of adenocarcinoma are similar to those seen in other GI primaries including mucinous, nonmucinous (including gland-forming and medullary types), and signet ring cell carcinomas. By definition, in order to be called a mucinous adenocarcinoma, the tumor must be composed of greater than 50% mucin. Similarly, signet ring cells must make up 50% of a tumor to be labeled a signet ring cell adenocarcinoma. Other tumors with metastatic potential can also arise in the appendix. A unique, if not exclusive, tumor of the appendix is the goblet cell carcinoid tumor and its variants (adenocarcinoma ex-goblet cell carcinoid tumor) [9,10]. Goblet cell carcinoid tumors are composed of small, ovoid nests, which generally contain numerous goblet cells, but can also display other cell types (including rare neuroendocrine cells and Paneth cells). This multidirectional differentiation is reflected in its previous characterization as "crypt cell carcinoma" or "adenocarcinoid tumor." In general, no mucosal precursor is identified, and the tumor appears to arise in the deep mucosa or submucosa infiltrating the appendiceal wall in a concentric pattern. Occasionally, frank carcinoma can arise in the background of more typical goblet cell carcinoid tumors, and when this occurs, the tumor has more recently referred to as adenocarcinoma ex goblet cell carcinoid tumor. With or without a frank carcinomatous component, goblet cell tumors can metastasize and are staged as an adenocarcinoma [11].

Grade refers to degree of differentiation of the tumor (morphologic/cytologic similarity to normal tissue of origin) and thus most tumors can be graded as low or high grade. Signet ring cell adenocarcinomas are considered high-grade adenocarcinomas by default. Figure 25.1 demonstrates features of high-grade adenocarcinomas.

Pseudomyxoma peritonei is a vague term that represents the clinical syndrome characterized by the development of peritoneal mucinous ascites. The term is not specific to lesions arising from appendiceal primaries (although most commonly the appendix is the origin) and should be used to describe a clinical finding only. There are a few commonly used classification systems utilized to grade pseudomyxoma peritonei. Unfortunately, there continues to be a lack of consensus among pathologists regarding which classification system is best. Previously, the most commonly used schema was designed by Ronnett and colleagues [12]. This system evaluated both the primary lesion as "appendiceal adenoma" (likely to be currently classified as "LAMN") or invasive mucinous adenocarcinoma from appendiceal or intestinal primary and qualitatively evaluated the peritoneal lesions (cellularity, architectural patterns and complexity, cytologic features, and mitotic activity). The peritoneal lesions were then categorized as disseminated peritoneal adenomucinosis (DPAM), peritoneal mucinous carcinomatosis (PMCA), or PMCA with intermediate or discordant features. DPAM showed scant epithelium within mucin characterized by strips of simple epithelium with only focal proliferation and/or rare mitotic figures associated with or without an appendiceal "adenoma." PMCA showed more abundant cellularity with proliferative epithelium and/or more complex or less differentiated components (glands, clusters, individual cells) and moderate to marked cytologic atypia associated with an appendiceal or intestinal adenocarcinoma. PMCA was "intermediate or discordant" if the peritoneal lesions showed features of both PMCA and DPAM but were derived from an adenocarcinoma or showed features of PMCA but were derived from an atypical appendiceal "adenoma."

The newer and more commonly used systems include low-grade and high-grade mucinous adenocarcinoma peritonei adopted by the World Health Organization and one that utilizes the criteria set forth in the seventh edition of the *AJCC Cancer Staging Manual* [11]. This latter approach highlights the importance of histologic grade using well, moderate, and poorly differentiated terminology, which is potentially more familiar to most pathologists and eliminates possible confusion associated with unfamiliar terms such as DPAM and PMCA (especially in the clinical setting).

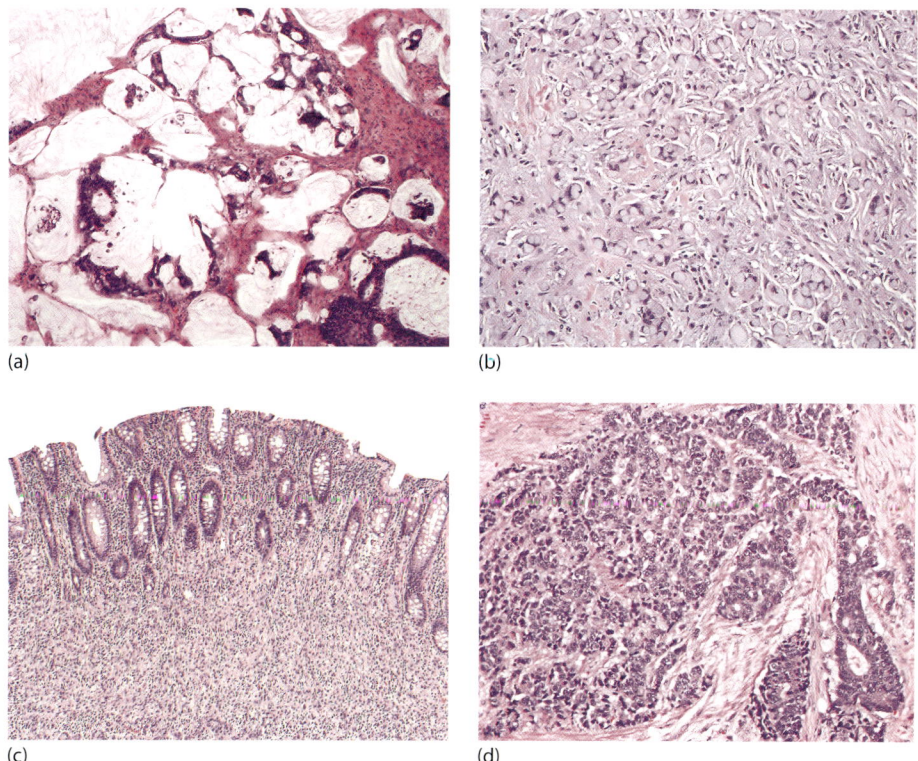

Figure 25.1 Appendiceal adenocarcinoma is categorized as poorly differentiated (high grade) when the tumor shows minimal gland formation and includes such morphologic patterns as signet ring cell adenocarcinoma. **(a)** Mucinous adenocarcinoma is characterized by neoplastic cells lining or floating in extracellular mucin (hematoxylin and eosin, 100×). Over 50% of the tumor must be composed of extracellular mucin. Limited gland formation, scattered single cells, and marked cytologic atypia place this tumor in a high-grade category. **(b)** In signet ring cell adenocarcinoma, numerous neoplastic cells, singularly or in small clusters, infiltrate a desmoplastic stroma (hematoxylin and eosin, 200×). The tumor cells have a prominent cytoplasmic mucin vacuole, which indents the nucleus, resembling a signet ring. **(c)** The tumor is composed of syncytial nests of neoplastic cells associated with infiltrating lymphocytes and is seen infiltrating into the cecum (hematoxylin and eosin, 100×). These features can be associated with high levels of microsatellite instability. This tumor had retained expression of DNA mismatch repair enzymes in the neoplastic cells, implying microsatellite stability. Although the tumor appears undifferentiated at low power, many cells showed intracytoplasmic mucin on routine hematoxylin and eosin staining, confirming adenocarcinoma. **(d)** The tumor is mostly arranged in solid sheets with little gland formation (lower right) within a desmoplastic stroma (hematoxylin and eosin, 100×).

The staging of appendiceal adenocarcinomas in the American Joint Committee on Cancer (AJCC) manual then separates into high grade (which includes moderate and poorly differentiated lesions) and low grade (which includes well-differentiated disease).

Though these binary divisions into low grade and high grade are simple to use, we recently utilized the SEER database to determine if moderately differentiated and poorly differentiated tumors behaved in a similar fashion. As expected, we found that grade was highly predictive of outcome. However, our data demonstrate three distinct survival curves based on histologic grade [1]. We would advocate that future studies should consider separating the moderate-grade tumors from the high-grade tumors as outcomes between these two groups are distinctly different. However, for the purposes of this chapter, we will discuss high-grade tumors as those including moderate and poorly differentiated appendiceal adenocarcinoma as that is what is most consistent in the literature.

DIAGNOSIS

At MD Anderson Cancer Center (MDACC), and other high-volume peritoneal surface malignancy centers, most patients have already undergone appendectomy and present with a diagnosis. All outside pathology reports and slides are reviewed by our dedicated pathologists to confirm the outside diagnosis. We use a three-tier system to designate the tumor grade as well differentiated, moderately differentiated, or poorly differentiated adenocarcinoma based on their microscopic characteristics.

Imaging/Staging

We review outside imaging and obtain new imaging as required. In general, we obtain computed tomography (CT) scan of the chest, abdomen, and pelvis with oral, intravenous, and rectal contrast with 5 mm maximum cuts. Patients with low-grade mucinous adenocarcinomas are very accurately evaluated with CT scans and can predict with >96% accuracy the ability to perform a complete CRS. Unfortunately, patients with high-grade adenocarcinomas are less well evaluated with CT scans. In this setting, the CT scan is far less reliable and tends to underestimate the volume of tumor actually present within the peritoneal cavity. PET/CT is not routinely obtained, but is selectively applied to address specific clinical questions. MRI may be obtained at the discretion of the attending surgeon, but typically are only obtained in situations of contrast allergy.

CT imaging is capable of reliably identifying peritoneal metastases that are >5 mm in size, below this cutoff, imaging is far less reliable [12,13]. CT findings consistent with peritoneal dissemination of disease include omental caking, serosal thickening, loss of normal tissue planes, solitary nodules, lymphadenopathy, mesenteric shortening, and ascites.

The role of diagnostic imaging in the selection of patients for CRS/HIPEC is aimed primarily at determining if a complete CRS can be performed. CT findings that should raise significant concerns about the ability/utility of CRS/HIPEC are as follows:

1. Evidence of extra-abdominal metastases
2. Significant retroperitoneal lymphadenopathy
3. Involvement of a large segment of the small intestine or small bowel mesentery
4. Ureteral obstruction
5. Significant disease burden around the porta hepatis
6. High estimated peritoneal carcinomatosis index (PCI)

CT findings of concern for small bowel involvement include mesenteric foreshortening, which can appear as cauliflowering of the small bowel mesentery. We routinely counsel patients that the CT findings will underestimate the true volume of disease >70% of the time when compared to findings at laparotomy/laparoscopy.

Tumor markers

We obtain baseline preoperative tumor markers including carcinoembryonic antigen (CEA), cancer antigen (CA) 19-9, and CA 125 levels as at least one marker will be elevated in up to 70% of patients. Elevated levels may allow for continued surveillance following CRS/HIPEC or response to systemic chemotherapy [13]. The relationship between elevated tumor markers and grade is not linear, and more elevated values do not necessarily correspond to a higher grade tumor. However, there are some emerging data to suggest that higher-grade tumors may have different patterns of tumor marker elevation. For example, significantly more patients with high-grade tumors had an elevation in CEA in a recent report from University of Pittsburgh [13]. Retrospective studies have evaluated the role of tumor markers in predicting outcomes and have met with varying success. The most consistent findings indicate that preoperative (baseline) elevation of CA 19-9 is associated with a decreased progression free survival [13,14] and is also indicative of not being able to obtain a complete cytoreduction [15,16]. Additionally, a return of elevated serum tumor markers to normal values following CRS/HIPEC is associated with improved outcomes.

MANAGEMENT OF NONMETASTATIC DISEASE

Patients with appendectomy specimens that are consistent with moderate or poorly differentiated adenocarcinoma, or that demonstrate the presence of signet ring cells are considered candidates for formal right colectomy. Patients with one of these high-grade lesions have a 20%–60% chance of harboring lymph node (LN) metastasis (Table 25.1). At the time of the right colectomy, we begin with diagnostic laparoscopy (DL) to formally assess the peritoneal cavity for evidence of peritoneal metastasis given the high rate of synchronous peritoneal carcinomatous (35%–80%) [18,19] (see Figure 25.2, algorithm). If there is no evidence of peritoneal metastasis, we move forward with laparoscopic or open right colectomy depending on the individual circumstances. We also routinely resect any omentum that was present in the area of the appendectomy or overlaying the right colon. We perform a right lower quadrant peritonectomy, removing the peritoneum in the vicinity of the cecum and previous appendectomy location. Halabi et al. [17] reviewed patients with high-grade appendiceal cancer treated at a single institution. The study identified LN metastases present in 44% of patients with high-grade disease. These patients with LN-positive disease fared significantly worse than those with negative LNs. Overall, the 5-year survival was 76% for LN-negative patients compared to 11% for LN-positive patients.

If the DL demonstrates evidence of peritoneal carcinomatosis, we obtain biopsies and abort the right colectomy unless there is concern for intestinal obstruction or perforation by the primary tumor. We then recommend the initiation of systemic chemotherapy (see systemic chemotherapy). Upon completion of systemic chemotherapy, we obtain restaging studies and potentially repeat the DL. If it appears that the patient is a good candidate for CRS and HIPEC (see "Surgical Intervention" section), we move forward with this and complete the right colectomy at the time of CRS/HIPEC.

MANAGEMENT OF PATIENTS WITH PERITONEAL DISSEMINATION

Physical exam and nutritional parameters

CRS/HIPEC can be associated with significant morbidity and acute decline in quality of life for 9–12 months after surgery. It is therefore imperative that an assessment of the patients' baseline physical functioning (ECOG performance scale) be made. Patients who have had a recent weight loss >20% of their body weight should be very carefully evaluated nutritionally as weight loss to this degree portends a difficult postoperative course. In one recent study, patients that were well nourished and undergoing CRS/HIPEC had an

Table 25.1 Lymph node positivity and survival according to histology in cancer of the appendix

Author (year)	Pathology	Number of patients	%LN positive	Median OS	3-year survival	5-year survival
Gupta et al. [28]	PMCA I/D	18	56	0.7 years	NA	NA
	PMCA	6	0	1.24 years	NA	NA
Omohwo et al. [29]	PMCA	56	NR	NA	68% CCR = 0	NA
					9% CCR > 1	
Chua et al. [30]	SRC	18	61	CRS/HIPEC 27 months Systemic chemo 15 months	NA	NA
El Halabi et al. [31]	PMCA	77	44	3.4 years	56%	40% 52% CCR = 0
Lieu et al. [21]	Poor	114	NR	2 years	NA	NA
	SRC	19	NR	2.5 years	NA	NA
	W/M with SRC	9	NR	12 years CCR = 0	NA	NA
Chua et al. [32]	PMCA I/D	140	17%			78% CRS/HIPEC
	PMCA	700				59% CRS/HIPEC
Turaga et al. [3]	Adeno		29%	48 months	NA	55%
	Mod	653				
	Poor	275				
	Mucinous		20%	61 months	NA	58%
	Mod	484				
	Poor	178				
	SRC		61%	24 months	NA	27%
	Mod	19				
	Poor	158				
Sirintrapun et al. [33]	High grade, no SRC	15	NR	2.9 years	42.4%	31.8%
	High-grade SRC/ mucin	20	NR	2.4 years	47.8%	35.8%
	High-grade SRC/ tissue					
Davison et al. [26]	AJCC Grade 2	55	17			61%
	AJCC Grade 3 (SRC)	27	72			23

Abbreviations: PMCA, peritoneal mucinous carcinoma; SRC, signet ring cell; CCR, completeness of cytoreduction score; CRS, cytoreductive surgery.

average length of stay of 15 versus 27.8 days for patients who were severely malnourished [18]. Likewise, well-nourished patients in this study had median overall survival (OS) of 22.4 months, versus 10.4 months in severely malnourished patients [18].

Nutritional parameters that we routinely consider are prealbumin, which gives a reasonable assessment of recent nutrition health. We also obtain albumin level as a more global marker of nutritional status. Significant deviations from normal should give great pause and consideration to preoperative nutritional supplementation. In patients that appear to be too deconditioned to tolerate a major abdominal operation, we recommend systemic chemotherapy only.

Chemotherapy

The type of chemotherapy, the optimal number of cycles, and the timing of chemotherapy (pre- or post-CRS/HIPEC) remain to be fully elucidated. The few retrospective studies that exist have demonstrated some conflicting results. Blackham et al. [19] and the Wake Forest group recently reported that postoperative systemic chemotherapy resulted in slightly better outcomes than preoperative systemic chemotherapy. In a recent analysis of 34 patients with PMCA, Bijelic et al. [20] found that patients who received preoperative systemic chemotherapy had a complete response rate of 29%, had a lower PCI, required fewer peritonectomies

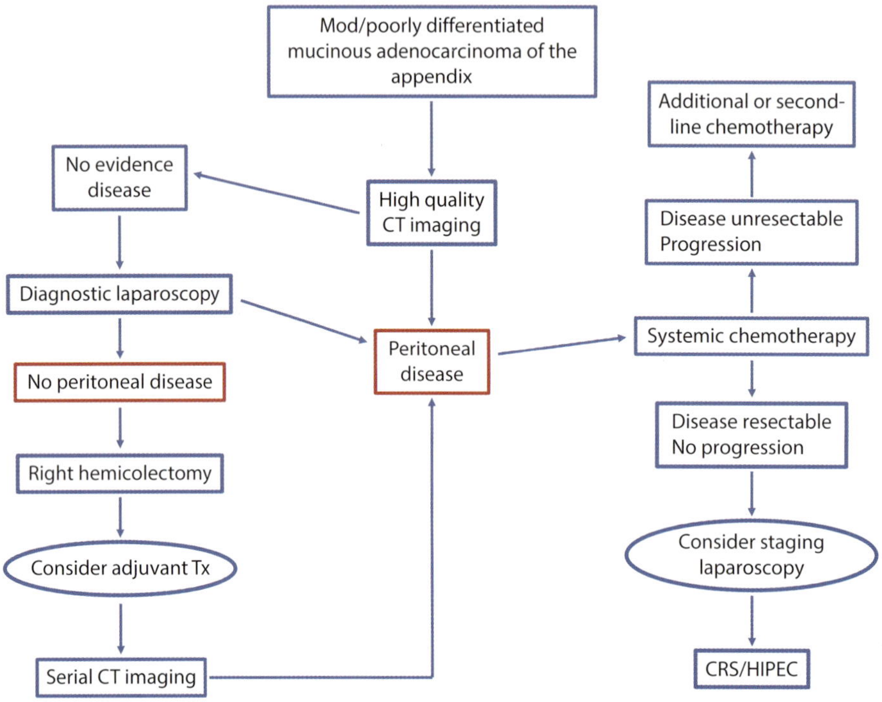

Figure 25.2 Treatment algorithm for high-grade appendix cancer. Following the diagnosis of high-grade appendiceal adenocarcinoma, high-quality imaging, if not already available, is obtained. If there is no evidence of peritoneal dissemination on this imaging, a diagnostic laparoscopy is performed to evaluate the peritoneal cavity for evidence of metastasis not seen on imaging. In the event that no peritoneal disease is identified, a right hemicolectomy is performed. Alternatively, if peritoneal disease is identified either on preoperative imaging or on diagnostic laparoscopy, systemic chemotherapy is initiated. Upon completion of systemic chemotherapy, the patient undergoes repeat staging, and based on the findings of these studies, cytoreductive surgery/hyperthermic intraperitoneal chemotherapy is performed when feasible.

and visceral resection, and had a higher rate of complete cytoreduction than those who had postoperative chemotherapy. As expected, a complete response was predictive of improved long-term outcomes.

If a patient presents to us with a known diagnosis of peritoneal dissemination of disease from a high-grade tumor, we review or obtain new staging studies. If the patient appears to be a good candidate for CRS/HIPEC, there is early involvement of both the peritoneal surface malignancy surgeons and the GI medical oncologist. Most of these patients are presented at the peritoneal multidisciplinary conference and consensus decisions made at that time. First-line systemic chemotherapy/targeted agents include 5-FU/oxaliplatin plus or minus bevacizumab.

Assuming patients have tolerated chemotherapy well, at the conclusion of their final cycle of chemotherapy, they undergo restaging studies with both CT imaging and serum tumor marker determination. Our experience at MDACC suggests that 44% of patients will demonstrate radiographic improvement in disease and 42% will have stable disease [21]. The remaining 14% will progress on chemotherapy, which would prompt a very cautious approach to subsequent CRS/HIPEC in that group. The median relapse-free survival (RFS) for this cohort was 6.9 months with a median OS of 1.7 years. However, those patients

who underwent a complete cytoreduction and HIPEC after systemic chemotherapy demonstrated improved RFS of 1.2 years and OS of 4.2 years [21]. In patients who have a completeness of cytoreduction score (CCR) = 0 resection, OS was 10.4 years.

In patients with peritoneal metastatic disease from high-grade appendiceal cancer, systemic chemotherapy was more frequently employed than for those patients with low-grade disease. For example, Turner et al. [22] evaluated 45 patients with high-grade appendiceal cancer with peritoneal dissemination. Twenty-six patients in this cohort underwent neoadjuvant chemotherapy, with FOLFOX + bevacizumab being most common, prior to CRS/HIPEC. The authors demonstrated a statistically significant increase in operative time of almost 2 hours. However, there was no significant adverse effect of preoperative chemotherapy with respect to complications or completeness of cytoreduction or length of stay. There was no improvement in survival in patients who had preoperative chemotherapy. Bijeclic et al. [20] reviewed 58 patients from the Washington Hospital Center experience, which did not reveal any adverse outcomes associated with preoperative chemotherapy. However, there was little benefit, which could be demonstrated. Our practice remains to administer preoperative chemotherapy in this cohort, though prospective studies are needed.

Diagnostic laparoscopy

If the patient has stability/improvement of disease on imaging and appears medically fit to undergo surgery, we perform a DL to formally evaluate the extent of intraperitoneal disease and access our ability to obtain a complete CRS. This helps to limit morbidity from an unnecessary laparotomy. Exclusionary findings at the time of DL are as follows:

1. Large volume peritoneal carcinomatosis that does not appear to be completely resectable
2. Extensive, infiltrative involvement of the small bowel or small bowel mesentery that will preclude safe resection
3. Extensive porta hepatis involvement
4. Extensive pelvic floor disease that would require a formal exenteration (i.e., cystectomy, proctectomy)

The technique for DL has been previously described. We typically perform a complete evaluation of the abdominal cavity using a video port and one instrument port, which are kept in the midline so that these can be resected with a midline incision at the time of CRS/HIPEC. Loose adhesions are taken down but an extensive adhesiolysis is not performed. The small bowel is manipulated to determine the degree of involvement. Additionally, the interface of the small bowel and the mesentery is a common location for disease, and this is inspected closely. Patients that have disease burden considered too extensive for complete cytoreduction are spared open exploration. A recent review of our patients demonstrated approximately 24% of patients that will be excluded from further CRS/HIPEC after undergoing DL, sparing them further unnecessary surgery.

SURGICAL INTERVENTION

Summary of current selection criteria for CRS/HIPEC

1. Partial response or stable disease during chemotherapy (based on imaging).
2. The volume of disease on imaging must appear to be completely resectable.
3. No evidence of extraperitoneal metastases.
4. No significant retroperitoneal or pericaval/periaortic lymphadenopathy.
5. No unresectable hepatic parenchymal metastases.
6. Patient fitness to undergo major operative intervention.
7. PCI less than 20 (relative).

Patients that meet inclusion criteria after this thorough evaluation and treatment are scheduled for CRS/HIPEC after medical clearance. The technique for CRS/HIPEC is addressed in more detail in a separate chapter. Briefly, our operation begins with a midline incision from xiphoid to pubis. If a previous laparoscopy was performed, we excise the scar tissue from prior surgery. We use a self-retaining retractor that provides traction under both costal margins and in both paracolic gutters. A complete omentectomy is performed. If disease involves the spleen, or if needed to completely remove the omentum, a splenectomy is performed. Following this, we proceed in a systematic fashion from the right upper quadrant in a clockwise fashion. Peritoneal surfaces are stripped, and visceral resection is performed as needed to remove all visible disease. Once all visible disease is removed, the perfusion is begun. A temporary closure of skin only is completed with inflow and outflow cannulas placed. HIPEC is performed using mitomycin C dosed at 20–25 mg/m^2 (we use 20 mg/m^2 for patients with prior systemic chemotherapy, which comprises the majority of patients with high-grade disease). Outflow temperatures are targeted to 41°C, and the patient is continuously agitated during the perfusion. We typically perfuse for 90 minutes. Once completed, GI continuity is restored for those patients who underwent a bowel resection.

On the horizon: Molecular characterization of appendiceal neoplasms

Though the molecular characteristics of appendiceal adenocarcinoma remain to be fully elucidated, there are some data to suggest that such characterization may be helpful in guiding treatment. For example, appendiceal and colorectal adenocarcinomas demonstrate distinct genetic signatures, indicating a difference in biology between the two entities [23]. Low-grade appendiceal adenocarcinomas tend to have a high rate of Kirsten rat sarcoma (KRAS) mutation (61%–91%), in contrast to high grade tumors, which rarely show KRAS mutation [24–27]. Likewise, high-grade tumors infrequently express GNAS mutations, in contrast to the high expression seen in low-grade lesions [24]. These differences imply that low-grade lesions do not progress to high-grade adenocarcinoma. Additionally, these initial studies show promise that appendiceal adenocarcinomas may soon be classified according to molecular characteristics, offering new insights into treatment strategies and prognostication.

OUTCOMES

Patients with high-grade tumors should be evaluated for potential surgical treatment in the form of CRS and HIPEC. Although outcomes in patients with high-grade disease do not match that of low-grade tumors, outcomes appear to be better than treatment with systemic chemotherapy alone (Table 25.1 for summary of outcomes). Complete cytoreduction and HIPEC is a standard practice in select patients with high-grade appendix cancer. Our institutional data demonstrate that in patients who undergo neoadjuvant oxaliplatin-based chemotherapy and subsequently undergo CCR0 resection and HIPEC have a median OS of 9 years. While this is in a very select group of patients whose biology is probably more favorable than most with high-grade adenocarcinoma, it does demonstrate what type of results can be obtained.

CONCLUSIONS

The importance of histology in appendiceal cancer cannot be overstated as can be seen by the dramatic difference in survival compared with low-grade tumors. However, select patients with high-grade disease should not be excluded from aggressive treatment. Patients that undergo CRS/HIPEC with a complete cytoreduction can still achieve favorable results compared to systemic chemotherapy alone, with 3-year survival seen in greater than 50% of patients. We recommend evaluation of patients with appendiceal cancer, particularly high-grade histology, at experienced centers that can offer a multidisciplinary approach to the treatment of these complex patients.

REFERENCES

1. Overman MJ, Fournier K, Hu, CH, Eng C, Taggart M, Royal R et al. Improving the AJCC/TNM staging for adenocarcinomas of the appendix: The prognostic impact of histological grade. *Annals of Surgery.* 2013;257(6):1072–1078.
2. McCusker ME, Coté TR, Clegg LX, Sobin LH. Primary malignant neoplasms of the appendix: A population-based study from the surveillance, epidemiology and end-results program, 1973–1998. *Cancer.* 2002;94(12):3307–3312.
3. Turaga KK, Pappas SG, Gamblin T. Importance of histologic subtype in the staging of appendiceal tumors. *Annals of Surgical Oncology.* 2012;19(5):1379–1385.
4. Shankar S, Ledakis P, El Halabi H, Gushchin V, Sardi A. Neoplasms of the appendix: Current treatment guidelines. *Hematology/Oncology Clinics of North America.* 2012;26(6):1261–1290.
5. Wolff M, Ahmed N. Epithelial neoplasms of the vermiform appendix (exclusive of carcinoid). II. Cystadeno mas, papillary adenomas, and adenomatous polyps of the appendix. *Cancer.* 1976;37(5):2511–2522.
6. Carr NJ, McCarthy WF, Sobin LH. Epithelial noncarcinoid tumors and tumor-like lesions of the appendix. A clinicopathologic study of 184 patients with a multivariate analysis of prognostic factors. *Cancer.* 1995;75(3):757–768.
7. Fenoglio-Preiser CM, Noffsinger AE, Stemmermann GN, Lantz PE, and Isaacson PG. *Gastrointestinal Pathology: An Atlas and Text,* 3rd edn., Philadelphia, PA: Lippincott Williams & Wilkins, 2007.
8. Misdraji J, Yantiss RK, Graeme-Cook FM, Balis UJ, Young RH. Appendiceal mucinous neoplasms: A clinicopathologic analysis of 107 cases. *American Journal of Surgical Pathology.* 2003;27(8):1089–1103.
9. Tang LH, Shia J, Soslow RA, Dhall D, Wong WD, O'Reilly E et al. Pathologic classification and clinical behavior of the spectrum of goblet cell carcinoid tumors of the appendix. *American Journal of Surgical Pathology.* 2008;32(10):1429–1443.
10. Bosman FT, World Health Organization, International Agency for Research on Cancer. *WHO Classification of Tumours of the Digestive System,* 4th edn., World Health Organization Classification of Tumours. Lyon, France: International Agency for Research on Cancer, 2010. 417p.
11. Edge SB, Byrd DR, Compton CC. In: Frederick MD, Greene L et al., eds., *AJCC Cancer Staging Handbook,* 7th edn., Chicago, IL: American Joint Committee on Cancer, 2010.
12. Ronnett BM, Zahn CM, Kurman RJ, Kass ME, Sugarbaker PH, Shmookler BM. Disseminated peritoneal adenomucinosis and peritoneal mucinous carcinomatosis. A clinicopathologic analysis of 109 cases with emphasis on distinguishing pathologic features, site of origin, prognosis, and relationship to "pseudomyxoma peritonei". *American Journal of Surgical Pathology.* 1995;19(12):1390–1408.
13. Wagner PL, Austin F, Sathaiah M, Magge D, Maduekwe U, Ramalingam L et al. Significance of serum tumor marker levels in peritoneal carcinomatosis of appendiceal origin. *Annals of Surgical Oncology.* 2013;20(2):506–514.
14. Carmignani CP, Hampton R, Sugarbaker CE, Chang D, Sugarbaker PH. Utility of CEA and CA 19–9 tumor markers in diagnosis and prognostic assessment of mucinous epithelial cancers of the appendix. *Journal of Surgical Oncology.* 2004;87(4):162–166.
15. Kusamura S, Hutanu I, Baratti D, Deraco M. Circulating tumor markers: Predictors of incomplete cytoreduction and powerful determinants of outcome in pseudomyxoma peritonei. *Journal of Surgical Oncology.* 2013;108(1):1–8.
16. Ross A, Sardi A, Nieroda C, Merriman B, Gushchin V. Clinical utility of elevated tumor markers in patients with disseminated appendiceal malignancies treated by cytoreductive surgery and HIPEC. *European Journal of Surgical Oncology.* 2010;36(8):772–776.
17. Halabi HE, Gushchin V, Francis J, Athas N, Macdonald R, Nieroda C et al. Prognostic significance of lymph node metastases in patients with high-grade appendiceal cancer. *Annals of Surgical Oncology.* 2012;19(1):122–125.
18. Vashi PG, Gupta D, Lammersfeld CA, Braun DP, Popiel B, Misra S, Brown KC. The relationship between baseline nutritional status with subsequent parenteral nutrition and clinical outcomes in cancer patients undergoing hyperthermic intraperitoneal chemotherapy. *Nutrition Journal.* 2013;12:118.
19. Blackham AU, Swett K, Eng C, Sirintrapun J, Bergman S, Geisinger KR et al. Perioperative systemic chemotherapy for appendiceal mucinous

carcinoma peritonei treated with cytoreductive surgery and hyperthermic intraperitoneal chemotherapy. *Journal of Surgical Oncology.* 2014;109(7).740–745.

20. Bijelic L, Kumar AS, Stuart OA, Sugarbaker PH. Systemic chemotherapy prior to cytoreductive surgery and HIPEC for carcinomatosis from appendix cancer: Impact on perioperative outcomes and short-term survival. *Gastroenterology Research and Practice.* 2012;2012:163284.

21. Lieu CH, Lambert LA, Wolff RA, Eng C, Zhang N, Wen S et al. Systemic chemotherapy and surgical cytoreduction for poorly differentiated and signet ring cell adenocarcinomas of the appendix. *Annals of Oncology.* 2012;23(3):652–658.

22. Turner KM, Hanna NN, Zhu Y, Jain A, Kesmodel SB, Switzer RA et al. Assessment of neoadjuvant chemotherapy on operative parameters and outcome in patients with peritoneal dissemination from high-grade appendiceal cancer. *Annals of Surgical Oncology.* 2013;20(4):1068–1073.

23. Levine EA, Blazer DG 3rd, Kim MK, Shen P, Stewart JH 4th, Guy C, Hsu DS. Gene expression profiling of peritoneal metastases from appendiceal and colon cancer demonstrates unique biologic signatures and predicts patient outcomes. *Journal of the American College of Surgeons.* 2012;214(4):599–606; discussion 606–607.

24. Alakus H, Babicky ML, Ghosh P, Yost S, Jepsen K, Dai Y et al. Genome-wide mutational landscape of mucinous carcinomatosis peritonei of appendiceal origin. *Genome Medicine.* 2014;6(5):43.

25. Nishikawa G, Sekine S, Ogawa R, Matsubara A, Mori T, Taniguchi H et al. Frequent GNAS mutations in low-grade appendiceal mucinous neoplasms. *British Journal of Cancer.* 2013;108(4):951–958.

26. Davison JM, Choudry HA, Pingpank JF, Ahrendt SA, Holtzman MP, Zureikat AH et al. Clinicopathologic and molecular analysis of disseminated appendiceal mucinous neoplasms: Identification of factors predicting survival and proposed criteria for a three-tiered assessment of tumor grade. *Modern Pathology.* 2014;27(11):1521–1539.

27. Raghav KP, Shetty AV, Kazmi SM, Zhang N, Morris J, Taggart M et al. Impact of molecular alterations and targeted therapy in appendiceal adenocarcinomas. *Oncologist.* 2013;18(12):1270–1277.

28. Gupta S, Parsa V, Adsay V, Heilbrun LK, Smith D, Shields AF et al. Clinicopathological analysis of primary epithelial appendiceal neoplasms. *Medical Oncology.* 2010;27(4):1073–1078.

29. Omohwo C, Nieroda CA, Studeman KD, Thieme H, Kostuik P, Ross AS et al. Complete cytoreduction offers longterm survival in patients with peritoneal carcinomatosis from appendiceal tumors of unfavorable histology. *Journal of the American College of Surgeons.* 2009;209(3):308–312.

30. Chua TC, Pelz JO, Kerscher A, Morris DL, Esquivel J. Critical analysis of 33 patients with peritoneal carcinomatosis secondary to colorectal and appendiceal signet ring cell carcinoma. *Annals of Surgical Oncology.* 2009;16(10):2765–2770.

31. El Halabi H, Gushchin V, Francis J, Athas N, Macdonald R, Nieroda C et al. The role of cytoreductive surgery and heated intraperitoneal chemotherapy (CRS/HIPEC) in patients with high-grade appendiceal carcinoma and extensive peritoneal carcinomatosis. *Annals of Surgical Oncology.* 2012;19(1):110–114.

32. Chua TC, Moran BJ, Sugarbaker PH, Levine EA, Glehen O, Gilly FN et al. Early- and long-term outcome data of patients with pseudomyxoma peritonei from appendiceal origin treated by a strategy of cytoreductive surgery and hyperthermic intraperitoneal chemotherapy. *Journal of Clinical Oncology.* 2012;30(20):2449–2456.

33. Sirintrapun SJ, Blackham AU, Russell G, Votanopoulos K, Stewart JH, Shen P et al. Significance of signet ring cells in high-grade mucinous adenocarcinoma of the peritoneum from appendiceal origin. *Human Pathology.* 2014;45(8):1597–1604.

26

Systemic therapy for appendiceal cancer

JENNIFER L. ZADLO AND CATHY ENG

INTRODUCTION

The role of systemic chemotherapy/biologic therapy in the treatment of appendiceal cancers is not well established and continues to be under investigation. A majority of available data consists of case series or reports or single-center retrospective reviews. Given the rarity of appendiceal cancers, the heterogeneous pathology, and relatively indolent biology, the ability to conduct large, prospective, randomized studies is very difficult and often unrealistic [1]. In this chapter, we will review the available literature and hope to provide insight on the role of systemic therapy for appendiceal cancer.

SYSTEMIC THERAPY FOR RESECTABLE DISEASE

The role of systemic therapy in the setting of resectable disease is still very unclear. At this time, there are limited roles for systemic therapy when the goal of treatment is cure [1]. A majority of patients who are deemed resectable at diagnosis proceed to receive cytoreductive surgery (CS) and hyperthermic intraperitoneal chemotherapy (HIPEC) [2,3]. Few studies have shown benefit of systemic chemotherapy/biologic therapy in the perioperative setting. Of the few studies that do exist, most are retrospective reviews, with a small sample size of very heterogeneous patients who may have received systemic chemotherapy/biologic therapy preoperatively/neoadjuvant, postoperative/adjuvant, or both. For the purposes of this chapter, preoperative and neoadjuvant are synonymous terms, as is postoperative and adjuvant with regard to systemic chemotherapy/biologic therapy.

Perioperative systemic treatment

In one of the earlier studies published, Smith and colleagues [4] report on their experience of pseudomyxoma peritonei (PMP) of appendiceal origin at Memorial Sloan Kettering Cancer Institute. From 1952 through 1989, 17 patients were identified with PMP originating from the appendix. All of the patients identified underwent cytoreductive surgical debulking. Ten patients were noted to have received chemotherapy; four patients received intraperitoneal (IP) chemotherapy and six patients with systemic chemotherapy. Of those patients who received systemic first-line chemotherapy, three of the six patients received a regimen consisting of semustine, 5-fluorouracil, vincristine, and streptozocin (MOF-Strep); three patients received monotherapy, one with 5-fluorouracil, one with melphalan, and one with cyclophosphamide [4].

The results of this study showed no significant difference in survival between patients who were treated with cytoreduction alone versus those who received systemic chemotherapy (p = 0.48) [4]. It is important to note that "patients who received chemotherapy" included all 10 patients who received any kind of chemotherapy—systemic or IP. Based on these results, the authors concluded that primary treatment for PMP is surgical debulking. Because no improvement in survival was seen with chemotherapy, the authors recommended that it should only be administered on a research protocol or when there is clinical tumor recurrence.

The results of a more recent and larger retrospective review of perioperative systemic chemotherapy for appendiceal mucinous carcinoma peritonei (MCP) were published by Blackham et al. [5]. This retrospective chart review included patients from two high-volume academic institutions from January 1997 through January 2011. This study separated low-grade MCP patients from high-grade MCP patients defined by the Bradley classification system [6]; low-grade MCP patients who received systemic chemotherapy where compared to low-grade MCP patients who underwent CS/HIPEC alone. The same substratification was evaluated in the high-grade MCP patients [5].

In the low-grade appendiceal MCP, 22 patients were treated with perioperative chemotherapy, 13 patients received preoperative systemic chemotherapy, and 9 patients received postoperative chemotherapy [5]. No patients with low-grade appendiceal MCP received both preoperative and postoperative chemotherapy. These 22 patients who received perioperative systemic chemotherapy were matched with 22 historical controls (treated without systemic chemotherapy) based on similar resection status, age, and nodal status [5].

Regimens containing a 5-fluorouracil backbone were most commonly chosen as systemic therapy in both the preoperative and postoperative settings [5]. 5-Fluorouracil plus oxaliplatin (FOLFOX) was the most common regimen administered with five patients (39%) and four patients (44%) in the preoperative and postoperative settings, respectively. The second most common regimen was 5-fluorouracil monotherapy administered to four patients (31%) and two patients (22%), in the preoperative and postoperative settings, respectively. 5-Fluorouracil plus irinotecan (FOLFIRI) was the third most common regimen, administered to two patients (15%) and one patient (11%) in the preoperative and postoperative settings, respectively. The addition of bevacizumab was more commonly seen in the preoperative setting (n = 7; 54%) than in the postoperative setting (n = 2; 22%). Patients who received preoperative chemotherapy received a median 4.5 months (range 1.5–18 months) of systemic treatment versus a median 4 months (range 3–6.5 months) in the postoperative arm [5].

There was no difference seen in median progression free survival (PFS) or median overall survival (OS) when comparing systemic chemotherapy versus no systemic chemotherapy in patients with low-grade MCP (p = 0.18 and p = 0.46, respectively) [5].

One hundred and nine patients were identified as high-grade appendiceal MCP, 70 (64%) of which received perioperative chemotherapy and 39 (36%) did not receive any systemic chemotherapy [5]. Thirty-seven (34%) received preoperative systemic treatment, 22 patients (20%) received postoperative systemic treatment, and 11 patients (10%) received both pre- and postoperative systemic treatments. The pattern of chemotherapy utilized in the high-grade appendiceal MCP patients was similar to that of the low-grade appendiceal MCP patients mentioned previously—regimens consisting of a 5-fluorouracil backbone. The most common systemic chemotherapy regimen was FOLFOX, followed by 5-fluorouracil monotherapy, and FOLFIRI. The median duration of treatment was 4 months (range 1.5–16 months) in those who received preoperative

systemic treatment versus a median of 6 months (range 1.5–17 months) duration for those who received postoperative systemic treatment [5].

Of the total 48 patients with high-grade appendiceal MCP who received preoperative systemic chemotherapy, no patients met Response Evaluation Criteria In Solid Tumors (RECIST) criteria for response [5]. A majority of patients (75%) achieved stable disease (SD), followed by 17% who progressed. Although no patient had a measurable response, 8% were considered to have achieved a clinical partial response (PR), as defined by a decrease in tumor markers and/or ascites. Thirty-three total patients received postoperative systemic chemotherapy. Eight patients (24%) developed recurrent or progression of disease while receiving treatment [5].

Overall, there was no difference in median PFS (p = 0.47) or median OS (p = 0.74) observed when comparing perioperative systemic chemotherapy to CS/HIPEC alone in patients with high-grade appendiceal MCP [5].

Within a subset of patients with high-grade appendiceal MCP, postoperative systemic chemotherapy was associated with a longer median PFS compared to preoperative systemic chemotherapy (p < 0.01) and HIPEC alone (p = 0.03) (postoperative systemic chemotherapy = 13.6 months, preoperative systemic chemotherapy = 6.8 months, and HIPEC alone = 7 months, respectively) [5]. There was also a trend toward a benefit in median OS in postoperative systemic chemotherapy patients versus preoperative (36.4 versus 16 months, p = 0.07) and HIPEC alone (36.4 versus 19.6 months, p = 0.14); however, these results were not statistically significant [5].

Patients who received both preoperative and postoperative chemotherapies had a similar median OS compared to those who received just preoperative systemic chemotherapy (p = 0.76) and a similar PFS to patients who received postoperative systemic chemotherapy alone (p = 0.24) [5].

The authors of this study concluded that there is a limited role for perioperative systemic chemotherapy in patients with low-grade appendiceal MCP treated with CS/HIPEC [5]. In patients with high-grade appendiceal MCP, preoperative chemotherapy should be reserved for patients who are borderline–resectable or nonresectable. Postoperative systemic chemotherapy was determined to be beneficial; however, management of high-grade appendiceal MCP should involve multidisciplinary management [5].

Neoadjuvant systemic therapy

Two retrospective studies have been conducted assessing systemic chemotherapy in patients with appendiceal cancer prior to CS/HIPEC—the first by Sugarbaker et al [7]. and the second by Bijelic et al [8].

Sugarbaker et al. [7], were the first to publish the results of a prospective study evaluating neoadjuvant systemic treatment in patients with disseminated peritoneal mucinous adenocarcinoma of appendiceal origin. Thirty-four patients received six cycles of FOLFOX or CapeOX, with or without the addition of bevacizumab prior to CS/HIPEC; 30 received FOLFOX, 4 patients received CapeOX, and 21 patients received the addition of bevacizumab [7].

After evaluation by computerized tomography (CT) scan, SD was reported in 22 patients (65%), 7 patients had progression (21%), and 5 patients (15%) achieved a PR [7]. Patients also underwent clinical, pathological, and histological evaluations. In contrast to CT results, operative findings found different responses—9 patients (26%) were thought to have SD, 17 patients progressed (50%), and 7 patients (21%) achieved a PR [7].

From a histological standpoint, 24 patients (71%) achieved SD, 7 patients (21%) achieved a PR, and 3 patients (9%) achieved a complete response (CR) [7]. With these results, the authors found a strong correlation between clinical and radiologic assessment by kappa statistics (K = 0.63, p < 0.001) and a statistically significant relationship between operative and histopathological response (K = 0.23, p < 0.004); however, other pairings were not significant [7].

The authors concluded that clinical and radiographic responses to neoadjuvant chemotherapy provided little useful data within the short duration of treatment and follow-up of this study [7]. Not only had this study demonstrated the difficulty in assessing patients clinically and radiographically for response, it also questioned the accuracy of these tools. The findings from this study, however, served as the neoadjuvant systemic treatment arm for patients included in the Bijelic study [7,8].

Bijelic et al. [8] conducted a retrospective review of patients with histologically confirmed PMCA of appendiceal origin who were thought to be candidates for CS/HIPEC at their time of referral at Washington Cancer Institute from January 2005 through December 2009. Fifty-eight patients were identified, 34 of which received systemic chemotherapy/biologic therapy for up to a maximum of 12 cycles prior to CS/HIPEC, and 24 patients who only underwent CS/HIPEC [8].

Of the 34 patients who received systemic preoperative treatment, all patients received a fluoropyrimidine plus oxaliplatin regimen with FOLFOX (n = 30) or XELOX (n = 4); bevacizumab was added in 21 (62%) cases [8]. Patients who received preoperative chemotherapy had a lower peritoneal carcinomatosis index score versus patients who did not receive preoperative chemotherapy (mean score 19 versus mean score 28, respectively; p = 0.0003). The mean number of peritonectomies and the mean number of visceral resections were lower in patients who received preoperative chemotherapy versus those who did not (mean peritonectomies with preoperative chemotherapy = 2.3 [range 0–5] versus without preoperative chemotherapy = 3.7 [range 1–5], respectively; p = 0.0032; mean number of visceral resections with preoperative chemotherapy = 2.7 [range 1–5] versus without preoperative chemotherapy 4.4 [range 2–7], respectively; p <0.001). This study also showed that those patients who received preoperative systemic treatment and achieved a complete or near CR to chemotherapy had a longer survival than those with no histological response (median survival not reached

versus 29.5 months, respectively; p = 0.033). Interestingly, median OS was only 37.2 months in patients who received preoperative chemotherapy versus 50.5 months for patients who did not receive preoperative chemotherapy; however, this was not statistically significant (p = 0.56) [8].

The role of neoadjuvant or preoperative chemotherapy has been well established as showing a benefit in other cancer types including breast [9], rectal [10], and gastroesophageal [11] cancers. The role of neoadjuvant chemotherapy is still unclear in appendiceal cancers. Neoadjuvant chemotherapy, however, does have several advantages and disadvantages.

Neoadjuvant chemotherapy allows practitioners to assess the clinical and/or radiographic response the tumor has to chemotherapy [1,9–11]. Tumor types more susceptible to chemotherapy may predict prognosis in certain tumor types. In the case of appendiceal cancer, there currently are no validated predictors of response. Some practitioners may follow the trend of various tumor markers, such as the carcinoembryonic antigen (CEA), cancer antigen/carbohydrate antigen (CA)-125, or CA 19-9; however, these do not predict radiographic response [1,12,13]. Practitioners may also use clinical signs to assess response to treatment. These include, but are not limited to, reduction in ascites and improvement in symptoms of abdominal fullness, nausea, fatigue, and pain [5,7,8].

Reduction in tumor volume and tumor burden is another advantage to neoadjuvant chemotherapy [1,5,9–11]. With adequate response to systemic chemotherapy, there is a better possibility for a less extensive surgical procedure to be performed and improved resectability with regard to surgical margins, organ preservation, and reduction in postoperative complications. In some appendiceal cancer cases, with a dramatic response to systemic chemotherapy/biologic therapy, patients may become candidates for CS/HIPEC who may have been deemed unresectable at diagnosis [12,14,15].

In the case of appendiceal cancer, it remains to be seen if neoadjuvant chemotherapy translates to an OS benefit. Generally, many patients who are recommended neoadjuvant systemic treatment often have more advanced disease at diagnosis and, therefore, may have a poorer prognosis at diagnosis. In contrast, low-grade appendiceal cancers have a rather indolent biology, thereby making assessment for OS benefit very difficult because results may be diluted over such a long follow-up period of time [1].

Adjuvant systemic therapy

Few studies have evaluated the role of systemic therapy for adjuvant treatment of appendiceal cancer, following standard CS/HIPEC.

A prospective phase II study of adjuvant thalidomide following CS/HIPEC for patients with peritoneal surface disease from colorectal and appendiceal cancer was conducted at Wake Forest Baptist Health under the direction of Shen and colleagues [16]. All were adult patients with peritoneal surface disease secondary to colorectal or appendiceal cancer. Patients received adjuvant thalidomide, starting with a 100 mg dose by mouth at bedtime for the first 28-day cycle, followed by an increase to 200 mg by mouth at bedtime for the second 28-day cycle, to a final dose of 300 mg by mouth at bedtime and continued as maintenance. A total of 26 patients were evaluable for response. The study population was split evenly between primary appendiceal (n = 14; 52%) and colorectal (n = 13; 48%) cancers as the primary site of origin. Also, approximately half of the patients received an R0/R1 resection (48%), and the other half (52%) received an R2 resection. In those patients with residual disease following CS/HIPEC, none achieved a partial or CR with adjuvant thalidomide. Median PFS was 42.3 months and the median OS was not reached for patients with R0/R1 resection versus a median PFS of 6.4 months and median OS of 29.8 months in patients with an R2 resection. As expected, the median PFS (29 months) and median OS (not reached) were longer in patients with a primary appendiceal cancer than those with a primary colorectal cancer (median PFS was 7 months; median OS was 30 months).

The most common Grade 3/4 toxicities seen among this group of patients included thromboembolism (8%), neurological disorders (16%), nausea (12%), and vomiting (8%). Nine patients (34%) withdrew from the study due to adverse drug reactions [16].

This study failed to show a benefit of adjuvant thalidomide following CS/HIPEC in peritoneal surface disease from primary colorectal and appendiceal cancers and, therefore, cannot be recommended. The results of this study are both difficult to apply to clinical practice as the population of patients was mixed between primary colorectal and primary appendiceal [16]. As already well established, colorectal cancer and appendiceal cancer have a different biology, disease course, and prognosis. To include both cancer types makes it more difficult, whether results would truly reflect each cancer type the same if they were evaluated independently. One must also consider the toxicity profile of thalidomide and the correlation with medication compliance. It does not appear that patient adherence to study medication was performed, which may have also impacted the results reported [16].

A case report by Chen and colleagues details the use of adjuvant FOLFOX for a patient with PMP of appendiceal origin [17]. The use of adjuvant FOLFOX following CS/HIPEC in patients with appendiceal cancer has been adapted from the adjuvant studies of FOLFOX in colorectal cancer patients.

SYSTEMIC THERAPY FOR UNRESECTABLE DISEASE

Currently, there is no standard systemic chemotherapy/biologic therapy recommended in the treatment of unresectable appendiceal cancer. Several retrospective chart reviews, case series and reports, and abstracts exist, investigating the efficacy of systemic chemotherapy/biologic therapy regimens in the treatment of unresectable appendiceal cancer. Current systemic regimens studied in this setting have been adopted from the treatment of metastatic colorectal cancer resembling a fluoropyrimidine backbone with the addition of oxaliplatin or irinotecan, with or without targeted biotherapies such as anti–vascular endothelial growth factor (VEGF) or anti–epidermal growth factor receptor (EGFR) monoclonal antibodies.

Farquharson et al. [12] were first to publish a study demonstrating a benefit of systemic chemotherapy in patients with advanced unresectable PMP. This phase II study evaluated tumor response, OS, toxicity, and quality of life (QOL) in patients receiving mitomycin-C 7 mg/m^2 intravenously (IV) day 1 and capecitabine 1250 mg/m^2 twice daily on days 1–14 of a 21-day cycle (cycle 1), alternating with capecitabine 1250 mg/m^2 twice daily on days 1–14 of a 21-day cycle (cycle 2). These 3-week cycles 1 and 2 were alternated until a total of 8 cycles were completed (MCap). Forty patients were treated from April 2003 through December 2006. Thirty-nine patients were evaluable for response, of which 15 (38%) showed a benefit from chemotherapy by demonstrating reduction in mucinous ascites or displaying SD after progressing on prior treatments. Tumor-related survival rates were 84% and 61%, respectively, at 1 and 2 years. Of note, 2 patients who were deemed unresectable at study entry underwent potentially curative CS following MCap administration and subsequent restaging. The MCap regimen was considered to be well tolerated, with Grade 3/4 toxicity events occurring in only 6% of 277 total cycles of chemotherapy; all were hand–foot syndrome. This study is an important benchmark, as it was the first to demonstrate the benefit of systemic chemotherapy, with mitomycin-C and capecitabine, in patients with advanced unresectable PMP [12].

Several years following, Shapiro and colleagues published the results of a retrospective chart review of chemotherapy-naïve patients with mucinous or signet ring cell adenocarcinoma or PMP of the appendix who were determined to be ineligible for CS with/without HIPEC by surgical consult [13]. Fifty-four patients were identified as having received ≥2 cycles of chemotherapy/biologic therapy from 2000 through 2005 at The University of Texas MD Anderson Cancer Center. A majority of patients (n = 21; 38.9%) received a regimen consisting of a fluoropyrimidine (5-fluorouracil or capecitabine) in combination with a platinum, followed by single agent fluoropyrimidine (n = 16; 29.6%). Other first-line regimens included gefitinib (n = 5; 9.3%), irinotecan plus a platinum (n = 4; 7.4%), 5-fluorouracil plus a platinum plus bevacizumab (n = 3; 5.6%), fluoropyrimidine plus irinotecan (n = 2; 3.7%), 5-fluorouracil plus a platinum plus cetuximab (n = 2; 3.7%), and FOLFIRI plus bevacizumab (n = 1; 1.8%). The overall response rate following a median 24-month (range, 2–66 months) follow-up was 56% (n = 30, 95% CI, 0.41–0.69); CR was noted in 2 patients (3.7%), PR in 11 patients (20.4%), and SD in 33 patients (61.1%); PFS was 7.57 months, 95% CI, and range 4.53–10.6. The median OS from the time of diagnosis was 56 months, with an estimated 3-year OS equal to 58.1%, 95% CI, 45.4%–74.3%. When the authors stratified for previous HIPEC, the 3-year OS was higher in the groups of patients who underwent previous HIPEC (73.4%, 95% CI, 54.1%–99.7%) versus patients who did not undergo previous HIPEC (50.6%, 95% CI, 35.6%–71.9%), p = 0.0495; however, no difference was detected for overall response rate. Too little surprise, when stratified for signet ring cell or poorly differentiated tumor types, both resulted in being negative prognostic indicators for OS. The results of this study demonstrated that systemic chemotherapy may provide a benefit in patients who are not optimal candidates for CS followed by HIPEC [13].

Lieu et al. focused their retrospective review specifically on those patients with poor prognostic factors—those with poorly differentiated histology, signet ring cell features, or both [18]. The authors identified 78 patients from September 1992 through January 2010 at the University of Texas MD Anderson Cancer Center who received first-line systemic chemotherapy/biologic therapy. A majority of patients (n = 48, 62%) received a platinum containing regimen with FOLFOX plus bevacizumab (n = 22), 5-fluorouracil/capecitabine plus oxaliplatin (n = 11), 5-fluorouracil/capecitabine plus cisplatin (n = 5), FOLFOX plus cetuximab (n = 2), or capecitabine plus carboplatin (n = 2). Thirteen patients (17%) received a first-line irinotecan containing regimen with FOLFIRI plus bevacizumab (n = 4), cisplatin plus irinotecan (n = 4), FOLFIRI (n = 3), or FOLFIRI plus cetuximab (n = 2). Other regimens used in the first-line setting included 5-fluorouracil/capecitabine monotherapy (n = 14), carboplatin plus paclitaxel (n = 2), and 5-fluorouracil plus doxorubicin (n = 1). The median OS was 1.7 years (95%, CI 1.4–2.3) and median PFS was 6.9 months (95%, CI 5.3–9.2). Overall response rate was 44%, with a majority of patients achieving SD (42%). With regard to specific systemic chemotherapy/biologic therapy regimens, no statistically significant difference was detected for OS, PFS, or response rate. Additionally, no benefit was observed from the addition of biologic agents, bevacizumab and cetuximab, for any endpoint. The authors concluded that, when achievable, complete cytoreduction should be considered. When systemic chemotherapy/biologic therapy is used, the ideal regimen is unclear, but a majority of patients received a fluoropyrimidine-based regimen [18].

Most recently, the results of a phase II, single-center, prospective, observational study were published by Pietrantonio and colleagues from Italy [15]. From July 2011 through September 2013, 20 patients with unresectable or recurrent PMP of appendiceal origin were administered FOLFOX-4 every 2 weeks for a maximum of 12 cycles. The median OS was 26.2 months (95%, CI 18.1–34.3) with a median PFS of 8 months (95%, CI 0–16.8). The overall response rate was 20%, with a majority of patients achieving SD (n = 9, 45%) followed by PR (n = 4, 20%); seven (35%) patients had disease progression. Of note, two patients were able to undergo laparotomy with complete cytoreduction, with one also receiving HIPEC. Based on these results, the authors concluded that FOLFOX-4 is active and tolerable in patients with PPM whose disease is relapsed or is deemed unresectable [15].

In an attempt to evaluate a stronger sample size, Tejani et al. [19] conducted a retrospective analysis evaluating the clinical efficacy of systemic chemotherapy regimens used in patients with advanced or metastatic appendiceal cancer. Patients were identified from the National Comprehensive Cancer Network Oncology Outcomes Database for colorectal cancer from eight participating member institutions. Due to the nature of this study, it is unknown if the patients included in this analysis were evaluated for candidacy of surgical resectability prior to receiving systemic chemotherapy. One hundred and twelve patients met the inclusion criteria for the study, a majority of which received a FOLFOX regimen (n = 37; 33%) with or without bevacizumab (n = 42; 37%). Other regimens included FOLFIRI with bevacizumab (n =15; 13%), without bevacizumab (n =6; 5%), and single agent 5-fluorouracil/capecitabine, or oxaliplatin, with or without bevacizumab. Best response was similar to that seen with other studies discussed. Median PFS was 1.2 years (95% CI, 1.0–1.8) and median OS was 2.1 years (95% CI, 1.0–2.3). Similar to other studies, shorter PFS and OS were seen in patients with nonmucinous histology and high-grade histology and shorter OS in patients who received nondebulking surgery. Because a majority of patients received a FOLFOX regimen, evaluating efficacy between different systemic regimens was not comparable. However, when comparing the addition of targeted therapy, omitting bevacizumab translated to a longer PFS than those that received a bevacizumab containing regimen (p = 0.01). Of importance, Tejani and colleagues grouped both well-differentiated and moderately differentiated histologies together, which may have clouded the results, as other studies differentiated between various histological subtypes [5,13,19,20].

Choe et al. [20] specifically assessed the role of combined systemic chemotherapy versus monotherapy in patients with unresectable appendiceal cancer. This retrospective chart review included 79 patients with unresectable appendiceal cancer treated at The University of Texas MD Anderson Cancer Center and Wake Forest Baptist Medical Center. Patients received either FOLFOX/CapeOX (n = 51; 65%), 5-fluorouracil/capecitabine monotherapy (n = 23; 29%), or FOLFIRI/CapeIRI (n = 5; 6%). After a median 9.9 years follow-up, median OS for the whole group was 45.3 months (95% CI; 36.4–54.2 months). When evaluated in a multivariate analysis, combination chemotherapy resulted in a longer median PFS compared to 5-fluorouracil/capecitabine monotherapy (9.2 months versus 6.5 months, respectively; HR, 0.21; 95% CI; 0.07–0.64; p = 0.006). There was no statistically significant difference in median OS. FOLFOX/CapeOX and FOLFIRI/CapeIRI demonstrated better response rates than 5-fluorouracil/capecitabine monotherapy (PR = 17%, 20%, 6%, respectively; SD = 61%, 40%, 37%, respectively; PD = 22%, 40%, 57%, respectively); however, this study was underpowered to differentiate superiority between the chemotherapy arms. Based on these results, the authors felt that combination chemotherapy regimens resulted in improved PFS [20]. However, a prospective randomized analysis should be conducted to validate these findings. (See Table 26.1 for a summary of studies presented.)

There have been documented cases, although uncommon, of patients deemed unresectable at diagnosis, offered systemic treatment, and demonstrated a robust response to treatment, making patients eligible for definitive CS/HIPEC. Two patients who were originally regarded as unresectable in the study by Farquharson and colleagues received eight cycles of MCap and, following restaging scans, received potentially curative CS [12]. Two patients (out of 20 patients evaluated) in the study of FOLFOX4 by Pietrantonio and colleagues achieved a substantial PR, with one patient going on to laparotomy and CS/HIPEC [15]. Bilen et al. [14] also documented their experience of four cases of patients with poorly differentiated appendiceal adenocarcinoma who demonstrated a pathologic CR to systemic chemotherapy/biologic therapy. Three of the cases proceeded to CS/HIPEC, while the fourth case underwent a different resection [14]. It is important to note that while these select patients received neoadjuvant/preoperative systemic therapy by definition, these patients were not originally thought to be curative by CS/HIPEC. However, upon receiving palliative systemic therapy, they had a dramatic response to treatment, rendering them surgically resectable cases.

Chemotherapy agents and their mechanism of action

As previously noted, the agents currently utilized for systemic treatment for appendiceal cancer are adapted from the agents and regimens studied in colorectal cancer. These agents include, but are not limited to, fluoropyrimidines (5-fluorouracil and capecitabine), oxaliplatin, irinotecan, bevacizumab, and cetuximab/panitumumab.

Among antineoplastic agents, 5-fluorouracil belongs to the class of antimetabolites. More specifically, it is a fluorinated analog of the pyrimidine uracil that interferes with both ribonucleic acid (RNA) and deoxyribonucleic acid (DNA) syntheses [21]. 5-Fluorouracil is a prodrug that must be converted via dehydrogenase enzymes to its active metabolites fluorodeoxyuridine monophosphate (F-dUMP) and fluorouridine triphosphate (F-UTP). F-dUMP is thought to be the more active metabolite with regard to cytotoxicity because of its ability to tightly bind and interfere with

Table 26.1 Systemic treatments for unresectable appendiceal cancer

Reference	Study design	Study population	Outcomes
Farquharson et al. [12] n = 40	Prospective, phase II MCap regimen	Advanced unresectable PMP	1-year tumor-related survival = 84% 2-year tumor-related survival = 61%
Shapiro et al. [13] n = 54	Retrospective, single institution	Unresectable mucinous or signet ring cell adenocarcinoma of PMP or appendiceal origin	PFS (median) = 7.57 months OS (median) = 56 months
Lieu et al. [18] n = 78	Retrospective, single institution	Poorly differentiated and/or signet ring cell appendiceal adenocarcinoma	PFS (median) = 6.9 months OS (median) = 1.7 years
Pietrantonio et al. [15] n = 20	Prospective, phase II FOLFOX regimen	Unresectable or recurrent PMP of appendiceal origin	PFS (median) = 8 months OS (median) = 26.2 months
Tejani et al. [19] n = 112	Retrospective	Advanced appendiceal cancer	PFS (median) = 1.2 years OS (median) = 2.1 years
Choe et al. [20] n = 79	Retrospective Fluoropyrimidine-based combination chemotherapy versus fluoropyrimidine monotherapy	Unresectable appendiceal epithelial neoplasms	PFS (median), all patients = 8.8 months OS (median), all patients = 45.3 months *PFS (median) longer in patients with combination chemotherapy (9.2 months) versus fluoropyrimidine monotherapy (6.5 months); p = 0.006
Eng et al. [31] n = 132	Retrospective Systemic chemotherapy with biologic therapy versus systemic chemotherapy alone	Unresectable appendiceal epithelial neoplasms	PFS (median), biologic therapy = 17 months PFS (median), no biologic therapy = 7 months; p = 0.007 OS (median), biologic therapy = 68 months OS (median), no biologic therapy = 50 months; p = 0.08

Abbreviations: PFS, progression free survival; OS, overall survival; PMP, pseudomyxoma peritonei.

thymidylate synthase (TS). With the inhibition of TS, thymidine cannot be formed from uracil, arresting this essential step in DNA synthesis. In contrast, the metabolite F-UTP exerts its mechanism of action on RNA. It is directly incorporated, in place of uracil, as an RNA base pair, halting RNA activity and synthesis [21].

When administered IV, 5-fluorouracil distributes widely into extracellular fluid, intestinal mucosa, liver, CSF, third space, and other tissues [21]. It may be administered as a rapid IV bolus infusion or as a prolonged continuous infusion. The efficacy and toxicity profile of 5-fluorouracil is largely based on whether the IV infusion is rapid or prolonged. With regard to colorectal cancers, the cytotoxic activity and tolerance have led to continuous-infusion-5-fluorouracil-based regimens such as modified FOLFOX and FOLFIRI [21].

Capecitabine is an orally active prodrug of 5-fluorouracil that mimics the mechanism of action and toxicity profile of continuous-infusion 5-fluorouracil [21,22]. Capecitabine is supplied as 150 and 500 mg tablets. The total daily dose is calculated based on a patient's body surface area and then divided twice daily and taken on a full stomach. Capecitabine is conventionally administered on days 1 through 14, of a 21-day cycle [21,22].

Common adverse reactions seen with capecitabine and continuous-infusion 5-fluorouracil are stomatitis, diarrhea, and palmar–plantar erythrodysesthesia (also referred to as hand–foot syndrome) [21,22]. These side effects can be managed with appropriate supportive care medications or dose reductions. Both capecitabine and 5-fluorouracil are considered to have minimal potential for causing chemotherapy-induced nausea and vomiting. While they are not interchangeable with regard to dosing, capecitabine and 5-fluorouracil are considered equally efficacious in the treatment of colorectal cancer. Organ dysfunction, cost considerations, drug interactions, individual toxicities, and the need for central venous access are reasons to consider when choosing one formulation over the other [21,22].

Oxaliplatin is another commonly used antineoplastic agent utilized in the systemic treatment of colorectal cancer and, therefore, commonly seen in the treatment of appendiceal cancer [23]. It is a third-generation platinum analog and a member of the alkylating agents. As an alkylating agent, oxaliplatin lends its cytotoxicity to the platinum compound that covalently binds to DNA, forming both inter- and intraplatinum–DNA cross-links. This inhibits both DNA replication and transcription, ultimately resulting in cell death [23].

Oxaliplatin is administered diluted as an IV infusion over 2 hours. Because it is classified as an irritant with vesicant-like properties, it may require a central catheter for administration, depending on institution-specific policies and procedures [23]. Common adverse reactions seen with oxaliplatin include anemia and thrombocytopenia, taste perversions, transaminitis, and hypersensitivity reactions. Unlike its predecessors, oxaliplatin has little nephrotoxicity and ototoxicity associated with its use. Oxaliplatin is considered a moderately emetogenic chemotherapy agent, requiring appropriate premedications. Also associated with oxaliplatin are two distinct types of peripheral neuropathy. One is a persistent neuropathy occurring with cumulative oxaliplatin dosing. This is a dose-limiting toxicity that presents as paresthesias that may interfere with daily activities such as writing, buttoning, and balance. If continued, it can lead to irreversible nerve damage and persistent symptoms. Unique to oxaliplatin is the second type of neuropathy that is acute, reversible, and exacerbated by cold temperatures. This type of neuropathy may include pharyngolaryngeal dysesthesias, jaw spasms, abnormal tongue sensations, or hypoesthesia of the hands or feet particularly when exposed to cold objects or stimuli [23].

The last of the antineoplastic agents utilized in the systemic treatment of colorectal and appendiceal cancer is irinotecan (also referred to as CPT-11), a topoisomerase I inhibitor [24]. More specifically, irinotecan is a prodrug that must undergo hepatic activation to the active metabolite SN-38. This active metabolite exerts its mechanism of action by reversibly binding to and inhibiting topoisomerase I. Because topoisomerase I is an enzyme involved relieving torsional strain of DNA during replication and transcription by generating single-strand breaks, inhibiting this enzyme prevents the relegation of the single-strand breaks. Ultimately, this will result in the accumulation of cleavable complexes and double-strand DNA breaks, which are unable to be repaired, leading to cell death [24].

A majority of the SN-38 active metabolite undergoes conjugation to an inactive glucuronide metabolite via an enzyme called UDP-glucuronosyl transferase 1A1 (also known as UTG1A1) [24]. While rare, patients homozygous for the UTG1A1*28 allele are unable to conjugate SN-38 to inactive metabolites, resulting in increased concentrations of SN-38 and subsequent irinotecan toxicities. Because hepatic metabolism is required to produce the active SN-38 metabolite, irinotecan manufacturer labeling has suggested empiric dose reductions for patients with underlying hepatic dysfunction [24].

Irinotecan is administered via IV infusion over 90 minutes, and when given in a regimen with continuous-infusion 5-fluorouracil (such as FOLFIRI), it is administered every 2 weeks [24]. Like oxaliplatin, irinotecan is categorized as a moderately emetogenic chemotherapy agent, requiring an appropriate antiemetic regimen prior to irinotecan administration. Aside from nausea and vomiting, irinotecan is also associated with alopecia, hyperbilirubinemia, mucositis, anemia, leukopenia, thrombocytopenia, neutropenia, and diarrhea. More specifically, irinotecan is associated with an acute onset diarrhea and a delayed or late onset diarrhea, each possessing a different mechanism for their toxicity. Early onset occurs during or within the first 24 hours of irinotecan administration. It is characterized as a cholinergic diarrhea, accompanied but other cholinergic symptoms such as rhinitis, hypersalivation, lacrimation, diaphoresis, facial flushing, and abdominal cramping. This cholinergic response is usually transient, but can also be treated with atropine. Late or delayed onset diarrhea normally occurs greater than 24 hours after irinotecan administration. The diarrhea may be prolonged and, if not properly managed, lead to dehydration, hospitalization, or death. Aside from treating with high-dose loperamide, fluid or electrolyte replacement may be warranted depending on the severity of diarrhea [24].

Biomarkers

As our knowledge of various biomarkers has expanded, so has our ability to evaluate their role in various cancer types. Several retrospective studies have been conducted evaluating the role various biomarkers play in appendiceal cancer [25,26].

In 2008, Logan-Collins and colleagues published their results of a retrospective chart review of VEGF expression in patients with peritoneal surface metastases secondary to appendiceal and colon cancer [25]. Thirty-five patients were identified from December 1999 through February 2004, with 32 patients with mucinous adenocarcinoma of the appendix and 3 patients with primary adenocarcinoma of the colon. Tumor specimens obtained from CS/IP hyperthermic perfusion were evaluated by immunohistochemistry for CD 34 counts (blood vessels) and VEGF expression [25].

This study demonstrated VEGF expression in 33 patients (94%). Investigators found that average VEGF expression correlated with OS, with survival being longer in patients with low VEGF expression versus those with high VEGF expression (24.9 versus 14.7 months, respectively; p = 0.017) [25]. For patients with recurrent tumors, this correlation was stronger (p = 0.002). Based on these results, the authors theorized that tumor cells are more angiogenic following surgery, when tumor burden has been swiftly reduced. They also supported the rationale for combining CS with antiangiogenic therapy [25].

Raghav et al. [26] retrospectively evaluated several molecular markers in 600 and 7 patients with adenocarcinoma of the appendix. The role of KRAS mutations is of particular interest as this may influence the decisions to include anti-EGFR therapy as a choice for systemic chemotherapy/biologic therapy regimens. One hundred and eight tumor samples were tests for KRAS mutations; 59 samples tested were KRAS mutated (55%), and 49 were KRAS wild type (45%). Of the 49 patients with KRAS wild-type tumors, only 20 received an anti-EGFR therapy with cetuximab (n = 16) or panitumumab (n = 4). Raghav et al. found no statistically significant difference in median OS for patients who received anti-EGFR therapy compared to those who did not (68.3 versus 51.7 months, respectively; p = 0.832). It is important to note that 25% of cases received anti-EGFR therapy as monotherapy, and a majority of patients received anti-EGFR therapy in the second- or third-line setting. The best radiologic response to anti-EGFR therapy was PR in seven patients and SD in three patients. Although a small sample size, the authors suggested further investigation on the use of targeted therapies such as EGFR inhibition [26].

Biologic therapy and mechanism of action

The first of the biologic treatments to be discussed is bevacizumab, a humanized monoclonal antibody against VEGF [27]. It exerts its mechanism of action by binding to the VEGF ligand and preventing it from binding to its receptors, VEGF receptor-1 and VEGF receptor-2. Because VEGF plays an important role in angiogenesis, inhibiting this pathway prevents the formation of new blood vessels, essentially starving cancer cells of a nutritious blood supply [27].

Bevacizumab can be administered IV over 30 minutes and can be added to regimens containing 5-fluorouracil, capecitabine, oxaliplatin, or irinotecan, without adding drastic side effects [27]. Because bevacizumab is a humanized monoclonal antibody, infusion-related reactions are uncommon, and preemptive premedication with histamine antagonists is not necessary. Other adverse reactions seen with bevacizumab include hypertension, headache, and impaired wound healing. Impaired wound healing is an important side effect to keep in mind when patients may be undergoing surgery or have incompletely healed wounds or fistulas. Uncommon, yet severe adverse reactions include hemorrhage, arterial and venous thromboembolism, and gastrointestinal perforation. It is important to be attentive to disease burden and location with regard to gastrointestinal perforation. Patients with appendiceal cancer often have a high disease burden contained within the abdominal cavity, amalgamated with the intestines, and there is a substantial risk of bowel perforation in patients with appendiceal cancer. These patients should be educated and monitored for signs of symptoms of bowel perforation, which include, but are not limited to, abdominal pain accompanied by constipation, nausea and vomiting, or fever [27].

More recently, ziv-aflibercept, another anti-VEGF inhibitor, has been studied in patients with colorectal cancer [28]. Ziv-aflibercept is a fully humanized fusion protein that inhibits angiogenesis by binding to and inhibiting VEGF-A, VEGF-B, and placental growth factors 1 and 2 [28]. This treatment, however, has not been studied in patients with appendiceal cancer, and the safety and efficacy of this treatment in patients with appendiceal cancer are unknown at this time.

Cetuximab and panitumumab are also monoclonal antibodies that have been studied in the systemic treatment of appendiceal cancer [29–30]. Both cetuximab and panitumumab bind to and inhibit ligand binding of the EGFR. The EGFR is a member of the Erb family of receptors and may also be referred to as HER1 or c-ErbB-1, which are located on both normal and tumor cells. By preventing ligand binding, cetuximab and panitumumab prevent subsequent downstream signaling pathways, resulting in inhibition of cell growth and induction of apoptosis. This mechanism of action, however, is only capable of being carried out in tumors that are KRAS wild type. In cells harboring a KRAS mutation, the KRAS protein is constantly active in signaling cell proliferation, regardless of EFGR activation on the surface. Therefore, these patients will not benefit from anti-EGFR therapy with cetuximab or panitumumab [29–30].

Not only do cetuximab and panitumumab share the same mechanism of action, they also share many adverse reactions [29,30]. The most common adverse reactions seen with these agents are hypomagnesemia, diarrhea, and acneform rash. The acneform rash may be macropapular and/or pustular and accompanied by xerosis, exfoliative dermatitis, secondary skin infections, and photosensitivity. This rash has an onset of 1–2 weeks following the first infusion and can be managed with appropriate skin care, supportive care medications, or dose reductions. Other toxicities may include hypertrichosis, keratitis, blepharitis, or skin fissures. One adverse reaction that is more severe and occurring with a higher incidence is infusion-related reaction, including anaphylactic reactions, bronchospasm, and hypotension in patients receiving cetuximab. Cetuximab is a recombinant human/mouse chimeric monoclonal antibody and, therefore, more likely to induce an IgE-mediated hypersensitivity reaction than its counterpart panitumumab, which is a fully human monoclonal antibody. All patients receiving cetuximab should receive premedication with an IV histamine-1 antagonist such as diphenhydramine. Patients should also be monitored for signs and symptoms of hypersensitivity reactions, such as fever, rash, hives, pruritus, diaphoresis, hypotension, flushing, rigors, angioedema, or pain during and after the cetuximab infusion. Depending on the severity of the hypersensitivity reaction, some patients may be candidates for cetuximab rechallenge with extensive premedications, prolonging the infusion time. For severe reactions, however, cetuximab should be discontinued, and panitumumab may be substituted [29,30].

Role of biologic therapy in surgically unresectable appendiceal carcinoma patients

Choe and colleagues retrospectively evaluated the role of systemic chemotherapy in combination with biologic therapy in 130 patients with unresectable appendiceal cancer [31]. Sixty-five (50%) received first-line chemotherapy in combination with biologic therapy; bevacizumab was included in regimens for 59 patients (91%), while an EGFR inhibitor was included in the regimens for 6 patients (9%). The incorporation of anti-VEGF therapy resulted in an improved median PFS and median OS (PFS, 9 versus 4 months, p = 0.047; OS, 76 versus 42 months, p = 0.03, for all histologic subtypes). Although further study with randomized prospective studies is warranted, this study showed a benefit by adding biologic therapy, notably anti-VEGF therapy to traditional chemotherapy in unresectable appendiceal cancer patients [31]. The authors concluded that anti-VEGF therapy should strongly be considered in the systemic treatment of appendiceal epithelial neoplasms, particularly, those with higher-grade histology.

Quality of life

Fewer studies have evaluated the impact of systemic chemotherapy on the QOL for patients with a rather indolent disease course. Eng et al. [32] presented their results of a prospective assessment on the impact of systemic therapy on QOL at the 2013 American Society of Clinical Oncology meeting. Fifty patients with unresectable appendiceal cancer were included. All patients received 5-fluorouracil-based systemic treatment, and 74% of them (n = 37) also received a biologic agent as part of their systemic regimen. EORTC (3.0) QLQ-C30 and QLQ-OV28 surveys and QOL scores were calculated at baseline and every 6 months. This study found no significant change from baseline in the global subscale (MME = 2.9095, p = 0.4422). Eng and colleagues concluded palliative systemic chemotherapy/biologic therapy in unresectable appendiceal cancer patients did not decrease QOL. Some improvement in symptoms of arthralgias, myalgias, and weakness was seen, as well as improvement in emotional well-being [32].

Farquharson et al. [12] also included an assessment of QOL in their phase II study of MCap in patients with unresectable PMP of appendiceal origin. Twenty-two (of a total of 29) patients from that study reported an improvement in their global health status during chemotherapy with systemic treatment with MCap [12].

More studies need to be conducted to evaluate the impact systemic treatment has on patients with unresectable appendiceal cancer.

DISCUSSION/FUTURE DIRECTIONS

After presentation of the published literature, it is clear that the role of systemic therapy in the treatment of appendiceal cancer should be tested in a prospective, randomized setting. Appendiceal cancer has long been classified and studied with other, more common types of cancer such as colorectal, ovarian, and primary peritoneal cancers [1]. Because appendiceal cancer is a rare disease with a substantial amount of heterogeneity, conclusive decisions are difficult to obtain. This scenario clouds the picture when deciding when to use systemic therapy and what chemotherapy and/or biologic therapy regimens and duration of therapy to choose.

Systemic chemotherapy is most commonly going to be reserved for patients who are not candidates for curative CS/HIPEC. This may include patients with extensive or advanced appendiceal cancer or patients whose performance status or comorbidities put them at risk for increased surgical morbidity and mortality. When systemic chemotherapy/biologic therapy is chosen, there are several challenges faced with the treatment regimen itself as well as in the assessment of the benefit that systemic treatment is providing to the patient [1,4].

First, systemic treatment of appendiceal cancer should include a fluoropyrimidine backbone with 5-fluorouracil or capecitabine, as these agents have most commonly been utilized in studies evaluating systemic treatment in patients with appendiceal cancer [7,12,13,15,18–20]. Only conflicting evidence of the addition of oxaliplatin, irinotecan, bevacizumab, or cetuximab/panitumumab has been presented, and none of the studies have included a large enough population of patients to accurately compare the addition of these agents. Therefore, the addition of chemotherapy/biologic therapy to the fluoropyrimidine backbone should be a discussion and decision of the treating physician based on patient specific factors.

Second, assessing systemic treatment response is also very difficult. Radiographically, this disease is difficult to appreciate [1]. Sugarbaker and colleagues found different response outcomes when patients were evaluated radiographically, histopathologically, and operatively to systemic therapy [7]. Because of the challenges in assessing responses radiographically, some practitioners measure and utilize tumor markers such as CEA, CA19-9, or CA-125 as surrogate markers to trend disease activity. These markers are not necessarily elevated in patients with appendiceal cancer and have not been validated to measure response; however, they may provide an indirect way of tracking disease activity or clinic response. Farquharson and colleagues found a statistically significant decline between pre- and posttreatment values of CEA ($p = 0.001$) and CA-125 ($p = 0.002$), but not CA19-9 [12]. Meanwhile, Shapiro and colleagues measured serum CEA and CA-125 pre- and postsystemic treatment in a subset of patients included in their study with unresectable appendiceal disease [13]. There was no statistically significant change in pre- and posttreatment CEAs, but there was a statistically significant decline in CA-125 from a median pretreatment of 57.4 U/mL to a median posttreatment level of 1.0 U/mL ($p = 0.006$), leading the authors to wonder if CA-125 is more indicative of treatment response than CEA [13].

This conflicting information has led practitioners to also consider clinic benefit as assessment of treatment response. Both Bijelic et al. [8] and Sugarbaker et al. [7] describe clinical response to treatment as a reduction in patient symptoms of abdominal fullness, bloating, and pain [5,7–8]. In the absence of radiographic or serum biomarker response, practitioners may rely on clinical response when deciding whether or not to continue systemic treatment.

Third, aside from questions surrounding efficacy of systemic treatment, this setting lacks data assessing of QOL and cost analysis. QOL has been underreported in the literature. Aside from the prospective study abstract by Eng and colleagues [32], the only mention of QOL has been as a secondary endpoint [12] or afterthought. The impact of cost of these systemic treatments on patient outcomes including OS, PFS, toxicity management, hospitalizations, and QOL is yet to be determined.

Colleagues at the University of Texas MD Anderson Cancer Center have opened a prospective, open-label, crossover trial of systemic chemotherapy in patients with metastatic well-differentiated mucinous appendiceal cancer with PMP. With the trial collecting data through 2017, it will likely be several years before the results are published; however, evaluating appendiceal cancer in a prospective study is a promising step toward more definitive answers in this rare disease [33]. A second randomized phase II trial validating the role of anti-VEGF therapy in combination with chemotherapy is planned for surgically unresectable and moderately and poorly differentiated appendiceal carcinoma patients.

CONCLUSION

Data supporting the use of systemic therapy in appendiceal cancer have been limited largely to retrospective studies, with a small, heterogeneous population of patients with mixed histology and treatment regimens. This has led to diluted results that are vague and ambiguous. There are few prospective studies, most of which are phase II. There is a strong demand for prospective, comparative studies designed to determine if systemic chemotherapy/biologic therapy improves patient-specific outcomes.

Currently, no standard of care exists with the use of systemic chemotherapy/biologic therapy. If chosen, systemic regimens should be carefully evaluated and selected based on tolerance, toxicity profile, organ dysfunction, performance status, and patient and practitioner preferences.

REFERENCES

1. Shankar S, Ledakis P, El Halabi H, Gushchin V, Sardi A. Neoplasms of the appendix: Current treatment guidelines. *Hematology/Oncology Clinics of North America*. 2012;26(6):1261–1290.
2. Sugarbaker PH. Patient selection and treatment of peritoneal carcinomatosis from colorectal and appendiceal cancer. *World Journal of Surgery*. 1995;19(2):235–240.
3. Sugarbaker PH. New standard of care for appendiceal epithelial neoplasms and pseudomyxoma peritonei syndrome? *The Lancet Oncology*. 2006;7(1):69–76.
4. Smith JW, Kemeny N, Caldwell C, Banner P, Sigurdson E, Huvos A. Pseudomyxoma peritonei of appendiceal origin. The memorial Sloan-Kettering cancer center experience. *Cancer*. 1992;70(2):396–401.
5. Blackham AU, Swett K, Eng C, Sirintrapun J, Bergman S, Geisinger KR et al. Perioperative systemic chemotherapy for appendiceal mucinous carcinoma peritonei treated with cytoreductive surgery and hyperthermic intraperitoneal chemotherapy. *Journal of Surgical Oncology*. 2014;109(7):740–745.
6. Bradley RF, Stewart JH IV, Russell GB, Levine EA, Geisinger KR. Pseudomyxoma peritonei of appendiceal origin: A clinicopathologic analysis of 101 patients uniformly treated at a single institution, with literature review. *The American Journal of Surgical Pathology*. 2006;30(5):551–559.

7. Sugarbaker PH, Bijelic L, Chang D, Yoo D. Neoadjuvant folfox chemotherapy in 34 consecutive patients with mucinous peritoneal carcinomatosis of appendiceal origin. *Journal of Surgical Oncology.* 2010;102(6):576–581.

8. Bijelic L, Kumar AS, Anthony Stuart O, Sugarbaker PH. Systemic chemotherapy prior to cytoreductive surgery and HIPEC for carcinomatosis from appendix cancer: Impact on perioperative outcomes and short-term survival. *Gastroenterology Research and Practice.* 2012;2012:6.

9. National Comprehensive Cancer Network. Breast Cancer (Version 3.2014). http://www.nccn.org/professionals/physician_gls/pdf/breast.pdf. Accessed September 1, 2014.

10. National Comprehensive Cancer Network. Rectal Cancer (Version 1.2015). http://www.nccn.org/professionals/physician_gls/pdf/rectal.pdf. Accessed September 1, 2014.

11. National Comprehensive Cancer Network. Gastric Cancer (Version 1.2014). http://www.nccn.org/professionals/physician_gls/pdf/gastric.pdf. Accessed September 1, 2014.

12. Farquharson AL, Pranesh N, Witham G, Swindell R, Taylor MB, Renehan AG et al. A phase II study evaluating the use of concurrent mitomycin C and capecitabine in patients with advanced unresectable pseudomyxoma peritonei. *British Journal of Cancer.* August 5, 2008;99(4):591–596.

13. Shapiro JF, Chase JL, Wolff RA, Lambert LA, Mansfield PF, Overman MJ et al. Modern systemic chemotherapy in surgically unresectable neoplasms of appendiceal origin. *Cancer.* 2010;116(2):316–322.

14. Bilen MA, Taggart MW, Fournier K, Ellis LM, Mansfield PF, Eng C et al. Pathologic complete response in poorly differentiated adenocarcinomas of the appendix: A case series. *Acta Oncologica.* 2013;52(5).1044–1046.

15. Pietrantonio F, Maggi C, Fanetti G, Iacovelli R, Di Bartolomeo M, Ricchini F et al. Folfox-4 chemotherapy for patients with unresectable or relapsed peritoneal pseudomyxoma. *The Oncologist.* August 1, 2014;19(8):845–850.

16. Shen P, Thomas CR, Fenstermaker J, Aklilu M, McCoy TP, Levine EA. Phase II trial of adjuvant oral thalidomide following cytoreductive surgery and hyperthermic intraperitoneal chemotherapy for peritoneal surface disease from colorectal/appendiceal cancer. (In English). *Journal of Gastrointestinal Cancer.* September 1, 2014;45(3):268–275.

17. Chen CF, Huang CJ, Kang WY, Hsieh JS. Experience with adjuvant chemotherapy for pseudomyxoma peritonei secondary to mucinous adenocarcinoma of the appendix with oxaliplatin/fluorouracil/leucovorin (Folfox4). *World Journal of Surgical Oncology.* 2008;6(1):118.

18. Lieu CH, Lambert LA, Wolff RA, Eng C, Zhang N, Wen S et al. Systemic chemotherapy and surgical cytoreduction for poorly differentiated and signet ring cell adenocarcinomas of the appendix. *Annals of Oncology.* March 1, 2012;23(3):652–658.

19. Tejani MA, ter Veer A, Milne D, Ottesen R, Bekaii-Saab T, Benson AB et al. Systemic therapy for advanced appendiceal adenocarcinoma: An analysis from the Nccn oncology outcomes database for colorectal cancer. *Journal of the National Comprehensive Cancer Network.* August 1, 2014;12(8):1123–1130.

20. Choe JH, Blackham AU, Overman MJ, Fournier KF, Royal RE, Gajula P et al. Combination systemic chemotherapy versus monotherapy in surgically unresectable appendiceal epithelial neoplasms. *Gastrointestinal Cancer Research.* In press.

21. Adrucil (fluorouracil injection) (prescribing information). Irvine, CA: Teva Parenteral Medicines, Inc; July 2007. http://bdipharma.com/msds/teva/adrucil_msds.pdf. Accessed September 1, 2014.

22. Xeloda (capecitabine) [prescribing information]. South San Francisco, CA: Genetech; December 2013. http://www.gene.com/download/pdf/xeloda_prescribing.pdf. Accessed September 1, 2014.

23. Eloxatin (oxaliplatin) [prescribing information]. Bridgewater, NJ: Sanofi-Aventis; July 2013. http://products.sanofi.us/eloxatin/eloxatin.html. Accessed September 1, 2014.

24. Camptosar (irinotecan) [prescribing information]. Kalamazoo, MI: Pharmacia and Upjohn Company; August 2010. http://labeling.pfizer.com/ShowLabeling.aspx?id=533. Accessed September 1, 2014.

25. Logan C, Jocelyn M, Lowy AM, Robinson-Smith TM, Kumar S, Sussman JJ, James LE, Ahmad SA. Vegf expression predicts survival in patients with peritoneal surface metastases from mucinous adenocarcinoma of the appendix and colon. (In English). *Annals of Surgical Oncology.* (March 1, 2008);15(3):738–744.

26. Raghav KPS, Shetty AV, Kazmi SMA, Zhang N, Morris J, Taggart M et al. Impact of molecular alterations and targeted therapy in appendiceal adenocarcinomas. *The Oncologist.* December 1, 2013;18(12):1270–1277.

27. Avastin (bevacizumab) [prescribing information]. South San Francisco, CA: Genentech Inc; December 2013. http://www.gene.com/download/pdf/avastin_prescribing.pdf. Accessed September 1, 2014.

28. Zaltrap (ziv-aflibercept) [prescribing information]. Bridgewater, NJ: Sanofi-Aventis; October 2013. http://products.sanofi.us/zaltrap/zaltrap.html. Accessed September 1, 2014.

29. Erbitux [package insert]. Princeton, NJ: Bristol-Myers Squibb; August 2013. http://pi.lilly.com/us/erbitux-uspi.pdf. Accessed September 1, 2014.

30. Vectibix (panitumumab) [prescribing information]. Thousand Oaks, CA: Amgen; May 2014. http://pi.amgen.com/united_states/vectibix/vectibix_pi.pdf. Accessed September 1, 2014.

31. Choe JH, Overman MJ, Fournier KF, Royal RE, Ohinata A, Rafeeq S et al. (2015). Improved survival with anti-VEGF therapy in the treatment of unresectable appendiceal epithelial neoplasms. *Annals of Surgical Oncology*, 1–7.

32. Eng C, Choe J, Overman MJ, Fournier KF, Phillips J, Baum G et al. Assessment of the impact of systemic chemotherapy (Sc) on the quality of life (Qol) in patients with metastatic unresectable appendiceal epithelial neoplasms (Aen). *ASCO Meeting Abstracts*. January 30, 2013;31(4 Suppl.):522.

33. The University of Texas MD Anderson Cancer Center. Crossover Trial of Systemic Chemotherapy in Patients With Metastatic Well-differentiated Mucinous Appendiceal Adenocarcinomas With Pseudomyxoma Peritonea. In: ClinicalTrials.gov. Bethesda, MD: National Library of Medicine (US). September 1, 2000–2014. Available from: https://clinicaltrials.gov/ct2/show/NCT01946854?term=appendiceal+cancer&state1=NA%3AUS%3ATX&rank=1. NLM Identifier: NCT01946854. Accessed September 1, 2014.

27

Toxicity and morbidity of IP drug therapy

COLETTE PAMEIJER

The morbidity and mortality associated with cytoreductive surgery (CRS) and heated intraperitoneal chemotherapy (HIPEC) stems largely from the surgical part of the procedure, rather than the intraperitoneal (IP) chemotherapy. Tumor burden, extent of surgery, duration of surgery, age, and blood loss have been significantly associated with morbidity from CRS and HIPEC [1–3]. The complications associated with IP chemotherapy can be significant, however, and can potentiate surgical complications. The specific chemotherapy agent, the targeted IP temperature, underlying patient physiology, and operative features all play a role in the risk of complications. Glehen et al. compared a group of patients who underwent HIPEC alone, without CRS, to patients who had both CRS and HIPEC. The morbidity of both CRS and HIPEC was 30.5% and of HIPEC alone 19.4%, indicating very real consequences from IP therapy independent of surgery [1]. Sorting out the cause and effect in this complex group of patients is challenging, and few centers have a large enough patient population to draw strong conclusions. Nevertheless, there are consistent findings in the literature, which will be reviewed in this chapter.

Hematologic toxicity is probably the easiest complication to ascribe to IP chemotherapy. An early report indicated a fairly low overall rate of hematologic toxicity, i.e., 2.5%, but a high associated mortality with 66% (four of six patients) of neutropenic patients dying. These patients all received HIPEC with mitomycin C (MMC) and early postop IP chemotherapy (EPIC) with 5-fluorouracil (5-FU), as well as timely support with granulocyte colony-stimulating factor (G-CSF). These patients had other significant gastrointestinal (GI), respiratory, and septic complications in addition to the neutropenia [4]. Subsequent reports identify varying rates of hematologic toxicity but much less mortality associated with neutropenia. Lambert et al. found that

neutropenia was not statistically significantly associated with an increased risk of mortality, or even an increased length of stay [5].

The question of optimal intra-abdominal temperature for perfusion creates heated debate. High temperatures may more effectively kill tumor cells but have also been associated with increased complications. Animal studies find a fairly narrow range of tolerance of hyperthermia, with rats subjected to intestinal hyperthermia at 46°C uniformly dying, most dying at 45°C but all surviving a temperature of 44°C [6]. The relationship between intra-abdominal temperature, core temperature, and complications specific to a chemotherapy agent is not clearly known. Some centers are more aggressive in cooling patients prior to perfusion and in maintaining core normothermia during perfusion. Core temperatures are often not reported; thus, it is difficult to draw any conclusions from the limited data available. Patients are typically cooled passively to 34°C–35°C, but acceptable core temperatures during perfusion range from 37°C to 39°C. Target outflow temperatures range from 40°C to 43°C depending on the surgeon and center, although the temperature achieved in any individual patient will depend on their body habitus and environmental measures, such as heating blankets over the abdomen and roller pump tubing.

Chemotherapy is believed to interfere with wound healing, supported by studies that demonstrate that chemotherapy interferes with collagen deposition and wound strength [7]. Animal studies evaluating the effect of hyperthermia with or without chemotherapy and comparing anastomotic strength have variable results, with some groups being equal (normothermia, hyperthermia, hyperthermia, and chemotherapy) [2,6] but others showing significantly less strength in the chemotherapy group [8]. These studies use different methods of testing the strength of the anastomosis, making comparisons difficult. The chemotherapy agent may also

Table 27.1 National Cancer Institute CTC terminology (v4)

Adverse event	Grades				
	1	2	3	4	5
Anemia	10 g/dL < LLN[a]	8–10 g/dL	6.5–8.0 g/dL	Life threatening, urgent intervention required	Death
Leukocytes	3,000/mm³ < LLN	2,000–3,000/mm³	1,000–2,000/mm³	<1,000/mm³	Death
Platelets	75,000 < LLN	50,000–75,000/mm³	25,000–50,000/mm³	<25,000/mm³	Death
Neutrophils	1,500/mm³ < LLN	1,000–1,500/mm³	500–1,000/mm³	<500/mm³	Death
Lymphocytes	800/mm³ < LLN	500–800/mm³	200–500/mm³	<200/mm³	Death
Acute kidney injury	Creatinine 1.5×–2× baseline	Creatinine 2×–3× baseline	Creatinine >3× baseline or >4 mg/dL	Life threatening, dialysis indicated	Death
Hyperglycemia	ULN[b]—160 mg/dL (fasting)	Fasting glucose 160–250 mg/dL	250–500 mg/dL	>500	Death
Hyponatremia	LLN—130 mmol/L	—	<130–120	<120, life threatening	Death
GI perforation	—	Symptomatic, medical intervention indicated	Severe symptoms, elective operative intervention	Life threatening, urgent operative intervention	Death
Fistula	Asymptomatic	Symptomatic, altered GI function	Symptomatic and severely altered function requiring IVF, tube feeds, or TPN	Life threatening	Death
Leak	Asymptomatic	Symptomatic, intervention indicated	Symptomatic + interfering with GI function	Life threatening	Death

[a] LLN = lower limit of normal.
[b] ULN = upper limit of normal.

make a difference, with cisplatin-treated animals having significantly weaker anastomoses than MMC-treated animals. These data are probably most useful for timing non-operative chemotherapy and less so for HIPEC.

What follows is a description of the most commonly used agents for IP therapy and complications specific to each. Toxicity is usually graded using the National Cancer Institute CTC Terminology [9], shown in Table 27.1. Grade 1 and 2 toxicities are considered mild; thus, this chapter will focus on grade 3, 4, and 5 toxicities, or their equivalent. It should be noted that the reporting of complications varies widely in the literature, in terms of defining the complications, whether they are grouped together (i.e., as hematologic toxicity) or specified (i.e., neutropenia), and whether they are actually graded or merely described.

MITOMYCIN C

MMC was chosen for IP therapy early on due to its high molecular weight and favorable pharmacokinetic profile, with a high AUC ratio between IP concentration times time and plasma concentration times time [10]. It is also compatible with many other drugs. The side effect profile of MMC is well described, though variably seen. Hematologic toxicity is the most common effect, with anemia, neutropenia, leukopenia, and thrombocytopenia all attributed to MMC. Bowel complications and renal injury are less common, but also noted.

The dosing of MMC is quite variable, as are the rates of morbidity. Higher total doses of MMC (over 60 mg) induce significant bone marrow suppression and are associated with significantly more adverse events [11]. Early experience suggested a 66% mortality rate with HIPEC-induced neutropenia [4], but collective experience has improved, and neutropenia has not been associated with an increased risk of mortality [3,5]. Table 27.2 outlines the experience of multiple centers with MMC. Neutropenia has been associated with the dose of MMC when adjusted for body surface area (BSA) and also female gender. There was a trend toward neutropenia in splenectomized patients, but this was not statistically significant [5]. The variable results in Table 27.2 make it clear that hematologic toxicity is not strictly related to dose of drug.

The impact of MMC on GI complications is more difficult to decipher. Multiple centers report anastomotic leaks,

Table 27.2 Frequency of complications with mitomycin C

Author	Patients	Dose MMC	Other drugs	Outflow temperature (°C)	Duration (minutes)	Grade 3/4 hematologic toxicity	Bowel toxicity	ATN
Glockzin et al. [33]	40	20 mg/m²	Doxorubicin 15 mg/m²	41–43	60	—	1 perforation (2.5%) 3 leak (7.5%)	
Lambert et al. [5]	117	10 mg/L		>40	90	47 (39%)		
Glehen et al. [1]	207	0.7 mg/kg 0.5 mg/kg	Cisᵇ 0.7 mg/kg	46–48 inflow	90	— 10	14 fistula (6.5%)	
Loggie et al. [46]	84			40.5	120	6 (7%) neutroᶜ 4 (4%) plt		
Smeenk et al. [3]	103	35 mg/m²		40–41	90	11 (11%)		
Verwaal et al. [47]	105	17.5 mg/m² 8.8 mg/m² boost q 30 minutes		>40	90	17% leuco 4% thrombo	7% fistula	6%
Loungnarath et al. [48]	27	0.5 mg/kg	Cis 0.7 mg/kg	42–42.5	90	—	3 leak (11%)	1 (4%)
Shen et al. [49]	109	10 mg/L		40.5	120	23 (21%) WBC 69 (63%) RBC		
Elias et al. [50]	27	5–10 mg/L		41–44	60	2 aplasia	5 fistula	
Jacquet et al. [51]	60	10 mg/L		46	120	4 hem tox (7%)	6 leak (10%) 5 perforation (8%)	
Facchiano et al. [52]ᵃ	5	75 mg	Cis 200 mg/m²	41–43	60–90	—	1 delayed gastric emptying	
Stephens et al. [53]	183	12.5 mg/m²♂ 10 mg/m²♀		42–43	90	9 (4%)	9 fistula (4.5%)	
Baratti et al. [44]	101	3.3 mg/m²/L	Cis 25 mg/m²/L	42.5	60	6 (6%)	7 leak/perforation (7%)	

a Malignant ascites.
b Cisplatin.
c Neutropenia.

bowel perforations, and fistulas, yet these occur in the setting of CRS, a morbid procedure by itself. GI complications are seen with other chemotherapeutic agents, and morbidity overall has repeatedly been associated with surgical factors such as extent of cytoreduction, number of anastomoses, blood loss, and duration of surgery. It is interesting to note that in a recent review from Wagner et al., [12] patients who had extensive CRS, defined as more than three organs resected or more than two anastomoses, had similar rates of GI complications as the comparison group with less extensive surgery, 3.3% and 2.3%, respectively [12]. Thus, with chemotherapy being equal, the extent of surgery does not seem to impact the rate of leak or fistula. There are likely operative details that are not captured in these reports, such as extent of lysis of adhesions, or extent of small bowel involvement. Until more (or better) data become available, it would seem that GI complications result from a combination of surgical factors and chemotherapy and occur in a small percentage of patients.

OXALIPLATIN

There is great interest in the use of IP oxaliplatin for patients with carcinomatosis from colorectal cancer, stemming from the results seen with systemic 5-FU, leucovorin, oxaliplatin (FOLFOX) therapy. Side effects from systemic oxaliplatin include neurotoxicity and hepatotoxicity. The use of IP oxaliplatin is complicated by the fact that oxaliplatin degrades in the presence of chlorine, necessitating 5% dextrose as a carrier solution. This limits compatibility with other drugs and also leads to significant metabolic changes during perfusion. Plasma glucose levels commonly exceed 300 or even 400 mg/dL during perfusion. This results in hyponatremia due to a shift of water to the extracellular space, with plasma sodium levels averaging 125 mmol/L by the completion of perfusion. It is important to note that at higher plasma glucose levels, the serum sodium decreases more rapidly [13]. Below 400 mg/dL, sodium levels will drop 1.6 meq/L for every 100 mg/dL increase in glucose. Once over 400 mg/dL, sodium levels will drop by 4 meq/L for every 100 mg/dL increase in glucose [14]. Plasma sodium levels will normalize in most patients by 72 hours after perfusion [15]. Patients will also develop a metabolic acidosis associated with elevated lactate levels. Lactate is a product of glycolysis, and the elevated lactate levels seen during perfusion with oxaliplatin are likely related to increased turnover of glucose and not anaerobic metabolism [13]. When reported, serum pH changes from 7.4 to 7.3 by the end of perfusion [13,16].

Overall, the morbidity and mortality associated with the use of oxaliplatin is not significantly different from that seen with MMC. Like MMC, the hematologic toxicity seen with oxaliplatin can be significant and is occasionally associated with mortality. In addition to neutropenia and sepsis, cerebral vascular accident due to thrombocytopenia has been reported [17]. Hematologic toxicity may be magnified by splenectomy. Votanopoulos et al. found that neutrophil and platelet toxicity occurred more frequently in patients who received oxaliplatin versus MMC, with a significant difference among patients who had a splenectomy as part of the cytoreduction. In other settings, splenectomy is associated with leukocytosis and thrombocytosis; thus, we might expect some protective effect from neutropenia and thrombocytopenia. In fact, the hematologic toxicities are more pronounced with splenectomy. It is unclear whether the increased toxicity with splenectomy is due to mechanical/pharmacokinetic differences, with increased dissection in the left upper quadrant and perhaps increased surface area for absorption of drug or is related to the function of the spleen itself [18].

As with MMC, some GI complications are seen in patients who receive oxaliplatin. The low incidence of perforation, anastomotic leak, and fistula is similar to that seen in patients who receive MMC, and interpretation of the data in light of a morbid surgical procedure carries the same pitfalls. The neurotoxicity seen with systemic oxaliplatin has rarely been seen, and only one center noted an increase in hepatic enzymes, qualifying as a grade 3 toxicity but not requiring any intervention [16]. Table 27.3 outlines the experience of several centers with oxaliplatin.

CISPLATIN

Cisplatin has significant cytotoxic activity against ovarian cancer, gastric cancer, and mesothelioma and is compatible with multiple other drugs. In the realm of GI malignancy, cisplatin is most commonly combined with MMC, doxorubicin, or paclitaxel and is rarely administered as a single agent. Cisplatin is often used in patients with ovarian cancer, via both IV and IP routes. The dosing of cisplatin varies widely, but a total dose >240 mg has been associated with major morbidity [19] including pancreatic fistula [20].

Much of the data related to IP cisplatin comes from Gyn Onc experience. The survival benefit of IP therapy over IV therapy was shown in several trials for women with ovarian cancer [21,22], despite the fact that a significant percentage of patients did not complete the scheduled six cycles of IP therapy (42%–58%) [21,23]. The most common reason for discontinuing IP therapy was catheter-related problems, with 34% of patients experiencing infection, blockage, leak, or access problems. Another 29% experienced nausea, vomiting, dehydration, renal, or metabolic problems related to therapy [23]. The tolerability of IP cisplatin varies and may depend on the concurrent IV therapy. Armstrong et al. [24] found significantly more adverse events in the IP group and a worse quality of life up to 6 weeks after treatment, although there were no quality of life differences by 1 year after treatment completion. In this study, subjects received IV paclitaxel in addition to the cisplatin. Alberts et al. [21] found that IP cisplatin was better tolerated than IV cisplatin, with fewer hematologic and ototoxic effects. Patients receiving IP therapy had significantly more abdominal pain, but this was controlled with either nonopioid or weak opioid drugs and typically resolved within 24 hours. In this study, women

Table 27.3 Frequency of complications with oxaliplatin

Author	# Patients	Ox[a] dose (mg/m^2)	Other drugs	Outflow temperature (°C)	Duration	Change in Na (meq/L)	Hematologic toxicity	GI
Rueth et al. [15]	20	300–400		41–42	30	139 → 127	3 Gr 3 Hgb (17%) 2 Gr 3 plt (8%)	
Stewart et al. [54]	12 3	200 250		40.6	120		9 Gr 3 lympho (75%) 1 Gr 5 plt 1 Gr 3 plt	
Votanopoulos et al. [18]	55	200		40	120		6 Gr 3/4 plt (11%) 8 neutro (14.5%)	
Glockzin et al. [33]	40	300	IV 5-FU 400 IV folic acid 20 mg/m^2	41–43	30		—	1 perforation (2.5%)
Ceelen et al. [16]	52	460	IV folate 20 IV 5-FU 400	41	30	136 → 125	—	2 leak (4%) 19 Gr 3 hepatic (36%)
Elias et al. [32]	106	360	Irinotecan 360 mg/m^2	43	30		11% neutro thrombo	24 fistula (23%)
Elias et al. [17]	30	460	IV 5-FU 400 LV[b] 20 mg/m^2	42–44	30		2 aplasia 1 Gr 5 plt	
De Somer et al. [13]	27	460		41	30	137 → 127	—	

a Oxaliplatin.
b LV = leucovorin.

received IV cyclophosphamide in addition to the cisplatin. Both studies used 100 mg/m^2 of cisplatin, and this remains the recommended dose.

Whether and how much the addition of heat may augment the toxicity of cisplatin is unclear. In an animal study, the addition of heat to IP cisplatin did not change the drug level in tumor or plasma, suggesting that the toxicity profile should be the same [25]. In reports of HIPEC with cisplatin, multiple drugs are used. The incidence of hematologic toxicity is similar between cisplatin combined with MMC and MMC alone (see Table 27.2). Kusamura et al. [19] describe their results in 209 patients using either cisplatin 25 mg/m^2/L and MMC 3.3 mg/m^2/L or cisplatin 43 mg/L and doxorubicin 15.25 mg/L for 60–90 minutes at 42°C–43°C outflow temperature. The complications are described for the group as a whole, but the incidence of grade 3 hematologic toxicity was only 1.4 %, with grade 3 or 4 renal toxicity of 2%. There were two patients who ultimately required hemodialysis and developed chronic renal failure. The group did find on univariate and multivariate analysis that a dose of cisplatin >240 mg significantly correlated with major morbidity, and no prior chemotherapy had borderline significance in increasing morbidity. In a later review from the same center, Baratti et al. [26] looked at 108 patients with mesothelioma who received cisplatin 45 mg/L and doxorubicin 15 mg/L for 90 minutes at 42.5°C. The rates of toxicity were higher, with 14 (12.9%) leak or perforation, 7 (6.5%) hematologic toxicity, and 10 (9.2%) renal toxicity. The mean dose of cisplatin was below 240 mg, and in this review the factors contributing to complications, such as prior chemotherapy, were not analyzed.

5-FLUOROURACIL

5-FU is an old drug and has been a standard component of chemotherapy regimens for GI cancer for decades. In addition to the IV route, 5-FU was delivered IP as early as the 1980s, with favorable tolerance and toxicity results [27]. 5-FU is not significantly synergized by heat and thus has been more commonly used as early postoperative chemotherapy. The toxicity associated with IP 5-FU includes chemical peritonitis and hematologic effects, although with a lower incidence of leukopenia and thrombocytopenia than IV 5-FU [27]. As with other drugs, the peritoneal barrier allows for higher doses of drug before toxicity is seen. In most recent reports, 5-FU is delivered IV with leucovorin, in conjunction with IP oxaliplatin as bidirectional chemotherapy. There is very recent interest, however, in HIPEC with 5-FU as an adjuvant in patients who are at high risk of peritoneal recurrence from colorectal cancer [28]. These are preliminary studies and, while promising, require validation.

OTHER AGENTS

Several other chemotherapeutic agents have been used for IP therapy, usually in more experienced centers and for less common histologies, or as part of multidrug regimens.

Doxorubicin was one of the first IP chemotherapy agents used in a clinical trial for peritoneal disease and was delivered postoperatively. Doxorubicin is a sclerosing agent, and with increasing doses (up to 50 mg), severe and prolonged abdominal pain developed during the treatment. The higher doses also resulted in peritoneal adhesions, which could interfere with additional IP treatment. The few responders in this study were women with small-volume disease [29]. Subsequent dose escalation studies identified 15 mg/m^2 as tolerable, [10] and this dose is very consistently reported by multiple centers. Doxorubicin is often combined with cisplatin and today is not used as a single agent. It is well tolerated, although if patients have received systemic doxorubicin, the total dose of this drug should be monitored to avoid cardiac complications.

Irinotecan, like oxaliplatin, has demonstrated survival benefit and is now considered second-line systemic therapy for patients with colorectal cancer. Irinotecan is a prodrug, however, and requires conversion to SN-38 in the liver, which is the active metabolite. Irinotecan is also not synergized by heat, [10] making it theoretically less attractive as a HIPEC agent. Despite these drawbacks, animal studies find pharmacokinetic advantages and greater efficacy of oxaliplatin and irinotecan delivered IP, rather than IV [30]. Irinotecan has been used IP with oxaliplatin, often in combination with IV 5-FU and leucovorin. The hematologic toxicity profile is similar to oxaliplatin, but overall complication rates are significantly higher in patients who receive both drugs [31]. In particular, the rate of fistula was much higher at 23% [32] and hematologic toxicity of up to 38% [31] compared to 0%–2.5% and 2.3%, respectively, in studies using IP oxaliplatin alone [31–33]. A Phase 1 clinical trial combining irinotecan and MMC found significant hematologic toxicity, with a maximum tolerated dose of only 100 mg/m^2 of irinotecan [34]. This increased toxicity with irinotecan has not yet been demonstrated to result in better survival.

Paclitaxel is widely used for mesothelioma and ovarian and gastric cancer, both IV and IP. Paclitaxel is not synergized by heat; thus, it is usually delivered in 1–2 L of solution instilled during closure of the abdomen, or postoperatively via an IP port. Several centers in Japan will place an IP catheter and port at the time of staging laparoscopy in order to deliver IP chemotherapy. Common consequences of IP therapy with paclitaxel include abdominal pain that is usually easily managed with analgesics and only occasional narcotics for some patients. True GI toxicity such as anastomotic leak or fistula is rarely reported with paclitaxel as a single agent, with only one enterocutaneous fistula described [35]. Hematologic toxicity is frequently described in a minority of patients. Anemia, leukopenia, and neutropenia have all been found, ranging from 3% to 14% in these often small studies. A significant component of the morbidity of nonoperative IP therapy relates to the catheter, as described earlier.

MANAGEMENT OF COMPLICATIONS

Many of the complications that arise after CRS and HIPEC, despite the complexity of the procedure, are really general surgical problems. The anastomotic leak or enterocutaneous fistula in a HIPEC patient is no different than in any other (complicated) patient. The risk of neutropenia, thrombocytopenia, and metabolic derangements associated with HIPEC should be minimized, so as not to compound other surgical problems.

The management of risk begins before surgery, with patient, drug, and dose selection. Several centers have more or less extensive criteria for CRS and HIPEC, which include performance status, white blood cells (WBC) and platelet counts, absence of extra-abdominal metastasis, and typically some assessment of the chance of resectability. More detailed criteria include an assessment of hepatic function as indicated by International Normalized Ratio, total bilirubin, alkaline phosphatase, and aspartate aminotransferase and adequate renal function. The drug of choice is another subject of great debate, but until more rigorous data are available, it remains the surgeon's preference. Disease histology should dictate the choice(s) of agents, with a patient's prior systemic chemotherapy experience taken into consideration. Many centers will reduce the dose of IP chemotherapy in the setting of prior systemic chemotherapy, poor performance status, very extensive surgery, or in elderly patients. Some of these criteria conflict with selection criteria for CRS and HIPEC, implying that cases are decided individually based on a multitude of factors including that center's experience. Drug doses are typically reduced by 25% for any of these criteria, although the duration of perfusion can also be adjusted. Table 27.4 summarizes the toxicity profile of the most commonly used agents for IP therapy.

The metabolic derangements associated with IP oxaliplatin demand active intervention by the anesthesia team during perfusion and ongoing close attention postoperatively. An insulin drip should be started before perfusion begins, with glucose and electrolyte measurements every 15 minutes during the perfusion to guide the rate of insulin infusion. Hyperglycemia will develop despite the insulin drip. The metabolic acidosis is a result of the hyperglycemia and does not usually require any separate intervention. Bicarbonate can be given for a base deficit of more than 5, and hypertonic saline should be administered for severe hyponatremia. Once perfusion is complete, electrolytes should be checked every 15–30 minutes until they stabilize and then daily [15,16].

Sodium thiosulfate was identified in the 1980s as an antidote to cisplatin. Sodium thiosulfate neutralizes cisplatin by irreversible binding of the drug and also acts as a diuretic that is believed to speed elimination of the drug. The concentration of active cisplatin in plasma and kidney tissue is significantly decreased in the presence of sodium thiosulfate [36]. The addition of sodium thiosulfate to cisplatin-containing regimens has reduced the incidence of nephrotoxicity and allows for higher doses of cisplatin to be administered. Without sodium thiosulfate, a dose of cisplatin 90 mg/m^2 produces nephrotoxicity, but with the addition of sodium thiosulfate, the dose of cisplatin can be escalated to 270 mg/m^2 without evidence of nephro- or myelotoxicity [37]. Sodium thiosulfate may also reduce ototoxicity. The incidence of either tinnitus or hearing loss in a large Southwest Oncology Group study was 12% in the group receiving IP cisplatin (vs. 29% in the IV group), in the absence of sodium thiosulfate [21]. A more recent review of patients undergoing HIPEC with cisplatin, who also received IV sodium thiosulfate, found no significant change in hearing sensitivity on audiometric testing [38]. While systemic exposure to cisplatin is limited with IP therapy, the sodium thiosulfate provides further protection for patients receiving cisplatin and should be incorporated into the treatment regimen.

Patients should have a daily complete blood count checked after HIPEC, until the counts are rising or stable for several days or for the first week after surgery. Neutropenia can develop between days 5 and 14 postoperatively and thrombocytopenia between days 7 and 11 [4]. Each center has their own criteria, but using the National Cancer Institute guidelines (Table 27.1), G-CSF can be started if the white blood cells count drops below 3000/mm^3, or if the absolute neutrophil count drops below 1000/mm^3, for grade 2 and grade 3 complications, respectively. Isolated thrombocytopenia is usually well tolerated, and in the absence of active bleeding or other complications, the platelet count will correct itself. Another factor that is not entirely within the surgeon's control but is worth noting is that grade 4 hematologic complications may be related to the duration of surgery. The duration of surgery is related to the severity of disease, usually measured with the peritoneal cancer index

Table 27.4 Toxicity profile of common IP chemotherapy agents

Agent	Hematologic	GI	Renal	Metabolic	Pain
Mitomycin C	X	X	X		
Oxaliplatin	X	X		X	
Cisplatin	X	X	X		X
5-Fluorouracil	X				X
Doxorubicin	X				X
Irinotecan	X	X			
Paclitaxel	X				X

(PCI) developed by Sugarbaker. Elias et al. [39] found that in a group of patients who all received the same dose of chemotherapy by BSA, those patients who developed a grade 4 hematologic complication (or grade 3–4 for platelets) had a significantly longer operation and higher PCI than those who did not develop aplasia (537 vs. 444 minutes and 19.5 vs. 15.3, respectively). They did not find any relation to the duration of preoperative chemotherapy. While the duration of surgery is determined by the disease, we can anticipate hematologic toxicity in the setting of prolonged surgery.

Anemia is a complication related largely to intraoperative blood loss, as well as bone marrow suppression from chemotherapy. The management can be as straightforward as transfusing packed red blood cells to maintain an acceptable hemoglobin level, but there are some longer-term issues to consider. There is a significant body of literature examining the impact of blood transfusion on cancer recurrence rates, particularly in the colorectal literature. A Cochrane Review of perioperative blood transfusion in patients undergoing curative resection of colorectal cancer (T1-3a/N0-1/M0) found 36 studies with 12,127 patients and determined that there is a negative effect of transfusion on recurrence rates, with an OR of 1.42 (95% CI 1.2–1.67) [40]. The data regarding blood transfusion in patients undergoing resection of hepatic metastasis of colorectal cancer are less decisive, although the study with the largest number of patients (1351) found a worse survival in patients receiving perioperative blood transfusion [41]. In the HIPEC literature, blood loss is reported more commonly than blood transfusion, and both vary widely. It is safe to estimate that at least one half of patients undergoing CRS/HIPEC will receive a perioperative blood transfusion. In this patient population with peritoneal metastasis and significant rates of blood transfusion, we have achieved significant survival gains. The immediate requirements of replacing operative blood loss and managing acute bone marrow suppression take precedence over longer-term concerns, and in the absence of any data in these patients, we can only speculate about the impact of blood transfusion on recurrence rates.

For less acute anemia, an erythropoietin-stimulating agent (ESA) can be considered. The use of ESAs in general has reduced the need for blood transfusion and has been associated with improvement in fatigue in patients with cancer. Early labeling of ESAs allowed for the initiation of treatment if the hemoglobin level was less than 11 g/dL. However, reports emerged that the use of ESAs may compromise outcome, with increased disease progression and worse survival. Some of these trials used ESAs to achieve hemoglobin levels over 12 g/dL, for a theoretical treatment benefit. The most recent meta-analysis included 60 studies with 15,323 patients and evaluated the impact of ESA use on survival, disease progression, and risk of venous thromboembolism (VTE). Studies included in the meta-analysis were randomized controlled trials of patients with cancer who received ESA and blood transfusion compared to no ESA (blood transfusion or supportive care only). The ESAs had a non-significant effect on mortality and disease progression but

posed a significant risk for VTE with an OR of 1.48 (95% CI 1.28–1.72) [42]. The current indications for ESAs approved by the Food and Drug Administration (FDA) state that therapy should be initiated in cancer patients if the hemoglobin is less than 10 g/dL and at least 2 additional months of chemotherapy are planned. Other than a dosing regimen, no recommendations are made for surgical patients. The boxed warning states that ESAs will shorten overall survival and increase the risk of recurrence in patients with breast, non–small cell lung, head and neck, lymphoid, and cervical cancers, but the supporting studies all targeted hemoglobin levels of 12–15 g/dL. Unfortunately, due to these concerns, prescribing physicians must now enroll in a program with the FDA in order to prescribe these drugs.

Besides the obvious rationale for preventing complications, there are longer-term implications of postoperative complications. Patients who have grade 3 or 4 complications have a shorter disease-free and overall survival. Major complications are associated with a PCI of >20, but the decreased survival occurs independent of PCI [43,44]. As high as the complication rates are, several centers with longer experience have found that their outcomes improve over time, with fewer complications, higher rates of complete cytoreduction, and longer patient survival [43,45]. Levine et al. found that their median survival times ranged from 16.4 to 40.7 months depending on the experience quintile [43]. The estimated learning curve for this procedure is about 100 cases, ranging from 50 to 140. Some of the learning curve is technical, but a significant part of the curve revolves around patient selection. The selection of patients who are good candidates for this procedure rests on the shoulders of the surgeon but involves a learning curve for referring physicians as well. This requires both buy-in and proper assessment of potential candidates, with timely referral to a specialty center.

CRS and IP chemotherapy has brought hope and longer survival to a group of patients previously thought untreatable. It is a demanding procedure, and significant time is spent planning before the patient comes to the operating room. Many factors play a role in patient outcome, and great attention to detail is of paramount importance. Successful centers will have a dedicated team of surgeons, anesthesiologists, oncologists, nurses, pharmacists, and perfusionists who do these procedures on a regular basis and are familiar with the potential consequences of this treatment.

ACKNOWLEDGMENT

Many thanks to Kim Walker for her invaluable assistance with the preparation of this chapter.

REFERENCES

1. Glehen O, Osinsky D, Cotte E, Kwiatkowski F, Freyer G, Isaac S et al. Intraperitoneal chemohyperthermia using a closed abdominal procedure and cytoreductive surgery for the treatment of peritoneal

carcinomatosis: Morbidity and mortality analysis of 216 consecutive procedures. *Annals of Surgical Oncology.* 2003;10(8):863–869.

2. Kuzu MA, Koksoy C, Kale T, Demirpence E, Renda N. Experimental study of the effect of preoperative 5-fluorouracil on the integrity of colonic anastomoses. *The British Journal of Surgery* 1998;85(2):236–239.

3. Smeenk RM, Verwaal VJ, Zoetmulder FA. Toxicity and mortality of cytoreduction and intraoperative hyperthermic intraperitoneal chemotherapy in pseudomyxoma peritonei—A report of 103 procedures. *European Journal of Surgical Oncology.* 2006;32(2):186–190.

4. Schnake KJ, Sugarbaker PH, Yoo D. Neutropenia following perioperative intraperitoneal chemotherapy. *Tumori.* 1999;85(1):11–16.

5. Lambert LA, Armstrong TS, Lee JJ, Liu S, Katz MH, Eng C et al. Incidence, risk factors, and impact of severe neutropenia after hyperthermic intraperitoneal mitomycin C. *Annals of Surgical Oncology.* 2009;16(8):2181–2187.

6. Shimizu T, Maeta M, Koga S. Influence of local hyperthermia on the healing of small intestinal anastomoses in the rat. *The British Journal of Surgery.* 1991;78(1):57–59.

7. Hendricks T, Martens MF, Huyben CM, Wobbes T. Inhibition of basal and TGF beta-induced fibroblast collagen synthesis by antineoplastic agents. Implications for wound healing. *British Journal of Cancer.* 1993;67(3):545–550.

8. Makrin V, Lev-Chelouche D, Even Sapir E, Paran H, Rabau M, Gutman M. Intraperitoneal heated chemotherapy affects healing of experimental colonic anastomosis: An animal study. *Journal of Surgical Oncology.* 2005;89(1):18–22.

9. National Cancer Institute. Common terminology criteria for adverse events v4.0 (CTCAE). Bethesda, MD: National Institues of Health, 2009. p. 196.

10. Sugarbaker PH, Mora JT, Carmignani P, Stuart OA, Yoo D. Update on chemotherapeutic agents utilized for perioperative intraperitoneal chemotherapy. *The Oncologist.* 2005;10(2):112–122.

11. Tuttle TM, Zhang Y, Greeno E, Knutsen A. Toxicity and quality of life after cytoreductive surgery plus hyperthermic intraperitoneal chemotherapy. *Annals of Surgical Oncology.* 2006;13(12):1627–1632.

12. Wagner PL, Austin F, Maduekwe U, Mavanur A, Ramalingam L, Jones HL et al. Extensive cytoreductive surgery for appendiceal carcinomatosis: Morbidity, mortality, and survival. *Annals of Surgical Oncology.* 2013;20(4):1056–1062.

13. De Somer F, Ceelen W, Delanghe J, De Smet D, Vanackere M, Pattyn P et al. Severe hyponatremia, hyperglycemia, and hyperlactatemia are associated with intraoperative hyperthermic intraperitoneal chemoperfusion with oxaliplatin. *Peritoneal Dialysis International.* 2008;28(1):61–66.

14. Hillier TA, Abbott RD, Barrett EJ. Hyponatremia: Evaluating the correction factor for hyperglycemia. *The American Journal of Medicine.* 1999;106(4):399–403.

15. Rueth NM, Murray SE, Huddleston SJ, Abbott AM, Greeno EW, Kirstein MN et al. Severe electrolyte disturbances after hyperthermic intraperitoneal chemotherapy: Oxaliplatin versus mitomycin C. *Annals of Surgical Oncology.* 2011;18(1):174–180.

16. Ceelen WP, Peeters M, Houtmeyers P, Breusegem C, De Somer F, Pattyn P. Safety and efficacy of hyperthermic intraperitoneal chemoperfusion with high-dose oxaliplatin in patients with peritoneal carcinomatosis. *Annals of Surgical Oncology.* 2008;15(2):535–541.

17. Elias D, Sideris L, Pocard M, Ede C, Ben Hassouna D, Ducreux M et al. Efficacy of intraperitoneal chemohyperthermia with oxaliplatin in colorectal peritoneal carcinomatosis. Preliminary results in 24 patients. *Annals of Oncology.* 2004;15(5):781–785.

18. Votanopoulos K, Ihemelandu C, Shen P, Stewart J, Russell G, Levine EA. A comparison of hematologic toxicity profiles after heated intraperitoneal chemotherapy with oxaliplatin and mitomycin C. *The Journal of Surgical Research.* 2013;179(1):e133–e139.

19. Kusamura S, Younan R, Baratti D, Costanzo P, Favaro M, Gavazzi C et al. Cytoreductive surgery followed by intraperitoneal hyperthermic perfusion: Analysis of morbidity and mortality in 209 peritoneal surface malignancies treated with closed abdomen technique. *Cancer.* 2006;106(5):1144–1153.

20. Kusamura S, Baratti D, Antonucci A, Younan R, Laterza B, Oliva GD et al. Incidence of postoperative pancreatic fistula and hyperamylasemia after cytoreductive surgery and hyperthermic intraperitoneal chemotherapy. *Annals of Surgical Oncology.* 2007;14(12):3443–3452.

21. Alberts DS, Liu PY, Hannigan EV, O'Toole R, Williams SD, Young JA et al. Intraperitoneal cisplatin plus intravenous cyclophosphamide versus intravenous cisplatin plus intravenous cyclophosphamide for stage III ovarian cancer. *The New England Journal of Medicine.* 1996;335(26):1950–1955.

22. Markman M, Bundy BN, Alberts DS, Fowler JM, Clark-Pearson DL, Carson LF et al. Phase III trial of standard-dose intravenous cisplatin plus paclitaxel versus moderately high-dose carboplatin followed by intravenous paclitaxel and intraperitoneal cisplatin in small-volume stage III ovarian carcinoma: An intergroup study of the Gynecologic Oncology Group, Southwestern Oncology Group, and Eastern Cooperative Oncology Group. *Journal of Clinical Oncology.* 2001;19(4):1001–1007.

23. Walker JL, Armstrong DK, Huang HQ, Fowler J, Webster K, Burger RA et al. Intraperitoneal catheter outcomes in a phase III trial of intravenous versus intraperitoneal chemotherapy in optimal

stage III ovarian and primary peritoneal cancer: A Gynecologic Oncology Group Study. *Gynecologic Oncology*. 2006;100(1):27–32.

24. Armstrong DK, Bundy B, Wenzel L, Huang HQ, Baergen R, Lele S et al. Intraperitoneal cisplatin and paclitaxel in ovarian cancer. *The New England Journal of Medicine*. 2006;354(1):34–43.

25. Zeamari S, Floot B, van der Vange N, Stewart FA. Pharmacokinetics and pharmacodynamics of cisplatin after intraoperative hyperthermic intraperitoneal chemoperdusion (HIPEC). *Anticancer Research*. 2003;23(2B):1643–1648.

26. Baratti D, Kusamura S, Cabras AD, Bertulli R, Hutanu I, Deraco M. Diffuse malignant peritoneal mesothelioma: Long-term survival with complete cytoreductive surgery followed by hyperthermic intraperitoneal chemotherapy (HIPEC). *European Journal of Cancer*. 2013;49(15):3140–3148.

27. Gianola FJ, Sugarbaker PH, Barofsky I, White DE, Meyers CE. Toxicity studies of adjuvant intravenous versus intraperitoneal 5-FU in patients with advanced primary colon or rectal cancer. *American Journal of Clinical Oncology*. 1986;9(5):403–410.

28. Shimizu T, Murata S, Sonoda H, Mekata E, Ohta H, Takebayashi K et al. Hyperthermic intraperitoneal chemotherapy with mitomycin C and 5-fluorouracil in patients at high risk of peritoneal metastasis from colorectal cancer: A preliminary clinical study. *Molecular Clinical Oncology*. 2014;2(3):399–404.

29. Ozols RF, Young RC, Speyer JL, Sugarbaker PH, Greene R, Jenkins J et al. Phase I and pharmacological studies of adriamycin administered intraperitoneally to patients with ovarian cancer. *Cancer Research*. 1982;42(10):4265–4269.

30. Elias D, Matsuhisa T, Sideris L, Liberale G, Drouard-Troalen L, Raynard B et al. Heated intra-operative intraperitoneal oxaliplatin plus irinotecan after complete resection of peritoneal carcinomatosis: Pharmacokinetics, tissue distribution and tolerance. *Annals of Oncology*. 2004;15(10):1558–1565.

31. Quenet F, Goere D, Mehta SS, Roca L, Dumont F, Hessissen M et al. Results of two bi-institutional prospective studies using intraperitoneal oxaliplatin with or without irinotecan during HIPEC after cytoreductive surgery for colorectal carcinomatosis. *Annals of Surgery*. 2011;254(2):294–301.

32. Elias D, Goere D, Blot F, Billard V, Pocard M, Kohneh-Shahri N et al. Optimization of hyperthermic intraperitoneal chemotherapy with oxaliplatin plus irinotecan at 43 degrees C after compete cytoreductive surgery: Mortality and morbidity in 106 consecutive patients. *Annals of Surgical Oncology*. 2007;14(6):1818–2184.

33. Glockzin G, von Breitenbuch P, Schlitt HJ, Piso P. Treatment-related morbidity and toxicity of CRS and oxaliplatin-based HIPEC compared to a mitomycin and doxorubicin-based HIPEC protocol in patients with peritoneal carcinomatosis: A matched-pair analysis. *Journal of Surgical Oncology*. 2013;107(6):574–578.

34. Cotte E, Passot G, Tod M, Bakrin N, Gilly FN, Steghens A et al. Closed abdomen hyperthermic intraperitoneal chemotherapy with irinotecan and mitomycin C: A phase I study. *Annals of Surgical Oncology*. 2011;18(9):2599–2603.

35. Munoz-Casares FC, Rufian S, Arjona-Sanchez A, Rubio MJ, Diaz R, Casado A et al. Neoadjuvant intraperitoneal chemotherapy with paclitaxel for the radical surgical treatment of peritoneal carcinomatosis in ovarian cancer: A prospective pilot study. *Cancer Chemotherapy and Pharmacology*. 2011;68(1):267–274.

36. Nagai N, Hotta K, Yamamura H, Ogata H. Effects of sodium thiosulfate on the pharmacokinetics of unchanged cisplatin and on the distribution of platinum species in rat kidney: Protective mechanism against cisplatin nephrotoxicity. *Cancer Chemotherapy and Pharmacology*. 1995;36(5):404–410.

37. Howell SB, Pfeifle CL, Wung WE, Olshen RA, Lucas WE, Yon JL et al. Intraperitoneal cisplatin with systemic thiosulfate protection. *Annals of Internal Medicine*. 1982;97(6):845–851.

38. Womack AM, Hayes-Jordan A, Pratihar R, Barringer DA, Hall JH, Jr., Gidley PW et al. Evaluation of ototoxicity in patients treated with Hyperthermic Intraperitoneal Chemotherapy (HIPEC) with cisplatin and sodium thiosulfate. *Ear and Hearing*. November–December 2014;35(6):e243–e247.

39. Elias D, Raynard B, Boige V, Laplanche A, Estphan G, Malka D et al. Impact of the extent and duration of cytoreductive surgery on postoperative hematological toxicity after intraperitoneal chemohyperthermia for peritoneal carcinomatosis. *Journal of Surgical Oncology*. 2005;90(4):220–225.

40. Amato A, Pescatori M. Perioperative blood transfusions for the recurrence of colorectal cancer. *The Cochrane Database of Systematic Reviews*. 2006;CD005033.

41. Kooby DA, Stockman J, Ben-Porat L, Gonen M, Jarnagin WR, Dematteo RP et al. Influence of transfusions on perioperative and long-term outcome in patients following hepatic resection for colorectal metastases. *Annals of Surgery*. 2003;237(6):860–869.

42. Glaspy J, Crawford J, Vansteenkiste J, Henry D, Rao S, Bowers P et al. Erythropoiesis-stimulating agents in oncology: A study-level meta-analysis of survival and other safety outcomes. *British Journal of Cancer*. 2010;102(2):301–315.

43. Levine EA, Stewart JH 4th, Shen P, Russell GB, Loggie BL, Votanopoulos KI. Intraperitoneal chemotherapy for peritoneal surface malignancy: Experience with 1,000 patients. *Journal of the American College of Surgeons*. 2014;218(4):573–585.

44. Baratti D, Kusamura S, Iusco D, Bonomi S, Grassi A, Virzi S et al. Postoperative complications after cytoreductive surgery and hyperthermic intraperitoneal chemotherapy affect long-term outcome of patients with peritoneal metastases from colorectal cancer: A two-center study of 101 patients. *Diseases of the Colon and Rectum.* 2014;57(7):858–868.

45. Chua TC, Yan TD, Saxena A, Morris DL. Should the treatment of peritoneal carcinomatosis by cytoductive surgery and hyperthermic intraperitoneal chemotherapy still be regarded as a highly morbid procedure?. *Annals of Surgery.* 2009;249(6):900–907.

46. Loggie BW, Fleming RA, McQuellon RP, Russell GB, Geisinger KR. Cytoreductive surgery with intraperitoneal hyperthermic chemotherapy for disseminated peritoneal cancer of gastrointestinal origin. *The American Surgeon.* 2000;66(6):561–568.

47. Verwaal VJ, van Ruth S, de Bree E, van Sloothen GW, van Tinteren H, Boot H et al. Randomized trial of cytoreduction and hyperthermic intraperitoneal chemotherapy versus systemic chemotherapy and palliative surgery in patients with peritoneal carcinomatosis of colorectal cancer. *Journal of Clinical Oncology.* 2003;21(20):3737–3743.

48. Loungnarath R, Causeret S, Bossard N, Faheez M, Sayag-Beaujard AC, Brigand C et al. Cytoreductive surgery with intraperitoneal chemohyperthermia for the treatment of pseudomyxoma peritonei: A prospective study. *Diseases of the Colon and Rectum.* 2005;48(7):1372–1379.

49. Shen P, Levine EA, Hall J, Case D, Russell G, Fleming R et al. Factors predicting survival after intraperitoneal hyperthermic chemotherapy with mitomycin C after cytoreductive surgery for patients with peritoneal carcinomatosis. *Archives of Surgery.* 2003;138(1):26–33.

50. Elias D, Blot F, El Otmany A, Antoun S, Lasser P, Boige V et al. Curative treatment of peritoneal carcinomatosis arising from colorectal cancer by complete resection and intraperitoneal chemotherapy. *Cancer.* 2001;92(1):71–76.

51. Jacquet P, Stephens AD, Averbach AM, Chang D, Ettinghausen SE, Dalton RR et al. Analysis of morbidity and mortality in 60 patients with peritoneal carcinomatosis treated by cytoreductive surgery and heated intraoperative intraperitoneal chemotherapy. *Cancer.* 1996;77(12):2622–2629.

52. Facchiano E, Scaringi S, Kianmanesh R, Sabate JM, Castel B, Flamant Y et al. Laparoscopic hyperthermic intraperitoneal chemotherapy (HIPEC) for the treatment of malignant ascites secondary to unresectable peritoneal carcinomatosis from advanced gastric cancer. *European Journal of Surgical Oncology.* 2008;34(2):154–158.

53. Stephens AD, Alderman R, Chang D, Edwards GD, Esquivel J, Sebbag G et al. Morbidity and mortality analysis of 200 treatments with cytoreductive surgery and hyperthermic intraoperative intraperitoneal chemotherapy using the coliseum technique. *Annals of Surgical Oncology.* 1999;6(8):790–796.

54. Stewart JH 4th, Shen P, Russell G, Fenstermaker J, McWilliams L, Coldrun FM et al. A phase I trial of oxaliplatin for intraperitoneal hyperthermic chemoperfusion for the treatment of peritoneal surface dissemination from colorectal and appendiceal cancers. *Annals of Surgical Oncology.* 2008;15(8):2137–2145.

28

Safety considerations and occupational hazards

JOEL M. BAUMGARTNER, KAITLYN J. KELLY, AND ANDREW M. LOWY

INTRODUCTION

Cytoreductive surgery with intraperitoneal chemotherapy (IPC) is the best available therapy for eligible patients with peritoneal surface malignancy. Cytotoxic agents most commonly used for IPC are mitomycin C (MMC), cisplatin, oxaliplatin, and doxorubicin. As discussed in previous chapters, IPC can be administered in the form of hyperthermic intraperitoneal chemotherapy (HIPEC) or early postoperative intraperitoneal chemotherapy (EPIC). Currently, the majority of centers performing IPC do so in the form of HIPEC and thus that will be the focus of this chapter.

Despite the general consensus on the delivery of IPC in the form of HIPEC over EPIC, there remains considerable institutional variation in the technique of HIPEC in terms of agents used, concentration of agent in the perfusion solution, duration of perfusion, and open or closed administration. Regardless of these variations in technique, there is a large volume of data demonstrating improvements in recurrence-free and disease-specific survival for patients with peritoneal surface malignancy treated with cytoreduction and HIPEC compared to historical controls [1–4]. As a result, the application and availability of cytoreduction and HIPEC has rapidly expanded worldwide. This therapy is now available at specialized centers in Asia, Australia, nearly all countries in Europe, and throughout the United States [5].

Despite the large volume of data published on therapeutic efficacy and morbidity and mortality associated with this therapy for patients, there are very limited data available on the risks of occupational exposure to healthcare personnel involved in the preparation and administration of HIPEC and in postoperative care of patients who have received it. The aims of this chapter are to define the potential risks of exposure to agents commonly used for HIPEC, to summarize existing data on occupational exposure during HIPEC, and to propose concrete guidelines that should be followed at centers performing HIPEC to minimize the risks of exposure to healthcare personnel.

HEALTH RISKS OF EXPOSURE TO CYTOTOXIC DRUGS

Risks of occupational exposure to antineoplastic/cytotoxic drugs include both acute and chronic toxicities. Examples of acute toxicity include irritation of the skin, eyes, and mucus membranes, hair loss, dizziness, nausea, and vomiting [6–8]. These toxicities are obvious when they occur and are often the result of spillage of or direct handling of cytotoxic agents without personal protective equipment (PPE). The Globally Harmonized System (GHS) is an internationally agreed upon system for the classification and labeling of hazardous chemicals that was developed by the United Nations. The GHS describes acute toxicities associated with hazardous substances, defined as adverse effects following oral, dermal, or inhalational exposure [9]. Table 28.1 summarizes the GHS warnings for cytotoxic agents commonly used in HIPEC. In 1985, global standards for the handling of cytotoxic drugs were implemented [10–12]. Since that time, there are essentially no published reports in the literature of acute toxicities related to occupational exposure to cytotoxic agents.

Table 28.1 Summary of mechanism of action and hazard classifications of agents commonly used in HIPEC

Agent	Mechanism	IARC grouping[a]	GHS[b] warnings
Mitomycin C	DNA cross-linking	2B	Fatal if swallowed
			Causes serious eye and skin irritation
			May cause respiratory irritation/drowsiness/dizziness
			Suspected of causing cancer
Cis-/oxaliplatin	DNA cross-linking	2A	Fatal if swallowed
			Causes serious eye damage
			May cause allergic skin reaction
			May cause cancer
			May cause organ damage
Doxorubicin	DNA	2A	Harmful if swallowed
			May cause genetic defects
			May damage fertility or the unborn child
			May cause cancer

[a] International Agency for Research on Cancer: (1) human carcinogens, (2A) probable human carcinogens, (2B) possible human carcinogens.

[b] Globally Harmonized System.

Potential chronic toxicities are not as well characterized but include carcinogenesis, mutagenesis, and teratogenesis or other reproductive dysfunction. Chronic toxicities may be related to repeat low-level exposure to cytotoxic agents that occur despite the proper use of PPE and standard safety precautions [13].

Carcinogenesis

The International Agency for Research on Cancer (IARC) has created a classification system for antineoplastic drugs. Group 1 agents are "human carcinogens," Group 2A are "probable human carcinogens," and Group 2B are "possible human carcinogens" [14]. Alkylating agents are classified as IARC Group 1 and are the type of cytotoxic drug most strongly associated with carcinogenesis. These include cyclophosphamide, ifosfamide, melphalan, dacarbazine, and temozolomide, among others. These agents act by placing alkyl groups on DNA in place of hydrogen ions. DNA alkylation results in cross-linking. Cross-linked DNA cannot uncoil and separate so it cannot be transcribed and cannot replicate.

Platinum-based agents are IARC Group 2A and are considered "alkylating-like" agents in that they similarly cross-link DNA and halt replication, but they do not do so by alkylation. Platinum-based agents act by forming permanent covalent bonds between DNA strands. The resultant cross-linking leads to interruption of transcription and replication and, eventually, apoptosis. Cisplatin was the first platinum-based agent brought into clinical use. Carboplatin and oxaliplatin followed. Similar to alkylating agents, platinum-based drugs are not specific for cancer cells and also affect rapidly dividing normal cells.

MMC is a cytotoxic antibiotic derived from fungus that also acts by cross-linking DNA in yet a different mechanism than alkylating agents and platinum-based compounds. MMC is classified as IARC Group 2B. Doxorubicin is a type of anthracycline antibiotic. Doxorubicin acts by intercalating into DNA between base pairs that causes uncoiling of the helical structure. This results in inhibition of DNA synthesis and apoptosis of rapidly dividing cells. Doxorubicin is classified as IARC Group 2A.

The carcinogenic effects of these cytotoxic agents have been demonstrated primarily in patients receiving therapeutic doses and in animal studies [15–20]. Only two published reports describe associations between alkylating and alkylating-like agents and hematologic and other malignancies in exposed healthcare workers [11,21,22]. These studies focused on nurses and pharmacists. Both were retrospective, and no causative link between exposure to cytotoxic agents and development of malignancy was demonstrated.

Mutagenesis

While no studies have shown a direct link between occupational exposure to cytotoxic agents and the development of malignancy, multiple studies have documented the presence of DNA damage and mutagenesis in healthcare personnel exposed to antineoplastic agents, including those agents used for the delivery of HIPEC [23–30]. The most recent of these, by Villarini and colleagues, documented an increase in primary DNA damage in leukocytes of nurses and pharmacists exposed to cytotoxic agents compared to nonexposed controls who were similar for age, gender, and smoking habits [23]. In this study, DNA damage correlated with degree of exposure and use of PPE was found to be protective, but did not completely eliminate exposure. The subjects in this study were exposed to multiple cytotoxic agents including cisplatin, doxorubicin, and MMC. Based on the type of DNA aberrations detected, the authors theorized that cross-linking drugs were the likely cause.

The consequences of this low-level DNA damage are not currently known, but multiple assays have been developed, including those measuring direct DNA damage, sister chromatid exchanges, chromosomal-level aberrations, and micronuclei [31]. Several studies have proposed biomonitoring of healthcare personnel exposed to cytotoxic agents with assays that measure DNA damage to determine the long-term effect and potentially direct future healthcare surveillance [23,24].

Teratogenicity/spontaneous abortion

The majority of studies demonstrating associations between occupational exposure to cytotoxic drugs and congenital malformations, stillbirths, or spontaneous abortions included healthcare workers exposed prior to 1985 [22,32–35]. Only one published study included workers exposed after 1985, and this study did not demonstrate an association between exposure and spontaneous abortion [36]. A more recent meta-analysis of these and other studies showed a slight increased risk of spontaneous abortion (OR 1.46; 95% CI 1.11–1.92) in female healthcare workers exposed to cytotoxic drugs, but no increased risk of stillbirth or congenital malformation [11].

RISKS OF OCCUPATIONAL EXPOSURE IN HIPEC

Given the toxicity associated with antineoplastic drugs used for IPC, there is potential risk to hospital personnel involved with transporting, handling, and administering the drugs and to those staff involved in caring for patients who have received such therapies. Since HIPEC is delivered in the operating room, the risk is theoretically highest to operating room staff. It should be noted that personnel in the operating room are trained to safely work with multiple other potential occupational hazards, including volatile anesthetic gases, flammable substances, electrical cautery devices, and blood-borne pathogens. Many of the same procedures and precautions can be applied to IPC to reduce the risk of exposure. However, there are several additional safety protocols that may reduce this risk. Universal precautions should be used when handling the bodily fluids of patients treated with IPC, as they should when handling any patient's bodily fluids. All chemoperfusion tubing should be tightly connected to adaptors and cannulas to avoid leakage. Open abdomen HIPEC procedures should utilize a protective cover over the open abdomen and a smoke evacuator to minimize vaporized drug inhalation. Closed HIPEC procedures should close the skin at the wound edge and catheter sites in a watertight fashion to minimize spillage. The closure should be tested with perfusate for leaks prior to chemoperfusion. Surgeons, scrub nurses, and trainees administering HIPEC in an open or closed fashion should double-glove and use eye protection in addition to standard operating room apparel. Large spills should be cleaned up with appropriate spill kits and protocols [37].

Several studies investigating the risk to operating room staff with HIPEC have found negligible exposure when these standard precautions are taken (Table 28.2). These studies have examined several potential sources of exposure to IPC, including airborne contamination from drug vaporization, transdermal contamination from direct contact with the drug (typically by glove permeability), and equipment surface contamination. Other hypothetical exposure sources include accidental injection or ingestion, which are rare enough to not warrant further discussion or investigation. Most studies of chemotherapy exposure to operating room staff have been done in open abdomen HIPEC techniques. Theoretically, the closed technique may impart a lower risk of chemotherapy exposure given the drugs are contained within a closed abdomen and direct exposure to the surgeon's (gloved) hand is therefore minimized. Alternatively, the closed technique could impart a higher exposure risk due to lack of smoke evacuator usage (typically used in the open technique) and spillage of chemotherapy through the temporary skin closure.

Airborne contamination

Two observational studies of MMC delivered through the open abdomen technique revealed no detectable airborne drug [38,39]. One of these studies sampled air 5 and 35 cm from the wound edge using methanol extraction [39], but this technique has been criticized [40], prompting a second study that validated the result of undetectable vaporized MMC. One in vitro study modeling open chemoperfusion technique using oxaliplatin found no detectable vaporized platinum [41]. This finding has been validated by two observational studies, which found no or low levels of vaporized platinum from various locations in the operating room [42,43]. The single study that measured detectable levels of airborne platinum found no detectable levels 5 m from the surgical field but found levels at the anesthesiologists' and the scrub nurses' stations (0.014 and 0.050 ng/m^3, respectively) [43]. These levels are comparable to atmospheric levels detected in urban areas of developed countries from automobile exhaust and highlight the increased sensitivity of measurement techniques of vaporized platinum compared to MMC [44].

Transdermal contamination

Given the low risk of exposure to vaporized drug with intraperitoneal administration, a more likely source of contamination is through direct contact with the chemotherapeutic agent and transdermal absorption. This risk is theoretically highest for surgeons using the open abdomen technique of intraperitoneal chemoperfusion where the surgeon's gloved hand manipulates the viscera as it is bathed in chemotherapy. Most studies investigating the transdermal route of contamination have investigated glove permeability to the drug. One in vitro study found impermeability to 18 antineoplastic drugs with nitrile rubber, latex, polyurethane, and neoprene gloves

Table 28.2 Summary of HIPEC safety studies

Study	Year	Drug	HIPEC technique	Vaporized drug conc.	Glove permeability drug penetration	Blood/urine drug conc.
Stuart et al. [39]	2002	MMC	Open	<0.5 ng/mL	0.01–0.28 µg (single glove)	Urine, <25 ng/mL
Schmid et al. [38]	2006	MMC	Open	<10.3 ng/m³	1/40 breakthrough (double glove) with 160 µg MMC	Plasma <1 µg/L
Korinth et al. [46]	2007	MMC	In vitro		1/40 breakthrough (double glove) at 0.4 mg/mL MMC	
Guerbet et al. [41]	2007	Oxaliplatin	In vitro	<1000 ng/L		
Näslund Andréasson et al. [49]	2010	Oxaliplatin	Open			Blood, <0.05 nmol/L Urine, <0.01 µg/L
Konate et al. [43]	2011	Oxaliplatin	Open	0.014–0.05 ng/m³a	2.0–2.2 ng (surgeon's hand, double glove)b	Urine, <1.5 to <5 ng/L
Schierl et al. [47]	2012	Cisplatin, Oxaliplatin	Open and closed		0.02–15 ng (inner surface of inner glove, double glove)	
Caneparo et al. [42]	2014	Cisplatin	Open	<10 ng/m³	<1 ng (skin, double glove)	Urine, <1 µg/L

Abbreviation: MMC, mitomycin C.
a Similar to platinum levels in air in urban areas of developed countries.
b Similar to platinum levels in the general population.

in most, but not all, circumstances [45]. Another study found a 10-fold range of permeability of MMC with different (single) gloves [39], but two other studies found only rare (1/40 experiments) breakthrough of MMC through double natural latex gloves at concentrations 100 times that used during typical HIPEC [38,46]. Two observational studies of glove permeability with platinums (oxaliplatin and cisplatin) in open abdomen HIPEC technique have been performed [42,43]. Both of these studies found low platinum levels on the inner surgeon glove (20–83.2 ng) and no or very low (2.0–2.2 ng) detectable platinum on the surgeon's hand itself. One study investigating closed HIPEC technique found low levels (<1 ng) of platinum on the outer surface of the inner glove and very low levels (0.01–0.2 ng) on the inner surface [47].

Equipment surface contamination

HIPEC administration requires use of a perfusion machine, reservoir, tubing, catheters, and drug container in addition to typical operating room equipment (surgical instruments, table, drapes, etc.). All of these pieces of equipment can potentially be contaminated with chemotherapy during HIPEC and be a source for personnel contamination. Studies investigating surface contamination of equipment in the operative room have been done in the open abdomen

technique using oxaliplatin or cisplatin. These studies have revealed relatively high levels of detectable platinum on the patient's abdomen, surgical instruments, operating room floor, surgeon's shoes, and the perfusion machine and reservoir [43,47]. One of these studies found higher levels on the perfusion reservoir when syringes were used rather than infusion bags, prompting the authors to recommend against using syringes to add chemotherapy to the perfusate [47]. This study also found detectable levels on the perfusion machine before chemoperfusion, suggesting contamination during storage from a prior procedure, which may put unsuspecting operating room personnel at risk when machines may be handled without gloves in storage. However, the study also noted the HIPEC device wipe levels were generally lower than that on the floors of local chemotherapy processing pharmacies.

Measured contamination in operating room staff

The most direct method of assessing risk of IPC to operating room personnel is by measuring blood or urine chemotherapy levels directly. This is particularly important as studies of occupational safety with intravenous chemotherapy administration have found measurable levels of chemotherapy in pharmacy technicians and nurses who have not even directly handled the drugs [12]. Multiple studies have examined urine or blood levels of chemotherapy in operating room staff after HIPEC. One study using MMC in an open abdomen technique found no detectable drug levels in the surgeon or perfusionist [39]. Another study found undetectable plasma levels of MMC in the surgeon after open chemoperfusion technique [38]. Plasma detection of MMC is preferable to urine as renal excretion of intact drug is low in humans [48]. Three studies investigating oxaliplatin found no or insignificant urine levels in operating room staff [42,43,49]. All three studies were performed at centers using an open chemoperfusion technique. One study found no detectable urine or blood levels in the surgeon and perfusionist [49]. Another study comprehensively tested the urine pre- and post-HIPEC of surgeons, anesthesiologist, operating room nurse, anesthesia nurse, housekeeper, and the transporter of drug from the pharmacy and found detectable levels (pre- and post-HIPEC) in some individuals, but these levels were similar to urine platinum levels in the general population as result of environmental exposure [43].

Risks to hospital staff outside of the operating room

Although operating room staff have the highest exposure risk to IPC, hospital staff outside the OR may also be at risk. This includes personnel handling the drugs (pharmacists, pharmacy technicians, nurses, shipping and receiving personnel, etc.) and personnel handling potentially contaminated bodily fluids. There are standard guidelines for personnel preparing, transporting, administering, storing, and disposing chemotherapy drugs that should be followed. In addition, patients receiving HIPEC theoretically excrete chemotherapy postoperatively in bodily fluids, placing additional hospital staff potentially at risk of exposure. This risk has not been fully investigated. Hospitals have differing policies on treatment of HIPEC patient bodily fluids. General guidelines for handling chemotherapy drugs and bodily fluids contaminated by them have been published by several occupational safety organizations, and these are summarized in Table 28.3.

Table 28.3 Summary of safety regulations and guidelines for chemotherapy drugs

Occupational safety and health administration (OSHA) [37]

Drug preparation in restricted, centralized, signed area with biologic safety cabinets (BSC).

Drug preparation personal protective equipment (PPE): powderless latex gloves (double glove if it does not interfere with individual's technique), lint-free disposable gowns, BSC or NIOSH-approved respirator (not surgical mask), eye protection (if splash, spray, or aerosols are generated).

Drug administration PPE: latex gloves, gowns, chemical splash goggles, NIOSH-approved respirator if aerosolized drug.

Patient excreta (especially urine) should be treated as potentially contaminated for 48 hours and dealt with personnel using latex gloves and disposable gowns.

Waste should be disposed in leak-proof plastic bags that are a different color than normal hospital waste bags.

Medical surveillance of workers potentially exposed: before job placement, periodically during employment, following acute exposures, at the time of job termination or transfer.

Spill kits: chemical splash goggles, two pairs of gloves, utility gloves, low-permeability gown, two 12″ × 12″ sheets of absorbent material, 250 mL and 1 L spill control pillows, "sharps" container, small scoop, two large waste-disposal bags.

National institute for occupational safety and health (NIOSH) [51]

Chemotherapy gloves and eye projection should be used when opening chemotherapy containers, and chemotherapy gloves should be used when transporting chemotherapy vials.

BSC should be used when preparing chemotherapy, and double gloves (changed every 30 minutes) and nonlinting/nonabsorbent gowns should be used when reconstituting and admixing drugs.

Double gloves, goggles, and gowns should be used when administering chemotherapy.

Place chemotherapy administration and clean up waste and disposables in yellow chemotherapy bins.

Spills: have spill kits in immediate area, use trained workers for large spill cleanup, and surgical masks are not effective for aerosol protection.

Medical surveillance: provided through workplace or private healthcare provider, monitor for blood in urine.

Joint commission standards related to hazardous drug management [52]

Standard EC.02.02.01: The hospital manages risks related to hazardous materials and waste.

The hospital minimizes risks associated with selecting, handling, storing, transporting, using, and disposing of hazardous chemicals.

The hospital minimizes risks associated with disposing of hazardous medications.

For managing hazardous materials and waste, the hospital has the permits, licenses, manifests, and material safety data sheets required by law and regulation.

The hospital labels hazardous materials and waste. Labels identify the contents and hazard warnings.

SUMMARY AND CONCLUSIONS

Based on the studies investigating the safety of HIPEC to operating room staff, there appears to be little occupational hazard associated with HIPEC. No significant detectable levels of chemotherapy in operating room staff performing HIPEC have been found in blood or urine. There is also no significant detectable vaporized drug, even with the open chemoperfusion technique. There is significant surface contamination to the operating room itself and to multiple pieces of equipment used during HIPEC. This is a potential source of occupational exposure, particularly since there seems to be some permeability of gloves to various chemotherapeutics.

The risks of chronic low-dose exposure to chemotherapy are unknown, but a growing body of evidence suggests that this type of exposure does cause DNA damage in exposed individuals. Thus, several safety procedures and protocols are recommended. Routine use of PPE including double gloves, disposable gowns, and eyewear is recommended, even for the closed HIPEC technique. Other standard occupational safety procedures for general chemotherapy handling should be followed per published guidelines. Medical surveillance is an important safety measure to identify early toxicities from occupational chemotherapy exposure and should be implemented per the guidelines described. Pregnant or nursing women and individuals actively pursuing pregnancy (men and women) should take extra precautions or consider eliminating involvement with IPC altogether [50]. If these procedures are followed, in addition to education of personnel involved in HIPEC therapy and those staff caring for patients who have received HIPEC, it can be performed with minimal risk to hospital staff.

REFERENCES

1. Chua TC, Moran BJ, Sugarbaker PH, Levine EA, Glehen O, Gilly FN et al. Early- and long-term outcome data of patients with pseudomyxoma peritonei from appendiceal origin treated by a strategy of cytoreductive surgery and hyperthermic intraperitoneal chemotherapy. *Journal of Clinical Oncology: Official Journal of the American Society of Clinical Oncology.* 2012;30:2449–2456.

2. Glehen O, Gilly FN, Boutitie F, Bereder JM, Quenet F, Sideris L et al. Toward curative treatment of peritoneal carcinomatosis from nonovarian origin by cytoreductive surgery combined with perioperative intraperitoneal chemotherapy: A multi-institutional study of 1,290 patients. *Cancer.* 2010;116:5608–5618.

3. Kuijpers AM, Mirck B, Aalbers AG, Nienjuijs SW, de Hingh IH, Wiezer MJ et al. Cytoreduction and HIPEC in the Netherlands: Nationwide long-term outcome following the Dutch protocol. *Annals of Surgical Oncology.* 2013;20:4224–4230.

4. Levine EA, Stewart JH 4th, Shen P, Russell GB, Loggie BL, Votanopoulos KI. Intraperitoneal chemotherapy for peritoneal surface malignancy: Experience with 1,000 patients. *Journal of the American College of Surgeons.* 2014;218:573–585.

5. Baratti D, Kusamura S, Deraco M. The Fifth International Workshop on Peritoneal Surface Malignancy (Milan, Italy, December 4–6, 2006): Methodology of disease-specific consensus. *Journal of Surgical Oncology.* 2008;98:258–262.

6. Pethran A, Schierl R, Hauff K, Grimm CH, Boos KS, Nowak D. Uptake of antineoplastic agents in pharmacy and hospital personnel. Part I: Monitoring of urinary concentrations. *International Archives of Occupational and Environmental Health.* 2003;76:5–10.

7. Valanis BG, Vollmer WM, Labuhn KT, Glass AG. Acute symptoms associated with antineoplastic drug handling among nurses. *Cancer Nursing.* 1993;16:288–295.

8. Valanis BG, Vollmer WM, Labuhn KT, Glass AG. Association of antineoplastic drug handling with acute adverse effects in pharmacy personnel. *American Journal of Hospital Pharmacy.* 1993;50:455–462.

9. UN. (2013). Globally Harmonized System of Classification and Labelling of Chemicals (GHS). Fifth revised edition. United Nations, New York and Geneva.

10. Connor TH, Anderson RW, Sessink PJ, Broadfield L, Power LA. Surface contamination with antineoplastic agents in six cancer treatment centers in Canada and the United States. *American Journal of Health-System Pharmacy (AJHP): Official Journal of the American Society of Health-System Pharmacists.* 1999;56:1427–1432.

11. Dranitsaris G, Johnston M, Poirier S, Schueller T, Milliken D, Green E et al. Are health care providers who work with cancer drugs at an increased risk for toxic events? A systematic review and meta-analysis of the literature. *Journal of Oncology Pharmacy Practice: Official Publication of the International Society of Oncology Pharmacy Practitioners.* 2005;11:69–78.

12. Sessink PJ, Boer KA, Scheefhals AP, Anzion RB, Bos RP. Occupational exposure to antineoplastic agents at several departments in a hospital. Environmental contamination and excretion of cyclophosphamide and ifosfamide in urine of exposed workers. *International Archives of Occupational and Environmental Health.* 1992;64:105–112.

13. Schreiber C, Radon K, Pethran A, Schierl R, Hauff K, Grimm CH et al. Uptake of antineoplastic agents in pharmacy personnel. Part II: Study of

work-related risk factors. *International Archives of Occupational and Environmental Health.* 2003;76:11–16.

14. IARC, ed. *Some Antiviral and Antineoplastic Drugs, and Other Pharmaceutical Agents*, Lyon, France: IARC, 2000.

15. Penn I. Malignancies induced by drug therapy: A review. *IARC Scientific Publications.* 1986;(78):13–27.

16. Puri HC, Campbell RA. Cyclophosphamide and malignancy. *Lancet.* 1977;1:1306.

17. Reichert D, Spengler U, Romen W, Henschler D. Carcinogenicity of dichloroacetylene: An inhalation study. *Carcinogenesis.* 1984;5:1411–1420.

18. Reimer RR, Hoover R, Fraumeni JF, Jr., Young RC. Acute leukemia after alkylating-agent therapy of ovarian cancer. *The New England Journal of Medicine.* 1977;297:177–181.

19. Sonneveld P, Kurth KH, Hagemeyer A, Abels J. Secondary hematologic neoplasm after intravesical chemotherapy for superficial bladder carcinoma. *Cancer.* 1990;65:23–25.

20. Hansen RJ, Nagasubramanian R, Delaney SM, Samson LD, Dolan ME. Role of O^6-methylguanine-DNA methyltransferase in protecting from alkylating agent-induced toxicity and mutations in mice. *Carcinogenesis.* 2007;28:1111–1116.

21. Gunnarsdottir HK, Aspelund T, Karlsson T, Rafnsson VV. Occupational risk factors for breast cancer among nurses. *International Journal of Occupational and Environmental Health.* 1997;3:254–258.

22. Skov T, Maarup B, Olsen J, Rorth M, Winthereik H, Lynge E. Leukaemia and reproductive outcome among nurses handling antineoplastic drugs. *British Journal of Industrial Medicine.* 1992;49:855–861.

23. Villarini M, Dominici L, Piccinini R, Fatigoni C, Ambrogi M, Curti G et al. Assessment of primary, oxidative and excision repaired DNA damage in hospital personnel handling antineoplastic drugs. *Mutagenesis.* 2011;26:359–369.

24. Cornetta T, Padua L, Testa A, Levoli E, Festa F, Tranfo G et al. Molecular biomonitoring of a population of nurses handling antineoplastic drugs. *Mutation Research.* 2008;638:75–82.

25. Falck K, Grohn P, Sorsa M, Vainio H, Heinonen E, Holsti LR. Mutagenicity in urine of nurses handling cytostatic drugs. *Lancet.* 1979;1:1250–1251.

26. Kopjar N, Kasuba V, Rozgaj R, Zeljezic D, Milic M, Ramic S et al. The genotoxic risk in health care workers occupationally exposed to cytotoxic drugs—A comprehensive evaluation by the SCE assay. *Journal of Environmental Science and Health Part A, Toxic/Hazardous Substances & Environmental Engineering.* 2009;44:462–479.

27. Laffon B, Teixeira JP, Silva S, Loureiro J, Torres J, Pásaro E et al. Genotoxic effects in a population of nurses handling antineoplastic drugs, and relationship with genetic polymorphisms in DNA repair enzymes. *American Journal of Industrial Medicine.* 2005;48:128–136.

28. Rekhadevi PV, Sailaja N, Chandrasekhar M, Mahboob M, Rahman MF, Grover P. Genotoxicity assessment in oncology nurses handling anti-neoplastic drugs. *Mutagenesis.* 2007;22:395–401.

29. Rombaldi F, Cassini C, Salvador M, Saffi J, Erdtmann B. Occupational risk assessment of genotoxicity and oxidative stress in workers handling anti-neoplastic drugs during a working week. *Mutagenesis.* 2009;24:143–148.

30. Testa A, Giachelia M, Palma S, Appolloni M, Padua L, Tranfo G et al. Occupational exposure to antineoplastic agents induces a high level of chromosome damage. Lack of an effect of GST polymorphisms. *Toxicology and Applied Pharmacology.* 2007;223:46–55.

31. Turci R, Sottani C, Spagnoli G, Minoia C. Biological and environmental monitoring of hospital personnel exposed to antineoplastic agents: A review of analytical methods. *Journal of Chromatography B: Analytical Technologies in the Biomedical and Life Sciences.* 2003;789:169–209.

32. Hemminki K, Kyyronen P, Lindbohm ML. Spontaneous abortions and malformations in the offspring of nurses exposed to anaesthetic gases, cytostatic drugs, and other potential hazards in hospitals, based on registered information of outcome. *Journal of Epidemiology and Community Health.* 1985;39:141–147.

33. Selevan SG, Lindbohm ML, Hornung RW, Hemminki K. A study of occupational exposure to antineoplastic drugs and fetal loss in nurses. *The New England Journal of Medicine.* 1985;313:1173–1178.

34. Stucker I, Caillard JF, Collin R, Gout M, Poyen D, Hemon D. Risk of spontaneous abortion among nurses handling antineoplastic drugs. *Scandinavian Journal of Work, Environment & Health.* 1990;16:102–107.

35. Valanis B, Vollmer WM, Steele P. Occupational exposure to antineoplastic agents: Self-reported miscarriages and stillbirths among nurses and pharmacists. *Journal of Occupational and Environmental Medicine/American College of Occupational and Environmental Medicine.* 1999;41:632–638.

36. Peelen S, Roeleveld N, Heederik D, Krombout H, Kort W. *Toxic Effects on Reproduction in Hospital Personnel.* The Hague, the Netherlands: Dutch Ministry of Social Affairs and Employment, 1999.

37. Controlling Occupational Exposure to Hazardous Drugs. Occupational Safety & Health Administration Technical Manual (OTM). Section VI: Chapter 2, 1999. https://www.osha.gov/dts/osta/otm/otm_vi/otm_vi_2.html. Accessed June 16, 2015.

38. Schmid K, Boettcher MI, Pelz JO, Meyer T, Korinth G, Angerer J et al. Investigations on safety of hyperthermic intraoperative intraperitoneal chemotherapy (HIPEC) with Mitomycin C. *European Journal of Surgical Oncology: The Journal of the European Society of Surgical Oncology and the British Association of Surgical Oncology.* 2006;32:1222–1225.

39. Stuart OA, Stephens AD, Welch L, Sugarbaker PH. Safety monitoring of the coliseum technique for heated intraoperative intraperitoneal chemotherapy with mitomycin C. *Annals of Surgical Oncology.* 2002;9:186–191.

40. Connor TH, Van Balen P, Sessink PJ. Monitoring for hazardous drugs in the operating room. *Annals of Surgical Oncology.* 2003;10:821–822; reply 822–823.

41. Guerbet M, Goulle JP, Lubrano J. Evaluation of the risk of contamination of surgical personnel by vaporization of oxaliplatin during the intraoperative hyperthermic intraperitoneal chemotherapy (HIPEC). *European Journal of Surgical Oncology: The Journal of the European Society of Surgical Oncology and the British Association of Surgical Oncology.* 2007;33:623–626.

42. Caneparo A, Massucco P, Vaira M, Maina G, Giovale E, Coggiola M et al. Contamination risk for operators performing semi-closed HIPEC procedure using cisplatin. *European Journal of Surgical Oncology: The Journal of the European Society of Surgical Oncology and the British Association of Surgical Oncology.* 2014;40:925–929.

43. Konate A, Poupon J, Villa A, Garnier R, Hasni-Pichard H, Mezzaroba D et al. Evaluation of environmental contamination by platinum and exposure risks for healthcare workers during a heated intraperitoneal perioperative chemotherapy (HIPEC) procedure. *Journal of Surgical Oncology.* 2011;103:6–9.

44. Kiilunen M, Aitio A. Platinum. In: Nordberg GF, Fowler BA, Nordberg M, Friberg LT, eds., *Handbook on the Toxicology of Metals*, 3rd edn., Amsterdam, the Netherlands: Elsevier, 2007. pp. 769–782.

45. Connor TH. Permeability of nitrile rubber, latex, polyurethane, and neoprene gloves to 18 antineoplastic drugs. *American Journal of Health-System Pharmacy (AJHP): Official Journal of the American Society of Health-System Pharmacists.* 1999;56:2450–2453.

46. Korinth G, Schmid K, Midasch O, Boettcher MI, Angerer J, Drexler H. Investigations on permeation of mitomycin C through double layers of natural rubber gloves. *The Annals of Occupational Hygiene.* 2007;51:593–600.

47. Schierl R, Novotna J, Piso P, Bohlandt A, Nowak D. Low surface contamination by cis/oxaliplatin during hyperthermic intraperitoneal chemotherapy (HIPEC). *European Journal of Surgical Oncology: The Journal of the European Society of Surgical Oncology and the British Association of Surgical Oncology.* 2012;38:88–94.

48. Sugarbaker PH, Mora JT, Carmignani P, Stuart OA, Yoo D. Update on chemotherapeutic agents utilized for perioperative intraperitoneal chemotherapy. *The Oncologist.* 2005;10:112–122.

49. Naslund Andreasson S, Anundi H, Thoren SB, Ehrsson H, Mahteme H. Is platinum present in blood and urine from treatment givers during hyperthermic intraperitoneal chemotherapy? *Journal of Oncology.* 2010;2010:649719.

50. Gonzalez-Moreno S, Gonzalez-Bayon L, Ortega-Perez G. Hyperthermic intraperitoneal chemotherapy: Methodology and safety considerations. *Surgical Oncology Clinics of North America.* 2012;21:543–557.

51. *Preventing Occupational Exposures to Antineoplastic and Other Hazardous Drugs in Health Care Settings,* Cincinnati, OH: NOISH, 2004.

52. *2014 Comprehensive Accreditation Manual for Hospitals,* Oakbrook Terrace, IL: The Joint Commission, 2014.

29

Role of CRS/HIPEC in the management of malignant ascites

KONSTANTINOS I. VOTANOPOULOS

INTRODUCTION

Malignant ascites is a dreaded complication of advanced abdominal cancer. Malignant ascites occurs when extensive peritoneal surface involvement has overwhelmed the ability of the peritoneum to properly absorb and redistribute the normally continuously produced peritoneal fluid. This protein-rich fluid will continue to increase in volume until the intra-abdominal pressure reaches a level high enough to deter further ascites production. Malignant ascites is a sign of late stages of disease, and therapeutic interventions are limited. Life expectancy is measured in weeks to a few months [1,2], with the only exception being patients with mucinous ascites from low-grade appendiceal (LGA) primaries. Medical therapy with diuretics is ineffective. Chemotherapy is usually administered with palliative intent and can result in a modest increase in life expectancy of up to 4–5 months, depending on the type of primary [3–5]. Delivery of chemotherapy to a patient with an inability to thrive due to mechanical pressure, often requires symptom control through either multiple paracenteses or placement of a peritoneal catheter for drainage. In our experience, the effects of both paracentesis and peritoneal catheters improve distension and dyspnea, at the expense of significant protein loss, fluid shifts, and infection. The effects are short lived as the ascites quickly reaccumulates, and cognitive and emotional quality of life continue to decline. Overall, current treatment options for patients with malignant ascites are limited to palliation [6,7]. Laparoscopic hyperthermic intraperitoneal chemotherapy (HIPEC) without cytoreductive surgery (CRS) can offer a palliative improvement by decreasing ascites, but it leaves the tumor burden unaddressed [8–10]. CRS followed by HIPEC addresses tumor burden, but recovery takes up to 3–6 months. Therefore, properly selecting patients with ascites for operative intervention is a fine balance between morbidity and quality of life. The following chapter presents a practical clinical approach for the surgical oncologist, of how to select patients with peritoneal disease and ascites for CRS/HIPEC or HIPEC alone.

PREOPERATIVE SELECTION ALGORITHM

All potential CRS/HIPEC patients are given a complete history and physical examination, preoperative tumor markers, and a CT scan of the chest, abdomen, and pelvis with IV contrast. Minimum eligibility criteria for CRS/HIPEC also include histologic or cytologic diagnosis of peritoneal carcinomatosis, resectable or resected primary lesion, debulkable peritoneal disease, absence of extra-abdominal disease, and complete recovery from previous radiation or chemotherapy treatments with an Eastern Cooperative Oncology Group functional status not higher than 2. CRS/HIPEC is performed with the closed technique. R0 and R1 resections are grouped together as complete cytoreductions, while those with residual macroscopic disease are characterized as R2 and are subdivided based on the size of residual disease (R2a ≤ 5 mm, R2b > 0.5 cm and ≤ 2 cm, R2c > 2 cm).

The selection of patients with ascites, however, must be even more stringent. Ascites indicates advanced disease, with a low chance of achieving a complete cytoreduction. Even though HIPEC without CRS can control ascites more than 90% of the time, without complete CRS, no patient with primary other than LGA will achieve long-term survival [11]. In order to determine which patients with ascites have higher chances to achieve a complete CRS, we have developed a scoring system. The ascites score (AS) is based on retrospective analysis of prior CRS procedures done at our institution over the past 20 years.

The AS is calculated by grading a preoperatively obtained CT of the abdomen and pelvis with the patient in supine

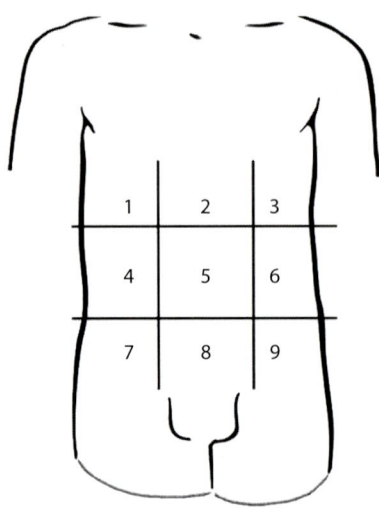

Figure 29.1 Abdominal regions used in the Ascites score calculation.

position. The abdominal cavity is divided into nine regions, similar to those used in calculating the peritoneal carcinomatosis index (except that the small bowel did not comprise of additional four regions). Each time ascites is present within a particular region, one point is assigned. Thus, preoperative ascites is graded on a scale ranging from 0 to 9, with 0 indicating the absence of ascites (Figure 29.1).

Our data indicated that patients with an AS greater than or equal to 4, regardless of primary, have no more than a 10% chance of complete CRS, while patients with an AS less than 4 have a 38% chance of an R0/R1 complete macroscopic CRS [11]. In order to identify and select this 38%, we prefer to treat non-LGA patients with AS < 4, either with upfront chemotherapy or staging laparoscopy followed by CRS/HIPEC, depending on the distribution and volume of peritoneal disease. In cases of AS ≥ 4, we routinely offer upfront chemotherapy with reevaluation post completion and repeat imaging (Scheme 29.1). We definitely do not recommend

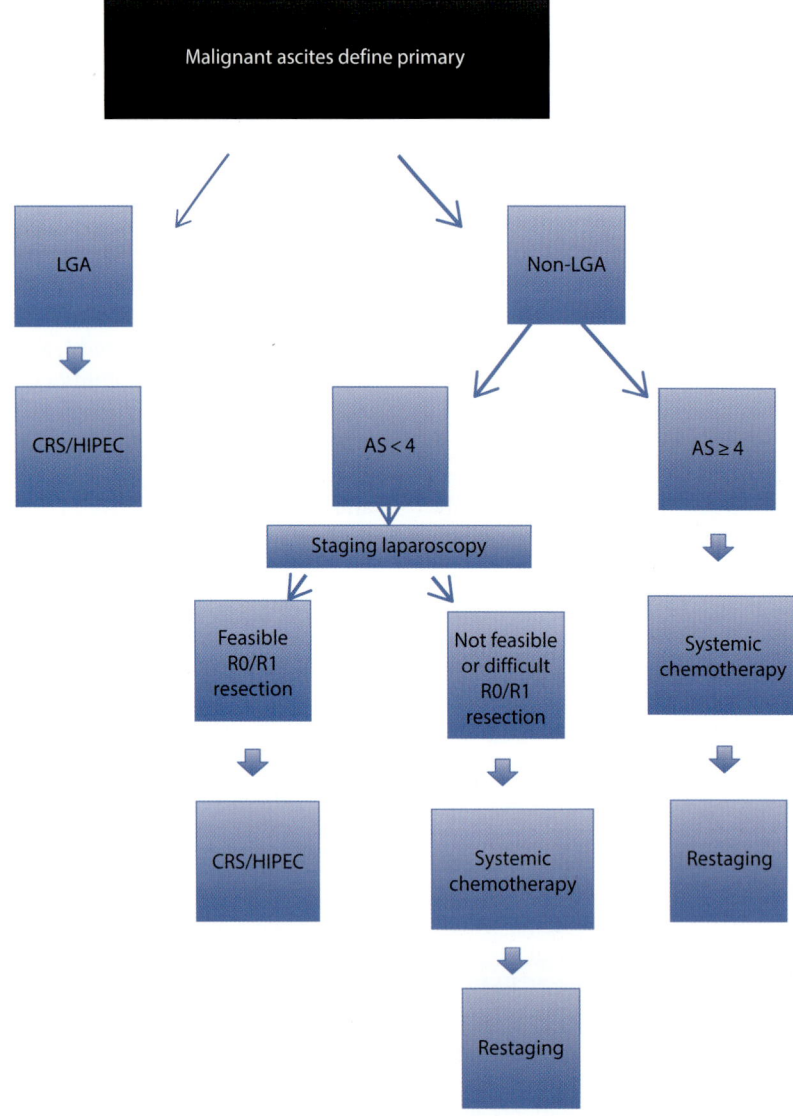

Scheme 29.1 Treatment algorithm of malignant ascites patients. LGA—low grade appendiceal primary. AS—ascites score.

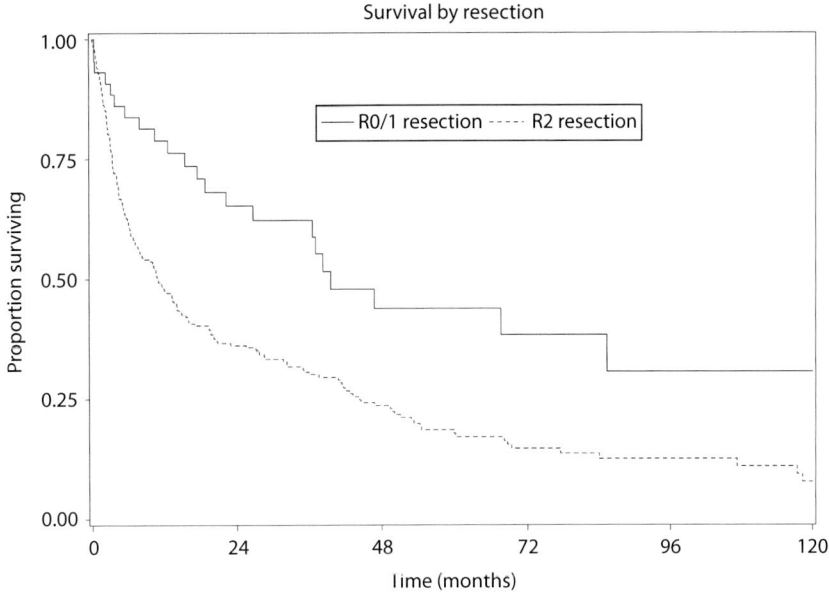

Figure 29.2 Survival based on type of resection in non-LGA patients with malignant ascites.

upfront CRS/HIPEC for AS ≥ 4 patients, given that the combination of incomplete CRS with a major complication can often result in a slow deterioration due to disease progression, without even the option of systemic chemotherapy being available.

In cases where a complete CRS is not feasible and ascites is interfering with quality of life, the patient will be treated with laparoscopic HIPEC with or without omentectomy, only for symptom control and without further organ resection. The default regimen that we currently use is mitomycin 40 mg (30 mg, followed by a 10 mg bolus at 1 hour) 120 minutes, heated at an inflow temperature of 42°C.

Given that not all ascites cases are the same, every effort to identify mucinous ascites from LGA primaries is of paramount importance. This can be accomplished with a combination of paracentesis for cytology, image-guided biopsies of index lesions, and diagnostic laparoscopy as a last resort. We do not routinely use the AS to decide which LGA primary will go for CRS/HIPEC, but we are still using it to provide the patient with a rough preoperative assessment of the chances to achieve a complete R0/R1 macroscopic CRS.

Patients with mucinous ascites from LGA primaries will be treated by exploratory laparotomy and cytoreduction regardless of volume of disease. The primary target is always a complete macroscopic CRS followed by HIPEC. In cases of incomplete macroscopic CRS, every effort is made to release the small bowel from implants that will potentially lead to future obstruction. In cases of more than 0.5 cm residual macroscopic disease, HIPEC is not usually delivered or given as a truncated session to control ascites. HIPEC will succeed ~90% in eliminating ascites within 3 months from the operation, but our experience is that for LGA-induced pseudomyxoma cases, the CRS itself without HIPEC may not be able to fully eliminate the production of ascites but will still decrease the volume of ascites to clinically asymptomatic levels in the majority

of patients. Therefore, HIPEC, in a physiologically marginal patient, may increase the morbidity of the procedure without necessarily providing a clinical benefit.

CONCLUSION

Malignant ascites is a sign of advanced disease and an indication of low chances to achieve a complete CRS. Non-LGA malignant ascites patients should be approached with a single question in mind: Is a complete cytoreduction feasible? In non-LGA patients with malignant ascites, incomplete macroscopic CRS offers no survival advantage and is also associated with a 3–6 months long deterioration in the quality of life, in a patient with equal or less life expectancy (Figure 29.2). Increased volume of disease in ascites patients requires extensive CRS, which is known to be associated with higher rates of incomplete cytoreduction and morbidity with associated loss of survival benefit [12–14]. Therefore, we propose that non-LGA ascites patients with AS < 4 be treated either with upfront chemotherapy or diagnostic laparoscopy, followed by possible CRS/HIPEC. In cases of AS ≥ 4, we routinely offer upfront chemotherapy with reevaluation post completion with repeat imaging. In cases where a complete CRS is not feasible and ascites is interfering with quality of life, laparoscopic HIPEC without debilitating incisions has a role of symptomatic control.

REFERENCES

1. Chu DZ, Lang NP, Thompson C, Osteen PK, and Westbrook KC. Peritoneal carcinomatosis in non-gynecologic malignancy. A prospective study of prognostic factors. *Cancer.* 1989;63:364–367.
2. Garrison RN, Kaelin LD, Galloway RH, and Heuser LS. Malignant ascites. Clinical and experimental observations. *Annals of Surgery.* 1986;203:644–651.

3. Oh SY, Kwon HC, Lee S, Lee DM, Yoo HS, Kim SH et al. A Phase II study of oxaliplatin with low-dose leucovorin and bolus and continuous infusion 5-fluorouracil (modified FOLFOX-4) for gastric cancer patients with malignant ascites. *Japan Journal of Clinical Oncology.* 2007;37:930–935.

4. Husain A, Bezjak A, Easson A. Malignant ascites symptom cluster in patients referred for paracentesis. *Annals of Surgical Oncology.* 2010;17:461–469.

5. Easson AM, Bezjak A, Ross S, and Wright JG. The ability of existing questionnaires to measure symptom change are paracentesis for symptomatic ascites. *Annals of Surgical Oncology.* 2007;14:2348–2357.

6. Adam RA, Adam YG. Malignant ascites: Past, present, and future. *Journal of the American College of Surgeons.* 2004;198:999–1011.

7. Sangisetty SL, Miner TJ. Malignant ascites: A review of prognostic factors, pathophysiology and therapeutic measures. *World Journal of Gastrointestinal Surgery.* 2012;4:87–95.

8. Valle M, Van der Speeten K, Garofalo A. Laparoscopic hyperthermic intraperitoneal peroperative chemotherapy (HIPEC) in the management of refractory malignant ascites: A multi-institutional retrospective analysis in 52 patients. *Journal of Surgical Oncology.* 2009;100:331–334.

9. Garofalo A, Valle M, Garcia J, and Sugarbaker PH. Laparoscopic intraperitoneal hyperthermic chemotherapy for palliation of debilitating malignant ascites. *European Journal of Surgical Oncology.* 2006;32:682–685.

10. Solass W, Giger-Pabst U, Zieren J, and Reymond MA. Pressurized intraperitoneal aerosol chemotherapy (PIPAC): Occupational health and safety aspects. *Annals of Surgical Oncology.* 2013;20:3504–3511.

11. Randle RW, Swett KR, Swords DS, Shen P, Stewart JH, Levine EA et al. Efficacy of cytoreductive surgery with hyperthermic intraperitoneal chemotherapy in the management of malignant ascites. *Annals of Surgical Oncology.* 2014;21: 1474–1479.

12. Ahmed S, Levine EA, Randle RW, Swett KR, Shen P, Stewart JH et al. Significance of diaphragmatic resections and thoracic chemoperfusion on outcomes of peritoneal surface disease treated with cytoreductive surgery (CRS) and hyperthermic intraperitoneal chemotherapy (HIPEC). *Annals of Surgical Oncology.* 2014;21:4226–4231.

13. Levine EA, Stewart JH, Shen P, Russell GB, Loggie BL, and Votanopoulos KI. Intraperitoneal chemotherapy for peritoneal surface malignancy: Experience with 1,000 patients. *Journal of the American College of Surgeons.* 2014;218:573–585.

14. Votanopoulos KI, Newman NA, Russell G, Ihemelandu C, Shen P, Stewart JH et al. Outcomes of Cytoreductive Surgery (CRS) with hyperthermic intraperitoneal chemotherapy (HIPEC) in patients older than 70 years; survival benefit at considerable morbidity and mortality. *Annals of Surgical Oncology.* 2013;20:3497–3503.

PART **6**

Novel and Experimental Approaches

30

Development of drug-loaded particles for intraperitoneal therapy

ZE LU, M. GUILLAUME WIENTJES, AND JESSIE L.-S. AU

ABBREVIATIONS

Cmax	Maximum concentration
CxT	Concentration–time product
EGFR	Epidermal growth factor receptor
IP	Intraperitoneal
MST	Median survival time
MTD	Maximally tolerated dose
NDDP	*cis-bis*-neodecanoato-*trans-R,R*-1,2-diaminocyclohexane platinum (II)
PBS	Phosphate-buffered saline
PLA	Poly(lactic acid)
PGA	Poly(glycolic acid)
PLGA	Poly(lactic-glycolic acid) copolymer
TPM	Tumor-penetrating microparticles

INTRODUCTION

Cancers originating from organs within the peritoneal cavity (pancreatic, ovarian, colorectal, gastric, liver) account for 250,000 new cases in the United States. Peritoneal metastases due to locoregional spread are common (e.g., 70% for ovarian, 50% for pancreatic, 32% for colon, ~20% for gastric) [1,2]. In the peritoneal cavity, tumors are disseminated by exfoliation of cells, which spread directly to pelvic and abdominal peritoneal surfaces. Movement of cells tends to follow the circulation of peritoneal fluid from the right pericolic gutter cephalad to the right hemidiaphragm. Tumors also spread to intestinal mesenteries, with omentum and mesentery as the common sites for peritoneal metastasis. Adhesions of tumors between loops of intestines

produce intestinal obstruction, whereas obstruction of the abdominal or diaphragmatic lymphatic drainage by tumor cells leads to decreased outflow of peritoneal fluid resulting in ascites [3,4]. Patients with malignant ascites suffer from abdominal distention, loss of appetite, shortness of breath, abdominal pain, low blood pressure, weakness, and fatigue and have short survival (e.g., 1.5–6 months).

Intraperitoneal (IP) therapy delivers high drug concentrations to tumors located in the peritoneal cavity. This treatment modality has been under development for several decades. The earlier clinical studies focused on 5-fluorouracil and methotrexate, whereas more recent studies have focused on using combinations of platinum and taxane analogs. Multiple studies have shown significant targeting advantage for IP therapy in cancer patients with peritoneal metastasis, with ratios of peritoneal cavity-to-systemic blood concentration–time product (CxT) ranging from 12 for cisplatin to 1000 for paclitaxel [5–11]. Adding IP chemotherapy to intravenous chemotherapy produces significantly longer progression-free and overall survival [12–15]; the most recent NCI-sponsored trial (GOG 172) showed a 16-month longer overall survival in stage III ovarian cancer patients with tumors of <1 cm diameter.

While the clinical data support the use of IP therapy, there are no approved IP products in the United States. A recent development is the monoclonal antibody catumaxomab, which, via its two binding arms specific for epithelial cell adhesion molecule and CD3 (T lymphocytes) and its Fc region, binds simultaneously to tumor cells, T cells, and antigen-presenting cells and causes cell death [16,17]. Catumaxomab was approved by the European

Commission for treatment of malignant ascites based on the prolongation in the puncture-free survival (i.e., duration over which paracentesis is not required; 46 days in catumaxomab-treated group vs. 11 days in control group) [18]. Because its antitumor activity depends on its ability to reach the binding sites on the cell surface, it is not known whether catumaxomab is effective against solid tumors where penetration/delivery of large molecules such as antibodies is likely to be more limited compared to small molecule drugs.

RATIONALE FOR PARTICULATE DRUG DELIVERY SYSTEMS FOR IP THERAPY

Particulate drug delivery systems have good safety profiles in humans, as shown by the several products approved for intravenous and intramuscular administration, including AmBisome® (amphotericin B liposomes), Doxil® (doxorubicin liposomes), Abraxane® (albumin-stabilized paclitaxel nanoparticles), Lupron® (leuprolide acetate), Trelstar® (triptorelin pamoate), and Risperdal® Consta® (risperidone).

The versatility of particulate drug delivery systems offers an opportunity to address the unmet need of IP therapeutics. By selecting suitable carrier materials, particulate drug delivery systems can be nontoxic, non-immunogenic, biocompatible, and biodegradable and thereby meet the requirement for clinical application. The properties of particulates can be modified to achieve the intended functions. For example, the particle size determines the clearance pathways and bigger particles have longer residence time in the peritoneal cavity. The drug release rate can be tuned by selecting the appropriate particle size, hydrophilicity/hydrophobicity, degradation time, and diffusivity of the carrier materials. The surface property can be modified with cationic charge for intracellular delivery, pegylation for prolonging the systemic circulation, ligand for receptor mediated drug delivery, or antibody for targeted delivery. The tunable drug release rate offers the opportunity to deliver the effective drug concentration at the time when tumor cells are susceptible to the drug actions (e.g., fast release for tumors with high growth fraction or cycling cells or slow release for slowly growing tumors).

The purpose of this chapter is to provide a review on the development of drug-loaded particles for IP therapy.

DRUG-LOADED PARTICLES FOR IP THERAPY: PRECLINICAL RESULTS

Most of the investigations of drug-loaded particles for IP therapy have used lipid and polymeric carriers. The studies include nano- and micron-size particles and surface-modified particles. As summarized later, these particle properties affect tumor targeting, systemic absorption, systemic and local toxicity, and antitumor efficacy. The in vivo studies

were typically conducted in rodents. The sizes quoted in this report refer to the diameter.

Nano- and micron-size liposomes

The lipid-based carrier, liposomes, is among the most studied in IP therapy. Liposomes are globular vesicles composed of an aqueous core and phospholipid bilayers and include small and large unilamellar liposomes and multilamellar liposomes. Due to the amphipathic nature, liposomes can be used as carriers for hydrophilic molecules with affinity to the hydrophilic head groups of phospholipid bilayers and the aqueous core and for hydrophobic molecules that intercalate into the fatty acid chains of the lipid bilayer. The properties of liposomes, e.g., size, charge, surface modification, and drug release rate, can be tailored to achieve the desired biological effects. For example, the control of liposome size is achieved by altering the preparation conditions such as freeze–thawing, sonication, and membrane filtration. The surface charge is controlled by choosing the correct mix of cationic, anionic, and neutral lipids. The stability is enhanced by including cholesterol, by avoiding unsaturated lipids and by using saturated lipids with higher glass transition temperatures. Surface modifications such as pegylation with polyethylene glycol reduce the opsonization by the reticuloendothelial system, and conjugation with tumor-targeting ligands enhances uptake in tumors.

Multiple examples have shown that the use of liposome carrier alters the systemic absorption and tissue distribution of IP therapeutics, with particle size being the major determinant [19–22]. A study using liposomes of four sizes (48, 170, 460, and 720 nm), each containing ^{14}C-labeled sucrose within the internal aqueous compartment, shows that (a) about 30% of the absorbed dose resided in the thoracic lymph with relatively high accumulation in the left mediastinal, parathymic, cisternal, and renal lymph nodes, indicating lymphatic drainage of submicron-size particles; (b) clearance of these liposomes from the peritoneal cavity was independent of particle size, indicating particle size is not rate limiting for the clearance of submicron-size particles; and (c) liposome size determines the distribution in lymph nodes and the systemic absorption. For the latter, the two smaller liposomes of 48 and 170 nm were not retained in lymph nodes and were mainly found in the lymph fluid, blood, lungs, liver, and spleen, whereas the largest liposomes of 720 nm showed the highest retention in lymph nodes. These findings indicate the size dependence of lymph node filtration and retention [22], with the small liposomes readily passing through the lymphatic ducts into the systemic circulation.

A later study evaluated the disposition of micron-size liposomes containing the ^{99m}technetium–hexamethyl-propyleneamineoxime complex (^{99m}Tc-HMPAO), at four different sizes (100, 400, 1000, and 3000 nm). The dose fraction of ^{99m}Tc-HMPAO recovered in peritoneal washes at 7 hours postinjection was >8 times higher for the liposomes compared to the free agent (ranged from 8% to 30% for liposomes vs. <1%) [23]. The second interesting observation is the recovery of the 3000 nm liposomes at/near the stomach, indicating a size threshold at which the liposomes would deposit on the peritoneal surface. The same finding was observed for large polymeric microparticles in mice and humans (e.g., 30 and 53 μm microparticles were deposited in the lower abdomen [24,25]). Third, consistent with the more extensive peritoneal retention, the appearance of ^{99m}Tc-HMPAO in blood was slower for the four liposome groups compared to the free agent (peak level at 2 vs. <0.5 hour). Fourth, among the liposomes, the smallest 100 nm liposomes showed eight times higher CxT in blood compared to three larger liposomes (all three yielded comparable CxT). The liposome size further affected the tissue distribution, with significantly higher accumulation in the kidneys and heart for the 100 nm liposomes and accumulation in the spleen for the 400 nm liposomes [23]. The higher CxT values in the blood for the 100 nm liposomes are consistent with their direct absorption into the systemic circulation as shown in the ^{14}C–sucrose study [22].

The aforementioned examples illustrate the critical role of liposome size on peritoneal retention and clearance and tissue distribution. However, the increased peritoneal retention does not necessarily improve treatment efficacy. For example, doxorubicin liposomes (150 nm) showed 30 times greater peritoneal retention (30% vs. 1% at 24 hours) but were no more effective in mice with IP colon C26 tumors compared to the free drug solution [26]. In a related study, IP doxorubicin liposomes (Doxil, 85 nm) were less effective compared to the intravenous treatment in mice with J6456 lymphoma ascites tumors; the investigators propose that the inferior activity of IP liposomes was in part due to the slow drug release from liposomes (15% in 24 hours) [27]. Comparison of three doxorubicin liposomes with different leakage rates (15.7%, 3.7%, and 0.4% leakage in 50% fetal bovine serum at 30 minutes) to the free drug solution shows that the high leakage liposomes produced superior activity, whereas the two low leakage liposomes produced inferior activity in Ehrlich ascites-bearing mice [28]. These examples indicate the importance of drug release or dosing rate in treatment efficacy (see more discussion under the section "In vitro–in vivo correlation").

Active tumor-targeting liposomes involve coating or covalently conjugating the targeting ligands, peptides, and antibodies on the liposome surface. These include epidermal growth factor receptor (EGFR)-targeted doxorubicin liposomes [29], folate receptor-targeted liposomes [30,31], DAL K29 antibody-conjugated methotrexate liposomes [32], and oligomannose-coated liposomes [33]. DAL K29 is an antigen expressed on the surface of human renal cancer cells. In mice bearing IP renal Caki-1 tumor, the DAL K29 antibody-conjugated methotrexate liposomes showed significantly higher activity compared to nontargeted liposomes or mixture of nontargeted liposomes plus free ligand [32]. In cultured human ovarian SKOV-3 cells, EGFR-targeted

doxorubicin liposomes showed significant higher receptor-mediated uptake and twofold greater cytotoxicity, compared to nontargeted liposomes. However, these targeting and efficacy advantages in cultured cells were not observed in vivo, where targeted and nontargeted liposomes yielded similar drug uptake in tumors and comparable treatment efficacy [29].

Polymeric nanoparticles

Biodegradable polymers are commonly used drug carriers. Among the synthetic biodegradable polymers, poly(lactide), poly(glycolide), and their copolymer poly(lactide-co-glycolide) have been used in the biomedical field since the 1960s. They do not induce inflammation or toxicity and break down to biocompatible and progressively smaller compounds, i.e., lactic acid or glycolic acid, which are further metabolized to carbon dioxide and water. These polymers are frequently used in IP studies. Other polymers are gelatin, albumin, and chitosan.

Polymeric nanoparticles generally have greater stability compared to liposomes. The tissue distribution, peritoneal retention, and lymph node accumulation of nanoparticles following IP administration is similar to that of liposomes in comparable sizes [34–40]. After IP administration in mice, about 80% of ^{14}C-labeled nanoparticles (250–300 nm) are found in the liver and spleen with particle aggregates observed in the lungs at early times (up to 1 hour) [36]. Systemic absorption of IP theophylline nanoparticles in rats is slower compared to the free drug solution in rats (peak blood concentration at 3 hours vs. 20 minutes for free drug solution) [41].

Polymeric nanoparticles can improve efficacy or reduce toxicity of chemotherapeutics. Compared to the respective free drug solutions, cisplatin nanoparticles showed improved efficacy in murine hepatic H22 tumors [42], etoposide-incorporated tripalmitin nanoparticles (387 nm) showed longer survival time [43], and vinblastine polybutyl-2-cyanoacrylate nanoparticles associated with vinblastine showed reduced bone marrow toxicity [44].

Several paclitaxel polymeric nanoparticle formulations have been evaluated [45–54]. A biodistribution study showed similar distribution in systemic tissues after intravenous or IP administration of paclitaxel nanoparticles (237 nm), except the intravenous treatment yielded higher accumulation in the lungs [47], probably due to the pulmonary first-pass effect. For efficacy, paclitaxel pH-responsive expansile nanoparticles that swell and release drug at pH <5 [49] were effective in preventing IP tumor implantation and prolonging survival. For active tumor targeting, paclitaxel-loaded nanoparticles coated with anti-HER2 monoclonal antibodies (Herceptin®, trastuzumab) yielded significantly longer survival in mice bearing metastatic HER2 overexpressing ovarian SKOV3 tumors, compared to a paclitaxel solution and nontargeted nanoparticles [47]. However, even though the nanoparticles yielded higher tumor accumulation compared to the free drug solution, there were no differences among targeted and nontargeted nanoparticles, suggesting that the therapeutic benefit of HER2-targeted liposomes was not due to enhanced delivery alone. Other nanoparticles such as hyaluronan-coated superparamagnetic iron oxide doxorubicin nanoparticles and folate receptor–targeted paclitaxel nanoparticles delayed tumor development, reduced tumor burden, and improved survival of mice bearing IP SKOV-3 ovarian tumor [53,55].

Polymeric microparticles

In general, polymeric microparticles yield longer peritoneal retention with reduced lymphatic clearance, and more sustained drug release, compared to polymeric nanoparticles [56]. IP distribution of polymeric microparticles (5–6 μm) is similar to the distribution of tumor cells with localization on the omentum and mesenteries [24], whereas larger microparticles (>30 μm) primarily localized in the lower abdomen [24,25].

Polymeric microparticles of several chemotherapeutics, e.g., cisplatin, 5-fluorouracil, mitoxantrone, and paclitaxel, offer higher tumor CxT, lower systemic absorption, greater efficacy, and/or lower toxicity compared to the respective free drug solution. For example, due to its small molecular size, cisplatin is rapidly absorbed into the systemic circulation and induces systemic side effects such as nephrotoxicity. These problems are overcome by using polymeric carriers. Cisplatin microparticles (47 μm, releasing the drug over 3 weeks) yielded higher and more sustained cisplatin concentrations in sarcoma180 tumor and ascites tumors but lower concentration in systemic organs and/or prolonged survival time [57–60]. 5-Fluorouracil microparticles (24 μm, releasing the drug over 3 weeks) yielded higher drug concentrations in IP tissues (especially in the omentum and mesenteries) and lower concentrations in systemic tissues and were more efficacious and less toxic in IP B-16 melanoma tumors [61–63]. CPT11 microparticles (10 μm diameter, releasing the drug over 3 weeks) showed gradual increases in plasma level due to sustained release [64]. Mitoxantrone microparticles (37 μm, releasing 30% of its drug content over 3 weeks) showed sustained drug levels in peritoneal fluid, lower local toxicity, and greater antitumor efficacy in Ehrlich ascites carcinoma [65–67]. Paclitaxel microparticles (14 μm, releasing drug over 2 weeks) were more efficacious compared to the Cremophor micelle solution [68].

Active tumor targeting was achieved in some situations. Conjugation of mesothelin-specific antibody to doxorubicin mesoporous silica microparticles yielded about 50% higher CxT in tumors compared to nontargeted microparticles [69]. Microparticles obtained by cross-linking hyaluronan (which binds to CD44 receptors) with cisplatin increased drug uptake by twofold to threefold selectively in CD44-expressing tumors and improved the survival of mice bearing IP A2780 ovarian tumors, compared to the free drug solution [70].

Drug delivery to the tumor core is necessary to prevent tumor regrowth and is important for treatment efficacy [71–74]. Studies in our group have focused on the determinants of drug delivery into peritoneal tumors and the methods to promote particle penetration. During IP therapy, drug delivery to peritoneal tumors is from two sources. Recirculation of drug absorbed from the peritoneal cavity via the systemic circulation is a minor source due to the relatively low concentration in the blood. The primary source is drug diffusion or convection through the interstitial space within a tumor mass. Studies have revealed differences of tumor penetration depths among chemotherapeutics, with the least penetration for doxorubicin (less than six cell layers or <0.06 mm) [75], followed by carboplatin (0.5 mm) [76] and cisplatin (1–2 mm) [77]. The limited drug penetration is likely the cause of limited treatment efficacy for patients with bulky tumors (>1 cm diameter [78–83]). Through a series of studies, we identified the major barrier to the transport of paclitaxel and doxorubicin is the high tumor cell density and subsequently established the tumor priming method to promote drug/particle penetration into solid tumors (i.e., use an apoptosis-inducing drug to transiently expand the interstitial space and promote the interstitial transport) [84–90]. Tumor priming is tumor selective due to the greater susceptibility of tumor cells to apoptosis compared to normal cells. We have since developed the two-component PLGA microparticles for IP therapy; these microparticles are designed to preferentially adhere to tumor surface and utilize the tumor priming technology. Both components of tumor-penetrating microparticles (TPM) are loaded with paclitaxel. The first component releases a small fraction of the dose to induce apoptosis, and the second component provides sustained drug delivery. Figure 30.1 shows the preferential localization of TPM on tumor surface (note the absence on the surface of peritoneum and other IP organs). Figure 30.2 shows that TPM yielded higher concentrations (>4 times higher maximum concentration [Cmax] and >16 times higher CxT), deeper drug penetration (e.g., >30 times higher levels at 0.5 mm from the tumor surface at day 7), and more sustained drug levels (>3 times) in tumors located on the omentum, compared to the Cremophor micelle solution of paclitaxel. Secondary to the sustained drug levels, a single dose of TPM was equally or more effective compared to multiple (four or eight) doses of the Cremophor micellar solution [24].

DRUG-LOADED PARTICLES FOR IP THERAPY: CLINICAL STUDIES

Several drug-loaded particles including liposomes, nanoparticles, and microparticles have advanced to clinical evaluation in IP therapy (Table 30.1). The chemotherapeutics include doxorubicin, platinum, and paclitaxel. For liposomes, the first were cardiolipin liposomes carrying doxorubicin, evaluated in 1989, followed by *cis-bis*-neodecanoato-*trans-R,R*-1,2-diaminocyclohexane

Rhodamine in PBS +
blank 4 µm particles

Lower abdomen
(injection site)

Mesentery

Mesentery

Small particles, 4 µm

Bar: 5 mm

4 µm rhodamine-
loaded particles

Large particles, 30 µm

Omentum

Bar: 5 mm

(a)

(b)

(c)

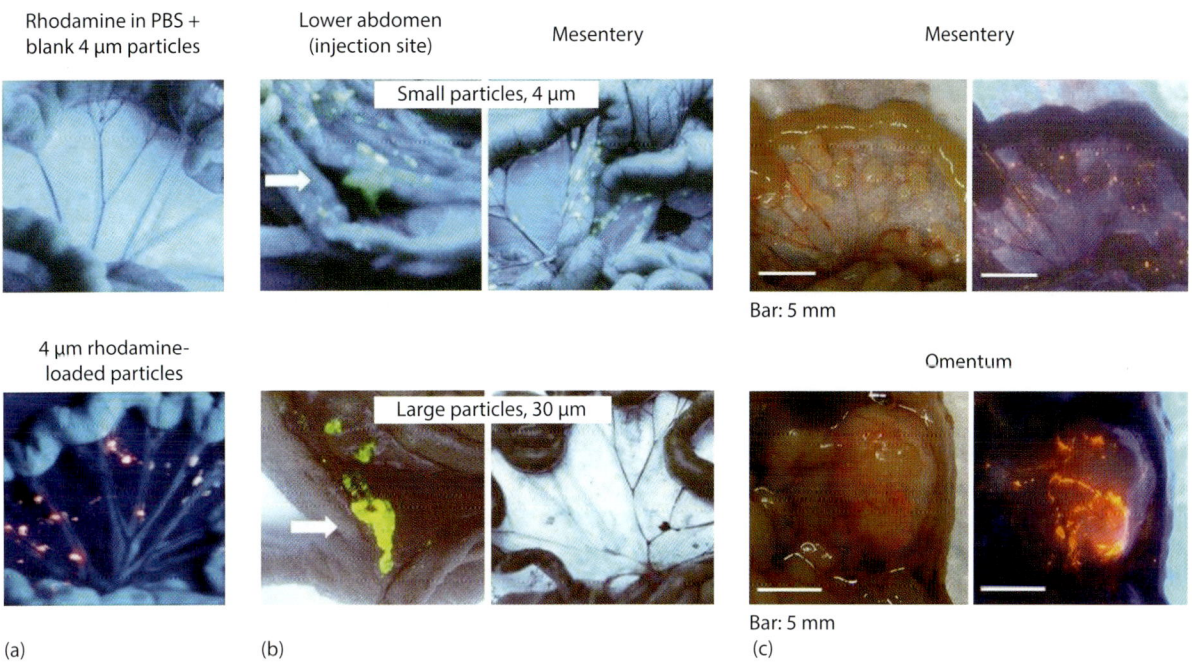

Figure 30.1 Intra-abdominal distribution of PLGA microparticles. **(a)** Distribution. Tumor-free mice were given IP injections of rhodamine dissolved in vehicle (0.01% Tween 80 in PBS) plus blank PLGA microparticles (top panel) or rhodamine-labeled microparticles (bottom panel). Rhodamine appears red under UV light. **(b)** Effect of particle size. Tumor-free mice were given IP injections of acridine orange–labeled microparticles with average diameters of 4 or 30 µm. Acridine orange appears yellow under UV light. The smaller particles were dispersed throughout the cavity and on the mesenteric membrane and omentum, which are common sites of local metastases of ovarian tumors. The larger particles were localized in the lower abdomen and were absent on the mesenteric membrane and omentum. Arrows indicate the subcutaneous injection sites. **(c)** Localization of 4 µm particles on tumors. Mice were implanted with IP human ovarian SKOV3 xenograft tumors. After tumors were established (day 42), a mouse was given an IP dose of rhodamine-labeled microparticles. Three days later, the animal was anesthetized and the abdominal cavity exposed. Photographs were taken in the region of omentum and mesentery under UV light (left panels) and room light (right panels). Note the large tumor on the omentum (~13 mm longest diameter) and multiple small tumors on the mesenteric membrane (1–3 mm longest diameter). Red color under UV light indicated localization of rhodamine-labeled particles on tumor surface. (Reprinted from Lu, Z. et al., *J. Pharmacol. Exp. Ther.*, 327, 673, 2008. With permission.)

platinum (II) (NDDP)-loaded liposomes in 2003. For polymeric microparticles, two cisplatin microparticles were evaluated in the mid-1990s, followed by paclitaxel microparticles (Paclimer®) in 2006. These earlier candidates are no longer under clinical development. Two paclitaxel nanoparticles, Abraxane and Nanotax®, are undergoing early clinical trials. In most clinical studies, IP therapy was administered in 2 L of physiological saline without drainage. One study evaluated peritoneal dialysis with a dwell time of 4 hours before drainage. As discussed in the following, drug-loaded particles generally show longer residence in the peritoneal cavity and slower systemic absorption relative to the free drug solution, resulting in a shift of dose-limiting toxicity from systemic toxicity to local toxicity such as peritonitis and abdominal pain. The particles, due to the slower and gated drug release, are generally better tolerated and show higher maximally tolerated doses (MTDs) compared to the free drug solution in a bolus presentation of the entire dose all at once, e.g., two times higher MTD for cisplatin microparticles that release 50% drug load in 1 day under sink conditions (200 vs. 100 mg) and 10 times higher

MTD for paclitaxel microparticles that release 1%–2% drug load per day (1200 vs. 125 mg/m² for the Cremophor micelle solution) [9,25,91].

A phase I trial in 15 patients with advanced ovarian cancer demonstrated that doxorubicin liposomes (900 nm) were better tolerated with a higher MTD (100 vs. 30–40 mg) compared to the free drug solution (which caused severe peritonitis) [92–95]. The lower toxicity may be due to the slow drug release from liposomes compared to the free drug solution where the entire dose was bioavailable all at once. For efficacy, three of four evaluable patients with small volume residual disease (<2 cm) showed tumor shrinkage, whereas none of the six evaluable patients with more bulky disease responded to liposomal doxorubicin, suggesting poor drug penetration into the tumor [95].

For platinated compounds, both liposomes and polymeric microparticles have been studied in patients. Multilamellar NDDP liposomes were evaluated in 16 patients with peritoneal carcinomatosis or sarcomatosis. The results showed (a) drug retention in the ascites fluid for up to 72 hours and sustained systemic absorption maintained for up to 120 hours,

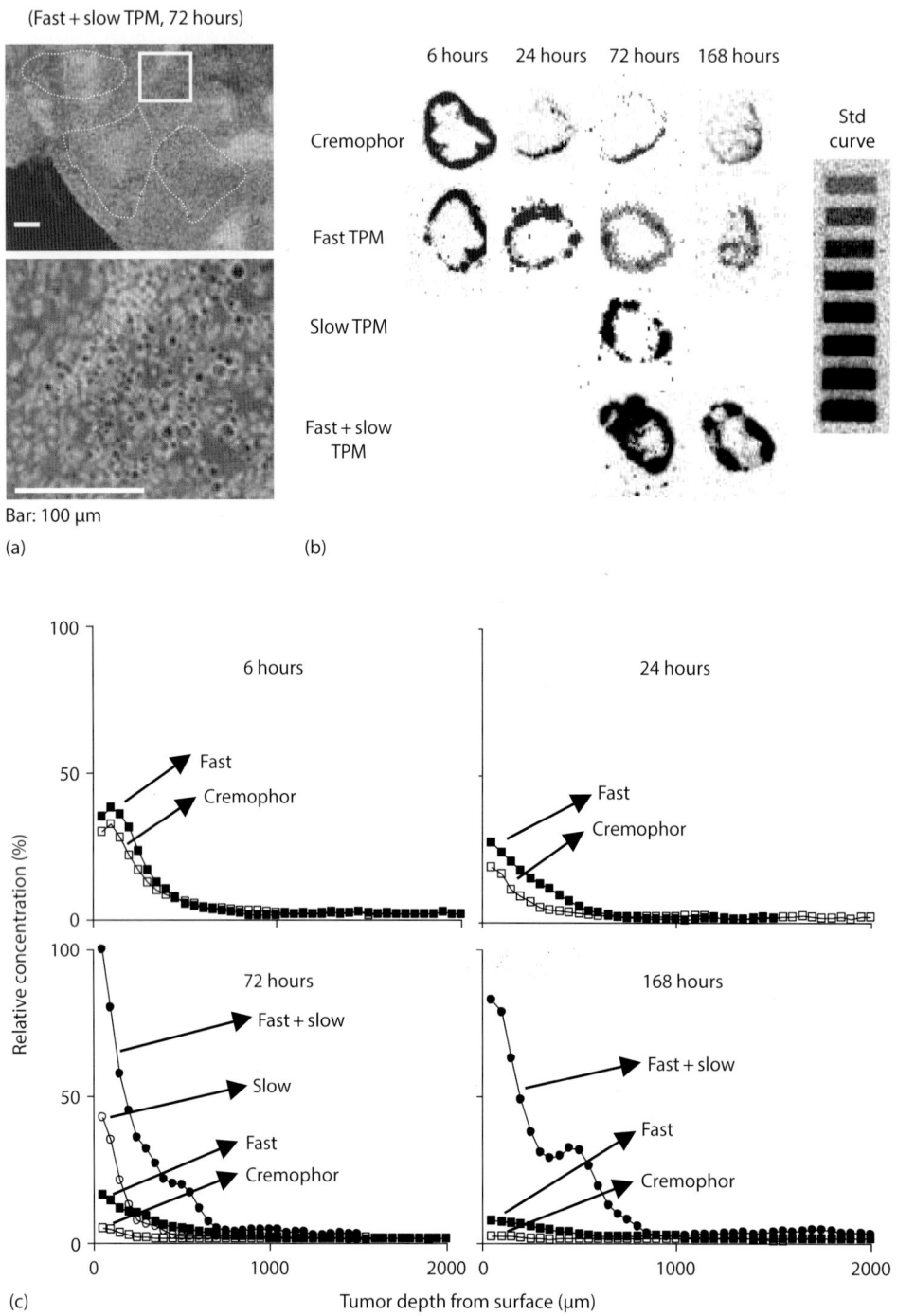

Figure 30.2 Spatial drug distribution in tumors. Mice bearing IP SKOV3 tumors were given IP injections of either the Cremophor micelle solution or the tumor-penetrating microparticles (TPMs) of ^{3}H-labeled paclitaxel. TPM comprised two components that release paclitaxel at different rates; the fast-release TPM released 70% drug load in 1 day, whereas the slow-release TPM released 1% per day. The doses of individual formulations were 20 mg/kg. The fast + slow TPM comprised 1:1 ratio of the two formulations. (a) TPM penetration into tumor interior. An omental tumor was removed from a mouse at 72 hours after treatment with two-component TPM, sectioned, and stained with hematoxylin and eosin. TPM appeared as black dots. Top panel shows areas with clusters of TPM (circumscribed with dotted lines). Bottom panel shows the enlarged picture of the boxed area. (b) Autoradiograms of tumor sections. (c) Concentration-depth profiles. Autoradiograms shown in (b) were processed to obtain measurements of total radioactivity using computer-assisted densitometric analysis. Radioactivity was expressed as paclitaxel equivalents, with the highest level set at 100%. (Reprinted from Lu, Z. et al., *J. Pharmacol. Exp. Ther.*, 327, 673, 2008. With permission.)

Table 30.1 Clinical development of IP drug-loaded particles

Particulate product	Diameter	Disease	Trial (ref.)
Doxorubicin liposomes	900 nm	Advanced ovarian cancer	Phase I/II completed in 1989 [95]
cis-bis-Neodecanoato-trans-R, R-1, 2-diaminocyclohexane) platinum II liposomes	1–3 μm	Peritoneal carcinomatosis or sarcomatosis	Phase I completed in 2003 [96]
Abraxane: albumin-stabilized paclitaxel nanoparticles	130 nm	Advanced cancer of the peritoneal cavity	Phase I, ongoing
Nanotax: paclitaxel nanocrystal	700–1200 nm	Refractory malignancies principally confined to the peritoneal cavity	Phase I, ongoing
Paclimer: paclitaxel polilactofate microparticles	53 μm	Refractory malignancies principally confined to the peritoneal cavity	Phase I completed in 2006 [25]
Cisplatin PLA microparticles	50–150 μm	Malignant ascites from cancers of the digestive organs	Phase I completed in 1993 [104]
Cisplatin PLA microparticles	100 μm	Recurrent ovarian cancer	Phase I completed in 1990 [91]

with 17–49 times greater CxT in peritoneal fluid compared to plasma and (b) higher platinum levels in the liver, omentum, and colon compared to other organs such as the heart, lung, spleen, and kidney within 24 hours of treatment. The dose-limiting toxicity was fatigue and abdominal pain at 450 mg/m². In comparison, the dose-limiting toxicity of the free drug solution was nephrotoxicity (without local toxicity at doses up to 270 mg/m², presumably due to rapid clearance and short residence in the peritoneal cavity). Out of 16 patients, 5 showed overall survival time of more than 3 years, suggesting activity of NDDP liposomes [96]. For microparticles, PLA microspheres of cisplatin (50–100 μm with about 50% and 70% released in 1 day and 3 weeks, respectively) were evaluated in 15 patients with malignant ascites originating from cancers of the digestive organs [59,97]. The doses used were 100 and 200 mg cisplatin, which maintained appreciable platinum concentrations for a week with minimal systemic absorption and yielded complete resolution of ascites in eight patients and partial resolution in five patients, for an overall response rate of 87%. A later study compared cisplatin microspheres against the free drug solution (200 vs. 100 mg, respectively) in 15 patients with recurrent ovarian cancer; the microparticle group showed lower peak but more sustained platinum concentrations in serum and ascites, and similar toxicity (grade 1/2 leukopenia and/or neutropenia occurred in two of five patients), compared to the free drug solution.

For paclitaxel, one microparticles and two nanoparticles have been evaluated in patients. The microparticles, Paclimer, used polilactofate polymer (copolymer of lactide and phosphate), containing about 10% paclitaxel, has an average size of 53 μm, and released the drug in ~90 days (~1%–2% per day) [98]. A phase I study in 12 patients with recurrent or persistent ovarian or primary peritoneal carcinoma showed that Paclimer was well tolerated at up to 1200 mg/m² paclitaxel, with 1 patient showing dose-limiting toxicity such as abdominal pain and ileus and bowel obstruction at the 900 mg/m² dose. The maintenance of low drug levels in the systemic circulation for at least 8 weeks posttreatment indicates sustained drug release. In comparison,

the Cremophor micelle formulation of paclitaxel caused significant abdominal pain at a fivefold lower dose of 175 mg/m² [99]. Laparoscopy at 7 months after Paclimer administration showed tissue adhesions, fat necrosis, foreign body giant cell reaction, and detectable residual polymer filaments in the lower part of the abdominal cavity [25]. Three patients who did not have measurable disease were tumor-free for at least 6 months.

Two nanoparticle products (Abraxane and Nanotax) are undergoing phase I clinical trials. Nanotax, a nanocrystal form of paclitaxel with volume-average diameter of 700–1200 nm, was evaluated in patients with refractory peritoneal cancers (mainly ovarian cancer) where the patient was first given an instillation of 500 mL physiological saline, followed by a bolus injection of Nanotax in physiological saline and then followed by instillation of saline (up to 2 L). Preliminary result showed Nanotax is well tolerated up to 275 mg/m². The Cmax in ascites fluid exceeded 1000 ng/mL, whereas the Cmax in plasma were >30 times lower (<35 ng/mL). This plasma Cmax is about 10 times lower compared to the historical results obtained from the Cremophor micelle solution of paclitaxel, indicating slower absorption of paclitaxel from Nanotax. For Abraxane, a human albumin–stabilized paclitaxel nanoparticles (130 nm diameter) approved for intravenous administration, patients with advanced cancer of the peritoneal cavity are given three weekly doses on a 28-day cycle; results are not yet available.

IN VITRO–IN VIVO CORRELATION

In vitro–in vivo correlation (IVIVC), i.e., relating an in vitro property of a dosage form to an in vivo property, has important implications in drug formulation design, optimization, quality control, and regulatory compliance. It has been widely used in bioequivalence studies where the drug dissolution/release in vitro is related to the in vivo pharmacokinetic parameters. In IP therapy, there is evidence that the in vitro drug release rate correlates with the in vivo treatment efficacy and toxicity, as follows:

For cisplatin microparticles prepared with various compositions of PLA and PLGA polymers, the MTD in mice increased progressively from 13.4 mg/kg for aqueous cisplatin solution to 34.6, 44.2, and 62.6 mg/kg for microparticles with increasingly slower release rate [100]. The CxT of platinum concentration in plasma correlated with the in vitro release profiles, with a linear relationship between the MTD and the half-time of drug release in phosphate-buffered saline (PBS) under sink condition ($R^2 = 0.99$). This IVIVC enabled the use of in vitro drug release rate to predict the systemic toxicity of cisplatin microparticles.

Another example is CPT11 microparticles, where a positive relationship was observed between higher in vitro release rate and in vivo efficacy in mice bearing IP P388 leukemia tumor [101].

Our group developed a method to use in vitro drug release from paclitaxel polymeric microparticles to simulate the initial burst and cumulative drug release of different treatments (different formulations and their combinations) in vivo [102]. This study was performed using the two-component TPM described in the section "Polymeric microparticles." We showed a correlation between toxicity and drug release rate, i.e., rapid drug release over a short duration (e.g., 1 day) is more toxic compared to fractionated release over days or weeks, presumably due to recovery from nonlethal damage. Next, we used the in vitro burst/cumulative release in PBS containing 0.1% w/v polysorbate 80 to simulate the in vivo drug release from microparticles with different particle sizes and release rates and demonstrated a linear relationship between the simulated in vivo release to the in vivo efficacy ($R^2 = 0.82$ and 0.86 for 1-day burst release and cumulative release at median survival time [MST], respectively) [102]. The results further indicate a temporal component of drug presentation, i.e., dosing rate, determines the treatment toxicity and efficacy; the threshold toxic 1-day release dose was 30 mg/kg; and the threshold drug amount in peritoneal cavity (cumulative amount at MST) required for disease-free cure was 40 mg/kg. Furthermore, while either fast- or slow-release microparticles had the highest dose efficiency (defined as survival extension per mg drug), cure was achieved only with their combinations indicating the benefits of using two dosing rates as a way to optimize IP drug delivery. We propose the combined use of slow- and fast-release microparticles enables the treatment of tumors with heterogeneous growth rates. This hypothesis was tested in two IP tumor models, i.e., the slow-growing ovarian SKOV3 tumors and the more-rapid-growing pancreatic Hs766T tumors (respective MST of 52 and 24 days for untreated mice). For the slow-growing tumor, the slow-release microparticles at 80 mg/kg showed better efficacy than the fast-release microparticles at 40 mg/kg (109 vs. 81 days MST), whereas the opposite was found for the rapidly growing tumors (i.e., better efficacy for the fast-release microparticles, 46 vs. 31 days MST) [24,102]. In comparison, a combination of fast- and slow-release microparticles at 120 mg/kg (1:2 fast/slow release) showed greatest efficacy in both tumor models (117 and 51 days MST for ovarian SKOV3 and pancreatic Hs766T, respectively).

SUMMARY AND PERSPECTIVES

Due to a lack of approved IP formulations, the earlier phase II and phase III clinical studies, conducted over more than 30 years, used off-label intravenous formulations. These clinical studies have shown that the utility and efficacy of IP therapy are limited by two problems. First, drug penetration into a tumor is usually restricted to the periphery. The impressive survival benefit applies mainly to patients with low bulk disease (e.g., tumors of <1 cm after surgical debulking) and is diminished in patients with larger tumors. Second, IP therapy is associated with morbidities (i.e., infection due to prolonged use of indwelling catheter and abdominal pain due to high local drug concentrations directly exposing the peritoneal organs and tissue) that have prevented widespread use of IP therapy as standard of care in spite of its demonstrated efficacy [15,103]. In our opinion, these are significant impediments that can be overcome by using drug-loaded particles due to their versatility. The lipid and polymeric particle delivery systems can be used to deliver both hydrophilic and hydrophobic drugs and can be made of different sizes. The drug release rate can be controlled so that the drug level in tumors is high enough to provide adequate control of the disease but at the same time below the threshold for producing significant local toxicity.

The preclinical and clinical studies on the development of IP drug-loaded particles to date have provided important information on the desired spatial and temporal properties. First, particle size is the major determinant of disposition and pharmacokinetics; smaller particles of 100 nm or less are readily absorbed into the systemic circulation, whereas larger particles show greater peritoneal retention and slower systemic absorption. On the other hand, there is a size threshold above which the particle distribution within the peritoneal cavity is hindered and results in particle precipitation on the peritoneal surface. The latter may lead to unfavorable tissue responses (e.g., adhesion, inflammation, necrosis) and, more important from the perspective of efficacy, prevent the spatial proximity to tumors. In view of the literature data showing significant retention of low micron-size particles (e.g., 1 μm, [23]) and the size of the lymphatic duct opening (i.e., 3 μm, [45]), we propose the optimal particle size for the purpose of enhancing peritoneal retention and avoiding precipitation is between 1 and 10 μm. Second, the treatment efficacy and toxicity depend on additional temporal factors such as the drug release/dosing rate. Defining the optimal drug release rate in order to maximize the therapeutic index is a formidable challenge as many of the processes that determine the treatment outcome are dynamic in nature. A slower drug release rate may reduce the toxicity and increase the MTD, but may also reduce the efficacy. In contrast, a rapid release rate may reduce the peritoneal retention advantage. Because a successful therapy requires that the drug is presented at the right concentration at the time the tumor cells are susceptible to drug actions, e.g., cycling but not noncycling cells are responsive to cycle-active agents, the optimal rate of drug release from particles is likely to depend on the drug action mechanisms as well as the tumor growth rate. From the standpoint of translating the preclinical findings to clinical applications, a further consideration is the unavoidable heterogeneous tumor growth rates in patients. One approach is to use mixtures of particles with different release rates in order to control both rapidly and slowly growing tumors.

REFERENCES

1. del Castillo CF, Warshaw L. Peritoneal metastases in pancreatic carcinoma. *Hepatogastroenterology*. 1993;40:430–432.
2. Beck W, Dalton WS. Mechanisms of drug resistance. In: DeVita VT, Hellman S, Rosenberg SA, eds., *Cancer: Principles & Practice of Oncology*, 4th edn., Philadelphia, PA: J.B. Lippincott Co., 1997. pp. 298–508.
3. Coates G, Bush RS, Aspin N. A study of ascites using lymphoscintigraphy with 99m Tc-sulfur colloid. *Radiology*. 1973;107:577–583.
4. Feldman GB, Knapp RC, Order SE, Hellman S. The role of lymphatic obstruction in the formation of ascites in a murine ovarian carcinoma. *Cancer Research*. 1972;32:1663–1666.
5. Nagel JD, Varossieau FJ, Dubbelman R, Bokkel Huinink WW, McVie JG. Clinical pharmacokinetics of mitoxantrone after intraperitoneal administration. *Cancer Chemotherapy and Pharmacology*. 1992;29:480–484.
6. Elferink F, van der Vijgh WJ, Klein I, Bokkel Huinink WW, Dubbelman R, McVie JG. Pharmacokinetics of carboplatin after intraperitoneal administration. *Cancer Chemotherapy and Pharmacology*. 1988;21:57–60.
7. Zimm S, Cleary SM, Lucas WE, Weiss RJ, Markman M, Andrews PA et al. Phase I/pharmacokinetic study of intraperitoneal cisplatin and etoposide. *Cancer Research*. 1987;47:1712–1716.
8. Speyer JL, Collins JM, Dedrick RL, Brennan MF, Buckpitt AR, Londer H et al. Phase I and pharmacological studies of 5-fluorouracil administered intraperitoneally. *Cancer Research*. 1980;40:567–572.
9. Markman M, Rowinsky E, Hakes T, Reichman B, Jones W, Lewis JL, Jr. et al. Phase I trial of intraperitoneal taxol: A Gynecoloic Oncology Group study. *Journal of Clinical Oncology*. 1992;10:1485–1491.
10. Markman M, Hakes T, Reichman B, Hoskins W, Rubin S, Jones W et al. Intraperitoneal therapy in the management of ovarian carcinoma. *Yale Journal of Biology and Medicine*. 1989;62:393–403.
11. Kerr DJ, Los G. Pharmacokinetic principles of locoregional chemotherapy. *Cancer Surveys*. 1993;17:105–122.
12. Gadducci A, Carnino F, Chiara S, Brunetti I, Tanganelli L, Romanini A et al. Intraperitoneal versus intravenous cisplatin in combination with intravenous cyclophosphamide and epidoxorubicin in optimally cytoreduced advanced epithelial ovarian cancer: A randomized trial of the Gruppo Oncologico Nord-Ovest. *Gynecologic Oncology*. 2000;76:157–162.
13. Markman M, Bundy BN, Alberts DS, Fowler JM, Clark-Pearson DL, Carson LF et al. Phase III trial of standard-dose intravenous cisplatin plus paclitaxel versus moderately high-dose carboplatin followed by intravenous paclitaxel and intraperitoneal cisplatin in small-volume stage III ovarian carcinoma: An intergroup study of the Gynecologic Oncology Group, Southwestern Oncology Group, and Eastern Cooperative Oncology Group. *Journal of Clinical Oncology*. 2001;19:1001–1007.
14. Armstrong DK, Bundy B, Wenzel L, Huang HQ, Baergen R, Lele S et al. Intraperitoneal cisplatin and paclitaxel in ovarian cancer. *New England Journal of Medicine*. 2006;354:34–43.
15. National Cancer Institute, 2006. http://www.cancer.gov/newscenter/pressreleases/IPchemotherapyrelease.
16. Sebastian M, Kuemmel A, Schmidt M, Schmittel A. Catumaxomab: A bispecific trifunctional antibody. *Drugs Today (Barcelona)*. 2009;45:589–597.
17. Linke R, Klein A, Seimetz D. Catumaxomab: Clinical development and future directions. *MAbs* 2010;2:129–136.
18. European Medicines Agency, 2015. http://www.ema.europa.eu/docs/en_GB/document_library/EPAR_Public_assessment_report/human/000972/WC500051808.pdf.
19. Arndt D, Zeisig R, Fichtner I, Teppke AD, Fahr A. Pharmacokinetics of sterically stabilized hexadecylphosphocholine liposomes versus conventional liposomes and free hexadecylphosphocholine in tumor-free and human breast carcinoma bearing mice. *Breast Cancer Research and Treatment*. 1999;58:71–80.
20. Kresta A, Shek PN, Odumeru J, Bohnen JM. Distribution of free and liposome-encapsulated cefoxitin in experimental intra-abdominal sepsis in rats. *Journal of Pharmacy and Pharmacology*. 1993;45:779–783.
21. Rosa P, Clementi F. Absorption and tissue distribution of doxorubicin entrapped in liposomes following intravenous or intraperitoneal administration. *Pharmacology*. 1983;26:221–229.
22. Hirano K, Hunt CA. Lymphatic transport of liposome-encapsulated agents: Effects of liposome size following intraperitoneal administration. *Journal of Pharmaceutical Sciences*. 1985;74:915–921.

23. Mirahmadi N, Babaei MH, Vali AM, Dadashzadeh S. Effect of liposome size on peritoneal retention and organ distribution after intraperitoneal injection in mice. *International Journal of Pharmaceutics*. 2010;383:7–13.

24. Lu Z, Tsai M, Lu D, Wang J, Wientjes MG, Au JL. Tumor-penetrating microparticles for intraperitoneal therapy of ovarian cancer. *Journal of Pharmacology and Experimental Therapeutics*. 2008;327:673–682.

25. Armstrong DK, Fleming GF, Markman M, Bailey HH. A phase I trial of intraperitoneal sustained-release paclitaxel microspheres (Paclimer) in recurrent ovarian cancer: A Gynecologic Oncology Group study. *Gynecologic Oncology*. 2006;103:391–396.

26. Mayhew E, Cimino M, Klemperer J, Lazo R, Wiernikowski J, Arbuck S. Free and liposomal doxorubicin treatment of intraperitoneal colon 26 tumor: Therapeutic and pharmacologic studies. *Selective Cancer Therapeutics*. 1990;6:193–209.

27. Cabanes A, Tzemach D, Goren D, Horowitz AT, Gabizon A. Comparative study of the antitumor activity of free doxorubicin and polyethylene glycol-coated liposomal doxorubicin in a mouse lymphoma model. *Clinical Cancer Research*. 1998;4:499–505.

28. Sadzuka Y, Hirama R, Sonobe T. Effects of intraperitoneal administration of liposomes and methods of preparing liposomes for local therapy. *Toxicology Letters*. 2002;126:83–90.

29. Lehtinen J, Raki M, Bergstrom KA, Uutela P, Lehtinen K, Hiltunen A et al. Pre-targeting and direct immunotargeting of liposomal drug carriers to ovarian carcinoma. *PLOS ONE*. 2012;7:e41410.

30. Chaudhury A, Das S, Bunte RM, Chiu GN. Potent therapeutic activity of folate receptor-targeted liposomal carboplatin in the localized treatment of intraperitoneally grown human ovarian tumor xenograft. *International Journal of Nanomedicine*. 2012;7:739–751.

31. Gabizon A, Tzemach D, Gorin J, Mak L, Amitay Y, Shmeeda H et al. Improved therapeutic activity of folate-targeted liposomal doxorubicin in folate receptor-expressing tumor models. *Cancer Chemotherapy and Pharmacology*. 2010;66:43–52.

32. Singh M, Ghose T, Mezei M, Belitsky P. Inhibition of human renal cancer by monoclonal antibody targeted methotrexate-containing liposomes in an ascites tumor model. *Cancer Letters*. 1991;56:97–102.

33. Matsui M, Shimizu Y, Kodera Y, Kondo E, Ikehara Y, Nakanishi H. Targeted delivery of oligomannose-coated liposome to the omental micrometastasis by peritoneal macrophages from patients with gastric cancer. *Cancer Science*. 2010;101:1670–1677.

34. Adlersberg L, Singer JM. The fate of intraperitoneally injected colloidal gold particles in mice. *Journal of Reticuloendothelial Society*. 1973;13:325–342.

35. Adlersberg L, Singer JM. Transfer of radioiodinated latex particles from the peritoneal cavity of mice to the mediastinum. *Journal of Reticuloendothelial Society*. 1972;12:565–591.

36. Sjoholm I, Edman P. Acrylic microspheres in vivo. I. Distribution and elimination of polyacrylamide microparticles after intravenous and intraperitoneal injection in mouse and rat. *Journal of Pharmacology and Experimental Therapeutics*. 1979;211:656–662.

37. Simeonova M, Ivanova T, Raikov Z, Konstantinov H. Tissue distribution of polybutylcyanoacrylate nanoparticles loaded with spin-labelled nitrosourea in Lewis lung carcinoma-bearing mice. *Acta Physiologica et Pharmacologica Bulgarica*. 1994;20:77–82.

38. Maincent P, Thouvenot P, Amicabile C, Hoffman M, Kreuter J, Couvreur P et al. Lymphatic targeting of polymeric nanoparticles after intraperitoneal administration in rats. *Pharmaceutical Research*. 1992;9:1534–1539.

39. Katsnelson BA, Degtyareva TD, Minigalieva II, Privalova LI, Kuzmin SV, Yeremenko OS et al. Subchronic systemic toxicity and bioaccumulation of Fe_3O_4 nano- and microparticles following repeated intraperitoneal administration to rats. *International Journal of Toxicology*. 2011;30:59–68.

40. Lu H, Li B, Kang Y, Jiang W, Huang Q, Chen Q et al. Paclitaxel nanoparticle inhibits growth of ovarian cancer xenografts and enhances lymphatic targeting. *Cancer Chemotherapy and Pharmacology*. 2007;59:175–181.

41. Radwan MA, Zaghloul IY, Aly ZH. In vivo performance of parenteral theophylline-loaded polyisobutylcyanoacrylate nanoparticles in rats. *European Journal of Pharmaceutical Sciences*. 1999;8:95–98.

42. Ding D, Zhu Z, Liu Q, Wang J, Hu Y, Jiang X et al. Cisplatin-loaded gelatin-poly(acrylic acid) nanoparticles: Synthesis, antitumor efficiency in vivo and penetration in tumors. *European Journal of Pharmaceutics and Biopharmaceutics*. 2011;79:142–149.

43. Reddy LH, Adhikari JS, Dwarakanath BS, Sharma RK, Murthy RR. Tumoricidal effects of etoposide incorporated into solid lipid nanoparticles after intraperitoneal administration in Dalton's lymphoma bearing mice. *AAPS Journal*. 2006;8:E254–E262.

44. Simeonova M, Ilarionova M, Ivanova T, Konstantinov C, Todorov D. Nanoparticles as drug carriers for vinblastine. Acute toxicity of vinblastine in a free form and associated to polybutylcyanoacrylate nanoparticles. *Acta Physiologica et Pharmacologica Bulgarica*. 1991;17:43–49.

45. Tsai M, Lu Z, Wang J, Yeh TK, Wientjes MG, Au JL. Effects of carrier on disposition and antitumor activity of intraperitoneal Paclitaxel. *Pharmaceutical Research*. 2007;24:1691–1701.

46. Roby KF, Niu F, Rajewski RA, Decedue C, Subramaniam B, Terranova PF. Syngeneic mouse model of epithelial ovarian cancer: Effects of nanoparticulate paclitaxel, Nanotax. *Advances in Experimental Medicine and Biology.* 2008;622:169–181.

47. Cirstoiu-Hapca A, Buchegger F, Lange N, Bossy L, Gurny R, Delie F. Benefit of anti-HER2-coated paclitaxel-loaded immuno-nanoparticles in the treatment of disseminated ovarian cancer: Therapeutic efficacy and biodistribution in mice. *Journal of Controlled Release.* 2010;144:324–331.

48. Kamei T, Kitayama J, Yamaguchi H, Soma D, Emoto S, Konno T et al. Spatial distribution of intraperitoneally administered paclitaxel nanoparticles solubilized with poly (2 methacryloxyethyl phosphorylcholine-co n-butyl methacrylate) in peritoneal metastatic nodules. *Cancer Science.* 2011;102:200–205.

49. Colson YL, Liu R, Southard EB, Schulz MD, Wade JE, Griset AP et al. The performance of expansile nanoparticles in a murine model of peritoneal carcinomatosis. *Biomaterials.* 2011;32:832–840.

50. Werner ME, Karve S, Sukumar R, Cummings ND, Copp JA, Chen RC et al. Folate-targeted nanoparticle delivery of chemo- and radiotherapeutics for the treatment of ovarian cancer peritoneal metastasis. *Biomaterials.* 2011;32:8548–8554.

51. Emoto S, Yamaguchi H, Kishikawa J, Yamashita H, Ishigami H, Kitayama J. Antitumor effect and pharmacokinetics of intraperitoneal NK105, a nanomicellar paclitaxel formulation for peritoneal dissemination. *Cancer Science.* 2012;103:1304–1310.

52. Gilmore D, Schulz M, Liu R, Zubris KA, Padera RF, Catalano PJ et al. Cytoreductive surgery and intraoperative administration of paclitaxel-loaded expansile nanoparticles delay tumor recurrence in ovarian carcinoma. *Annals of Surgical Oncology.* 2013;20:1684–1693.

53. Tong L, Chen W, Wu J, Li H. Folic acid coupled nano-paclitaxel liposome reverses drug resistance in SKOV3/TAX ovarian cancer cells. *Anticancer Drugs.* 2014;25:244–254.

54. Cai Y, Zhang X. Pharmacokinetics of carbon nanoparticle-paclitaxel suspension for use in intraperitoneal chemotherapy. *Hepatogastroenterology.* 2013;60:1998–2003.

55. El-Dakdouki MH, Xia J, Zhu DC, Kavunja H, Grieshaber J, O'Reilly S et al. Assessing the in vivo efficacy of doxorubicin loaded hyaluronan nanoparticles. *ACS Applied Materials & Interfaces.* 2014;6:697–705.

56. Yoshikawa H, Nakao Y, Takada K et al. Targeted and sustained delivery of aclarubicin to lymphatics by lactic acid-oligomer microsphere in rat. *Chemical & Pharmaceutical Bulletin (Tokyo).* 1989;37:802–804.

57. Tamura T, Fujita F, Tanimoto M, Koike M, Suzuki A, Fujita M et al. Anti-tumor effect of intraperitoneal administration of cisplatin-loaded microspheres to human tumor xenografted nude mice. *Journal of Controlled Release.* 2002;80:295–307.

58. Kumagai S, Sugiyama T, Nishida T, Ushijima K, Yakushiji M. Improvement of intraperitoneal chemotherapy for rat ovarian cancer using cisplatin-containing microspheres. *Japan Journal of Cancer Research.* 1996;87:412–417.

59. Hagiwara A, Takahashi T, Kojima O, Yamaguchi T, Sasabe T, Lee M et al. Pharmacologic effects of cisplatin microspheres on peritoneal carcinomatosis in rodents. *Cancer.* 1993;71:844–850.

60. Tokuda K, Natsugoe S, Shimada M, Kumanohoso T, Baba M, Takao S et al. Design and testing of a new cisplatin form using a base material by combining poly-D,L-lactic acid and polyethylene glycol acid against peritoneal metastasis. *International Journal of Cancer.* 1998;76:709–712.

61. Hagiwara A, Sakakura C, Shirasu M, Yamasaki J, Togawa T, Takahashi T et al. Therapeutic effects of 5-fluorouracil microspheres on peritoneal carcinomatosis induced by Colon 26 or B-16 melanoma in mice. *Anticancer Drugs.* 1998;9:287–289.

62. Hagiwara A, Sakakura C, Tsujimoto H, Imanishi T, Ohgaki M, Yamasaki J et al. Selective delivery of 5-fluorouracil (5-FU) to i.p. tissues using 5-FU microspheres in rats. *Anticancer Drugs.* 1997;8:182–188.

63. Hagiwara A, Takahashi T, Sawai K, Sakakura C, Tsujimoto H, Imanishi T et al. Pharmacological effects of 5-fluorouracil microspheres on peritoneal carcinomatosis in animals. *British Journal of Cancer.* 1996;74:1392–1396.

64. Machida Y, Onishi H, Kurita A, Hata H, Morikawa A, Machida Y. Pharmacokinetics of prolonged-release CPT-11-loaded microspheres in rats. *Journal of Controlled Release.* 2000;66:159–175.

65. Luftensteiner CP, Schwendenwein I, Paul B, Eichler HG, Viernstein H. Evaluation of mitoxantrone-loaded albumin microspheres following intraperitoneal administration to rats. *Journal of Controlled Release.* 1999;57:35–44.

66. Luftensteiner CP, Schwendenwein I, Eichler HG, Paul B, Wolfl G, Viernstein H. Toxicity of a particulate formulation for the intraperitoneal application of mitoxantrone. *International Journal of Pharmaceutics.* 1999;180:251–260.

67. Jameela SR, Latha PG, Subramoniam A, Jayakrishnan A. Antitumour activity of mitoxantrone-loaded chitosan microspheres against Ehrlich ascites carcinoma. *Journal of Pharmacy and Pharmacology.* 1996;48:685–688.

68. Yang M, Yu T, Wood J, Wang YY, Tang BC, Zeng Q et al. Intraperitoneal delivery of paclitaxel by poly(ether-anhydride) microspheres effectively

suppresses tumor growth in a murine metastatic ovarian cancer model. *Drug Delivery and Translational Research.* 2014;4:203–209.

69. Macura SL, Steinbacher JL, Macpherson MB, Lathrop MJ, Sayan M, Hillegass JM et al. Microspheres targeted with a mesothelin antibody and loaded with doxorubicin reduce tumor volume of human mesotheliomas in xenografts. *BMC Cancer.* 2013;13:400.

70. Li SD, Howell SB. CD44-targeted microparticles for delivery of cisplatin to peritoneal metastases. *Molecular Pharmacology.* 2010;7:280–290.

71. Durand RE. Slow penetration of anthracyclines into spheroids and tumors: A therapeutic advantage? *Cancer Chemotherapy and Pharmacology.* 1990;26:198–204.

72. Erlanson M, Daniel-Szolgay E, Carlsson J. Relations between the penetration, binding and average concentration of cytostatic drugs in human tumour spheroids. *Cancer Chemotherapy and Pharmacology.* 1992;29:343–353.

73. Baguley BC, Finlay GJ. Pharmacokinetic/cytokinetic principles in the chemotherapy of solid tumours. *Clinical and Experimental Pharmacology and Physiology.* 1995;22:825–828.

74. Jain RK. Delivery of molecular medicine to solid tumors. *Science.* 1996;271:1079–1080.

75. Ozols RF, Locker GY, Doroshow JH, Grotzinger KR, Myers CE, Young RC. Pharmacokinetics of adriamycin and tissue penetration in murine ovarian cancer. *Cancer Research.* 1979;39:3209–3214.

76. Los G, Verdegaal EM, Mutsaers PH, McVie JG. Penetration of carboplatin and cisplatin into rat peritoneal tumor nodules after intraperitoneal chemotherapy. *Cancer Chemotherapy and Pharmacology.* 1991;28:159–165.

77. Los G, Mutsaers PH, Lenglet WJ, Baldew GS, McVie JG. Platinum distribution in intraperitoneal tumors after intraperitoneal cisplatin treatment. *Cancer Chemotherapy and Pharmacology.* 1990;25:389–394.

78. Gitsch E, Sevelda P, Schmidl S, Salzer H. First experiences with intraperitoneal chemotherapy in ovarian cancer. *European Journal of Gynaecological Oncology.* 1990;11:19–22.

79. Recio FO, Piver MS, Hempling RE, Driscoll DL. Five-year survival after second-line cisplatin-based intraperitoneal chemotherapy for advanced ovarian cancer. *Gynecologic Oncology.* 1998;68:267–273.

80. Piver MS, Recio FO, Baker TR, Driscoll D. Evaluation of survival after second-line intraperitoneal cisplatin-based chemotherapy for advanced ovarian cancer. *Cancer.* 1994;73:1693–1698.

81. Barakat RR, Sabbatini P, Bhaskaran D, Revzin M, Smith A, Venkatraman E et al. Intraperitoneal chemotherapy for ovarian carcinoma: Results of long-term follow-up. *Journal of Clinical Oncology.* 2002;20:694–698.

82. Topuz E, Saip P, Aydmer A, Salihoglu Y, Berkman S, Bengisu E. Intraperitoneal cisplatin-mitoxantrone and intravenous ifosfamide combination as first-line treatment of ovarian cancer. *European Journal of Gynaecological Oncology.* 1998;19:265–270.

83. Alberts DS, Liu PY, Hannigan EV, O'Toole R, Williams SD, Young JA et al. Intraperitoneal cisplatin plus intravenous cyclophosphamide versus intravenous cisplatin plus intravenous cyclophosphamide for stage III ovarian cancer. *New England Journal of Medicine.* 1996;335:1950–1955.

84. Zheng JH, Chen CT, Au JL, Wientjes MG. Time- and concentration-dependent penetration of doxorubicin in prostate tumors. *AAPS PharmSciTech* 2001;3:E15.

85. Kuh HJ, Jang SH, Wientjes MG, Weaver JR, Au JL. Determinants of paclitaxel penetration and accumulation in human solid tumor. *Journal of Pharmacology and Experimental Therapeutics.* 1999;290:871–880.

86. Jang SH, Wientjes MG, Au JL. Enhancement of paclitaxel delivery to solid tumors by apoptosis-inducing pretreatment: Effect of treatment schedule. *Journal of Pharmacology and Experimental Therapeutics.* 2001;296:1035–1042.

87. Chen CT, Au JL, Wientjes MG. Pharmacodynamics of doxorubicin in human prostate tumors. *Clinical Cancer Research.* 1998;4:277–282.

88. Lu D, Wientjes MG, Lu Z, Au JL. Tumor priming enhances delivery and efficacy of nanomedicines. *Journal of Pharmacology and Experimental Therapeutics.* 2007;322:80–88.

89. Jang SH, Wientjes MG, Au JL. Determinants of paclitaxel uptake, accumulation and retention in solid tumors. *Investigational New Drugs.* 2001;19:113–123.

90. Au JLS, Li D, Gan Y, Gao X, Johnson AL, Johnston J et al. Pharmacodynamics of immediate and delayed effects of paclitaxel: Role of slow apoptosis and intracellular drug retention. *Cancer Research.* 1998;58:2141–2148.

91. Sugiyama T, Kumagai S, Nishida T, Ushijima K, Matsuo T, Yakushiji M et al. Experimental and clinical evaluation of cisplatin-containing microspheres as intraperitoneal chemotherapy for ovarian cancer. *Anticancer Research.* 1998;18:2837–2842.

92. Ozols RF, Young RC, Speyer JL, Sugarbaker PH, Greene R, Jenkins J et al. Phase I and pharmacological studies of adriamycin administered intraperitoneally to patients with ovarian cancer. *Cancer Research.* 1982;42:4265–4269.

93. Rahman A, White G, More N, Schein PS. Pharmacological, toxicological, and therapeutic evaluation in mice of doxorubicin entrapped in cardiolipin liposomes. *Cancer Research.* 1985;45:796–803.

94. Rahman A, Carmichael D, Harris M, Roh JK. Comparative pharmacokinetics of free doxorubicin and doxorubicin entrapped in cardiolipin liposomes. *Cancer Research.* 1986;46:2295–2299.

95. Delgado G, Potkul RK, Treat JA, Lewandowski GS, Barter JF, Forst D et al. A phase I/II study of intra-peritoneally administered doxorubicin entrapped in cardiolipin liposomes in patients with ovarian cancer. *American Journal of Obstetrics & Gynecology.* 1989;160:812–817.

96. Verschraegen CF, Kumagai S, Davidson R, Feig B, Mansfield P, Lee SJ et al. Phase I clinical and pharmacological study of intra-peritoneal *cis-bis*-neodecanoato(trans-R, R-1, 2-diaminocyclohexane)-platinum II entrapped in multilamellar liposome vesicles. *Journal of Cancer Research and Clinical Oncology.* 2003;129:549–555.

97. Hagiwara A, Takahashi T, Sasabe T, Ito M, Lee M, Sakakura C et al. Toxicity of a new dosage format, cisplatin incorporated in lactic acid oligomer micro-spheres, in mice. *Anticancer Drugs.* 1992;3:237–244.

98. Harper E, Dang W, Lapidus RG, Garver RI, Jr. Enhanced efficacy of a novel controlled release pacli-taxel formulation (PACLIMER delivery system) for local-regional therapy of lung cancer tumor nodules in mice. *Clinical Cancer Research.* 1999;5:4242–4248.

99. Markman M, Francis P, Rowinsky E, Hakes T, Reichman B, Jones W et al. Intraperitoneal Taxol (paclitaxel) in the management of ovarian cancer. *Annals of Oncology.* 1994;5(Suppl. 6):S55–S58.

100. Tamura T, Imai J, Tanimoto M, Matsumoto A, Suzuki A, Horikiri Y et al. Relation between dissolution profiles and toxicity of cisplatin-loaded microspheres. *European Journal of Pharmaceutics and Biopharmaceutics.* 2002;53:241–247.

101. Machida Y, Onishi H, Morikawa A, Machida Y. Antitumor characteristics of irinotecan-containing microspheres of poly-d,l-lactic acid or poly(d,l-lactic acid-co-glycolic acid) copolymers. *STP Pharma Sciences.* 1998;8:175–181.

102. Tsai M, Lu Z, Wientjes MG, Au JL. Paclitaxel-loaded polymeric microparticles: Quantitative relation-ships between in vitro drug release rate and in vivo pharmacodynamics. *Journal of Controlled Release.* 2013;172:737–744.

103. Walker JL, Armstrong DK, Huang HQ, Fowler J, Webster K, Burger RA et al. Intraperitoneal cath-eter outcomes in a phase III trial of intravenous versus intraperitoneal chemotherapy in optimal stage III ovarian and primary peritoneal cancer: A Gynecologic Oncology Group Study. *Gynecologic Oncology.* 2006;100:27–32.

104. Hagiwara A, Takahashi T, Sawai K, Sakakura C, Tsujimoto H, Osaki K et al. Clinical trials with intra-peritoneal cisplatin microspheres for malignant ascites—a pilot study. *Anticancer Drug Design.* 1993;8:463–470.

31

Biomaterials and drug delivery systems for intraperitoneal chemotherapy

BO SUN AND YOON YEO

INTRODUCTION

The mainstay of current peritoneal malignancy treatment is surgical debulking of visible tumors and postsurgical chemotherapy to remove residual microscopic tumors [1,4,77]. Recently, intraperitoneal (IP) chemotherapy has been pursued in postsurgical management of peritoneal malignancies, due to the promise of a high local concentration and a longer half-life of a drug in the peritoneal cavity, which provides a unique opportunity for the locoregional treatment of the IP malignances [23,65,66]. Part of the IP-administered drugs are absorbed to systemic circulation, but it occurs at a slower rate than those administered intravenously [53,64,75]; therefore, IP dosage forms can also serve as a depot for sustained systemic drug delivery. IP chemotherapy has proven significantly more effective than intravenous (IV) therapy in several clinical studies [1,4,68]. Accordingly, the National Cancer Institute issued a clinical alert to recommend IP chemotherapy for stage III patients with optimally debulked ovarian cancer in 2006 [74].

On the other hand, several challenges remain to be overcome before IP chemotherapy to make a standard protocol for postsurgical management of peritoneal malignancies. For example, IP-administered drugs show limited penetration into tumors [67], thus necessitating the use of high IP doses. The high IP doses in turn account for increased toxicities such as myelotoxicity, neurotoxicity, nephrotoxicity, nausea, vomiting,

and abdominal pain [74,115,126]. Cumulative toxicities reduce options for subsequent rounds of therapy [3]. Moreover, complications related to IP administration, such as discomfort due to prolonged infusion, catheter implantation, and peritoneal adhesion, result in poor quality of life and, thus, high rate of dropout prior to the completion of planned treatment [4,115].

While the long list of challenges seems discouraging, this leaves the formulation scientists with several questions: Can drug delivery systems help overcome any of these problems? What are the unique requirements for IP drug delivery? What needs to be done and what has been done to improve drug delivery to the peritoneal cavity? In this chapter, we intend to address these questions by reviewing recent literature concerning IP drug delivery. We will discuss experimental approaches to improve the effectiveness of IP chemotherapy, focusing on the biomaterials used as drug carriers and various dosage forms that have been reported to date. The chapter will conclude with a discussion of remaining challenges and future perspectives.

MATERIALS FOR IP DELIVERY SYSTEMS

Requirements for IP drug carriers

Typical first-line chemotherapeutic agents such as paclitaxel (PTX), docetaxel (DTX), and cisplatin are low-molecular-weight drugs (<20 kDa), which are absorbed through the peritoneal capillaries and enter the systemic circulation in a few hours [53,64,75]. The short residence time not only compromises the effectiveness of local chemotherapy but also requires frequent or continuous dosing, culminating in complications related to catheters and infection [84]. For the delivery of low-molecular-weight drugs, it is therefore important to attenuate fast systemic absorption and maintain a high local concentration of a drug. Ideally, the IP drug carriers should provide a sustained drug release to maintain the local drug concentration within an effective range over several weeks. The sustained local delivery of chemotherapy is also found beneficial for avoiding tumor repopulation, which can occur during drug-free cycles in conventional intermittent therapy [110]. In addition, it is desirable that the carriers are degraded into molecules that are readily absorbed and cleared from the body by the time the loaded drug is exhausted so that surgical removal of empty carriers may not be necessary.

While the primary goal of the IP delivery system is to remain in the peritoneal cavity and provide a local reservoir of a drug for a prolonged period, such an effort often faces a challenge due to the sensitivity of the peritoneal cavity to foreign materials. The peritoneal cavity is responsible for protecting the body from breaches in the integrity of the gut; therefore, it is armed with powerful innate and adaptive immune mechanisms [31]. When confronted by an insult, peritoneal mesothelial cells, polymorphonuclear neutrophils, and the resident peritoneal-associated lymphoid tissues interact with one another via chemical signaling to produce inflammatory responses to the foreign materials [31]. Due to this sensitivity, some biomaterials typically considered biocompatible are found to induce significant inflammatory responses such as peritoneal adhesions [25,120]. Therefore, in designing an IP drug delivery system, it is necessary to apply more stringent criteria for the selection of biomaterials for formulations.

Biomaterials for IP drug delivery

A list of polymers used for other biomedical applications is a good starting point for selection of drug carrier materials. In particular, biomaterials used for peritoneal adhesion prevention are great candidates for IP drug delivery. Several natural and synthetic polymers have been used clinically and experimentally as physical barrier devices, as reviewed elsewhere in detail [122].

NATURAL POLYMERS

Polysaccharides such as hyaluronic acid (HA) [9,10,79, 87,117], cellulose derivatives [11,58,79], dextran [39,44,81], and chitosan [85,86,120] have been explored for IP application. The popularity of these polysaccharides stems from the biocompatibility proven in various biomedical applications. The polysaccharides are chemically modified into reactive precursors, which can form cross-linkable hydrogels upon application [43,120,121]. For example, HA is modified into two types of precursors—one with adipic acid dihydrazide

and the other oxidized to have aldehydes, which instantly form a hydrogel upon contact [9]. The polysaccharide-based hydrogels are enzymatically degraded; therefore, the degradation rate can be controlled by combining polymers with different enzyme susceptibility. For example, the degradation rate of HA gel in the peritoneal cavity was extended by replacing one of the gel precursors with cellulose derivatives, which were not degraded by human enzymes [43]. For the delivery of hydrophobic drugs, it is likely necessary to balance the hydrophobicity and hydrophilicity of the polymer [5]. For this purpose, it is conceivable to modify the polymer with hydrophobic moieties to increase the compatibility between drugs and polymers [41,56]. Chitosan has also been widely explored as a local depot of chemotherapeutic agents, where various stimuli (light, pH, temperature) are employed as a trigger to form a hydrogel in situ [99].

SYNTHETIC POLYMERS

Synthetic polymers used for the prevention of peritoneal adhesion and IP chemotherapy include polylactic acid (PLA), poly(lactide-co-glycolide) (PLGA), polyethylene glycol (PEG), poly(Ɛ-caprolactone) (PCL), and their block copolymers [16,51,79,93,96,101]. Most of these polymers are commercially available at reasonable prices. In particular, PLGA is widely used as a drug carrier [112] or a device [70,116] because of its track record in the approved products and the well-known biodegradability and biocompatibility [122]. An advantage of synthetic polymers over natural polymers is that it is relatively easier to control the molecular weight, monomer composition, and structure of the polymer; therefore, there is greater flexibility in delivering various types of drugs [93,101].

DOSAGE FORMS FOR IP DRUG DELIVERY

The most common form of IP chemotherapy is the repurposed IV solutions. To increase the drug retention in the peritoneal cavity, viscous polymer solutions, micro- or nanoparticle formulations, implantable polymeric depots, and hydrogel-based systems have been explored [63,106,121,122].

Solutions

PTX is poorly water-soluble and, thus, requires a solubility enhancer. An equal parts mixture of ethanol and Cremophor EL (polyethoxylated castor oil) is used to solubilize PTX in Taxol® [78,105]. Alternative solubilization strategies are pursued to reduce toxicities related to Cremophor EL. For example, PTX and randomly methylated-β-cyclodextrin (RAME-β-CD) form water-soluble inclusion complexes, which does not precipitate upon dilution and stay stable after 24-hour storage at ambient temperature or 2 hours at 41.5°C [8]. When used for hyperthermic peritoneal perfusion, PTX/RAME-β-CD complexes showed 40-fold higher plasma concentration than Taxol in a rat model [6] and delayed the growth of peritoneal carcinomatosis [7].

The authors argued that PTX/RAME-β-CD complexes had a greater ability to penetrate into IP tumors than Taxol, which entrapped PTX in surfactant micelles and thus limited direct tumor exposure of the drug [6].

A viscous solution of hydroxyethyl starch was used for the IP delivery of PTX [72] and DTX [73]. Sprague Dawley rats were administered IP with the taxane compounds using 6% hydroxyethyl starch (hetastarch) or 1.5% dextrose peritoneal dialysis solution as a carrier. Fluid clearance and mean taxane concentrations in plasma were lower when the drugs were delivered with hetastarch solution than with the peritoneal dialysis solution. Importantly, the total amount of drug remaining in the peritoneal cavity was significantly higher with hetastarch solution [72,73]. These studies demonstrate that hetastarch solution helped retain taxane compounds in the peritoneal cavity and reduce systemic exposure to the drugs.

Micro- or nanoparticles

A tumor-penetrating microparticle (TPM) loaded with PTX was designed for IP drug delivery [63]. The TPM system consisted of two types of particles. One was priming TPM, which encapsulated PTX in a low-molecular-weight PLGA (lactic acid/glycolic acid [LA/GA] = 50:50) and released the drug rapidly to "prime" the tumors, i.e., to expand the interstitial space via apoptosis induction and enhance the penetration of the second type of particles into tumors. The second component called sustaining TPM encapsulated PTX in a high-molecular-weight PLGA (LA/GA = 75:25) and, thus, provided sustained drug release to kill tumor cells. TPMs were able to retain in the peritoneal cavity for a longer time and achieve greater therapeutic effect and lower toxicity than Taxol [63]. The tumor-priming technology was later used to promote the delivery of survivin siRNA, which targeted a gene encoding survivin, an antiapoptotic protein associated with metastases and poor prognosis of patients with gastric and colorectal cancers [113]. Here, siRNA was encapsulated in PEGylated cationic liposomes (PCat) that were administered IP after TPM treatment of IP tumors. The combination of PTX-loaded TPM and PCat–siSurvivin was more effective than each treatment in suppressing tumor growth due to the synergy of the two treatments: TPM enhancing the penetration of PCat–siSurvivin into peritoneal tumors and PCat–siSurvivin reducing survivin expression and augmenting TPM-induced antiproliferation and apoptosis [113].

A nanocrystal (NC) form (submicron drug particles stabilized by surfactants and/or polymers) of PTX has been used in conjunction with hyperthermia for IP chemotherapy [20]. PTX NCs were produced using Pluronic F127 as a stabilizer and administered to rats bearing peritoneal tumors via IP perfusion at 41.5°C for 45 minutes. The PTX NCs showed similar antitumor activity as Taxol with relatively low apparent toxicity [20]. Unlike Taxol, the blood level of PTX continued to increase even after the discontinuation of NC hyperthermic intraperitoneal chemotherapy (HIPEC),

which suggests the long-term residence of NCs in the peritoneal cavity due to their mucoadhesive properties [20].

Polymeric micelles have been used for delivery of multiple drugs to IP tumors [16]. A combination of three drugs with distinct mechanisms of action—PTX as a cytotoxic drug, cyclopamine as an inhibitor of hedgehog signaling to reverse taxane resistance, and gossypol as a proapoptotic compound—was encapsulated in poly(ethylene glycol)-block-poly(ε-caprolactone) micelles for codelivery to tumors. Simultaneous encapsulation of three drugs in a single polymeric micelle was possible as they have similarly poor water solubility [16]. The three-drug loaded micelles were able to disaggregate 3D spheroids of ES-2 human ovarian cancer cells, whereas micelles with a single drug or two-drug combination showed negligible effects on tumor spheroids. In mouse models of IP xenograft, the IP administered three-drug micelles reduced tumor burden to a greater extent than PTX alone and vehicles controls [16]. Following debulking and induction of apoptosis of IP tumors with the three-drug micelles, secondary micelles with a near-infrared fluorescence probe, DiR, were systemically administered to visualize and help remove residual tumors (Figure 31.1) [12]. Here, the secondary micelles were conjugated with a peptide having high affinity for apoptotic tissues (externalized phosphatidylserine) so that the secondary micelles could specifically visualize apoptotic tumors [12]. A similar approach was used for systemic administration of drug combinations and visualization of residual tumors [13,14].

While the particle systems in the aforementioned examples are intended for local drug delivery, they also provide a useful tool for lymphatic or systemic drug delivery. Particles administrated in the peritoneal cavity are drained into lymphatic circulation (Figure 31.2) [34,106]. Within the lymphatic system, particles smaller than 50 nm pass through lymph nodes and reach systemic circulation via thoracic lymph ducts [34]. Kohane et al. reported that even larger PLGA nanoparticles (265 nm) entered systemic circulation from the peritoneal cavity in less than 2 days, ending up in the spleen and the liver [51]. On the other hand, larger particles (>500 nm) are trapped in lymph nodes. Therefore, depending on the particle size, nanoparticles can serve as a sustained systemic delivery system or for targeting cancer cells spreading via lymphatics.

Conversely, microparticles (1–100 μm) are retained longer in the peritoneal cavity and, thus, have a greater potential to enhance local availability of a drug in the peritoneal cavity and attenuate systemic drug absorption than nanoparticles [63,106] (Figure 31.2). However, the long-term residence of microparticles in the peritoneal cavity can cause inflammatory tissue responses and peritoneal adhesions [51], which may offset the benefits of the localized medicine. For this reason, a combination of nanoparticles and hydrogels was proposed as an alternative option. Here, nanoparticles served as a sustained drug delivery system and hydrogels prevented premature clearance of nanoparticles from the peritoneal cavity [117]. Additionally, the hydrogel prevented the retained polymeric nanoparticles from causing adhesions [117].

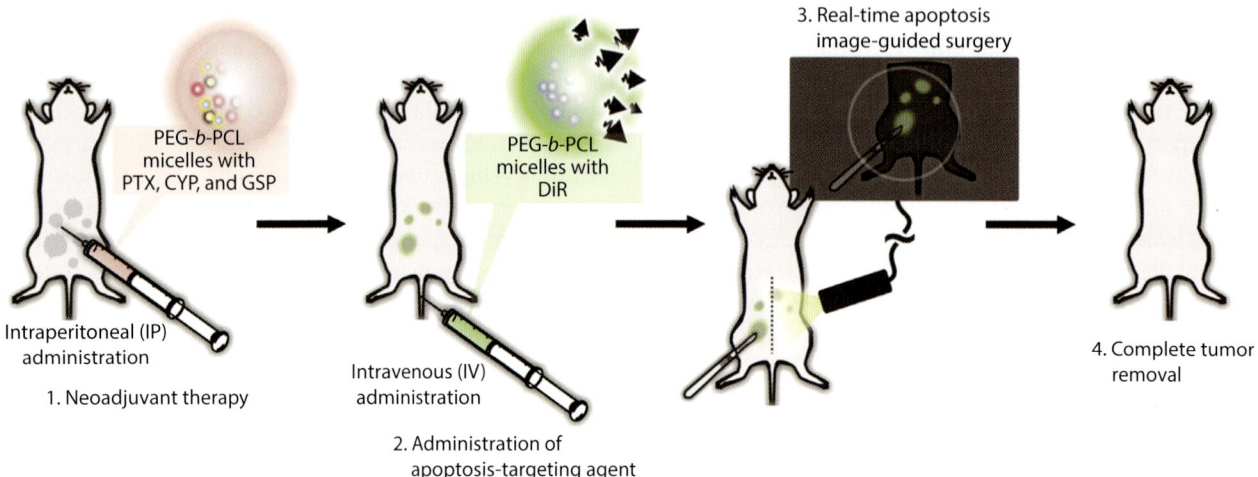

Figure 31.1 Schematic illustration of two-step strategy for neoadjuvant therapy, apoptosis-targeted optical imaging, and intraoperative surgical guidance, enabled by a tandem of poly(ethylene glycol)-block-poly(ε-caprolactone) micelles. (Reprinted from Cho, H. et al., *PLOS ONE*, 9, e89968, 2014, per Creative Commons Attribution (CC BY) license.)

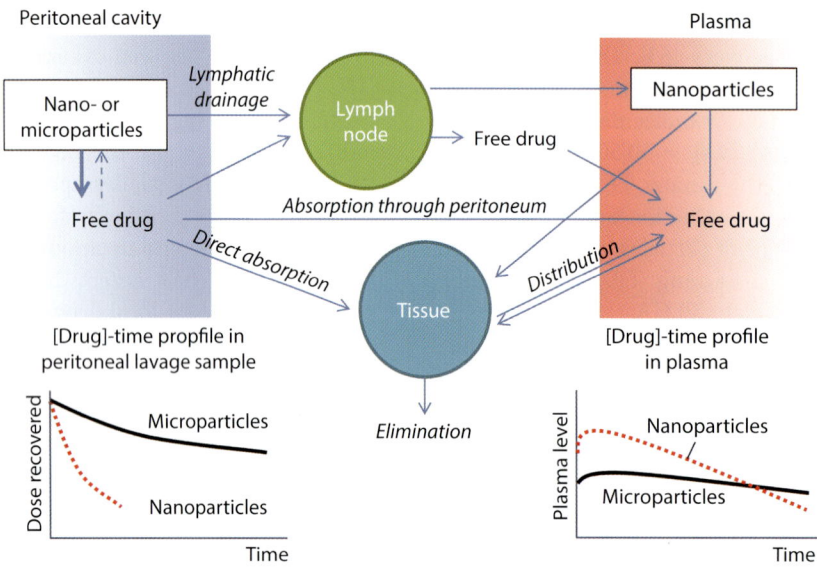

Figure 31.2 A model of kinetic processes during intraperitoneal (IP) administration of nano- or microparticles. Nanoparticles are drained through the lymphatic system, reaching systemic circulation, or trapped in the lymph nodes depending on the size. Microparticles tend to stay in the peritoneal cavity. Free drugs released from particles are absorbed directly to IP tissues or systemic circulation. Consequently, microparticles can maintain a higher drug concentration in the peritoneal cavity than nanoparticles, whereas nanoparticles yield a higher rate and extent of systemic absorption than microparticles. (Modified from Tsai, M. et al., *Pharm. Res.*, 24, 1691, 2007.)

Implantable depots

Chitosan–phospholipid implantable formulations have been developed for sustained and localized delivery of taxane compounds to ovarian tumors in the peritoneal cavity [109,111,124]. The films were composed of chitosan and egg phosphatidylcholine (ePC) (chitosan–ePC film) blended with PLA-*b*-PEG [28], PLA-*b*-PEG/PLA [61], or PLGA nanoparticles [36] containing PTX. PTX release from the nanoparticle/chitosan–ePC films was evaluated in lysozyme-containing phosphate-buffered saline (PBS) [28], cell culture medium [36], or ascitic fluid [61]. PTX

was released over 3 months with no significant initial burst release as the chitosan–ePC matrix swelled and degraded by lysozyme [28,36,61]. Animals implanted with chitosan–ePC films IP showed no signs of fibrous encapsulation or inflammation around the implant area over 2–4 weeks, indicating good biocompatibility of the implants [36]. The maximum tolerable dose (MTD) of PTX was 280 mg/kg/week when delivered with the nanoparticle/chitosan–ePC film, much higher than Taxol with the MTD of 20 mg/kg/week [111]. The PTX/nanoparticle/chitosan–ePC film significantly enhanced the antitumor efficacy as compared to Taxol at total dose of 60 mg/kg [109,111]. It is noticeable that continuous sustained delivery of PTX by PTX/nanoparticle/chitosan–ePC film (60 mg/kg) was superior to intermittent Taxol administration (20 mg/kg every 7 days (q7d) × 3 schedule) at an equivalent dose and administration route (IP) in suppressing tumor growth and extending animal survival [109]. Moreover, intermittent Taxol administration resulted in a significant increase of tumor proliferation indices as compared with nontreated controls, which indicates potential repopulation of tumors during treatment-free intervals [109]. In contrast, PTX/nanoparticle/chitosan–ePC film is thought to increase tumor responsiveness to the treatment by continuously exposing the tumors to high concentration of PTX by localizing the drug source in the peritoneal cavity [109]. In addition, PTX/nanoparticle/chitosan ePC film did not induce the expression of multidrug resistance (MDR) gene (MDR1) in vivo, whereas intermittent Taxol administration caused significant MDR1 expression [35]. These results demonstrate the benefits of local sustained drug delivery to IP tumors.

Injectable hydrogels

The implantable films are an effective way of localizing chemotherapy in the peritoneal cavity, but the fact that it requires surgical implantation poses challenges in administration and patient compliance [29]. Therefore, the implantable film was replaced with an injectable depot (PoLigel), composed of a water-soluble chitosan derivative, ePC, and a fatty acid analog [29]. This mixture formed a gel at physiological temperature via hydrophobic interaction between the water-soluble chitosan and acyl chains of ePC, reinforced by their interactions with the fatty acid analog [29]. Biocompatibility of the PoLigel depended on the type of fatty acid analog lauric aldehyde was better tolerated than lauric chloride when injected subcutaneously in mice and observed over 4 weeks [21]. PoLigel was used for sustained and localized delivery of DTX to murine models of SKOV3 ovarian cancer [124,125]. DTX loaded in PoLigel (DTX/PoLigel) showed constant release kinetics over 2 weeks with a minimal initial burst release in 0.01 M PBS (pH 7.4) containing lysozyme and albumin [124]. DTX/PoLigel IP administered to mice maintained constant DTX levels in plasma and peritoneal tissues over 2 weeks without causing significant toxicity or inflammation [124]. Tumor burden was reduced by >70% in DTX/PoLigel-treated group as compared with saline control [124]. Similar to the PTX/nanoparticle/chitosan–ePC film [109], DTX/PoLigel achieved a greater antitumor effect than intermittent Taxol injections, which was partly attributed to antiangiogenic effect of local DTX, continuously released by PoLigel [22]. In addition to local tumors, the IP administrated DTX/PoLigel was capable of delivering DTX to subcutaneous tumors distant from the peritoneal cavity [125]. This result demonstrates that IP sustained and localized delivery platform can treat not only local tumors but also metastasis distal to the site of administration via the systemically absorbed drug. The PoLigel was also used for codelivery of

DTX and cepharanthine, where the latter inhibited MDR due to drug efflux transporters and helped manage refractory ovarian cancer with the MDR phenotype [123].

Another type of injectable gel used for IP chemotherapy is a thermosensitive hydrogel based on PLGA-b-PEG-b-PLGA triblock copolymers [127]. These polymers are soluble in water, form a free-flowing solution at low temperature (e.g., 4°C), but spontaneously gels at body temperature to create a water-insoluble gel called ReGel® [127]. ReGel (23w/w%) injected subcutaneously into rats maintained the gel structure for 2 weeks but degraded into a viscous liquid and gradually resorbed in the next 2 weeks. The hydrophobic segments (PLGA) formed hydrophobic regions in the gel, in which poorly water-soluble drugs could be encapsulated. ReGel loaded with PTX (OncoGel™) released ~40% of the loaded PTX in the first 10 days and continuously released the remaining payload in the next 40 days. In subcutaneous injection and the FDA modified biocompatibility tests, ReGel caused no signs of inflammation and significant toxicities, confirming its biocompatibility [127]. OncoGel has been evaluated in local therapy of solid tumors through preclinical and clinical studies and considered a promising adjuvant therapy for ovarian cancer [26]. ReGel was recently evaluated as a carrier of a three-drug combination (PTX and two protein inhibitors) for IP chemotherapy [15]. The three-drug loaded ReGel (Triogel) IP injected as a free-flowing solution formed a depot at body temperature and released drugs at an equal rate according to gel erosion. The IP administered Triogel showed greater antitumor efficacy and lower systemic toxicity than IP or IV administrated PEG-b-PLA micelles with the same payloads in ES-2 ovarian cancer xenograft model [15]. These results demonstrated the potential of Triogel as a multidrug carrier for IP chemotherapy of ovarian cancer.

While the PoLigel or ReGel form gels through noncovalent interactions between polymer chains, polymers with functional groups that can react in situ and form covalent cross-linking to make hydrogels are also used for IP drug delivery [24]. The HA derivatives that formed in situ hydrogels via hydrazone bond (see the section "Natural polymers") were evaluated for the prevention of postsurgical adhesion as a physical adhesion barrier and/or drug carrier, showing excellent biocompatibility in the peritoneal cavity and effectiveness in adhesion prevention [117–119,121] Accordingly, the in situ cross-linkable HA hydrogels have also been evaluated as an IP drug delivery system for local therapy of cancers in the peritoneal cavity [5,27].

CHALLENGES IN IP CHEMOTHERAPY

The aforementioned examples illustrate that various drug delivery systems deliver standard anticancer drugs to the peritoneal cavity and help manage peritoneal malignancies by providing sustained drug release and maintaining high local drug concentration. However, several challenges remain to be addressed before IP chemotherapy becomes a standard therapeutic option in the clinic.

Drug release in peritoneal environment

The volume of peritoneal fluid in a healthy adult is about 50 mL with a turnover rate of 4–5 mL/h, whereas blood volume is ~5 L [95]. The protein content of peritoneal fluid is 25% of that in the blood [114]. Although malignancies may raise the protein level and accelerate the turnover in the ascites, the relatively small volume of the peritoneal fluid poses challenges to the IP delivery of poorly water-soluble drugs. Our previous effort to deliver PTX with HA-based hydrogel provides an example of such a challenge [5]. Here, PTX was mixed in HA hydrogel precursor solutions in the form of Taxol or concentrated DMSO solution and administered IP to tumor-bearing mice so that the precursors could form a hydrogel in situ [5]. Upon dilution in the gel precursor solutions, the concentrated PTX/DMSO solution started to form micrometer-scale precipitates (PPTs), whereas Taxol maintained the micelle size (14 nm) [5]. The large particle size of the former and HA hydrogel helped maintain PTX in the peritoneal cavity over 2 weeks. However, the prolonged retention of PPT–hydrogel did not translate to an improved antitumor effect, due to the large size of PPTs and, thus, limited dissolution of PTX [5]. This result indicates that hydrogel as a delivery medium helps localize drug in the peritoneal cavity but does not prevent precipitation of poorly water-soluble drug, limiting its availability to the local tumors.

A potential solution to this problem may be to reduce the particle size to facilitate drug dissolution; however, it should not be as small as Taxol micelles as they are not retained in the hydrogel [5]. Therefore, the challenge is to produce drug particles with an optimal size, large enough to remain in the gel but small enough to allow continuous and unhindered drug dissolution. There are several methods to produce drug particles in a specific size range [19]. For example, nanocrystallization is a technique to produce crystalline particles of poorly water-soluble drugs in the nanometer range (i.e., NCs). Due to the size and, thus, the high surface-area-to-volume ratio, NCs can increase the dissolution rate of drug particles [82]. The unique advantage of NCs is that they are mainly composed of drug molecules and create little concern for the safety of excipients [98]. A minimal amount of surface stabilizers are, however, needed to prevent aggregation of NCs during their lifetime [108]. For example, ionic surfactants such as sodium cholate, sodium deoxycholate, and sodium lauryl sulfate are used to stabilize NCs via electrostatic repulsion. Alternatively, NCs are stabilized with amphiphilic polymers that establish a steric barrier against aggregation [98]. Another strategy is to use proteins as stabilizers [62]. Serum proteins, such as human serum albumin (HSA), can serve as a stabilizer due to their ability to adsorb onto hydrophobic surfaces and therefore provides steric hindrance to NC aggregation and growth [47,94]. Moreover, serum proteins can interact with cell membrane to facilitate cellular uptake of anticancer drugs in tumors [54]. We have recently used PTX NCs stabilized with HSA for IP delivery with hydrogels (Figure 31.3) and

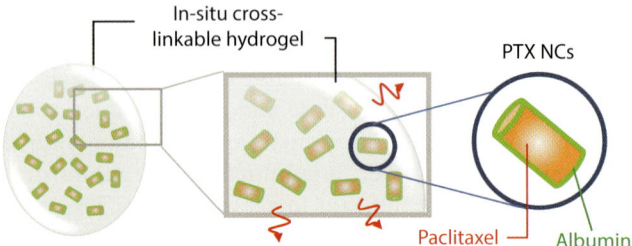

Figure 31.3 Schematic illustration of an injectable depot system, composed of an in situ cross-linkable hydrogel and albumin-stabilized paclitaxel nanocrystals.

observed that the NC–hydrogel hybrid system had a superior antitumor activity than Taxol at an equivalent total dose in a murine model of IP tumors.

Tumor specificity and penetration

Reduced blood flow, increased interstitial fluid pressure, and high collagen density interfere with drug transport into solid tumors [104]. In addition, hyaluronan [52] and stromal cells [48] in the tumor extracellular matrix aggravate the difficulty in drug penetration into tumors. While the tumor penetration is a general issue in chemotherapy of solid tumors [71], IP delivery faces a greater challenge than IV or intratumoral administrations in tumor penetration because IP-administered drugs mostly approach the tumor tissue from the periphery rather than the interior of the tumors (Figure 31.4). In vitro studies using multicellular layers [30,57,59,102] and tumor spheroids [37,76] have shown that limited drug penetration results in constant tumor exposure to a suboptimal level of drug, making an important mechanism for tumor resistance against chemotherapy. An approach to address this challenge is to loosen up the tumor matrix prior to chemotherapy to alleviate the drug penetration barrier [45,55]. This strategy involved two-step chemotherapy with an interval, where the first treatment with proapoptotic agent like PTX-induced reduction in cell density of solid tumors and allowed the subsequent dose to reach the interior of the tumors. This study provided a proof of concept for the development of TPM for IP delivery of anticancer drugs or siRNA to peritoneal malignances (see the section "Micro- or nanoparticles") [63,113]. Manipulating tumor microenvironment is another way of improving delivery and intratumoral distribution of a drug or a nanoparticulate drug delivery system [42]. For example, local mild hyperthermia was applied to tumors to improve vasculature permeability, perfusion, and interstitial fluid flow [60]. Local hyperthermia at 41°C increased tumor vasculature permeability and allowed liposomes (~85 nm) to extravasate into the interstitial space (Figure 31.5) [60]. This effect may explain the increasing popularity and positive clinical outcomes of IP chemotherapy combined with hyperthermia (HIPEC) [18,32,40,46,88,92,97,103]. Recently,

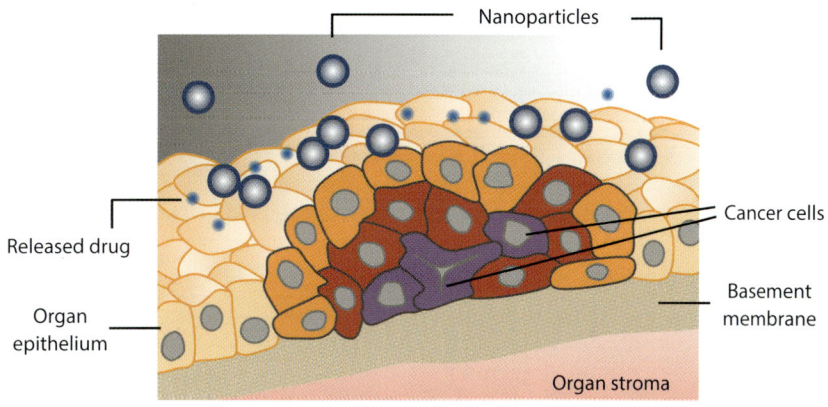

Figure 31.4 Schematic illustration of poor penetration of an intraperitoneally administered drug. Drug approaching tumors from the peritoneal cavity has a limited depth of penetration, which aggravates with increasing carrier size.

several new approaches have been proposed to improve drug delivery to the interior of solid tumors [13,90]. These approaches facilitate drug penetration into tumors by enhancing interactions between drug carriers and tumor stroma [91], preventing intracellular sequestration of a drug [80] or addressing hypoxic region of tumors prior to standard chemotherapy [89]. Although these studies have not been presented in the context of IP chemotherapy, it is worthwhile to explore their applicability in the treatment of peritoneal malignances.

Tissue responses to carrier materials

EFFECTS OF CARRIER MATERIALS ON PERITONEAL TISSUES

As mentioned in the section "Requirements for IP drug carriers," careful selection of biomaterials as a drug carrier is particularly important for IP application because of the high sensitivity of the peritoneal cavity to foreign insults. Biomaterials generally considered biocompatible or wildly used in other biomedical applications have caused inflammatory responses and peritoneal adhesion upon IP application. For example, PLGA microparticles (5 µm) induced adhesions 2 weeks after IP injection in mice [51]. This problem worsened with increasing molecular weight of the polymer [51]. A photo-cross-linkable chitosan derivative, which showed no attractive interactions or proliferative effect on mesothelial cells and macrophages in vitro, caused extensive and persistent peritoneal adhesions in animals receiving it as a hydrogel in the peritoneal cavity [120]. It was later learned that the parent chitosan had the same effect in vivo [120]. Both chitosans had significant proinflammatory properties, which might have been tolerated in other locations but not in the peritoneal cavity.

EFFECTS OF CARRIER MATERIALS ON TUMORS

Drug carriers, once they are proven biocompatible, are often used under an assumption that they have no other roles than delivering the payload to the body. Our recent studies suggest otherwise. We have delivered platinum into the peritoneal cavity using HA nanoparticles and hydrogels IP in mice for local chemotherapy of ovarian cancer. We find that they do not show a greater antitumor efficacy than platinum solution but rather cause a slight increase in tumor burdens at later time points, which suggests a potential involvement of empty carriers and degradation products in the growth of residual tumors. This hypothesis is supported by various biological roles of HA. HA is an indispensable extracellular matrix macromolecule for cell migration, differentiation, and proliferation [128]. Endogenous HA is implicated in the invasion and growth of several tumor cells [50,69,107,128]. CD44, a well-known receptor of HA, is found at the surface of various tumor cells and positively correlated with poor prognosis of ovarian cancer patients [49]. HA concentration in tumor stroma is considered an essential indicator of tumor aggressiveness and overall survival [2,33]. However, the role of exogenous HA in tumor invasion and growth remains controversial. Picaud et al. reported that HA–carboxymethyl cellulose membrane had no effect on the proliferation of tumor cells in vitro and in vivo [83]. Similarly, HA-based antiadhesion membrane was found to have no influence on metastasis of colon cancer in a human xenograft/nude mouse model [38]. On the other hand, Tan et al. reported that HA solution promoted proliferation and motility of colorectal tumor cell lines and increased peritoneal tumor load as compared with nontreated control group, confirming its positive role on metastatic potential of colorectal tumors [100]. Although the exact effect of HA-based biomaterials on IP tumors and its role remain to be investigated, the mixed results beg a question—if the drug carrier is indeed biologically inert and does no harm after it remains in the body after complete exhaustion of the payload. This means that in designing a new drug carrier, one should consider not only the biocompatibility of the material but also its biological effects on residual tumors, which may not be readily predicted from routine toxicity testing.

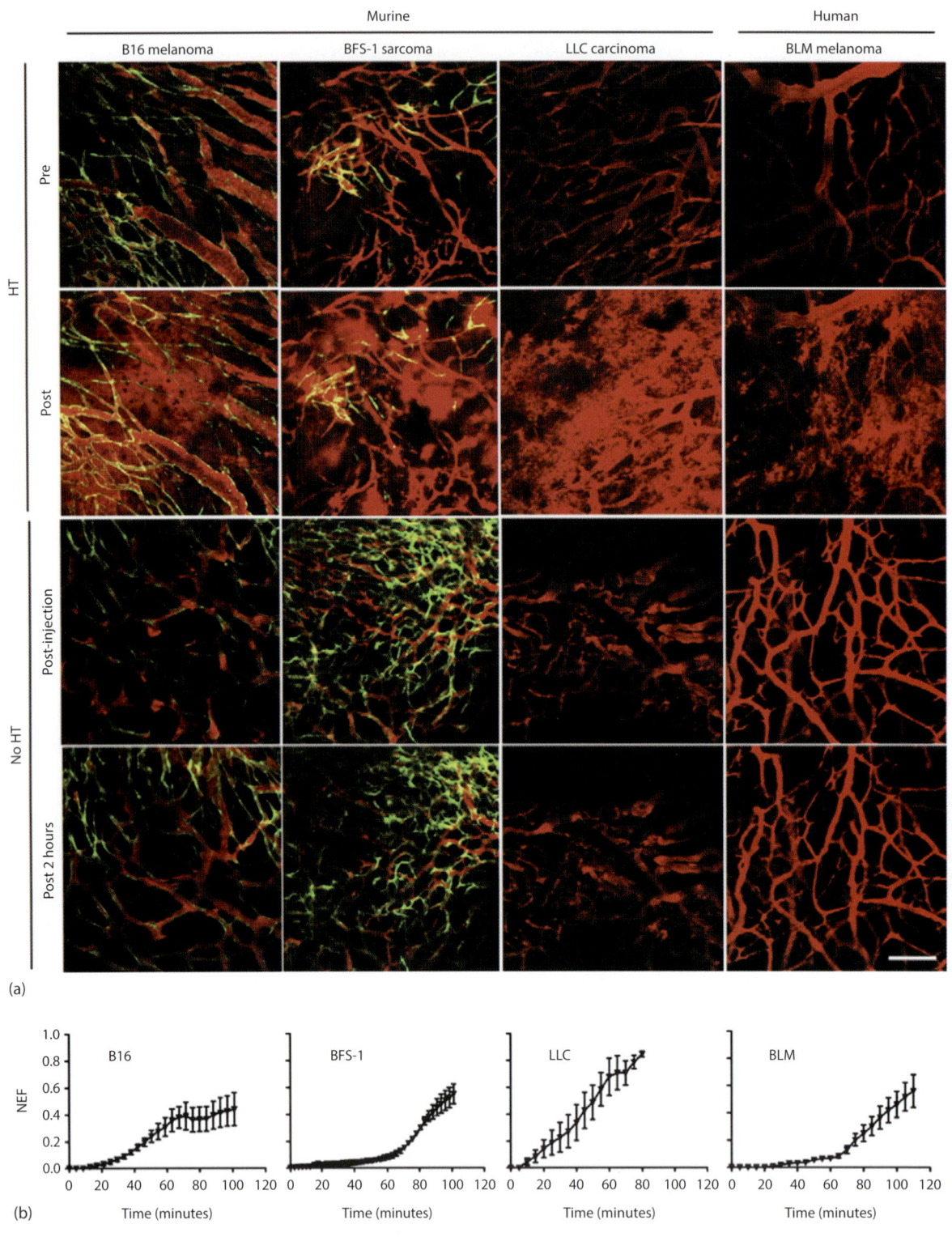

Figure 31.5 (a) Liposome (red) extravasation through tumor vasculature (green) with or without mild hyperthermia for 1 hour. **(b)** Quantification of liposome extravasation through tumor vasculature in four tumor models under local mild hyperthermia at 41°C for 1 hour. NEF, normalized extravascular fluorescence. Bar, 200 μm. (Reprinted from *J. Control. Release*, 167, Li, L., ten Hagen, T.L., Bolkestein, M., Gasselhuber, A., Yatvin, J., van Rhoon, G.C., Eggermont, A.M., Haemmerich, D., and Koning, G.A., Improved intratumoral nanoparticle extravasation and penetration by mild hyperthermia, 130–137, Copyright 2013, with permission from Elsevier.)

CONCLUSION

The premise of IP chemotherapy in the treatment of malignant diseases confined in the peritoneal cavity lies in the theoretical potential for increased exposure of the tumors to anticancer drugs and improved toxicity to local tumors [67]. Although the proof of concept has been demonstrated in several clinical trials, current practice of IP chemotherapy leaves plenty of room for improvement in delivery methods. Solutions, micro- or nanoparticles, implantable depots, and in situ cross-linkable hydrogels have been evaluated in the context of IP chemotherapy, achieving varying levels of success in preclinical studies. Due to the unique biological environment of the peritoneal cavity, several challenges remain to be overcome before the IP drug delivery systems can benefit patients to the full potential. Despite the needs and gravity of the challenges, there are surprisingly few players in the field of IP drug delivery systems. It means that this is a prime time to explore opportunities in IP drug delivery.

REFERENCES

1. Alberts DS, Liu PY, Hannigan EV, O'Toole R, Williams SD, Young JA et al. Intraperitoneal cisplatin plus intravenous cyclophosphamide versus intravenous cisplatin plus intravenous cyclophosphamide for stage III ovarian cancer. *New England Journal of Medicine*. 1996;335:1950–1955.
2. Anttila MA, Tammi RH, Tammi MI, Syrjanen KJ, Saarikoski SV, Kosma VM. High levels of stromal hyaluronan predict poor disease outcome in epithelial ovarian cancer. *Cancer Research*. 2000;60:150–155.
3. Armstrong, Deborah K. Relapsed ovarian cancer: Challenges and management strategies for a chronic disease. *Oncologist* 2002;7:20–28.
4. Armstrong DK, Bundy B, Wenzel L, Huang HQ, Baergen R, Lele S, Copeland LJ, Walker JL, Burger RA. Intraperitoneal cisplatin and paclitaxel in ovarian cancer. *New England Journal of Medicine*. 2006;354:34–43.
5. Bajaj G, Kim MR, Mohammed SI, Yeo Y. Hyaluronic acid-based hydrogel for regional delivery of paclitaxel to intraperitoneal tumors. *Journal of Controlled Release*. 2012;158:386–392.
6. Bouquet W, Ceelen W, Adriaens E, Almeida A, Quinten T, De Vos F, Pattyn P, Peeters M, Remon JP, Vervaet C. In vivo toxicity and bioavailability of Taxol and a paclitaxel/β-cyclodextrin formulation in a rat model during HIPEC. *Annals of Surgical Oncology*. 2010;17:2510–2517.
7. Bouquet W, Deleye S, Staelens S, De Smet L, Van Damme N, Debergh I, Ceelen WP, De Vos F, Remon JP, Vervaet C. Antitumour efficacy of two paclitaxel formulations for hyperthermic intraperitoneal chemotherapy (HIPEC) in an in vivo rat model. *Pharmaceutical Research*. 2011;28:1653–1660.
8. Bouquet W, Ceelen W, Fritzinger B, Pattyn P, Peeters M, Remon JP, Vervaet C. Paclitaxel/β-cyclodextrin complexes for hyperthermic peritoneal perfusion—Formulation and stability. *European Journal of Pharmaceutics and Biopharmaceutics*. 2007;66:391–397.
9. Bulpitt P, Aeschlimann D. New strategy for chemical modification of hyaluronic acid: Preparation of functionalized derivatives and their use in the formation of novel biocompatible hydrogels. *Journal of Biomedical Materials Research*. 1999;47:152–169.
10. Burns JW, Skinner K, Colt J, Sheidlin A, Bronson R, Yaacobi Y, Goldberg EP. Prevention of tissue injury and postsurgical adhesions by precoating tissues with hyaluronic acid solutions. *Journal of Surgical Research*. 1995;59:644–652.
11. Caicco MJ, Zahir T, Mothe AJ, Ballios BG, Kihm AJ, Tator CH, Shoichet MS. Characterization of hyaluronan–methylcellulose hydrogels for cell delivery to the injured spinal cord. *Journal of Biomedical Materials Research Part A*. 2013;101:1472–1477.
12. Cho H, Cho CS, Indig GL, Lavasanifar A, Vakili MR, Kwon GS. Polymeric micelles for apoptosis-targeted optical imaging of cancer and intraoperative surgical guidance. *PLOS ONE*. 2014;9:e89968.
13. Cho H, Indig GL, Weichert J, Shin H-C, Kwon GS. In vivo cancer imaging by poly(ethylene glycol)-b-poly(ε-caprolactone) micelles containing a near-infrared probe. *Nanomedicine*. 2012;8:228–236.
14. Cho H, Kwon GS. Polymeric micelles for neoadjuvant cancer therapy and tumor-primed optical imaging. *ACS Nano*. 2011;5:8721–8729.
15. Cho H, Kwon GS. Thermosensitive poly-(d,l-lactide-co-glycolide)-block-poly(ethylene glycol)-block-poly-(d,l-lactide-co-glycolide) hydrogels for multi-drug delivery. *Journal of Drug Targeting*. 2014;22:669–677.
16. Cho H, Lai TC, Kwon GS. Poly(ethylene glycol)-block-poly(epsilon-caprolactone) micelles for combination drug delivery: Evaluation of paclitaxel, cyclopamine and gossypol in intraperitoneal xenograft models of ovarian cancer. *Journal of Controlled Release*. 2013;166:1–9.
17. Choi IK, Strauss R, Richter M, Yun CO, Lieber A. Strategies to increase drug penetration in solid tumors. *Frontiers in Oncology*. 2013;3:193.
18. Cui HB, Ge H-E, Bai X-Y, Zhang W, Zhang Y-Y, Wang J, Li X, Xing L-P, Guo S-H, Wang Z-Y. Effect of neoadjuvant chemotherapy combined with hyperthermic intraperitoneal perfusion chemotherapy on advanced gastric cancer. *Experimental and Therapeutic Medicine*. 2014;7:1083–1088.

19. D'Addio SM, Prud'homme RK. Controlling drug nanoparticle formation by rapid precipitation. *Advanced Drug Delivery Reviews.* 2011;63:417–426.

20. De Smet L, Colin P, Ceelen W, Bracke M, Van Bocxlaer J, Remon J, Vervaet C. Development of a nanocrystalline paclitaxel formulation for HIPEC treatment. *Pharmaceutical Research.* 2012;29:2398–2406.

21. De Souza R, Zahedi P, Allen CJ, Piquette-Miller M. Biocompatibility of injectable chitosan–phospholipid implant systems. *Biomaterials* 2009;30:3818–3824.

22. De Souza R, Zahedi P, Moriyama EH, Allen CJ, Wilson BC, Piquette-Miller M. Continuous docetaxel chemotherapy improves therapeutic efficacy in murine models of ovarian cancer. *Molecular Cancer Therapeutics.* 2010;9:1820–1830.

23. Dedrick RL, Myers CE, Bungay PM, De Vita VT, Jr. Pharmacokinetic rationale for peritoneal drug administration in the treatment of ovarian cancer. *Cancer Treatment Reports.* 1978;62:1–11.

24. Deligkaris K, Tadele TS, Olthuis W, van den Berg A. Hydrogel-based devices for biomedical applications. *Sensors and Actuators B.* 2010;147:765–774.

25. Dufrane D, van Steenberghe M, Goebbels R-M, Saliez A, Guiot Y, Gianello P. The influence of implantation site on the biocompatibility and survival of alginate encapsulated pig islets in rats. *Biomaterials.* 2006;27:3201–3208.

26. Elstad NL, Fowers KD. OncoGel (ReGel/paclitaxel)—Clinical applications for a novel paclitaxel delivery system. *Advanced Drug Delivery Reviews.* 2009;61:785–794.

27. Emoto S, Yamaguchi H, Kamei T, Ishigami H, Suhara T, Suzuki Y, Ito T, Kitayama J, Watanabe T. Intraperitoneal administration of cisplatin via an in situ cross-linkable hyaluronic acid-based hydrogel for peritoneal dissemination of gastric cancer. *Surgery Today.* 2014;44:919–926.

28. Grant J, Blicker M, Piquette-Miller M, Allen C. Hybrid films from blends of chitosan and egg phosphatidylcholine for localized delivery of paclitaxel. *Journal of Pharmaceutical Sciences.* 2005;94:1512–1527.

29. Grant J, Lee H, Soo PL, Cho J, Piquette-Miller M, Allen C. Influence of molecular organization and interactions on drug release for an injectable polymer-lipid blend. *International Journal of Pharmaceutics.* 2008;360:83–90.

30. Grantab R, Sivananthan S, Tannock IF. The penetration of anticancer drugs through tumor tissue as a function of cellular adhesion and packing density of tumor cells. *Cancer Research.* 2006;66:1033–1039.

31. Hall JC, Heel KA, Papadimitriou JM, Platell C. The pathobiology of peritonitis. *Gastroenterology.* 1998;114:185–196.

32. Helm JH, Miura JT, Glenn JA, Marcus RK, Larrieux G, Jayakrishnan TT, Donahue AE, Gamblin TC, Turaga KK, Johnston FM. Cytoreductive surgery and hyperthermic intraperitoneal chemotherapy for malignant peritoneal mesothelioma: A systematic review and meta-analysis. *Annals of Surgical Oncology.* 2015;22:1686–1693.

33. Hiltunen EL, Anttila M, Kultti A, Ropponen K, Penttinen J, Yliskoski M, Kuronen AT, Juhola M, Tammi R, Tammi M, Kosma VM. Elevated hyaluronan concentration without hyaluronidase activation in malignant epithelial ovarian tumors. *Cancer Research.* 2002;62:6410–6413.

34. Hirano K, Hunt CA. Lymphatic transport of liposome-encapsulated agents: Effects of liposome size following intraperitoneal administration. *Journal of Pharmaceutical Sciences.* 1985;74:915–921.

35. Ho EA, Soo PL, Allen C, Piquette-Miller M. Impact of intraperitoneal, sustained delivery of paclitaxel on the expression of p-glycoprotein in ovarian tumors. *Journal of Controlled Release.* 2007;117:20–27.

36. Ho EA, Vassileva V, Allen C, Piquette-Miller M. In vitro and in vivo characterization of a novel biocompatible polymer–lipid implant system for the sustained delivery of paclitaxel. *Journal of Controlled Release.* 2005;104:181–191.

37. Ho WY, Yeap SK, Ho CL, Rahim RA, Alitheen NB. Development of multicellular tumor spheroid (MCTS) culture from breast cancer cell and a high throughput screening method using the MTT assay. *PLOS ONE.* 2012;7:e44640.

38. Hubbard SC, Burns JW. Effects of a hyaluronan-based membrane (Seprafilm) on intraperitoneally disseminated human colon cancer cell growth in a nude mouse model. *Diseases of the Colon & Rectum.* 2002;45:334–341; discussion 341–344.

39. Hudson SP, Langer R, Fink GR, Kohane DS. Injectable in situ cross-linking hydrogels for local antifungal therapy. *Biomaterials.* 2010;31:1444–1452.

40. Ihemelandu C, Bijelic L, Sugarbaker PH. Iterative cytoreductive surgery and hyperthermic intraperitoneal chemotherapy for recurrent or progressive diffuse malignant peritoneal mesothelioma: Clinicopathologic characteristics and survival outcome. *Annals of Surgical Oncology.* 2014;14:14.

41. Ilevbare GA, Liu H, Edgar KJ, Taylor LS. Impact of polymers on crystal growth rate of structurally diverse compounds from aqueous solution. *Molecular Pharmaceutics.* 2013;10:2381–2393.

42. Ishida T, Kiwada H. Alteration of tumor microenvironment for improved delivery and intratumor distribution of nanocarriers. *Biological and Pharmaceutical Bulletin.* 2013;36:692–697.

43. Ito T, Yeo Y, Highley CB, Bellas E, Benitez CA, Kohane DS. The prevention of peritoneal adhesions by in situ cross-linking hydrogels of hyaluronic acid and cellulose derivatives. *Biomaterials.* 2007;28:975–983.

44. Ito T, Yeo Y, Highley CB, Bellas E, Kohane DS. Dextran-based in situ cross-linked injectable hydrogels to prevent peritoneal adhesions. *Biomaterials.* 2007;28:3418–3426.

45. Jang SH, Wientjes MG, Au JL. Enhancement of paclitaxel delivery to solid tumors by apoptosis-inducing pretreatment: Effect of treatment schedule. *Journal of Pharmacology and Experimental Therapeutics.* 2001;296:1035–1042.

46. Jarvinen P, Ristimaki A, Kantonen J, Aronen M, Huuhtanen R, Jarvinen H, Lepisto A. Comparison of serial debulking and cytoreductive surgery with hyperthermic intraperitoneal chemotherapy in pseudomyxoma peritonei of appendiceal origin. *International Journal of Colorectal Disease.* 2014;29:999–1007.

47. Jeyachandran YL, Mielczarski E, Rai B, Mielczarski JA. Quantitative and qualitative evaluation of adsorption/desorption of bovine serum albumin on hydrophilic and hydrophobic surfaces. *Langmuir.* 2009;25:11614–11620.

48. Johansson A, Ganss R. Remodeling of tumor stroma and response to therapy. *Cancers.* 2012;4:340–353.

49. Kayastha S, Freedman AN, Piver MS, Mukkamalla J, Romero-Guittierez M, Werness BA. Expression of the hyaluronan receptor, CD44S, in epithelial ovarian cancer is an independent predictor of survival. *Clinical Cancer Research.* 1999;5:1073–1076.

50. Kimata K, Honma Y, Okayama M, Oguri K, Hozumi M, Suzuki S. Increased synthesis of hyaluronic acid by mouse mammary carcinoma cell variants with high metastatic potential. *Cancer Research.* 1983;43:1347–1354.

51. Kohane DS, Tse JY, Yeo Y, Padera R, Shubina M, Langer R. Biodegradable polymeric microspheres and nanospheres for drug delivery in the peritoneum. *Journal of Biomedical Materials Research Part A.* 2006;77:351–361.

52. Kohli AG, Kivimae S, Tiffany MR, Szoka FC. Improving the distribution of Doxil® in the tumor matrix by depletion of tumor hyaluronan. *Journal of Controlled Release.* 2014;20:105–114.

53. Krasner CN, Roche M, Horowitz NS, Supko JG, Lee SI, Oliva E. Case 11–2006. *New England Journal of Medicine.* 2006;354:1615–1625.

54. Kratz F, Elsadek B. Clinical impact of serum proteins on drug delivery. *Journal of Controlled Release.* 2012;161:429–445.

55. Kuh HJ, Jang SH, Wientjes MG, Weaver JR, Au JL. Determinants of paclitaxel penetration and accumulation in human solid tumor. *Journal of Pharmacology and Experimental Therapeutics.* 1999;290:871–880.

56. Kwon S, Park JH, Chung H, Kwon IC, Jeong SY, Kim I-S. Physicochemical characteristics of self-assembled nanoparticles based on glycol chitosan bearing 5 beta-cholanic acid. *Langmuir.* 2003;19:10188–10193.

57. Kyle AH, Huxham LA, Yeoman DM, Minchinton AI. Limited tissue penetration of taxanes: A mechanism for resistance in solid tumors. *Clinical Cancer Research.* 2007;13:2804–2810.

58. Leach RE, Burns JW, Dawe EJ, Smith Barbour MD, Diamond MP. Reduction of postsurgical adhesion formation in the rabbit uterine horn model with use of hyaluronate/carboxymethylcellulose gel. *Fertility and Sterility.* 1998;69:415–418.

59. Lee JH, Na K, Song SC, Lee J, Kuh HJ. The distribution and retention of paclitaxel and doxorubicin in multicellular layer cultures. *Oncology Reports.* 2012;27:995–1002.

60. Li L, ten Hagen TL, Bolkestein M, Gasselhuber A, Yatvin J, van Rhoon GC, Eggermont AM, Haemmerich D, Koning GA. Improved intratumoral nanoparticle extravasation and penetration by mild hyperthermia. *Journal of Controlled Release.* 2013;167:130–137.

61. Lim SP, Cho J, Grant J, Ho E, Piquette-Miller M, Allen C. Drug release mechanism of paclitaxel from a chitosan–lipid implant system: Effect of swelling, degradation and morphology. *European Journal of Pharmaceutics and Biopharmaceutics.* 2008;69:149–157.

62. Lu Y, Wang ZH, Li T, McNally H, Park K, Sturek M. Development and evaluation of transferrin-stabilized paclitaxel nanocrystal formulation. *Journal of Controlled Release.* 2014;176:76–85.

63. Lu Z, Tsai M, Lu D, Wang J, Wientjes MG, Au JLS. Tumor-penetrating microparticles for intraperitoneal therapy of ovarian cancer. *Journal of Pharmacology and Experimental Therapeutics.* 2008;327:673–682.

64. Marchettini P, Stuart AO, Mohamed F, Yoo D, Sugarbaker PH. Docetaxel: pharmacokinetics and tissue levels after intraperitoneal and intravenous administration in a rat model. *Cancer Chemotherapy and Pharmacology.* 2002;49:499–503.

65. Markman M. Intraperitoneal drug delivery of antineoplastics. *Drugs.* 2001;61:1057–1065.

66. Markman M, Rowinsky E, Hakes T, Reichman B, Jones W, Lewis JL, Jr. et al. Phase I trial of intraperitoneal taxol: A Gynecologic Oncology Group study. *Journal of Clinical Oncology.* 1992;10:1485–1491.

67. Markman M. Intraperitoneal antineoplastic drug delivery: Rationale and results. *The Lancet Oncology.* 2003;4:277–283.

68. Markman M, Bundy BN, Alberts DS, Fowler JM, Clark-Pearson DL, Carson LF, Wadler S, Sickel J. Phase III trial of standard-dose intravenous cisplatin plus paclitaxel versus moderately high-dose carboplatin followed by intravenous paclitaxel and intraperitoneal cisplatin in small-volume stage III ovarian carcinoma: An intergroup study of the Gynecologic Oncology Group, Southwestern Oncology Group, and Eastern Cooperative Oncology Group. *Journal of Clinical Oncology.* 2001;19:1001–1007.

69. McBride WH, Bard JB. Hyaluronidase-sensitive halos around adherent cells. Their role in blocking lymphocyte-mediated cytolysis. *Journal of Experimental Medicine.* 1979;149:507–515.

70. Middleton JC, Tipton AJ. Synthetic biodegradable polymers as orthopedic devices. *Biomaterials.* 2000;21:2335–2346.

71. Minchinton AI, Tannock IF. Drug penetration in solid tumours. *Nature Reviews Cancer.* 2006;6:583–592.

72. Mohamed F, Marchettini P, Stuart OA, Sugarbaker PH. Pharmacokinetics and tissue distribution of intraperitoneal paclitaxel with different carrier solutions. *Cancer Chemotherapy and Pharmacology.* 2003;52:405–410.

73. Mohamed F, Stuart OA, Sugarbaker PH. Pharmacokinetics and tissue distribution of intraperitoneal docetaxel with different carrier solutions. *Journal of Surgical Research.* 2003;113:114–120.

74. NCI. 2006. NCI Clinical announcement on intraperitoneal therapy for ovarian cancer. http://ctep.cancer.gov/highlights/docs/clin_annc_010506.pdf. Accessed on September 9, 2014.

75. Nemes KB, Abermann M, Bojti E, Grezal G, Al-Behaisi S, Klebovich I. Oral, intraperitoneal and intravenous pharmacokinetics of deramciclane and its *N*-desmethyl metabolite in the rat. *Journal of Pharmacy and Pharmacology.* 2000;52:47–51.

76. Nicholson KM, Bibby MC, Phillips RM. Influence of drug exposure parameters on the activity of paclitaxel in multicellular spheroids. *European Journal of Cancer.* 1997;33:1291–1298.

77. Ozols RF, Bundy BN, Greer BE, Fowler JM, Clarke-Pearson D, Burger RA, Mannel RS, DeGeest K, Hartenbach EM, Baergen R. Phase III trial of carboplatin and paclitaxel compared with cisplatin and paclitaxel in patients with optimally resected stage III ovarian cancer: A Gynecologic Oncology Group Study. *Journal of Clinical Oncology.* 2003;21:3194–3200.

78. Panchagnula R. Pharmaceutical aspects of paclitaxel. *International Journal of Pharmaceutics.* 1998;172:1–15.

79. Park SN, Jang HJ, Choi YS, Cha JM, Son SY, Han SH, Kim JH, Lee WJ, Suh H. Preparation and characterization of biodegradable anti-adhesive membrane for peritoneal wound healing. *Journal of Materials Science. Materials in Medicine.* 2007;18:475–482.

80. Patel KJ, Lee C, Tan Q, Tannock IF. Use of the proton pump inhibitor pantoprazole to modify the distribution and activity of doxorubicin: A potential strategy to improve the therapy of solid tumors. *Clinical Cancer Research.* 2013;19:6766–6776.

81. Patenaude M, Hoare T. Injectable, mixed natural-synthetic polymer hydrogels with modular properties. *Biomacromolecules.* 2012;13:369–378.

82. Patravale VB, Date AA, Kulkarni RM. Nanosuspensions: A promising drug delivery strategy. *Journal of Pharmacy and Pharmacology.* 2004;56:827–840.

83. Picaud L, Thibault B, Mery E, Ouali M, Martinez A, Delord J-P, Couderc B, Ferron G. Evaluation of the effects of hyaluronic acid-carboxymethyl cellulose barrier on ovarian tumor progression. *Journal of Ovarian Research.* 2014;7:40.

84. Poveda A, Salazar R, Campo JM, Mendiola C, Cassinello J, Ojeda B, Arranz JA, Oaknin A, García-Foncillas J, Rubio MJ, Martín AG. Update in the management of ovarian and cervical carcinoma. *Clinical and Translational Oncology.* 2007;9:443–451.

85. Prasitsilp M, Jenwithisuk R, Kongsuwan K, Damrongchai N, Watts P. Cellular responses to chitosan in vitro: The importance of deacetylation. *Journal of Materials Science. Materials in Medicine.* 2000;11:773–778.

86. Risbud M, Bhonde M, Bhonde R. Chitosan-polyvinyl pyrrolidone hydrogel does not activate macrophages: Potentials for transplantation applications. *Cell Transplantation.* 2001;10:195–202.

87. Rodgers KE, Johns DB, Girgis W, Campeau J, diZerega GS. Reduction of adhesion formation with hyaluronic acid after peritoneal surgery in rabbits. *Fertility and Sterility* 1997;67:553–558.

88. Safra T, Grisaru D, Inbar M, Abu-Abeid S, Dayan D, Matceyevsky D, Weizman A, Klausner JM. Cytoreduction surgery with hyperthermic intraperitoneal chemotherapy in recurrent ovarian cancer improves progression-free survival, especially in BRCA-positive patients—A case-control study. *Journal of Surgical Oncology.* 2014;24:23688.

89. Saggar JK, Tannock IF. Activity of the hypoxia-activated pro-drug TH-302 in hypoxic and perivascular regions of solid tumors and its potential to enhance therapeutic effects of chemotherapy. *International Journal of Cancer.* 2014;134:2726–2734.

90. Saggar JK, Yu M, Tan Q, Tannock IF. The tumor microenvironment and strategies to improve drug distribution. *Frontiers in Oncology.* 2013;3:154.

91. Sagnella SM, Duong H, MacMillan A, Boyer C, Whan R, McCarroll JA, Davis TP, Kavallaris M. Dextran-based doxorubicin nanocarriers with improved tumor penetration. *Biomacromolecules.* 2014;15:262–275.

92. Sammartino P, Sibio S, Biacchi D, Cardi M, Mingazzini P, Rosati MS, Cornali T, Sollazzo B, Atta JM, Di Giorgio A. Long-term results after proactive management for locoregional control in patients with colonic cancer at high risk of peritoneal metastases. *International Journal of Colorectal Disease.* 2014;29:1081–1089.

93. Santovena A, Farina JB, Llabres M, Zhu Y, Dannies P. Pharmacokinetics analysis of sustained release hGH biodegradable implantable tablets using a mouse model of human ovarian cancer. *International Journal of Pharmaceutics*. 2010;388:175–180.

94. Seo JH, Dembereldorj U, Park J, Kim M, Kim S, Joo S-W. Facile internalization of paclitaxel on titania nanoparticles in human lung carcinoma cells after adsorption of serum proteins. *Journal of Nanoparticle Research*. 2012;14:1–8.

95. Sherwood L. *Human Physiology: From Cells to Systems*, Belmont, CA: Thomson/Brooks/Cole, 2007.

96. Shin HC, Cho H, Lai TC, Kozak KR, Kolesar JM, Kwon GS. Pharmacokinetic study of 3-in-1 poly(ethylene glycol)-block-poly(D, L-lactic acid) micelles carrying paclitaxel, 17-allylamino-17-demethoxygeldanamycin, and rapamycin. *Journal of Controlled Release*. 2012;163:93–99.

97. Suidan RS, St Clair CM, Lee SJ, Barlin JN, Roche KCL, Tanner EJ, Sonoda Y, Barakat RR, Zivanovic O, Chi DS. A comparison of primary intraperitoneal chemotherapy to consolidation intraperitoneal chemotherapy in optimally resected advanced ovarian cancer. *Gynecologic Oncology*. 2014;17:468–472.

98. Sun B, Yeo Y. Nanocrystals for the parenteral delivery of poorly water-soluble drugs. *Current Opinion in Solid State & Materials Science*. 2012;16(6):295–301.

99. Ta Thu H, Dass CR, Dunstan DE. Injectable chitosan hydrogels for localised cancer therapy. *Journal of Controlled Release*. 2008;126:205–216.

100. Tan B, Wang JH, Wu QD, Kirwan WO, Redmond HP. Sodium hyaluronate enhances colorectal tumour cell metastatic potential in vitro and in vivo. *British Journal of Surgery*. 2001;88:246–250.

101. Tang Q, Wang Y, Huang R, You Q, Wang G, Chen Y, Jiang Z, Liu Z, Yu L, Muhammad S, Wang X. Preparation of anti-tumor nanoparticle and its inhibition to peritoneal dissemination of colon cancer. *PLOS ONE*. 2014;9:e98455.

102. Tannock IF, Lee CM, Tunggal JK, Cowan DS, Egorin MJ. Limited penetration of anticancer drugs through tumor tissue: A potential cause of resistance of solid tumors to chemotherapy. *Clinical Cancer Research*. 2002;8:878–884.

103. Teo MC, Tan GHC, Lim C, Chia CS, Tham CK, Soo KC. Colorectal peritoneal carcinomatosis treated with cytoreductive surgery and hyperthermic intraperitoneal chemotherapy: The experience of a tertiary asian center. *Asian Journal of Surgery*. 2014;21:1–9.

104. Torosean S, Flynn B, Axelsson J, Gunn J, Samkoe KS, Hasan T, Doyley MM, Pogue BW. Nanoparticle uptake in tumors is mediated by the interplay of vascular and collagen density with interstitial pressure. *Nanomedicine*. 2013;9:151–158.

105. Trissel LA. Pharmaceutical properties of paclitaxel and their effects on preparation and administration. *Pharmacotherapy*. 1997;17:133S–139S.

106. Tsai M, Lu Z, Wang J, Yeh T-K, Wientjes MG, Au JLS. Effects of carrier on disposition and antitumor activity of intraperitoneal paclitaxel. *Pharmaceutical Research*. 2007;24:1691–1701.

107. Turley EA, Tretiak M. Glycosaminoglycan production by murine melanoma variants in vivo and in vitro. *Cancer Research*. 1985;45:5098–5105.

108. Van Eerdenbrugh B, Van den Mooter G, Augustijns P. Top-down production of drug nanocrystals: Nanosuspension stabilization, miniaturization and transformation into solid products. *International Journal of Pharmaceutics*. 2008;364:64–75.

109. Vassileva V, Moriyama EH, De Souza R, Grant J, Allen CJ, Wilson BC, Piquette-Miller M. Efficacy assessment of sustained intraperitoneal paclitaxel therapy in a murine model of ovarian cancer using bioluminescent imaging. *British Journal of Cancer*. 2008;99:2037–2043.

110. Vassileva V, Allen CJ, Piquette-Miller M. Effects of sustained and intermittent paclitaxel therapy on tumor repopulation in ovarian cancer. *Molecular Cancer Therapeutics*. 2008;7:630–637.

111. Vassileva V, Grant J, De Souza R, Allen C, Piquette-Miller M. Novel biocompatible intraperitoneal drug delivery system increases tolerability and therapeutic efficacy of paclitaxel in a human ovarian cancer xenograft model. *Cancer Chemotherapy and Pharmacology*. 2007;60:907–914.

112. Wang F, Saidel GM, Gao J. A mechanistic model of controlled drug release from polymer millirods: Effects of excipients and complex binding. *Journal of Controlled Release*. 2007;119:111–120.

113. Wang J, Lu Z, Yeung BZ, Wientjes MG, Cole DJ, Au JLS. Tumor priming enhances siRNA delivery and transfection in intraperitoneal tumors. *Journal of Controlled Release*. 2014;178:79–85.

114. Watson MS. *Oxford Handbook of Palliative Care*, New York: Oxford University Press, 2009.

115. Wenzel LB, Huang HQ, Armstrong DK, Walker JL, Cella D. Health-related quality of life during and after intraperitoneal versus intravenous chemotherapy for optimally debulked ovarian cancer: A Gynecologic Oncology Group Study. *Journal of Clinical Oncology*. 2007;25:437–443.

116. Wu L, Ding J. In vitro degradation of three-dimensional porous poly(d,l-lactide-co-glycolide) scaffolds for tissue engineering. *Biomaterials*. 2004;25:5821–5830.

117. Yeo Y, Ito T, Bellas E, Highley CB, Marini R, Kohane DS. In situ cross-linkable hyaluronan hydrogels containing polymeric nanoparticles for preventing postsurgical adhesions. *Annals of Surgery*. 2007;245:819–824.

118. Yeo Y, Adil M, Bellas E, Astashkina A, Chaudhary N, Kohane DS. Prevention of peritoneal adhesions with an in situ cross-linkable hyaluronan hydrogel delivering budesonide. *Journal of Controlled Release.* 2007;120:178–185.

119. Yeo Y, Bellas E, Highley CB, Langer R, Kohane DS. Peritoneal adhesion prevention with an in situ cross-linkable hyaluronan gel containing tissue-type plasminogen activator in a rabbit repeated-injury model. *Biomaterials.* 2007;28:3704–3713.

120. Yeo Y, Burdick JA, Highley CB, Marini R, Langer R, Kohane DS. Peritoneal application of chitosan and UV-cross-linkable chitosan. *Journal of Biomedical Materials Research Part A.* 2006;78A:668–675.

121. Yeo Y, Highley CB, Bellas E, Ito T, Marini R, Langer R, Kohane DS. In situ cross-linkable hyaluronic acid hydrogels prevent post-operative abdominal adhesions in a rabbit model. *Biomaterials.* 2006;27:4698–4705.

122. Yeo Y, Kohane DS. Polymers in the prevention of peritoneal adhesions. *European Journal of Pharmaceutics and Biopharmaceutics.* 2008;68:57–66.

123. Zahedi P, De Souza R, Huynh L, Piquette-Miller M, Allen C. Combination drug delivery strategy for the treatment of multidrug resistant ovarian cancer. *Molecular Pharmaceutics.* 2010;8:260–269.

124. Zahedi P, De Souza R, Piquette-Miller M, Allen C. Chitosan–phospholipid blend for sustained and localized delivery of docetaxel to the peritoneal cavity. *International Journal of Pharmaceutics.* 2009;377:76–84.

125. Zahedi P, Stewart J, De Souza R, Piquette-Miller M, Allen C. An injectable depot system for sustained intraperitoneal chemotherapy of ovarian cancer results in favorable drug distribution at the whole body, peritoneal and intratumoral levels. *Journal of Controlled Release.* 2012;158:379–385.

126. Zeimet AG, Reimer D, Radl AC, Reinthaller A, Schauer C, Petru E, Concin N, Braun S, Marth C. Pros and cons of intraperitoneal chemotherapy in the treatment of epithelial ovarian cancer. *Anticancer Research.* 2009;29:2803–2808.

127. Zentner GM, Rathi R, Shih C, McRea JC, Seo M-H, Oh H, Rhee BG, Mestecky J, Moldoveanu Z, Morgan M, Weitman S. Biodegradable block copolymers for delivery of proteins and water-insoluble drugs. *Journal of Controlled Release.* 2001;72:203–215.

128. Zhang L, Underhill CB, Chen L. Hyaluronan on the surface of tumor cells is correlated with metastatic behavior. *Cancer Research.* 1995;55:428–433.

32

Intraperitoneal nonviral nucleic acid delivery in the treatment of peritoneal cancer

GEORGE R. DAKWAR, STEFAAN S.C. DE SMEDT, AND KATRIEN REMAUT

INTRODUCTION

Peritoneal carcinomatosis is a secondary cancer in the peritoneal cavity that originates from gynecological or nongynecological organs. Due to the late stage of discovery, these peritoneal metastases are often widely spread in the peritoneal cavity and difficult to treat. Current treatment is based on cytoreductive surgery followed by intravenous (IV) administration of conventional chemotherapeutic agents. However, complete surgical removal is often not possible. Also, remaining tumor cells can spread and lead to the formation of new metastasis. Therefore, the majority of patients unfortunately develop disease recurrence and relapse. Intraperitoneal (IP) administration has shown several advantages over the IV one, due to the ability to inject higher concentrations of anticancer agents into the site of action (i.e., the peritoneal cavity), with limited systemic side effects [10]. Also here, however, the IP administration of cytostatics suffers from the fact that the action of the currently used cytostatics is not tumor-specific and not long lasting.

The rapid progress that has been made during the last 20 years in medical sciences led to the development of new strategies in the treatment of cancer [30,72]. Gene therapy, for example, enables to specifically express or silence genes, thereby minimizing side effects that are often observed with the conventional chemotherapy. Given this, IP gene therapy is an attractive strategy to target tumors within the peritoneal cavity, taking advantage of the direct administration to the tumor site and also the selectivity that could be achieved in gene targeting. Therefore, IP nucleic acid delivery could prove to be useful to specifically target the metastases in the peritoneum. In this chapter we will provide a brief introduction on the delivery of nucleic acids into tumor cells confined within the peritoneal cavity, with a focus on the mechanism of action of lipidic and polymeric carriers that have been administered IP. It should be noted that none of these delivery systems has received FDA approval yet.

DELIVERY OF NUCLEIC ACIDS FOR THE TREATMENT OF PERITONEAL CARCINOMATOSIS

Plasmid DNA

Plasmid DNA (pDNA) is a powerful tool to induce the expression of proteins and offers great opportunities for cancer treatment. Plasmids are circular, double-stranded DNA molecules that can be engineered to carry any gene of interest and can range between 1 and 1000 kilo base pair (kbp) in size. The rationale behind using DNA as a therapeutic agent is to take advantage of the body's cell machinery to produce the encoded proteins at the site of action, thereby overcoming the need to produce and repeatedly administer highly purified proteins [7]. Generally speaking, the encoded proteins that result from the expression of a therapeutic gene can act either on intracellular or extracellular targets when the formed proteins are released outside the cells and act on neighboring or distant cells [70]. In most applications using nonviral gene delivery, the resulting gene expression is transient (e.g., limited in function of time). Alternatively, stable long-lasting gene expression can be obtained when a mutated gene is replaced with the wild-type one.

To ensure biological activity of DNA-based therapeutics, the genetic material should enter the nucleus of the target cell and later on be transcribed into messenger RNA (mRNA) and translated into active protein. There are however several barriers for the delivery of DNA into cells, which will be discussed later in this chapter.

DNA FOR CANCER THERAPY

The use of DNA for cancer therapy can be accomplished by targeting tumor cells directly or indirectly. Direct targeting includes the expression of tumor suppressors and the delivery of suicide genes. Tumor suppressor genes control the cell division rate of normal cells, preventing them to divide excessively and form tumor tissue. Cancer cells carrying mutated tumor suppression genes can be treated by the DNA-induced expression of correct tumor suppressor genes, resulting in cell cycle arrest or death. The most common tumor suppressors are P53, PTEN, ARF, and APC [52,57,69,88]. Also the delivery of suicide genes is being used to specifically kill cancer cells. Once delivered into the nucleus of cancer cells, suicide genes encode for enzymes that allow to metabolize a prodrug into a cytotoxin that is capable of diffusing into neighboring cells. Suicide genes can also directly encode for toxins, such as the diphtheria toxin A (DT-A), which inhibits protein synthesis thereby causing cell death. Indirect strategies include immunotherapy and chemoprotection. Chemoprotection is a process by which bone marrow cells are infected with viruses that protect them from the toxic effects of chemotherapy [49]. Immunotherapy aims to activate a local and systemic immune response against cancer cells and is thought to be the least toxic approach in cancer therapy [50,83]. As an example for immunotherapy, genes encoding for anti-inflammatory cytokines can be incorporated into pDNA and delivered into cells to enhance the immune response against cancer cells [16]. Alternatively, dendritic cells can be challenged with tumor-specific antigens, after which they activate the immune system to specifically target the tumor cells where the antigens were derived from. Finally, pDNA can also be used as a precursor to form short hairpin RNA (shRNAs) that can be processed by the cell to small interfering RNA (siRNA). Unlike pDNA, siRNA is used to downregulate the expression of the target proteins in a process called RNA interference (RNAi) as will be discussed in the following text.

RNAi

In 1998, Fire and Mello reported the discovery of double-stranded RNA (dsRNA) that is capable to knockdown gene activity [20]. siRNA is a 21–23-nucleotide dsRNA that binds to a complementary mRNA sequence in the cytoplasm of cells, causing degradation of the desired mRNA and consequently a decrease in the expression of the corresponding protein [17]. In principle, siRNA can be designed to be complementary for any mRNA sequence. For cancer applications, genes involved in apoptotic and proliferative pathways are subject to silencing in order to treat tumors that are resistant to chemotherapy or nonresectable tumors [64]. Currently, several RNAi-based drugs are in clinical trials, including treatments against solid tumors and advanced cancer [37]. As mentioned earlier, another type of RNAi uses shRNAs that are synthesized in living cells after the delivery of plasmids or viral or bacterial vectors into cells encoding for these shRNAs [63]. shRNAs consist of two complementary 19–22 (bp) RNA sequences linked by a short loop, which is similar in structure to the natural microRNA (miRNA), and are processed intracellular into functional siRNA.

RNAi FOR CANCER THERAPY

The last two decades have witnessed a revolution in genomics and proteomics during which tens of molecular pathways involved in proliferation of cancer cells were identified. These include immune evasion, angiogenesis, and metastasis. Theoretically, knockdown of every gene should be possible; however, for successful and specific gene knockdown, it is important to screen targets that are overexpressed by cancer cells. As we will discuss later in the section "Current in vivo use of plasmid DNA for IP carcinomatosis," RNAi opens the opportunity for designing personalized medicine [29], since it can influence the expression or knockdown of a specific gene in a particular cancer patient. To date, the most common RNAi targets that are related to cancer are the multidrug resistance (MDR) proteins [5]. MDR is a situation in which cancer cells develop resistance against anticancer drugs by several mechanisms such as decreased drug uptake, increased drug efflux, and induction of DNA repair mechanisms. For instance, P-glycoprotein (P-gp) is a transporter protein encoded by the MDR-1 gene that pumps drugs into the extracellular space before reaching the target. It has been shown that P-gp is overexpressed in several cancer types following chemotherapeutic treatment, making it an attractive target for RNAi [44]. Another common example of MDR-encoded protein is survivin, a member of the inhibitor of apoptosis (IAP) protein family, since it is upregulated in solid tumors and has been involved with drug resistance [2,79]. Recently, codelivery of conventional anticancer chemotherapeutics and siRNA has received tremendous attention to overcome cancer resistance [12].

Mechanisms of DNA and RNAi

The aim of DNA therapy is to bring wild-type genes into the nucleus of cells or to correct mutated genes. The second requires a process called homologous recombination by which new exogenously administered DNA sequences can be introduced into the genome of a living cell [9]. Homologous recombination is considered a rare event;

therefore, most of the DNA therapies are based on transient delivery of the DNA sequence into the nucleus. Once in the nucleus, the DNA can be transcribed into mRNA, which relocates to the cytoplasm where it is translated into the corresponding proteins (Figure 32.1b2, step 8). The extent by which the delivered gene is expressed depends on the number of DNA copies being transcribed. It has been suggested that the minimum number of copies required to measure gene expression ranges from 75 to 4000 [11,28]. For RNAi medicines, however, the site of action is the cytoplasm of the cell. Briefly, in the cytoplasm of the cell, a protein complex known as RNA-induced silencing complex (RISC) mediates the cleavage of one RNA strand, while the other guide strand is involved in degrading the targeted mRNA (Figure 32.1b1, steps 5–7). Double-stranded siRNAs can be produced endogenously (by cells) or chemically synthesized and applied. Exogenously administered RNA can either interact with the RISC complex immediately as double strand or after cleavage by an enzyme known as RNAse III Dicer [14]. The mechanism by which shRNA is processed within the cells is very similar to that of siRNA. Shortly, after its transcription in the nucleus, it is exported to the cytosol where it interacts with Dicer, which in turn converts shRNA into siRNA and binds to the RISC complex as described earlier [55].

Naked nucleic acids suffer from instability and are prone to enzymatic degradation in the biological environment. Moreover, naked nucleic acids are rapidly excreted by kidney filtration and are not able to interact with biological membranes due to their anionic charge. Hence, naked nucleic acids suffer from low transfection efficiency [48,75] and are complexed with viral or nonviral carriers to optimize their cellular delivery, as discussed in the following text.

Viral and nonviral vectors for nucleic acids delivery

Viruses are infectious agents that can internalize into the host cell and take advantage of its cellular machinery to replicate its own genetic material and to infect other cells [38]. Different viruses have been exploited to deliver therapeutic DNA and siRNA into cells [78,80]. Importantly, viruses are genetically modified before their use in vivo, by removing the pathogenic part and replacing it with the desired therapeutic nucleic acid [8], without changing its structural properties and ability to infect other cells [38]. The nonpathogenic virus is then called a viral vector and can be used for in vivo transfection. Despite their high transfection efficiency [78], several limitations have been reported when viral vectors were used. First of all, acute immune response and toxicity continue to be a major concern for viral vectors [60]. Also, viral vectors are generally produced in small quantities and scaling up the process would come with a large cost [59]. Finally, due to size limitations of the viral vectors, not all genes can be carried by the virus [59].

The drawbacks of viral vectors made scientists think of other safer and possibly cheaper alternatives. Over the past

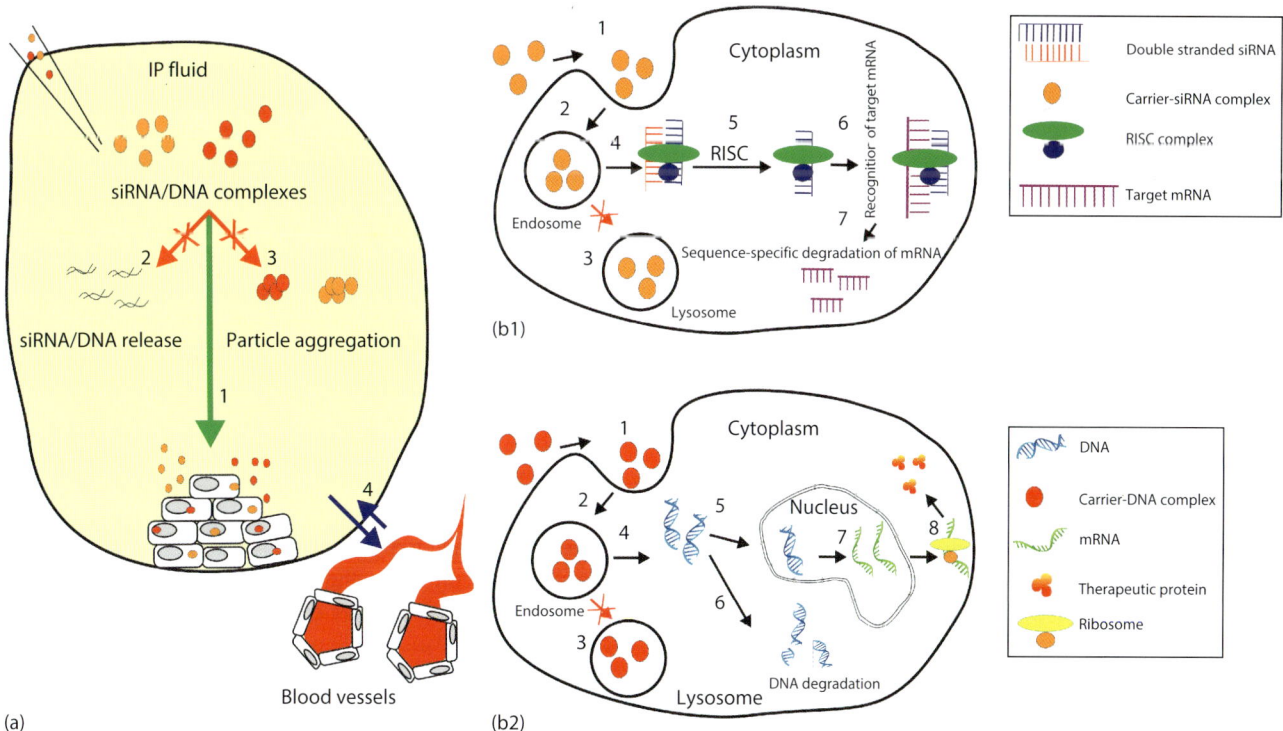

Figure 32.1 Schematic overview of the different barriers in nonviral nucleic acid delivery: (a) IP extracellular barriers and (b) intracellular barriers for (1) siRNA and (2) plasmid DNA.

decade, nonviral vectors have been widely investigated for DNA and siRNA delivery into cells both in vitro and in vivo. In this respect, nonviral vectors possess several advantages over their viral counterparts. They are relatively safe and do not induce a strong immune response. Also, they can be more easily prepared in large quantities [1,23]. Nevertheless, the application of nonviral nucleic acid delivery systems is still limited due to low cellular uptake and poor transfection efficiency [60].

Most nonviral nucleic acid delivery systems are based on polymeric or lipidic nanosized carriers. Nanotechnology in general and nano-based drug delivery in particular have played a vital role in cancer therapy [18,68,73]. The ultimate goal for nonviral nucleic acid delivery systems is to obtain site-specific delivery of therapeutic nucleic acids and release these nucleic acids in a controlled fashion, in order to maximize the treatment efficacy while minimizing side effects [43,53]. It has been shown that complexation or encapsulation of nucleic acids with lipid-based or polymer-based nanoparticles significantly enhances their uptake into tumor cells. In the majority of the cases, negatively charged nucleic acids are added to positively charged lipid or polymer particles, taking advantage of the electrostatic interactions to form liposome/nucleic acid complexes (lipoplexes) or polymer/nucleic acid complexes (polyplexes). These complexes generally have a positive charge and a size range between 80 and 600 nm.

Barriers for IP DNA and siRNA delivery

Clinical applications of nonviral DNA and siRNA carriers are still hampered by inefficient in vivo delivery. To obtain the desired therapeutic effect of nucleic acids, several extra- and intracellular barriers should be overcome, which will largely depend on the administration route of the complexes.

For efficacious IP nucleic acid delivery, nonviral vectors should meet several requirements on both the extracellular (Figure 32.1a) and intracellular (Figure 32.1b1 and b2) level. Following IP administration, nonviral vectors are present in the peritoneal fluid. Hence, they should remain stable in this IP fluid until the target cells are reached (Figure 32.1a, step 1). Nonviral vectors can however interact with components of the peritoneal fluid, especially proteins. This potentially leads to (1) aggregation of the vectors (Figure 32.1a, step 3) and (2) premature release of the cargo (i.e., nucleic acid) (Figure 32.1a, step 2), which results in the loss of transfection efficiency [13]. In this regard, the stability of different nanosized particles should be studied in the extracellular fluids they will reside in, namely, the peritoneal fluid in the case of IP delivery [13]. Also, the ascites fluid is being investigated to understand and develop different clinical strategies for the treatment of peritoneal cancer [39]. Ideally, nonviral vectors should protect nucleic acids from interaction with different molecules in the biological fluids without inducing immune responses [6]. Extracellular stability is a prerequisite to ensure interaction

of the nonviral vectors with biological membranes of cells, which is essential toward reaching the site of action and to ensure good intracellular uptake. To enhance extracellular stability, carriers are often grafted with polyethylene glycol (PEG) chains to minimize binding of proteins, thereby preventing aggregation and recognition by the mononuclear phagocyte system. However, PEGylation has several disadvantages, especially on the intracellular level. It is known that the PEG chains can limit the interaction of carriers with intracellular organelles, such as the endosomal membrane. This on its turn prevents or seriously lowers endosomal escape of the carriers and thus the amount of nucleic acids that can be successfully delivered [40]. Also, we have shown that PEGylation may interfere with the electrostatic interactions formed between the negatively charged nucleic acid and the positively charged carrier, resulting in a more rapid premature release of the cargo in the biological fluid [13]. It is therefore clear that a good balance should be reached between extracellular stability of the carriers and the ability to still efficiently deliver the nucleic acids in the intracellular environment. Also, carriers intended for IP delivery should remain in the peritoneum for a sufficiently long time, without relocation to the blood stream (Figure 32.1a, step 4). Which physicochemical properties are best to prevent leakage from the nanocarriers through the peritoneal/plasma barrier remains to be elucidated.

Once a carrier has reached its target cell, it should enter the cells, which mostly occurs through endocytosis (Figure 32.1b1 and b2, step 1). Following uptake by cells via endocytosis, delivery vectors are present in the early endosome (Figure 32.1b1 and b2, step 2), which mature to late endosome and eventually deliver their content to lysosomes. To avoid degradation in the lysosomal compartment (Figure 32.1b1 and b2, step 3), the delivery vector needs to destabilize the endosomal membrane, leading to the release of the cargo into the cytoplasm of the cell, in a process that is known as endosomal escape (Figure 32.1b1 and b2, step 4) [84]. It is often argued that endosomal escape is the most critical step in nucleic acid delivery. In the case of siRNA delivery, the cytoplasm is the intracellular site where the RISC machinery can be engaged (Figure 32.1b1, step 5) and eventually recognize the target mRNA leading to its degradation (Figure 32.1b1, steps 6 and 7). DNA vectors, however, have to efficiently migrate through the cytoplasm of the cell toward the nucleus in addition to the endosomal escape (Figure 32.1b2, step 5). Then, crossing the nuclear membrane is required for DNA to be transcribed (Figure 32.1b2, step 7) and translated (Figure 32.1b2, step 8) into the encoded proteins [15,46]. It is generally accepted that the nuclear membrane is one of the most difficult intracellular barriers to overcome for DNA delivery. Also, degradation of DNA in the cytoplasm of the cells should be avoided (Figure 32.1b2, step 6).

Despite the progress that has been made over the last decade in overcoming the aforementioned extracellular and intracellular challenges in nonviral nucleic acid delivery, their translation into clinical oncology is still premature.

In the following section, we will review the nonviral DNA and siRNA delivery systems that were investigated in vivo for their ability to target tumors confined within the peritoneal cavity following IP administration up to date.

CURRENT IN VIVO USE OF PLASMID DNA FOR IP CARCINOMATOSIS

Table 32.1 summarizes the current in vivo studies that have been performed with pDNA for the treatment of IP carcinomatosis up to date. As mentioned earlier, pDNA aims to induce the expression of deficient proteins, suicide genes or proteins that stimulate the host immune system, with the goal to target tumor cells. Some studies also made use of reporter proteins such as luciferase, to explore the suitability of DNA carriers to reach tumor cells. For example, Zhang et al. performed a proof of concept study of a delivery system for its ability to express luciferase in peritoneal tumors in vivo, without investigating its effect on tumor growth. They studied "stabilized plasmid–lipid particles" composed of DOPE, the cationic lipid dioleoydimethylammonium chloride (DODAC), and C8 ceramide-PEG (C8 Cer-PEG) in an IP human melanoma B16 tumor model. C8 Cer-PEG was chosen to PEGylate the lipid nanoparticles, because of its ability to diffuse out of the nanoparticles with a certain kinetic, ensuring good PEGylation in the extracellular biofluids, while the de-PEGylation over time restores the intracellular trafficking of the complexes. This is in contrast to the commonly used DSPE-PEG, which results in stable PEGylation that ensures good extracellular stability but interferes on the level of cellular uptake and endosomal escape [25]. The authors reported high expression of luciferase in B16 tumors 24 hours following IP injection [89]. In a study by Louis et al., the widely used linear polymer polyethylenimine (L-PEI) was used to deliver DNA expressing luciferase in mice bearing SKOV-3 human ovarian cancer cells. Multiple IP injections of PEI/DNA complexes resulted in high transgene expression, without any toxicity signs [45].

Immunotherapy is receiving increasing attention in the treatment of cancer. In this respect, several cytokines have been suggested to induce immune response, particularly IL-12 [65]. Fewell et al. synthesized PEG-PEI-cholesterol lipopolymers complexed with IL-12 plasmid and tested its ability to induce an anticancer immune response in mice bearing ovarian adenocarcinomas tumors. The authors reported a significant increase in murine IL-12 and interferon-γ (IFN-γ) in ascites fluid and an increased survival of the animals. Additionally, a significant decrease was noted in vascular endothelial growth factor, which plays an important role in ascites formation. As expected, when combined with chemotherapy, an additional increase in the survival of the treated mice was observed [19]. These successful in vivo experiments paved the way to clinical trials in humans. A phase I clinical trial was carried out on women diagnosed with chemotherapy-resistant ovarian cancer. In this study, 13 patients received 4 increasing doses of the formulated plasmid, namely, 0.6, 3, 12, or 24 mg × m^{-2}, once every 4 weeks, via IP infusion. No major side effects were reported, except for fever and abdominal pain. High levels of IL-12 plasmid and (IFN-γ) were measured in the peritoneal fluid but not in serum during the treatment, suggesting that this IL-12 delivery system is suitable for local delivery and treatment of recurrent ovarian cancer [4]. Recently, the results of a phase II clinical trial addressing the toxicity and antitumor activity of the formulation in 20 platinum-resistant patients were published [3]. Briefly, patients received a weekly IP infusion of the IL-12 plasmid containing lipopolymer at a dose of 24 mg × m^{-2}. Common adverse effects were reported including fatigue, fever, chills, abdominal pain, nausea, vomiting, anemia, thrombocytopenia, and leukopenia. No patients with partial or complete response were reported. In summary, seven patients had stable disease, nine had progressive disease, and six had survival progression-free survival for 6 months. Therefore, the authors deduced that the treatment had insufficient and limited biological activity in platinum-resistant ovarian cancer patients [3]. To this end, a phase I clinical trial is ongoing to evaluate the efficacy and toxicity of combined therapy of the IL-12 formulation (gene therapy) with a liposomal doxorubicin formulation (conventional chemotherapy) in ovarian cancer patients.

Colon cancer is among the most common diseases in the world, with about 50,000 deaths in the United States [37]. The difficulty in treating colon cancer is due to rapid spread and metastases. Vesicular stomatitis virus matrix protein (VSVMP) has been shown to block nuclear export by interacting with the nucleoporin Nup 98, an important component of the nuclear pore complex, leading to the inhibition of host gene expression and the induction of apoptosis [85]. Guo et al. synthesized and investigated heparin–polyethyleneimine (HPEI) nanogels complexed with plasmids encoding for VSVMP (pVSVMP) for their ability to induce apoptosis in C-26 colon carcinoma cells. HPEI/pVSVMP nanogels efficiently inhibited peritoneal metastasis of C-26 colon carcinoma in mice following IP injection and prolonged their survival [26]. Worth mentioning is the fact that IV administration of HPEI/pVSVMP nanogels resulted in rapid degradation of the complexes and their excretion through urine. Therefore, the data demonstrate a clear advantage of the IP route for the treatment of colon carcinoma when compared with the systemic one. In another study, the same research group used the same HPEI nanogels to deliver filamin A–interacting protein 1-like (FILIP1L). FILIP1L plays a role in regulating angiogenesis, apoptosis and proliferation of tumor cells. Interestingly, it has been proposed that FILIP1L is absent in ovarian cancer cell lines [54]. When tested in SKOV-3 IP ovarian carcinomatosis model, HPEI-incorporating plasmids expressing FILIP1L suppressed tumor growth and decreased tumor weight about 72% compared to the control group [87].

Table 32.1 Summary of in vivo studies evaluating intraperitoneal delivery of nanoparticles for cancer DNA therapy

Gene type	Carrier	Cancer model	Results	References
Luciferase DNA (reporter gene)	Stabilized plasmid–lipid particles coated with diffusible ceramide-poly(ethylene-glycol)	B16BL-6 human melanoma cells were seeded in the peritoneal cavity of C57BL/6 mice.	High luciferase expression in tumor tissue compared to healthy tissue.	[89]
Luciferase DNA (reporter gene)	Linear polyethylenimine	SKOV-3 IP ovarian carcinomatosis.	Dose-dependent significant level of transgene expression, preferentially in tumors compared to other organs, without toxicity.	[45]
pmIL-12 (immunotherapy)	Polyethylenimine covalently attached to methoxy polyethylene glycol and cholesteryl chloroformate	ID8 IP Ovarian cancer that lead to peritoneal carcinomatosis. *Phase I*: 13 women with chemotherapy-resistant recurrent ovarian cancer. *Phase II*: 20 patients with platinum-resistant recurrent ovarian cancer.	*In vivo:* Suppression of ascites accumulation, dramatic decrease in VEGF levels, no signs of toxicity. *Phase I*: High levels of IFN-γ in PF but not in serum. *Phase II*: Seven patients had a stable disease, nine patients had progressive disease and six had a progression-free survival.	[3,4,19]
pVSVMP	Heparin conjugated to polyethylenimine	C-26 colon carcinoma.	The treatment prevented growth of abdominal metastasis and increased the life span of the treated mice.	[26]
FILIP1LΔC103	Heparin conjugated to polyethylenimine	SKOV-3 IP ovarian carcinomatosis.	Significant inhibition of ovarian cancer, reduction in angiogenesis, decrease in cell proliferation, and increase in tumor apoptosis.	[87]
hTNF-α	PEG-SS-P[Asp(DET)]	SUIT-2 IP human pancreatic carcinoma.	High antitumor activity without renal and hepatic toxicity.	[42]
(GM-CSF) (immunotherapy)	(PEG)-b-P[Asp(DET)]/P[Asp(DET)]	SUIT-2 IP human pancreatic carcinoma.	Efficient uptake in tumor nodules and prolongation of the survival rate in treated mice.	[61]
Plasmid expressing shRNA against claudin-3 (CLDN3) (short hairpin RNA)	Poly(lactic-co-glycolic acid) (PLGA)	SKOV-3 IP ovarian carcinomatosis.	Efficient downregulation of CLDN3, tumor suppression, reduction in tumor weight, and increase in tumor apoptosis.	[77]
Diphtheria toxin (DT-A) (suicide therapy)	Cationic biodegradable poly(β-amino ester)	Epithelial ovarian cancer.	Reduction in tumor mass and increase in survival rate. Tumor suppression was superior over cisplatin and paclitaxel treatment.	[35,36]
pRad51-DT-A (suicide therapy)	Linear polyethylenimine (jetPEI)	IP HeLa tumor cells.	Efficient inhibition of malignant ascites, fourfold decrease in tumor mass, 90% increase in the mean survival time of treated mice.	[33,34]

As mentioned in the section "Barriers for IP DNA and siRNA delivery," the use of PEG poses a challenge for the drug delivery community, especially within the field of nucleic acid delivery. It is becoming more common to coat different nanoparticles with PEG chains that can be detached upon trigger or diffuse spontaneously out of the complexes in function of time [67]. Addressing this point, Kumagai et al. compared the toxicity and gene expression efficiency of two block copolymers that are able to form nanosized micelles. The first is poly(ethyleneglycol)-block-poly (PEG-P[Asp(DET)]) and the second is PEG-SS-P[Asp(DET)] containing a disulfide bond (S–S) between the cationic polymer and the PEG chains. The idea behind the disulfide bond is to trigger detachment of the PEG chains upon exposure to the intracellular reducing environment of the cells and consequently facilitate interactions with intracellular organelles. When both polymers loaded with pDNA encoding for human tumor necrosis factor-α (hTNF-α) were IP injected in mice bearing a peritoneally disseminated cancer model, higher antitumor activity was observed for the polymer containing S–S bonds, without any differences in toxicity [42]. Similarly, in a study carried out by the same research group, a mixture of block/homomixed polymers was used to prepare micelles. More specifically, poly{N′-[N-(2-aminoethyl)-2-aminoethyl]aspartamide} P[Asp(DET)] and (PEG)-b-P[Asp(DET)] were compared to (PEG)-b-P[Asp(DET)] alone for their ability to express luciferase in mice with peritoneal dissemination following IP administration. The mixture showed 12-fold higher luciferase expression 24 hours after the injection. Additionally, antitumor activity of the mixed polymer loaded with granulocyte macrophage colony stimulating factor in mice as well as in cynomolgus monkeys was observed following IP injection via the activation of natural killer cells [61].

Within the frame of gene therapy, delivery of suicide DNA to epithelial ovarian cancer cells has also been investigated. To date, several attempts have been reported. Langer and coworkers have developed a DNA construct that contains the diphtheria toxin A (DT-A) and a recombinase, to regulate gene expression on both the transcriptional and recombination level. This construct was delivered into ovarian cancer cells and inhibited tumor growth in mice [71]. Huang et al. showed that IP administration of cationic biodegradable poly(β-amino ester) to deliver DNA encoding for diphtheria toxin A (DT-A) in mice bearing metastatic ovarian cancer tumors not only inhibited tumor growth and prolonged the survival of mice but also was more efficient in terms of tumor suppression than the conventional anticancer agents paclitaxel and cisplatin [35]. Taking advantage of the DT-A toxin, Hine et al. proved that the fusion of the recombinase Rad51 promoter, which is overexpressed in many tumors, to the DT-A gene results in a specific killing of tumors and thus is an attractive strategy for cancer treatment [32]. Later on, Hine et al. brought evidence for the efficiency of the system in vivo. In this study, a Rad-51-luciferase construct was IP delivered using a cationic linear PEI, known as jetPEI, in mice bearing HeLa cells xenografts. Due to the luciferase expression it was possible to specifically detect tumors, with an in vivo bioluminescent camera, while no bioluminescence was detected in healthy mice. Furthermore, the treatment decreased tumor mass by fourfold, which was accompanied with a reduction in malignant ascites and a 90% increase in the life span of the treated mice compared to the control mice [33]. Finally, the study recommends to use pRad51-Luc-DT-A/jetPEI to image and treat different types of cancer.

As explained earlier, plasmids can also be used to express shRNA that is further processed by the cell into siRNA. Therefore, plasmid delivery can also be used to downregulate specific proteins. Claudin-3 (CLDN3) is a tight junction, integral membrane protein that is overexpressed in ovarian tumors, but not in healthy ovarian tissue. CLDN3 overexpression eventually leads to invasion and survival of ovarian tumors [56,64]. Hence, downregulation of CLDN3 offers an attractive strategy for cancer treatment. Sun et al. developed a plasmid expressing shRNA against CLDN3 and encapsulated the plasmids within biodegradable poly(lactic-co-glycolic acid) (PLGA) nanoparticles. Following 12 IP administrations to nude mice bearing SKOV-3 ovarian cancer, a significant reduction in the tumor weight of 67.4% compared to the control was measured [77].

CURRENT IN VIVO USE OF RNAi FOR IP CARCINOMATOSIS

As mentioned earlier, since its discovery, siRNA has attracted remarkable attention for cancer applications. In general, RNAi aims to downregulate cancer-related proteins that are often overexpressed in cancer cells and contribute to their invasiveness and increased proliferation. Table 32.2 summarizes the siRNA-based therapies that have been explored in vivo so far. In an attempt to downregulate the expression of focal adhesion kinase (FAK), which plays an important role in survival, migration, and invasion of cancer cells [42], FAK siRNA complexed with 1,2-dioleoyl-sn-glycero-3-phosphatidylcholine (DOPC) liposomes was IP injected in mice bearing an ovarian cancer model. This treatment reduced the mean tumor weight by 44%–72% in three cell lines [27]. Similarly, the same research group employed the same ovarian cancer model in mice, evaluating the ability of interleukin-8 (IL-8) siRNA-DOPC complexes to suppress IL-8 activity. IL-8 is a proangiogenic cytokine that is overexpressed in many human cancers. The authors reported a significant reduction in the tumor weight that varies between 32% and 52% in the tested cell lines, proposing that IL-8 gene silencing decreases tumor growth via an antiangiogenic mechanism [51].

As mentioned earlier, the downregulation of claudin-3 (CLDN3) offers possibilities for anticancer treatments. Huang et al. investigated whether the siRNA-induced knockdown of CLDN3 prevented the growth of metastasis in a mice model derived from ovarian surface epithelial ID8 cells. Interestingly, IP injection of lipoplexes containing

Table 32.2 Summary of in vivo studies evaluating intraperitoneal delivery of nanoparticles for cancer RNAi therapy

siRNA against	Carrier	Cancer model	Results	References
Focal adhesion kinase (FAK)	DOPC liposomes	Human ovarian cancer using three cell lines SKOV-3ip1, HeyA8 (taxane sensitive), and HeyA8MDR (taxane resistant) in nude mice.	Reduction in tumor weight by 44%–72% depending on the cell line, synergistic effect when siRNA was combined with docetaxel.	[27]
IL-8	DOPC liposomes	Human ovarian cancer using three cell lines SKOV-3ip1, HeyA8 (taxane sensitive), and SKOV-3ip2.TR (taxane resistant) in nude mice.	Reduction in tumor weight 32%–52% depending on the cell line, Synergistic effect when siRNA was combined with docetaxel.	[51]
CLDN3	Lipidoid	ID8 IP Ovarian cancer.	Suppression of tumor growth, reduction in ascites, without any toxicity following multiple administrations.	[34,35]
NEDD1	Atelocollagen	HSC-60 IP gastric cancer in scid mice.	Significant increase in the life span of the treated mice.	[22]
ID4	Cell-penetrating peptides (CPPs)	OVCAR-8 IP tumors.	Remarkable prolongation in survival, 80% of the animals survived at least 60 days without inducing immune response following one injection every 3 days for 30 days.	[66]
Survivin	Liposomes composed of DOTAP DOPE PEG and cholesterol	H766T IP pancreatic human metastatic xenograft.	Efficient knockdown of survivin was possible only when combined with paclitaxel.	[84]
PARP-1	Lipidoid	Genetically defined murine ovarian cancer.	High specificity of the treatment, prolongation of the survival of mice.	[24]

siRNA against CLDN3 to mice significantly decreased not only tumor growth but also the development of ascites, indicating that suppression of metastasis occurred [34].

Likewise, Fujita et al. proposed an atelocollagen delivery system loaded with siRNA against NEDD1, a centrosomal protein that associates with the gamma-tubulin ring complex protein and plays an important role in regulating the metaphase of the cell cycle [31]. NEDD1 downregulation prolonged the survival of mice bearing a gastric and peritoneal metastasis model from ascites tumors [22]. In addition to CLDN3, IL-8, and FAK, inhibition of oncogenes is also an attractive strategy to suppress tumors. Briefly, oncogenes are genes that tend to cause cancer and are mutated or overexpressed in tumor cells [47]. In a study by Ren et al., an inhibitor of DNA binding 4 (ID4) was characterized and shown to be overexpressed on the surface of human ovarian cancer cells. In the same study, the authors demonstrate in vitro and in vivo silencing when nanocomplexes of cell-penetrating peptides containing siRNA against ID4 were injected IP to mice with disseminated intra-abdominal tumors, every 3 days for 30 days. The treatment remarkably increased the survival rate of 80% of the animals, with the ability to live 60 days or even more, without inducing a strong immune response [66]. Recently, survivin, a member of the IAP protein family, is receiving increased attention in cancer therapy, since it is upregulated in solid tumors [2]. In an attempt to knockdown survivin expression in mice bearing a metastatic human pancreatic tumor model, Wang et al. investigated the ability of liposomes composed of 1,2-dioleoyl-3-trimethylammoniumpropane (DOTAP), 1,2-dioleoyl-sn-glycero-3-phosphoethanolamine (DOPE) and 1,2-distearoyl-sn-glycero-3-phosphoethanolamine-N-[methoxy(polyethylene glycol)-2000 (DSPE-PEG) complexed with siRNA against survivin. The study revealed that these complexes successfully decreased the expression of survivin but only when they were coadministered with the conventional chemotherapeutic paclitaxel (PTX) [86]. The data presented in the study thus encourage the codelivery of siRNA and other chemotherapeutic agents to tumors.

Other RNAi strategies are especially useful for personalized medicine purposes. BRCA1 is a tumor suppressor that is mutated in about 5% of the ovarian cancer population, leading to defects in the DNA repair process, such as mutations in chromosomal rearrangements [58,76]. On the contrary, poly(ADP-ribose) polymerase-1 (PARP-1) is involved in preventing DNA damage and genomic stability [41]. It has been postulated that orally administered PARP-1 inhibitors in patients with BRCA mutations resulted in antitumor activity [21]. When PARP-1 siRNA was IP delivered using lipid-like nanostructures called "lipidoids" in mice bearing disseminated BRCA1-deficient murine ovarian carcinoma allografts, a significant cell growth inhibition and extended survival of the treated mice was noticeable [24].

CONCLUDING REMARKS AND FUTURE PROSPECTIVE

In this chapter, we restricted our discussion on IP injection of nonviral vectors to deliver nucleic acids into tumors residing in the peritoneal space. IP delivery of nucleic acids is indeed an attractive approach to target peritoneal carcinomatosis. Although several nonviral gene delivery systems carrying pDNA or siRNA have proven antitumor effect to some extent, none of the tested formulations have been approved for use in clinical oncology so far. Translation into the clinic still awaits a new class of formulations that can overcome both the intracellular and extracellular barriers as discussed in the preceding text. The main problem in optimizing nonviral gene delivery systems is the lack of knowledge on the relation between the physicochemical properties of delivery systems (e.g., charge and size) and their obtained therapeutic effect. Also, carrier properties that assure stability on the extracellular level (for example, surface PEGylation) still often interfere with the intracellular performance of the same carrier. It should be noted that the efficiency of a delivery system can greatly depend on the extracellular barriers that are encountered and thus on the administration route. It is crucial to evaluate and optimize gene delivery vehicles with the intended administration route in mind. For IP delivery, this implies that carrier properties should be studied in the IP fluid. In an attempt to perform reliable measurements in more complex biological fluids, we have proven that advanced microscopy techniques such as fluorescence correlation spectroscopy and single particle tracking enable to monitor the disassembly and aggregation of nonviral vectors in undiluted biological fluids [13]. By employing these powerful techniques, we can simulate the in vivo situation and screen for formulations that show minimal aggregation properties while keeping the maximal amount of their siRNA or pDNA load in the IP fluid. For local IP delivery, it should be noted that having colloidal stable particles in the IP cavity is not the only requirement for optimal tumor targeting. It has been reported that nanosized vectors are rapidly cleared from the peritoneal cavity following IP administration compared to microparticles [81] (Figure 32.1a, step 4). This rapid absorption from the peritoneal cavity to the systemic circulation, most likely seriously limits the amount of complexes that actually reach and enter the tumor target cells. The rapid clearance of nanoparticles from the IP cavity has however also been exploited in some studies, where the IP route is being used for systemic gene delivery, to target systemic tumors. In a study by Aigner and coworkers, siRNA against c-erbB2/neu (HER-2) receptor complexed with PEI was injected IP into mice bearing subcutaneous SKOV-3 tumors and exhibited a remarkable reduction in tumor growth, whereas no reduction in tumor growth was observed following injection of naked siRNA [82]. In this case, the IP delivery is thus used as a depot system, from which systemic delivery of nanoparticles is aimed.

In the vast majority of the studies we reviewed, it is important to stress out the fact that long-term biological activity by silencing or overexpressing genes was obtained only after multiple administrations of the formulations to the IP cavity. Therefore, future strategies will most likely also depend on delivery systems that can increase the residence time of nonviral nucleic acid delivery systems in the IP cavity, with limited distribution to the systemic circulation. In this respect, sustained release of nonviral vectors from an injectable depot system might be an advantage, due to the ability to maintain stable gene silencing or expression for a prolonged period of time. It is expected that the constantly increasing knowledge on possible gene targets in tumor cells will continue to fine-tune the use of pDNA and siRNA delivery to IP carcinomatosis. Also, nucleic acid delivery will play a major role in personalized cancer treatments as screening methods allow more and more cancer-associated genes to be identified on a person-to-person basis. Finally, the combination of nucleic acids with conventional chemotherapeutics can also contribute to the translation of IP gene therapy to the clinic.

REFERENCES

1. Al-Dosari MS, Gao X. Nonviral gene delivery: Principle, limitations, and recent progress. *AAPS Journal*. 2009;11(4):671–681.
2. Altieri DC. Survivin, cancer networks and pathway-directed drug discovery. *Nature Reviews Cancer*. 2008;8(1):61–70.
3. Alvarez RD, Sill MW, Davidson SA, Muller CY, Bender DP, DeBernardo RL, Behbakht K, Huh WK. A phase II trial of intraperitoneal EGEN-001, an IL-12 plasmid formulated with PEG-PEI-cholesterol lipopolymer in the treatment of persistent or recurrent epithelial ovarian, fallopian tube or primary peritoneal cancer: A Gynecologic Oncology Group study. *Gynecologic Oncology*. 2014;133(3):433–438.
4. Anwer K, Barnes MN, Fewell J, Lewis DH, Alvarez RD. Phase-I clinical trial of IL-12 plasmid/lipopolymer complexes for the treatment of recurrent ovarian cancer. *Gene Therapy*. 2010;17(3):360–369.
5. Baguley BC. Multidrug resistance in cancer. *Methods in Molecular Biology*. 2010;596:1–14.
6. Barbalat R, Ewald SE, Mouchess ML, Barton GM. Nucleic acid recognition by the innate immune system. *Annual Review of Immunology*. 2011;29:185–214.

7. Blau HM, Springer ML. Gene therapy—A novel form of drug delivery. *New England Journal of Medicine.* 1995;333(18):1204–1207.
8. Bouard D, Alazard-Dany D, Cosset FL. Viral vectors: From virology to transgene expression. *British Journal of Pharmacology.* 2009;157(2):153–165.
9. Capecchi MR. Altering the genome by homologous recombination. *Science.* 1989;244(4910):1288–1292.
10. Ceelen WP, Flessner MF. Intraperitoneal therapy for peritoneal tumors: Biophysics and clinical evidence. *Nature Reviews Clinical Oncology.* 2010;7(2):108–115.
11. Cohen RN, van der Aa MA, Macaraeg N, Lee AP, Szoka FC, Jr. Quantification of plasmid DNA copies in the nucleus after lipoplex and polyplex transfection. *Journal of Controlled Release.* 2009;135(2):166–174.
12. Creixell M, Peppas NA. Co-delivery of siRNA and therapeutic agents using nanocarriers to overcome cancer resistance. *Nano Today.* 2012;7(4):367–379.
13. Dakwar GR, Zagato E, Delanghe J, Hobel S, Aigner A, Denys H, Braeckmans K, Ceelen W, De Smedt FC, Remaut K. Colloidal stability of nano-sized particles in the peritoneal fluid: Towards optimizing drug delivery systems for intraperitoneal therapy. *Acta Biomaterialia.* 2014;10(7):2965–2975.
14. De Paula D, Bentley MV, Mahato RI. Hydrophobization and bioconjugation for enhanced siRNA delivery and targeting. *RNA.* 2007;13(4):431–456.
15. Dinh AT, Pangarkar C, Theofanous T, Mitragotri S. Understanding intracellular transport processes pertinent to synthetic gene delivery via stochastic simulations and sensitivity analyses. *Biophysical Journal.* 2007;92(3):831–846.
16. Dranoff G. Cytokines in cancer pathogenesis and cancer therapy. *Nature Reviews Cancer.* 2004;4(1):11–22.
17. Elbashir SM, Harborth J, Lendeckel W, Yalcin A, Weber K, Tuschl T. Duplexes of 21-nucleotide RNAs mediate RNA interference in cultured mammalian cells. *Nature.* 2001;411(6836):494–498.
18. Farokhzad OC, Langer R. Impact of nanotechnology on drug delivery. *ACS Nano.* 2009;3(1):16–20.
19. Fewell JG, Matar MM, Rice JS, Brunhoeber E, Slobodkin G, Pence C, Worker M, Lewis DH, Anwer K. Treatment of disseminated ovarian cancer using nonviral interleukin-12 gene therapy delivered intraperitoneally. *Journal of Gene Medicine.* 2009;11(8):718–728.
20. Fire A, Xu S, Montgomery MK, Kostas SA, Driver SE, Mello CC. Potent and specific genetic interference by double-stranded RNA in *Caenorhabditis elegans. Nature.* 1998;391(6669):806–811.
21. Fong PC, Boss DS, Yap TA, Tutt A, Wu PJ, Mergui-Roelvink M et al. Inhibition of poly(ADP-ribose) polymerase in tumors from BRCA mutation carriers. *New England Journal of Medicine.* 2009;361(2):123–134.
22. Fujita T, Yanagihara K, Takeshita F, Aoyagi K, Nishimura T, Takigahira M et al. Intraperitoneal delivery of a small interfering RNA targeting NEDD1 prolongs the survival of scirrhous gastric cancer model mice. *Cancer Science.* 2013;104(2):214–222.
23. Gao X, Kim KS, Liu DX. Nonviral gene delivery: What we know and what is next. *AAPS Journal.* 2007;9(1):E92–E104.
24. Goldberg MS, Xing DY, Ren Y, Orsulic S, Bhatia SN, Sharp PA. Nanoparticle-mediated delivery of siRNA targeting Parp1 extends survival of mice bearing tumors derived from Brca1-deficient ovarian cancer cells. *Proceedings of the National Academy of Sciences of the United States of America.* 2011;108(2):745–750.
25. Gomes-da-Silva LC, Fonseca NA, Moura V, MC Pedroso de Lima, Simoes S, Moreira JN. Lipid-based nanoparticles for siRNA delivery in cancer therapy: Paradigms and challenges. *Accounts of Chemical Research.* 2012;45(7):1163–1171.
26. Gou M, Men K, Zhang J, Li Y, Song J, Luo S et al. Efficient inhibition of C-26 colon carcinoma by VSVMP gene delivered by biodegradable cationic nanogel derived from polyethyleneimine. *ACS Nano.* 2010;4(10):5573–5584.
27. Halder J, Kamat AA, Landen CN, Han LY, Lutgendorf SK, Lin YG et al. Focal adhesion kinase targeting using in vivo short interfering RNA delivery in neutral liposomes for ovarian carcinoma therapy. *Clinical Cancer Research.* 2006;12(16):4916–4924.
28. Hama S, Akita H, Iida S, Mizuguchi H, Harashima H. Quantitative and mechanism-based investigation of post-nuclear delivery events between adenovirus and lipoplex. *Nucleic Acids Research.* 2007;35(5):1533–1543.
29. Hamburg MA, Collins FS. The path to personalized medicine. *New England Journal of Medicine.* 2010;363(4):301–304.
30. Hanahan D, Weinberg RA. Hallmarks of cancer: The next generation. *Cell.* 2011;144(5):646–674.
31. Haren L, Remy MH, Bazin I, Callebaut I, Wright M, Merdes A. NEDD1-dependent recruitment of the gamma-tubulin ring complex to the centrosome is necessary for centriole duplication and spindle assembly. *Journal of Cell Biology.* 2006;172(4):505–515.
32. Hine CM, Seluanov A, Gorbunova V. Use of the Rad51 promoter for targeted anti-cancer therapy. *Proceedings of the National Academy of Sciences of the United States of America.* 2008;105(52):20810–20815.

33. Hine CM, Seluanov A, Gorbunova V. Rad51 promoter-targeted gene therapy is effective for in vivo visualization and treatment of cancer. *Molecular Therapy*. 2012;20(2):347–355.

34. Huang YH, Bao YH, Peng WD, Goldberg M, Love K, Bumcrot DA, Cole G, Langer R, Anderson DG, Sawicki JA. Claudin-3 gene silencing with siRNA suppresses ovarian tumor growth and metastasis. *Proceedings of the National Academy of Sciences of the United States of America*. 2009;106(9):3426–3430.

35. Huang YH, Zugates GT, Peng WD, Holtz D, Dunton C, Green JJ et al. Nanoparticle-delivered suicide gene therapy effectively reduces ovarian tumor burden in mice. *Cancer Research*. 2009;69(15):6184–6191.

36. Jemal A, Siegel R, Ward E, Hao Y, Xu J, Murray T, Thun MJ. Cancer statistics, 2008. *CA: A Cancer Journal for Clinicians*. 2008;58(2):71–96.

37. Kanasty R, Dorkin JR, Vegas A, Anderson D. Delivery materials for siRNA therapeutics. *Nature Materials*. 2013;12(11):967–977.

38. Kay MA. State-of-the-art gene-based therapies: The road ahead. *Nature Reviews Genetics*. 2011;12(5):316–328.

39. Kipps E, Tan DSP, Kaye SB. Meeting the challenge of ascites in ovarian cancer: New avenues for therapy and research. *Nature Reviews Cancer*. 2013;13(4):273–282.

40. Knop K, Hoogenboom R, Fischer D, Schubert US. Poly(ethylene glycol) in drug delivery: Pros and cons as well as potential alternatives. *Angewandte Chemie-International Edition*. 2010;49(36):6288–6308.

41. Krishnakumar R, Kraus WL. The PARP side of the nucleus: Molecular actions, physiological outcomes, and clinical targets. *Molecular Cell*. 2010;39(1):8–24.

42. Kumagai M, Shimoda S, Wakabayashi R, Kunisawa Y, Ishii T, Osada K, Itaka K, Nishiyama N, Kataoka K, Nakano K. Effective transgene expression without toxicity by intraperitoneal administration of PEG-detachable polyplex micelles in mice with peritoneal dissemination. *Journal of Controlled Release*. 2012;160(3):542–551.

43. Langer R. Drug delivery and targeting. *Nature*. 1998;392(6679):5–10.

44. Lee TB, Park JH, Min YD, Kim KJ, Choi CH. Epigenetic mechanisms involved in differential MDR1 mRNA expression between gastric and colon cancer cell lines and rationales for clinical chemotherapy. *BMC Gastroenterology*. 2008;8:(33).

45. Louis MH, Dutoit S, Denoux Y, Erbacher P, Deslandes E, Behr JP, Gauduchon P, Poulain L. Poulain. Intraperitoneal linear polyethylenimine (L-PEI)-mediated gene delivery to ovarian carcinoma nodes in mice. *Cancer Gene Therapy*. 2006;13(4):367–374.

46. Lukacs GL, Haggie P, Seksek O, Lechardeur D, Freedman N, Verkman AS. Size-dependent DNA mobility in cytoplasm and nucleus. *Journal of Biological Chemistry*. 2000;275(3):1625–1629.

47. Luo J, Solimini NL, Elledge SJ. Principles of cancer therapy: Oncogene and non-oncogene addiction. *Cell*. 2009;136(5):823–837.

48. Malek A, Merkel O, Fink L, Czubayko F, Kissel T, Aigner A. In vivo pharmacokinetics, tissue distribution and underlying mechanisms of various PEI(-PEG)/siRNA complexes. *Toxicology and Applied Pharmacology*. 2009;236(1):97–108.

49. McCormick F. Cancer gene therapy: Fringe or cutting edge? *Nature Reviews Cancer*. 2001;1(2):130–141.

50. Mellman I, Coukos G, Dranoff G. Cancer immunotherapy comes of age. *Nature*. 2011;480(7370):480–489.

51. Merritt WM, Lin YG, Spannuth WA, Fletcher MS, Kamat AA, Han LY et al. Effect of interleukin-8 gene silencing with liposome-encapsulated small interfering RNA on ovarian cancer cell growth. *Journal of the National Cancer Institute*. 2008;100(5):359–372.

52. Minaguchi T, Mori T, Kanamori Y, Matsushima M, Yoshikawa H, Taketani Y, Nakamura Y. Growth suppression of human ovarian cancer cells by adenovirus-mediated transfer of the PTEN gene. *Cancer Research*. 1999;59(24):6063–6067.

53. Moghimi SM, Hunter AC, Murray JC. Long-circulating and target-specific nanoparticles: Theory to practice. *Pharmacological Reviews*. 2001;53(2):283–318.

54. Mok SC, Wong KK, Chan RKW, Lau CC, Tsao SW, Knapp RC, Berkowitz RS. Molecular-cloning of differentially expressed genes in human epithelial ovarian-cancer. *Gynecologic Oncology*. 1994;52(2):247–252.

55. Moore CB, Guthrie EH, Huang MT, Taxman DJ. Short hairpin RNA (shRNA): Design, delivery, and assessment of gene knockdown. *Methods in Molecular Biology*. 2010;629:141–158.

56. Morin PJ. Claudin proteins in ovarian cancer. *Disease Markers*. 2007;23(5–6):453–457.

57. Morin PJ, Vogelstein B, Kinzler KW. Apoptosis and APC in colorectal tumorigenesis. *Proceedings of the National Academy of Sciences of the United States of America*. 1996;93(15):7950–7954.

58. Moynahan ME, Chiu JW, Koller BH, Jasin M. Brca1 controls homology-directed DNA repair. *Molecular Cell*. 1999;4(4):511–518.

59. Nagasaki T, Shinkai S. The concept of molecular machinery is useful for design of stimuli-responsive gene delivery systems in the mammalian cell. *Journal of Inclusion Phenomena and Macrocyclic Chemistry*. 2007;58(3–4):205–219.

60. Nguyen J, Szoka FC. Nucleic acid delivery: The missing pieces of the puzzle? *Accounts of Chemical Research*. 2012;45(7):1153–1162.

61. Ohgidani M, Furugaki K, Shinkai K, Kunisawa Y, Itaka K, Kataoka K, Nakano K. Block/homo polyplex micelle-based GM-CSF gene therapy via intraperitoneal administration elicits antitumor immunity against peritoneal dissemination and exhibits safety potentials in mice and cynomolgus monkeys. *Journal of Controlled Release.* 2013;167(3):238–247.

62. Paddison PJ, Caudy AA, Bernstein E, Hannon GJ, Conklin DS. Short hairpin RNAs (shRNAs) induce sequence-specific silencing in mammalian cells. *Genes & Development.* 2002;16(8):948–958.

63. Pai SI, Lin YY, Macaes B, Meneshian A, Hung CF, Wu TC. Prospects of RNA interference therapy for cancer. *Gene Therapy.* 2006;13(6):464–477.

64. Rangel LBA, Agarwal R, D'Souza T, Pizer ES, Alo PL, Lancaster WD, Gregoire L, Schwartz DR, Cho KR, Morin PJ. Tight junction proteins claudin-3 and claudin-4 are frequently overexpressed in ovarian cancer but not in ovarian cystadenomas. *Clinical Cancer Research.* 2003;9(7):2567–2575.

65. Robertson MJ, Ritz J. Interleukin 12: Basic biology and potential applications in cancer treatment. *Oncologist.* 1996;1(1 & 2):88–97.

66. Ren Y, Cheung HW, von Maltzhan G, Agrawal A, Cowley GS, Weir BA et al. Targeted tumor-penetrating siRNA nanocomplexes for credentialing the ovarian cancer oncogene ID4. *Science Translational Medicine.* 2012;4(147):147ra112.

67. Romberg B, Hennink WE, Storm G. Sheddable coatings for long-circulating nanoparticles. *Pharmaceutical Research.* 2008;25(1):55–71.

68. Ross JS, Schenkein DP, Pietrusko R, Rolfe M, Linette GP, Stec J, Stagliano NE, Ginsburg GS, Symmans WF, Pusztai L, Hortobagyi GN. Targeted therapies for cancer 2004. *American Journal of Clinical Pathology.* 2004;122(4):598–609.

69. Roth JA, Nguyen D, Lawrence DD, Kemp BL, Carrasco CH, Ferson DZ et al. Retrovirus-mediated wild-type p53 gene transfer to tumors of patients with lung cancer. *Nature Medicine.* 1996;2(9):985–991.

70. Sandhu JS, Keating A, Hozumi N. Human gene therapy. *Critical Reviews in Biotechnology.* 1997;17(4):307–326.

71. Sawicki JA, Anderson DG, Langer R. Nanoparticle delivery of suicide DNA for epithelial ovarian cancer therapy. *Ovarian Cancer: State of the Art and Future Directions in Translational Research.* 2008;622:209–219.

72. Schaller MD, Parsons JT. Focal adhesion kinase: An integrin-linked protein tyrosine kinase. *Trends in Cell Biology.* 1993;3(8):258–262.

73. Schroeder A, Heller DA, Winslow MM, Dahlman JE, Pratt GW, Langer R, Jacks T, Anderson DG. Treating metastatic cancer with nanotechnology. *Nature Reviews Cancer.* 2012;12(1):39–50.

74. Scott AM, Wolchok JD, Old LJ. Antibody therapy of cancer. *Nature Reviews Cancer.* 2012;12(4):278–287.

75. Soutschek J, Akinc A, Bramlage B, Charisse K, Constien R, Donoghue M et al. Therapeutic silencing of an endogenous gene by systemic administration of modified siRNAs. *Nature.* 2004;432(7014):173–178.

76. Stratton JF, Gayther SA, Russell P, Dearden J, Gore M, Blake P, Easton D, Ponder BAJ. Contribution of BRCA1 mutations to ovarian cancer. *New England Journal of Medicine.* 1997;336(16):1125–1130.

77. Sun CT, Yi T, Song XR, Li SZ, Qi XR, Chen XC, Lin HG, He X, Li ZY, Wei YQ, Zhao X. Efficient inhibition of ovarian cancer by short hairpin RNA targeting claudin-3. *Oncology Reports.* 2011;26(1):193–200.

78. Thomas CE, Ehrhardt A, Kay MA. Progress and problems with the use of viral vectors for gene therapy. *Nature Reviews Genetics.* 2003;4(5):346–358.

79. Tolcher AW, Quinn DI, Ferrari A, Ahmann F, Giaccone G, Drake T, Keating A, de Bono JS. A phase II study of YM155, a novel small-molecule suppressor of survivin, in castration-resistant taxane-pretreated prostate cancer. *Annals of Oncology.* 2012;23(4):968–973.

80. Tomar RS, Matta H, Chaudhary PM. Use of adeno-associated viral vector for delivery of small interfering RNA. *Oncogene.* 2003;22(36):5712–5715.

81. Tsai M, Lu Z, Wang J, Yeh TK, Wientjes MG, Au JLS. Effects of carrier on disposition and antitumor activity of intraperitoneal paclitaxel. *Pharmaceutical Research.* 2007;24(9):1691–1701.

82. Urban-Klein B, Werth S, Abuharbeid S, Czubayko F, Aigner A. RNAi-mediated gene-targeting through systemic application of polyethylenimine (PEI)-complexed siRNA in vivo. *Gene Therapy.* 2005;12(5):461–466.

83. Vanneman M, Dranoff G. Combining immunotherapy and targeted therapies in cancer treatment. *Nature Reviews Cancer.* 2012;12(4):237–251.

84. Varkouhi AK, Scholte M, Storm G, Haisma HJ. Endosomal escape pathways for delivery of biologicals. *Journal of Controlled Release.* 2011;151(3):220–228.

85. von Kobbe C, van Deursen JM, Rodrigues JP, Sitterlin D, Bachi A, Wu X, Wilm M, Carmo-Fonseca M, Izaurralde E. Vesicular stomatitis virus matrix protein inhibits host cell gene expression by targeting the nucleoporin Nup98. *Molecular Cell.* 2000;6(5):1243–1252.

86. Wang J, Lu Z, Yeung BZ, Wientjes MG, Cole DJ, Au JLS. Tumor priming enhances siRNA delivery and transfection in intraperitoneal tumors. *Journal of Controlled Release.* 2014;178:79–85.

87. Xie C, Gou ML, Yi T, Deng HX, Li ZY, Liu P, Qi XR, He X, Wei YQ, Zhao X. Efficient inhibition of ovarian cancer by truncation mutant of FILIP1L gene delivered by novel biodegradable cationic heparin-polyethyleneimine nanogels. *Human Gene Therapy.* 2011;22(11):1413–1422.

88. Yang CT, You L, Yeh CC, Chang JW, Zhang F, McCormick F, Jablons DM. Adenovirus-mediated p14(ARF) gene transfer in human mesothelioma cells. *Journal of the National Cancer Institute.* 2000;92(8):636–641.

89. Zhang YP, Sekirov L, Saravolac EG, Wheeler JJ, Tardi P, Clow K, Leng E, Sun R, Cullis PR, Scherrer P. Stabilized plasmid-lipid particles for regional gene therapy: Formulation and transfection properties. *Gene Therapy.* 1999;6(8):1438–1447.

33

Immunotherapy of peritoneal carcinomatosis

MICHAEL A. STRÖHLEIN AND MARKUS M. HEISS

IMMUNE COMPETENCE IN THE COMPARTMENT OF THE PERITONEAL CAVITY

The peritoneum and the associated immunocompetent components provide a local microenvironment, which is able to promote proliferation, differentiation, and recruitment of lymphocytes and unspecific immunity to generate a state of effective immune response against cellular or viral pathogens. In the peritoneal cavity, 45% monocytes/macrophages (CD68+), 45% T-lymphocytes (CD2+), 8% NK-cells, and 2% dendritic cells (DCs) have been reported [1]. A high percentage of the peritoneal CD4+ (92%) and CD8+ (73%) were also found to be CD45RO+, which indicated the memory and effector T-cell phenotype.

An inverse ratio of CD4+ to CD8+ T-cells with respect to those of the peripheral blood, with a predominance of CD8+ T-cells, was reported. These findings exhibit the anti-inflammatory Th2 phenotype in human normal peritoneum.

The mesenchymal cells of the peritoneum also create substantial immunocompetence. After suitable stimulation, mesenchymal cells were found to secrete proinflammatory mediators like interleukin-1, interleukin-6, prostaglandin E2, monocyte colony–stimulating factor, granulocyte colony–stimulating factor, granulocyte monocyte colony–stimulating factor, and vascular epithelial growth factor (VEGF). Human peritoneal mesothelial cells were found to express HLA-DR molecules and upregulation of ICAM-1 in tissue culture conditions after interferon (IFN)-gamma stimulation, containing an extended capacity to present antigens to autologous T-lymphocytes, also promoting anti-CD3-induced T-cell proliferation. These findings were supported by the secretion of IL-2, IL-15, and IFN-gamma in further laboratory experiments [2].

In summary, a high level of immunocompetence in antigen presentation and T-cell activation characterizes the peritoneal cavity to qualify for local compartment immunotherapy.

Although peritoneal carcinomatosis represents a far advanced tumor disease, the distribution of single cells or tumor cell clusters on an extended surface of the peritoneum is another attractive point for locally administered immunotherapy (Table 33.1). The same is true for patients with malignant ascites, where single tumor cells or clusters of few tumor cells represent an easily accessible target. In contrast to chemotherapy, the efficacy of immune therapies is not dependent on the cell cycle or pharmacokinetic parameters, as tumor cells can also be attacked in a dormant cell phase.

UNSPECIFIC IMMUNOTHERAPY/ CYTOKINES

Despite the variety of immunocompetent cells obviously included in the peritoneal cavity, the anti-inflammatory Th2 phenotype was found to be predominant in physiological conditions. Therefore, polarization to a more cellular phenotype by unspecific immunomodulation was tried. The streptococcal preparation OK-432 was tested in a rat model to have immunostimulatory activity on natural killer cells, lymphokine-activated killer (LAK) cells, and T-lymphocytes. Locoregional administration of OK-432 was found to be effective in single patients with malignant ascites from gastric cancer, which was associated with an

Table 33.1 Overview of immunotherapeutic approaches in peritoneal carcinomatosis

Concept	Mode of action	Clinical effects
Unspecific immunomodulation • OK-432 • Flt3 ligand	Modulation of cellular immune reactions by induction of the predominant Th1 phenotype	Induction of Th1 cells Decrease of ascites in single patients
Cytokines • Interleukin-2 • Interferon-γ	Direct unspecific stimulation of NK- and T-cells	Significant reduction of tumor masses in animal models and single patients/severe side effects
Monoclonal antibodies	Specific binding of tumor antigens ADCC	Limited efficacy as a single agent
Radionucleotide antibody conjugates	Specific targeting of tumor cells for local microradiation	Clinical efficacy in ascites in single patients
Bispecific antibodies	Specific targeting of tumor cells and simultaneous activation of effector cells	Reduction of ascites reaccumulation
Trifunctional antibodies	Specific targeting of tumor cells, stimulation of T-cells, simultaneous activation of accessory cells	Clinical responses in >60% of patients with PC Stop of ascites accumulation Induction of long-term immunity

upregulation of Th1 responses [3]. Induction of predominant Th1 type T-helper cells was further increased by combining OK-432 with interleukin-2. Another concept was the intraperitoneal (i.p.) application of fms-like tyrosine kinase-3-ligand (Flt3-L), a truncated glycoprotein that increases DCs and monocytes. Increased interleukin-12 as a sign of enhanced cellular immunity together with a maturational shift toward the monocyte-derived DC phenotype was observed [4]. Clinical efficacy against peritoneal carcinomatosis was only limited to a special group of immunoreactive patients, which were able to overcome factors like tumor-related immunosuppression within OK-432 or Flt3-L treatment. Nevertheless, these attempts demonstrated the potential of induction of a more predominant Th1 phenotype together with stimulation of innate components of the immune system like natural killer cells and macrophages.

STIMULATION OF IMMUNOCOMPETENT CELLS BY DEFINED CYTOKINES

Since 1980, a variety of cytokines and correlating receptors were characterized to dramatically increase the antitumor cytotoxicity of defined subsets of immune cells. Interleukin-2, which is able to unspecifically stimulate T-lymphocytes and to induce LAK cells, was intensively investigated. Another concept was the generation of tumor-infiltrating lymphocytes (TIL), which represented highly specific T-cells expanded out of solid tumor masses. In several animal experiments, application of interleukin-2-generated LAK cells resulted in significant reduction of i.p. tumor masses [5,6]. Clinical interleukin-2 regimens were finally limited by severe side effects or technical problems during isolation and expansion of TIL but clearly demonstrated the power of T-cell responses in peritoneal carcinomatosis of ovarian and colon carcinoma [7]. Clinical responses in single patients were also reported in patients with malignant ascites due to peritoneal carcinomatosis after i.p. treatment

by IFN alpha [8]. However, unspecific immune stimulation was accompanied by severe side effects, which finally limited the clinical treatment concepts.

ANTIBODY CONSTRUCTS

The possibility to direct immunotherapy against defined molecular targets was the key feature for all antibody treatment concepts. However, the major drawback of conventional monoclonal antibodies (mAbs) was the lack of a direct antitumor effector component. One possibility to overcome this problem was to use of radionucleotide-conjugated antibodies for locoregional treatment in peritoneal carcinomatosis to direct toxic radiation against tumor cells after specific binding of tumor antigens. For example, iod-131, indium-111-, and yttrium-90-labeled human IgM or IgG constructs provided efficacy in animal experiments and clinical models, which were clearly superior to any kind of radiotherapy, focusing the significance of locoregional i.p. therapy against peritoneal carcinomatosis [9–11].

Presently, promising concepts of antibody therapy are based on antibody-induced involvement of immune effector cells. Direct activation of immunocompetent cells against defined tumor antigens led to the concept of bispecific antibodies, representing engineered antibody proteins, which are able to bind tumor antigens by one binding site and to bind and activate immune cells by the second binding site (Figure 33.1). Wunderlich et al. demonstrated significant destruction of tumor cells by using an anti-CD3 × anti-FR (fetal receptor of the ovarian cancer cell) bispecific antibody in combination with LAK cells [12]. Clinical efficacy was reported in patients with peritoneal carcinomatosis and malignant ascites by treatment with the bispecific antibody anti-HEA125 × anti-CD3, which was shown to redirect T-lymphocytes toward carcinoma cells and to induce tumor cell lysis in vitro. In treated patients, a decrease or stabilization of ascites accumulation was reported.

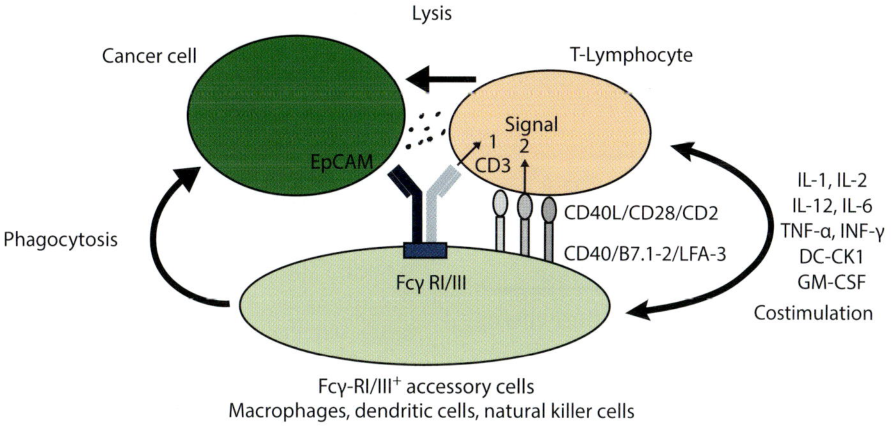

Figure 33.1 Catumaxomab mode of action. The mouse IgG2a arm binds to the human EpCAM. The rat IgG2b-binding site activates CD3-positive T-lymphocytes. A third functional binding site within the hybrid Fc-region selectively binds to and activates Fcg-receptor type I (CD64), type IIa (CD16), and type III (CD16) positive accessory cells (23), resulting in the restimulation of T-lymphocytes as a self-supporting system.

EpCAM IN CANCER TREATMENT

The human epithelial cell adhesion molecule (EpCAM, CD326) represents a membrane-embedded protein that mediates epithelium-specific cell-to-cell adhesion [13]. Investigations on the expression of EpCAM on normal human tissue showed that the protein could primarily be detected on epithelial tissue including pancreas, colon, lung, bile ducts, and breast, whereas EpCAM-negative tissue includes bone marrow, lymphocytes, endothelium, heart, ovary, muscle, and mesenchymal tissue [14,15]. The high frequency of its overexpression on epithelial tumors qualifies EpCAM as a smart target for anticancer therapy. High-level EpCAM expression was found in gastric cancer, colon cancer, prostate cancer, and lung cancer [16]. Treatment of head and neck cancer and breast cancer cell lines with EpCAM-specific antisense or siRNAs resulted in the partial or complete reduction of cell migration, proliferation and invasive capacity [17,18].

TRIFUNCTIONAL ANTIBODIES: CATUMAXOMAB, MODE OF ACTION

The basic principle of mAb-based cancer therapy is the specific binding to a distinct antigen on the tumor cell surface, which can activate specific responses against tumor cells like growth inhibition due to cell cycle arrest, inhibition of invasion and metastatic spread, inhibition of angiogenesis, sensitization to chemo- and/or radiotherapy, induction of apoptosis, growth factor antagonism, or secondary immune functions. mAbs recruit accessory cells via their Fc region, and these contribute to the observed immunological antitumor effect (e.g., antibody dependent cellular cytotoxicity).

Efforts to enhance mAbs' immunological efficacy led to the elaboration of bispecific antibodies [19], which are antibody-like proteins with two different antigen-binding sites. They are able to target tumor cells via a tumor-specific antigen and simultaneously immune effector cells, e.g., T-cells.

Unlike intact classical monospecific mAbs, bispecific molecules redirect cytotoxic T-cells against tumor cells, but they lack the constant Fc region necessary to activate Fcg-receptor-positive accessory cells [19–22].

Trifunctional antibodies overcome this problem and therefore represent the most advanced antibody development: Catumaxomab is a biologically engineered, hybrid-hybridoma-derived, trifunctional mAb consisting of a mouse immunoglobulin G (IgG)2a chain and a rat IgG2b chain [23]. The antibody is characterized by three binding sites: The mouse IgG2a arm binds to the human EpCAM. The rat IgG2b-binding site binds to human CD3 on T-lymphocytes; and a third functional binding site within the hybrid Fc-region selectively binds to and activates Fcγ-receptor-type I (CD64)-, Fcγ-receptor-type IIa (CD16)-, and Fcγ-receptor-type III (CD16)-positive accessory cells [23], Figure 33.1.

The simultaneous activation of different immune cell types locally at the tumor site results in efficient killing of tumor cells. The antibody-mediated phagocytosis of tumor cells by accessory cells is supposed to result in processing and presentation of tumor antigens [24–28]. Simultaneous accessory cell and T-cell binding and their mutual stimulation via costimulatory receptor molecules and cytokines augment their activation and induce the second signal in the T-cell for physiological T-cell activation.

The unique mechanism of trifunctional antibodies resulted in efficient destruction of tumor cells by several killing mechanisms: T-cell-mediated lysis through perforin and granzyme B, cytotoxicity by T-cell-secreted cytokines (i.e., TNF-α and IFN-γ), and phagocytosis via activation of accessory cells [24–28].

In a syngeneic mouse tumor model, treatment with trAbs did not only cause killing of the primary cancer but also induced immunity against the cancer: A second tumor challenge without further treatment with trAbs survived, whereas all untreated control mice developed cancer [25]. In patients with PC, trifunctional antibodies were able to induce an increase of specific tumor-reactive CD4+ and

CD8+ T-lymphocytes after i.p. therapy and restimulation by injection of trifunctional antibodies, autologous PBMC, and irradiated autologous tumor cells [29].

SPECIFIC RATIONALE OF INTRAPERITONEAL CATUMAXOMAB THERAPY IN PERITONEAL CARCINOMATOSIS

Peritoneal carcinomatosis is characterized by diffuse tumor spread of malignant cells found either in the cavity or directly at the peritoneum. Since the peritoneal cavity is easily accessible by interventional catheters, a locoregional immune therapy is able to induce an effect directly at the site of proposed tumor growth. Systemic side effects are minimized by this intracompartment therapy. The i.p. therapy with trifunctional antibodies is supposed to take place in a so-called immunological privileged site. Regarding the i.p. immune capacity (lymph nodes, Peyer plaques, peritoneal macrophages), induction of tumor-specific effector cells is likely to be simplified, and even the reversal of a T-cell energy into an activational process seems to be possible. Malignant ascites also contains all different immune cells needed for action of the proposed tri-cell complex. Additionally, a systemic effect through the induction of cell-mediated antitumor immunity with subsequent spreading of tumor-specific T-cells may be possible (in the sense of a cell-mediated immunity after "tumor vaccination").

Another important factor for i.p. catumaxomab therapy against peritoneal carcinomatosis is based on the mesenchymal origin of the peritoneal surface [30]. There is no physiological EpCAM expression on the mesenchymal cells. This factor enables tumor cells of peritoneal carcinomatosis to be specifically targeted by catumaxomab via the anti-EpCAM binding arm [31].

CLINICAL TRIALS WITH CATUMAXOMAB

The clinical application of trifunctional antibodies was firstly investigated in a pilot study of eight patients with PC, which demonstrated the diminishing of ascites accumulation with no need for further paracentesis, which was associated with a complete tumor cell killing [32].

The clinical safety and feasibility were investigated in a phase I/II study, which was designed to explore the tolerability and efficacy of catumaxomab, as well as to identify the maximal tolerated dose (MTD) administered i.p. in 23 patients with malignant ascites due to ovarian cancer. Most of the adverse events (AEs) were in context with the proposed immunological mechanism of action (e.g., fever, nausea/vomiting, abdominal pain) [33]. Reversible elevation of liver parameters as a result of immunological cholangitis was measured, as the EpCAM antigen is expressed on normal bile duct epithelium. A cytokine-release syndrome with a substantial increase of interleukin-6 and TNF-alpha was observed [33].

The clinical treatment effect was to be confirmed by a randomized phase II/III study in EpCAM-positive cancer patients with symptomatic malignant ascites requiring therapeutic ascites puncture. Patients were randomized to the treatment groups in a 2:1 ratio (catumaxomab/control) stratified by cancer entity (ovarian and nonovarian). Patients in the catumaxomab group received four i.p. infusions of catumaxomab, whereas control patients were treated with paracentesis only. The primary endpoint was puncture-free survival, defined as the time to first therapeutic ascites puncture or death, whichever occurs first [34]. A total of 258 patients were included into the study with 129 patients in each stratum (ovarian cancer patients and nonovarian cancer).

Gastric cancer patients were the largest subgroup (51.2%). Intraperitoneal therapy with catumaxomab resulted in a significant improvement of puncture-free-survival time (37 days for catumaxomab vs. 14 days for control [gastric cancer 44 vs. 15 days]; $p < 0.0001$) and time to next puncture (80 vs. 15 days [gastric cancer 118 vs. 15 days]; $p < 0.0001$). Prolonged time to progression (110 vs. 34 days; gastric cancer 110 vs. 35 days; $p < 0.0001$) and overall survival (gastric cancer 71 vs. 44 days; $p = 0.0313$) indicate effects on the underlying tumor. Gastric cancer patients benefited most from catumaxomab. Catumaxomab was well tolerated. The most commonly reported AEs in the catumaxomab group were cytokine release–related symptoms (pyrexia, nausea, and vomiting) and abdominal pain, which was consistent in ovarian and nonovarian cancer patients. These events were generally mild to moderate in intensity and mostly fully reversible [34].

Based on this study, in 2009, the European Medicines Agency's Committee for Medicinal Products for Human Use approved catumaxomab for the i.p. treatment of malignant ascites in EpCAM-positive carcinomas [35]. To date, catumaxomab is still the only bispecific antibody construct to be approved for clinical application in patients.

Treatment of peritoneal carcinomatosis without significant malignant ascites was investigated in a multicenter phase I/II study in patients with peritoneal carcinomatosis due to colon, gastric, or pancreatic cancer. A total of 24 patients were treated with 4 i.p. applications of escalating catumaxomab doses. The MTD was found at 10–20–50 and 200 μg catumaxomab for the four i.p. infusions.

Most frequent side effects were nausea/vomiting, abdominal pain, and fever and comparable to the results of previous studies. No intensive care unit treatment was necessary. A matched-pair analysis compared the survival with patients receiving conventional treatment. Patients were matched regarding sex, age, tumor surgery, chemotherapy, and extent of peritoneal carcinomatosis. The median survival after diagnosis of PC was 180 days in the matched-pair population treated conventionally versus 502 days in the catumaxomab group [36].

In addition to the i.p. therapy trials for patients with peritoneal carcinomatosis, the development program for catumaxomab included a new concept for the prevention of peritoneal carcinomatosis in patients with high-risk gastric cancer.

The first study was a single-arm, open-label, single-center phase I feasibility study in patients with intra-abdominal epithelial carcinomas in order to investigate intraoperative and early postoperative therapy. Primary endpoint was safety and tolerability. A total of 12 patients (8 gastric, 3 pancreatic, 1 colon cancer) were included. Intraoperative treatment was well tolerated up to 20 µg of i.p. catumaxomab without dose limiting toxicities. During follow-up of 30 months, only one patient presented with an intra-abdominal tumor recurrence after complete resection of gastric cancer and local peritoneal carcinomatosis so far. The vast majority of observed AEs belonged once again to the pattern of well-known cytokine release–related symptoms overlapping with common postoperative reactions after major gastrointestinal surgery [30].

Another study was a multicenter, phase II, two-arm randomized study: A total of 55 patients were randomized during D2 procedure to surgery alone or surgery + catumaxomab treatment consisting of 1 intraoperative and 4 postoperative i.p. infusions with ascending doses on day 7, 10, 13, and 16. This adjuvant treatment was well tolerated; the most frequent AEs were anemia, pyrexia, systemic inflammatory response syndrome, and abdominal pain. Unfortunately, the study was not powered to provide valuable efficacy data on time to relapse or survival.

TUMOR STEM CELLS, VACCINATION, AND PREDICTIVE BIOMARKERS IN CATUMAXOMAB IMMUNOTHERAPY

Catumaxomab was also shown to induce relevant activity against tumor stem cells after i.p. immunotherapy in patients with malignant ascites. Peritoneal fluid samples from 258 patients with malignant ascites randomized to catumaxomab or control groups in the phase II/III study mentioned earlier were investigated for molecular effects of catumaxomab treatment. After catumaxomab treatment, the number of tumor cells and VEGF levels decreased, whereas the CD4+ and CD8+ T-cell activation increased substantially after treatment. Notably, CD133(+)/EpCAM(+) cancer stem cells vanished from the catumaxomab samples but not from the control samples. In vitro investigations indicated that catumaxomab eliminated tumor cells in a manner associated with release of proinflammatory Th1 cytokines [37].

Catumaxomab enhanced T-cell activation [CD69, CD107A (LAMP1), HLA-DR, and PD-1(PDCD1) expression] and stimulated inflammatory CD4(+) TH1 and CD8(+) TH1 to release IFN-γ but failed to trigger TH17 cells. Engagement of CD16-expressing cells caused upregulation of TRAIL (TNSF10) and costimulatory CD40 and CD80 molecules. CatmAb promoted tumor cell death associated with ATP release and strongly synergized with oxaliplatin for the exposure of the three hallmarks of immunogenic cell death (calreticulin, HMGB1, and ATP) [38].

Moreover, the relative lymphocyte count (RLC) was identified as a biomarker for the treatment effect of catumaxomab on survival of malignant ascites patients. A RLC >13% was found to be a significant prognostic biomarker.

The role of RLC in the context of i.p. immunotherapy was discussed as a rapid and simple marker of the balance between antitumor immune activity and tumor-induced immunosuppression [39,40].

SUMMARY

The trifunctional antibody catumaxomab showed clinically meaningful activity after i.p. administration in patients with malignant ascites due to EpCAM expressing epithelial cancers. To date, catumaxomab is the only drug for specific and targeted treatment of malignant ascites in patients with peritoneal carcinomatosis. This observation is outstanding, as it is accompanied by complete destruction of tumor cells by a unique mode of action. Moreover, it is the only approved drug for ascites treatment.

The concept of i.p. catumaxomab treatment has been established as a feasible EpCAM-targeted immunotherapy in peritoneal carcinomatosis. Since i.v. chemotherapy does not necessary contain i.p. efficacy, i.p. catumaxomab contains reasonable options for local control and therapy of PC and malignant ascites.

This statement is especially true in patients with advanced peritoneal carcinomatosis, who are not suitable for surgical peritonectomy and HIPEC. Here, systemic chemotherapy together with i.p. catumaxomab will offer new treatment opportunities.

Further perspectives include the efficacy of catumaxomab against tumor stem cells and the selection of optimal patients and the optimal time point for treatment by prognostic biomarkers like RLC.

REFERENCES

1. Kubicka U, Olszewski WL, Tarnowski W, Bielecki K, Ziolkowska A, Wierzbicki Z. Normal human immune peritoneal cells: Subpopulations and functional characteristics. *Scandinavian Journal of Immunology*. 1996;44:157–163.
2. Jayne DG, Perry SL, Morrison E, Farmery SM, Guillou PJ. Activated mesothelial cells produce heparin-binding growth factors: Implications for tumour metastases. *British Journal of Cancer*. 2000;82:1233–1238.
3. Yamaguchi Y, Ohshita A, Kawabuchi Y, Hihara J, Miyahara E, Noma K et al. Locoregional immunotherapy of malignant ascites from gastric cancer using DTH-oriented doses of the streptococcal preparation OK-432: Treatment of Th1 dysfunction in the ascites microenvironment. *International Journal of Oncology*. 2004;24:959–966.

4. Freedman RS, Vadhan-Raj S, Butts C, Savary C, Melichar B, Verschraegen C et al. Pilot study of Flt3 ligand comparing intraperitoneal with subcutaneous routes on hematologic and immunologic responses in patients with peritoneal carcinomatosis and mesotheliomas. *Clinical Cancer Research: An Official Journal of the American Association for Cancer Research.* 2003;9:5228–5237.

5. Eggermont AM, Sugarbaker PH. Lymphokine-activated killer cell and interleukin-2 inhibitors: Their role in adoptive immunotherapy. *Cellular Immunology.* 1987;107:384–394.

6. Ottow RT, Steller EP, Sugarbaker PH, Wesley RA, Rosenberg SA. Immunotherapy of intraperitoneal cancer with interleukin 2 and lymphokine-activated killer cells reduces tumor load and prolongs survival in murine models. *Cellular Immunology.* 1987;104:366–376.

7. Perrin P, Cassagnau E, Burg C, Patry Y, Vavasseur F, Harb J et al. An interleukin 2/sodium butyrate combination as immunotherapy for rat colon cancer peritoneal carcinomatosis. *Gastroenterology.* 1994;107:1697–1708.

8. Sartori S, Nielsen I, Tassinari D, Trevisani L, Abbasciano V, Malacarne P. Evaluation of a standardized protocol of intracavitary recombinant interferon alpha-2b in the palliative treatment of malignant peritoneal effusions. A prospective pilot study. *Oncology.* 2001;61:192–196.

9. Andersson H, Lindegren S, Back T, Jacobsson L, Leser G, Horvath G. Radioimmunotherapy of nude mice with intraperitoneally growing ovarian cancer xenograft utilizing 211At-labelled monoclonal antibody MOv18. *Anticancer Research.* 2000;20:459–462.

10. Kinuya S, Li XF, Yokoyama K, Mori H, Shiba K, Watanabe N et al. Intraperitoneal radioimmunotherapy in treating peritoneal carcinomatosis of colon cancer in mice compared with systemic radioimmunotherapy. *Cancer Science.* 2003;94:650–654.

11. Muto MG, Finkler NJ, Kassis AI, Howes AE, Anderson LL, Lau CC et al. Intraperitoneal radioimmunotherapy of refractory ovarian carcinoma utilizing iodine-131-labeled monoclonal antibody OC125. *Gynecologic Oncology.* 1992;45:265–272.

12. Wunderlich JR, Mezzanzanica D, Garrido MA, Neblock DS, Daddona PE, Andrew SM et al. Bispecific antibodies and retargeted cellular cytotoxicity: Novel approaches to cancer therapy. *International Journal of Clinical & Laboratory Research.* 1992;22:17–20.

13. Litvinov SV, Velders MP, Bakker HA, Fleuren GJ, Warnaar SO. Ep-CAM: A human epithelial antigen is a homophilic cell-cell adhesion molecule. *The Journal of Cell Biology.* 1994;125:437–446.

14. Amann M, Brischwein K, Lutterbuese P, Parr L, Petersen L, Lorenczewski G et al. Therapeutic window of MuS110, a single-chain antibody construct bispecific for murine EpCAM and murine CD3. *Cancer Research.* 2008;68:143–151.

15. Went PT, Lugli A, Meier S, Bundi M, Mirlacher M, Sauter G et al. Frequent EpCam protein expression in human carcinomas. *Human Pathology.* 2004;35:122–128.

16. Went P, Vasei M, Bubendorf L, Terracciano L, Tornillo L, Riede U et al. Frequent high-level expression of the immunotherapeutic target Ep-CAM in colon, stomach, prostate and lung cancers. *British Journal of Cancer.* 2006;94:128–135.

17. Munz M, Kieu C, Mack B, Schmitt B, Zeidler R, Gires O. The carcinoma-associated antigen EpCAM upregulates c-myc and induces cell proliferation. *Oncogene.* 2004;23:5748–5758.

18. Osta WA, Chen Y, Mikhitarian K, Mitas M, Salem M, Hannun YA et al. EpCAM is overexpressed in breast cancer and is a potential target for breast cancer gene therapy. *Cancer Research.* 2004;64:5818–5824.

19. Peipp M, Valerius T. Bispecific antibodies targeting cancer cells. *Biochemical Society Transactions.* 2002;30:507–511.

20. Baeuerle PA, Kufer P, Lutterbuse R. Bispecific antibodies for polyclonal T-cell engagement. *Current Opinion in Molecular Therapeutics.* 2003;5:413–419.

21. Haas C, Krinner E, Brischwein K, Hoffmann P, Lutterbuse R, Schlereth B et al. Mode of cytotoxic action of T cell-engaging BiTE antibody MT110. *Immunobiology.* 2009;214:441–453.

22. Kufer P, Lutterbuse R, Baeuerle PA. A revival of bispecific antibodies. *Trends in Biotechnology.* 2004;22:238–244.

23. Lindhofer H, Mocikat R, Steipe B, Thierfelder S. Preferential species-restricted heavy/light chain pairing in rat/mouse quadromas. Implications for a single-step purification of bispecific antibodies. *Journal of Immunology.* 1995;155:219–225.

24. Lindhofer H, Menzel H, Gunther W, Hultner L, Thierfelder S. Bispecific antibodies target operationally tumor-specific antigens in two leukemia relapse models. *Blood.* 1996;88:4651–4658.

25. Ruf P, Lindhofer H. Induction of a long-lasting antitumor immunity by a trifunctional bispecific antibody. *Blood.* 2001;98:2526–2534.

26. Zeidler R, Mayer A, Gires O, Schmitt B, Mack B, Lindhofer H et al. TNFalpha contributes to the antitumor activity of a bispecific, trifunctional antibody. *Anticancer Research.* 2001;21:3499–3503.

27. Zeidler R, Mysliwietz J, Csanady M, Walz A, Ziegler I, Schmitt B et al. The Fc-region of a new class of intact bispecific antibody mediates activation of

accessory cells and NK cells and induces direct phagocytosis of tumour cells. *British Journal of Cancer*. 2000;83:261–266.

28. Zeidler R, Reisbach G, Wollenberg B, Lang S, Chaubal S, Schmitt B et al. Simultaneous activation of T cells and accessory cells by a new class of intact bispecific antibody results in efficient tumor cell killing. *Journal of Immunology*. 1999;163:1246–1252.

29. Strohlein MA, Siegel R, Jager M, Lindhofer H, Jauch KW, Heiss MM. Induction of anti-tumor immunity by trifunctional antibodies in patients with peritoneal carcinomatosis. *Journal of Experimental & Clinical Cancer Research*. 2009;28:18.

30. Strohlein MA, Heiss MM. Intraperitoneal immunotherapy to prevent peritoneal carcinomatosis in patients with advanced gastrointestinal malignancies. *Journal of Surgical Oncology*. 2009;100:329–330.

31. Strohlein MA, Heiss MM. Immunotherapy of peritoneal carcinomatosis. *Cancer Treatment and Research*. 2007;134:483–491.

32. Heiss MM, Strohlein MA, Jager M, Kimmig R, Burges A, Schoberth A et al. Immunotherapy of malignant ascites with trifunctional antibodies. *International Journal of Cancer*. 2005;117:435–443.

33. Burges A, Wimberger P, Kumper C, Gorbounova V, Sommer H, Schmalfeldt B et al. Effective relief of malignant ascites in patients with advanced ovarian cancer by a trifunctional anti-EpCAM x anti-CD3 antibody: A phase I/II study. *Clinical Cancer Research: An Official Journal of the American Association for Cancer Research*. 2007;13:3899–3905.

34. Heiss MM, Murawa P, Koralewski P, Kutarska E, Kolesnik OO, Ivanchenko VV et al. The trifunctional antibody catumaxomab for the treatment of malignant ascites due to epithelial cancer: Results of a prospective randomized phase II/III trial. *International Journal of Cancer*. 2010;127:2209–2221.

35. Seimetz D, Lindhofer H, Bokemeyer C. Development and approval of the trifunctional antibody catumaxomab (anti-EpCAMxanti-CD3) as a targeted cancer immunotherapy. *Cancer Treatment Reviews*. 2010;36:458–467.

36. Ströhlein MA, Lordick F, Rüttinger D, Grützner KU, Schemanski OC, Jäger M et al. Immunotherapy of peritoneal carcinomatosis with the antibody catumaxomab in colon, gastric, or pancreatic cancer: An open-label, multicenter, phase I/II trial. *Onkologie*. 2011;34:101–110.

37. Jager M, Schoberth A, Ruf P, Hess J, Hennig M, Schmalfeldt B et al. Immunomonitoring results of a phase II/III study of malignant ascites patients treated with the trifunctional antibody catumaxomab (anti-EpCAM x anti-CD3). *Cancer Research*. 2012;72:24–32.

38. Goere D, Flament C, Rusakiewicz S, Poirier-Colame V, Kepp O, Martins I et al. Potent immunomodulatory effects of the trifunctional antibody catumaxomab. *Cancer Research*. 2013;73:4663–4673.

39. Heiss MM, Strohlein MA, Bokemeyer C, Arnold D, Parsons SL, Seimetz D et al. The role of relative lymphocyte count as a biomarker for the effect of catumaxomab on survival in malignant ascites patients: Results from a phase II/III study. *Clinical Cancer Research: An Official Journal of the American Association for Cancer Research*. 2014;20:3348–3357.

40. Strohlein MA, Lefering R, Bulian DR, Heiss MM. Relative lymphocyte count is a prognostic parameter in cancer patients with catumaxomab immunotherapy. *Medical Hypotheses*. 2014;82:295–299.

34

The promise of oncolytic viral therapy for the treatment of peritoneal surface malignancies

JOHN H. STEWART, IV AND LAUREN GILLORY

RATIONALE FOR ONCOLYTIC VIRAL THERAPY

The previous chapters of this book have evaluated current treatment modalities for the treatment of peritoneal surface malignancies including systemic chemotherapy and hyperthermic intraperitoneal chemotherapy (HIPEC). However, our group and others have focused on the use of oncolytic viral agents as a novel approach to providing therapy to patients who are ineligible for HIPEC due to the volume of disease at presentation or poor performance status.

All trials of HIPEC to date have demonstrated a strong correlation between the completeness of cytoreduction and survival. Presently, two classification systems are used to describe the extent of cytoreduction. The resection classification system used at Wake Forest includes complete (R0, no gross disease with negative microscopic margins; R1, no gross disease with positive microscopic margins) versus incomplete (R2a-c) cytoreduction. A resection classification of R2a indicates residual tumor of up to 5 mm, R2b designates 6–20 mm of gross disease, and R2c identifies more than 20 mm gross residual disease. Data from our institution, and others, demonstrate a significant survival advantage for patients undergoing R0/R1 resection compared to those with R2 resections [1–5]. When it is not possible to perform a significant cytoreduction, HIPEC is rarely indicated; the 1-year survival in these individuals is exceedingly low. A recent study of 56 patients with peritoneal carcinomatosis demonstrated a 79% 2-year survival rate in patients undergoing complete cytoreduction and HIPEC, while those

undergoing incomplete cytoreduction had a 2-year survival of only 44.7% [1]. Similarly, Yonemura et al. demonstrated a 40% 3-year survival in patients with gastric carcinomatosis treated with complete cytoreduction and HIPEC. This is a dramatic improvement over the 3-year survival rate of 10% seen in a similar group of patients treated with HIPEC only [6]. In our experience, patients undergoing R0 resection followed by intraperitoneal heated chemotherapy experienced 3-year survival rates of 72.4%, while those undergoing R1, R2a, R2b, and R2c resections experienced 5-year survival rates of 50%, 44%, 22.2%, and 9.3%, respectively [1].

Due to the extent of surgery necessary to obtain optimal cytoreduction, the morbidity and mortality of HIPEC are significant [1,7,8]. Current morbidity rates experienced by centers performing HIPEC range between 27% and 56%. The most common complications of HIPEC include abscess, fistula, prolonged ileus, pneumonia, and hematologic toxicity. The national mortality rate for HIPEC has been reported to be between 0% and 11% [1]. Given the significant risks associated with this procedure, it is necessary to select patients who will derive the maximal benefit with lower risks of postoperative morbidity and mortality. As a result, many patients with poor performance status or high-volume disease are not candidates for the extensive cytoreduction that is necessary to derive the full benefit of HIPEC.

We therefore propose an alternative approach to peritoneal surface malignancies that utilizes the cytolytic effects of oncolytic viruses while leveraging their impact on antitumor immunity. Many groups to date have studied oncolytic viruses as promising anticancer agents due to their ability to preferentially kill malignant cells while sparing normal cells. A key finding in recent years is that direct cytolysis of cancer cells by oncolytic viruses initiate immune responses that are essential for therapeutic efficacy. The work contained herein will review current progress in the field of oncolytic viral therapy and its potential application to the treatment of peritoneal surface malignancies.

MOLECULAR BASIS FOR VIRAL SELECTIVITY

Among the hallmarks of a malignant cell are hyperproliferation, diminished growth factor requirements, the activation of aberrant growth signaling pathways, and the loss of anchorage-dependent growth. A balance exists between the proliferative and antiviral signaling pathways in cellular homeostasis. Although cells respond to growth factors, they are also able to respond to antiviral signals that are generally antiproliferative. A flurry of proliferative events occurs during molecular carcinogenesis including overexpression of epithelial and platelet-derived growth factors, as well as transforming growth factor alpha. In addition, mutations in the p53 tumor suppressor gene and Ras pathways have been shown to drive dysregulated cellular proliferation at the expense of antiviral signaling pathways. Thus, many cancer cells have defective antiviral defenses. During oncolytic viral infections, normal cells produce interferon, which activates protective antiviral signaling in surrounding cells (see Figure 34.1). Consequently, proliferative pathways are inhibited and the infected index normal cells die, while the surrounding normal cells survive. Cancer cells, however, support viral replication after infection due to the overexpression of the proliferative pathways such as Ras at

the expense of the antiviral signaling pathways including protein kinase R (PKR). Therefore, surrounding cancer cells are susceptible to cell death after viral infection.

With this understanding, oncolytic viral therapy has grown as a potential treatment for a number of histologies. The field's growth has been guided by three overarching principles. First, cancer cells downregulate their antiviral responses during molecular carcinogenesis. Second, cancer cells vary in their susceptibility to virus depending on which of the proliferative pathways are activated and which antiviral pathways are suppressed. Finally, there are a number of potential oncolytic viruses in various stages of development including herpes simplex virus (HSV), adenovirus, vaccinia virus, vesicular stomatitis virus (VSV), measles virus, Newcastle disease virus (NDV), influenza A virus, and reovirus.

SPECIFIC ONCOLYTIC VIRUSES

Herpes simplex viruses

HSV is a double-stranded DNA virus that contains about 80 viral genes. These genes allow for multiple manipulations that aid in its development as an oncolytic agent. The first selective replication-competent HSV, as reported by Martuza et al., employed a thymidine kinase (TK)-deficient oncolytic HSV mutant in the treatment of glioblastoma multiforme [9]. Given the significant neuropathogenicity associated with the first generation of the TK-deficient oncolytic HSVs, subsequent work focused on developing an HSV that featured deletion of both copies of the γ34.5 gene to reduce neurovirulence and enhance tumor specificity. ICP34.5, the gene product of the γ34.5 gene, is necessary for HSV to replicate in normal neurons; however, it is not required

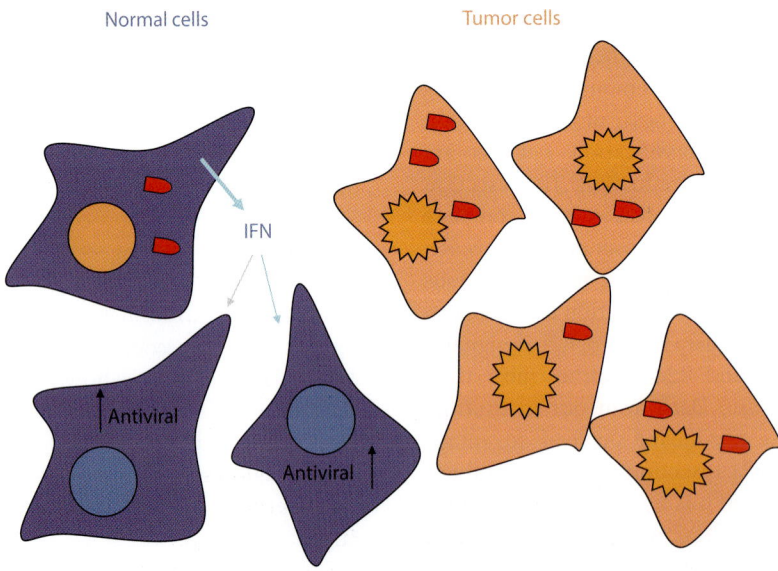

Figure 34.1 Normal cells, when infected with oncolytic viruses, produce interferons. The resultant antiviral responses in surrounding cells protect them from the virus' cytopathic effects. On the other hand, cancer cells lack antiviral signaling and are therefore susceptible to the cytopathic effects of oncolytic viruses.

for production of infectious progeny in cancer cells. An open reading frame mutation of the γ34.5 gene thus confers specificity for oncolytic HSV [10,11]. Another target of genetic engineering to confer specificity is the UL39 gene, which encodes the large subunit of ribonucleotide reductase (ICP6) [12,13]. Although nondividing cells require ICP6 for efficient viral growth, those with abundant deoxyribose nucleotide triphosphates pools or mutated p16 do not require this protein. Therefore, mutation of the UL39 gene results in selective replication in cancer cells [14]. Subsequent generations of oncolytic HSV have been engineered with multiple gene mutations/deletions. For example, the G207 HSV has deletions that inactivate ICP34.5 as well as a *lacZ* gene insertion that inactivates the UL39 gene [15,16]. Current oncolytic HSVs have been developed to also include therapeutic transgenes including GM-CSF and Fas ligand [17,18].

Adenovirus

Adenoviruses, members of the Adenoviridae family, are the most commonly used viral oncolytic agents in clinical trials due to its ability to infect a wide variety of cell types [19,20]. In theory, adenoviral infection and replication continues until complete tumor eradication has been achieved. Additionally, the adenoviral genome can be readily manipulated, and it will accommodate insertion of large and/or multiple therapeutic genes for augmented antitumor effects [21–23]. Finally, clinical-grade recombinant oncolytic Ad stocks can be manufactured at high yields and titers [19].

Several clinical trials of oncolytic adenovirus therapies have been reported [19,24,25]. The ONYX-015 (Pfizer Corp., Groton, CT) adenovirus was the first replication-selective oncolytic adenovirus used in clinical trials [26,27]. This oncolytic virus, which contains a deletion of the gene encoding the p53-inactivating protein E1B, specifically kills tumor cells with p53 mutations [28]. To date, more than 18 clinical trials have been conducted with ONYX-015 against a variety of cancers, including colorectal and ovarian carcinomas [19,29]. However, the antitumor efficacy of ONYX-015 as a single agent was disappointing in the majority of these trials [24,30].

Vaccinia viruses

Vaccinia virus, an enveloped DNA virus, has been developed as the backbone of many oncolytic viral strains [31], due to its demonstrated tumor-selective replication and its ability to target host cell cycle, apoptotic pathways, and immune response [32–34]. In addition, its use as a vaccine vector against smallpox has led to a comprehensive understanding of its immune-activating capacity.

Although recent clinical trials with GM-CSF expressing oncolytic vaccinia virus have demonstrated the role of antitumor immunity as a means of enhancing therapeutic activity [35–37], approaches with other cytokines have produced less promising preclinical results due to a variety of reasons including the induction of immunosuppressive monocyte-derived suppressor cells and the upregulation of antiviral immunity [38–41]. Alternative approaches that serve as the focus of current investigation include viral expression of monoclonal antibodies, chemokines, and decoys to prometastatic molecules [42–45].

Vesicular stomatitis virus

VSV, the prototypical member of the family Rhabdoviridae, is a potent inducer of apoptosis with many types of tumor cells susceptible to infection and killing by VSV [44,46–53]. Furthermore, VSV is highly sensitive to the antiviral effects of IFN and therefore replicates selectively in cancer cells that have defects in the IFN pathway. The selectivity of VSV for cancer cells can be enhanced by introducing mutations in the matrix (M) protein. The M protein of VSV is a multifunctional protein that plays a major role in virus assembly as well as in the inhibition of host gene expression. The inhibition of host gene expression suppresses the antiviral responses of host cells. This inhibition occurs at multiple levels, including transcription, nuclear–cytoplasmic RNA transport, and translation [54–56]. The inhibitory effects of M protein on host gene expression are genetically separable from its virus assembly functions, so that a number of different mutations render the M protein defective in its ability to inhibit host gene expression without compromising its ability to function in virus assembly [57,58]. Because the inhibition of host gene expression suppresses the production of IFNs and other antiviral proteins in infected cells, mutations in the M protein allow infected cells with intact IFN signaling to mount antiviral responses. As a result, normal cells, which have intact antiviral responses, are able to produce IFN and other antiviral cytokines in response to infection with M protein mutant VSV, thereby enhancing the virus' specificity for cancer cells.

Our group has generated genetically engineered recombinant viruses derived from cDNA clones containing M protein mutations, such as the M51R virus, which contains a single M51R amino acid substitution in the M protein, that is selective for cancer cells [46]. Such M protein mutants appear to be strong candidates for oncolytic viral therapy as they are attenuated for replication in normal tissues, but replicate as well as recombinant virus with wild-type (wt) M protein (rwt virus) in cancers that have defective antiviral responses. Future work in the field will evaluate the impact of additional mutations on the antitumor effects of VSV.

Measles virus

The measles virus is a negative-strand RNA virus. Burkitt's and Hodgkin's lymphomas have been reported to spontaneously resolve following wt measles infections, thus supporting its role as a potential oncolytic agent [59,60]. The measles virus genome contains six genes encoding the phosphoprotein and nucleocapsid, M, fusion (F), hemagglutinin (H), and large proteins, as well as the two accessory C and V proteins [61]. The binding of H protein to a cellular receptor induces conformational changes to both H and F proteins resulting in pH-independent membrane fusion. As a result, the viral H and F glycoproteins are expressed on the cell surface of cells infected by the measles virus thus facilitating cell-to-cell fusion that is triggered via H glycoprotein recognition of the viral receptor on neighboring cells [62]. This cell-to-cell interaction results in the formation of giant multinucleated cell aggregates (syncytia) that ultimately undergo apoptotic death in a number of cancer lines [63,64].

Newcastle disease virus

NDV, a member of the Paramyxoviridae family, is an enveloped negative-stranded RNA virus. As with the vast majority of oncolytic viruses, NDV selectively replicates in human cancer cells that have developed defects in the interferon signaling pathway. The virus has been given intravenously, intraperitoneally, and intratumorally in preclinical studies with human tumor xenograft models. These studies demonstrated evidence of oncolytic activity with few systemic side effects [65–69].

An attenuated Newcastle virus strain, PV701 virus, was recently tested in a phase I clinical trial. The virus was administered intravenously (5.9×10^9–24×10^9 plaque-forming units [pfu]/m^2 every 28 days) in 79 patients with solid tumors. Interestingly, the toxicity of this treatment decreased after the initial treatment. The side effects were generally mild and limited to fever, flu-like symptoms, and hypotension. The maximum tolerated dose following a single infusion was established at 12×10^9 pfu/m^2, and subsequent infusions were tolerated up to 120×10^9 pfu/m^2. Twenty three percent of the patients eligible for response assessment maintained stable disease from 4 months to >30 months after treatment with one patient achieving a complete response [70].

The intravenous delivery of NDV was optimized to include a 3-hour infusion for the first dose compared with the 10- and 30-minute infusions administered in the aforementioned trial with subsequent doses infused over 1 hour. Eighteen patients were enrolled in this phase I trial in which six doses were given per 3-week cycle. The first dose was safely escalated to 24×10^9 pfu/m^2, and doses 2–6 were safely escalated to 120×10^9 pfu/m^2. This infusion technique resulted in better tolerability as well as fewer infusion reactions [71].

A recent prospective, randomized phase III evaluated the clinical utility of a NDV-infected autologous tumor cell vaccine after hepatic metastasectomy for colorectal cancer. Although there were no differences in overall and disease-free survival, subgroup analysis revealed significant overall (p = 0.042) and disease-free survival (p = 0.047) advantages for vaccinated patients in the colon cancer cohort in the intention-to-treat analysis [72].

Influenza virus

Influenza virus is a negative-sense, single-stranded RNA virus that belongs to the Orthomyxoviridae family. Unlike other RNA viruses, orthomyxovirus genomes are transcribed and replicated in the nucleus of the infected cell. The oncolytic potential of influenza can be traced to a 1904 report that described a complete remission of leukemia in a woman who had been stricken by the flu. Interestingly, there have been no subsequent reports of influenza virus–mediated tumor regression.

Because the influenza virus lacks oncolytic specificity, recent efforts have focused on engineering the virus for optimal oncolytic effect through manipulation of the NS-1 protein [73,74]. Inhibition of the NS-1 protein, an influenza virulence factor that counteracts PKR, prevents the propagation of influenza virus in normal cells. On the other hand, the Ras pathway is frequently activated during molecular carcinogenesis thereby inhibiting PKR. This results in an ineffective antiviral response in cancer cells, thus rendering them susceptible to the oncolytic effects of the influenza virus. Current reports have demonstrated antitumor activity on a variety of malignancies including colon cancer [75,76].

Reovirus

This double-stranded RNA virus is a member of the Reoviridae [77]. The genome of this oncolytic virus is comprised of 10 segments, and it is therefore difficult to generate recombinant versions of this virus that can be modified with attachment proteins or therapeutic genes [78]. Preclinical work has shown that cellular events favoring reovirus-mediated apoptosis include downregulation of nuclear factor kappa-light-chain-enhancer of activated B cells (NF-κB) through elevation of β-catenin expression in HEK293 and HCT116 colon cancer cell lines as well as TNF-related apoptosis-inducing ligand (TRAIL)-induced apoptosis [79,80]. Additional studies have reported that reovirus activates human dendritic cells to promote innate antitumor immunity [81]. Current work is focused on clinical trials of reovirus against a variety of histologies including colorectal cancer [82].

FUTURE DIRECTIONS

At present, we do not know what proportion of metastatic peritoneal tumors will be sensitive to oncolytic viruses. Furthermore, there is no information on the molecular determinants of virus resistance or immune signature of these tumors. As highlighted in past meetings of the NIH Recombinant DNA Advisory Committee, it is important to determine the proportion of human metastatic colorectal tumors that are susceptible to the oncolytic effects of viral agents prior to moving this therapy to the clinical setting. It is unclear what proportion of metastatic peritoneal tumors that we see in the clinical setting are susceptible to the oncolytic effects of M51R VSV [53]. Determining the proportion of patient tumors that are sensitive to each oncolytic virus will provide critical information for the rational design of clinical trials, as it is not possible to perform proper power calculations without these data. As an extension to this barrier, the molecular determinants of virus resistance for this type of tumor are not known. The application of cDNA microarray studies to clinical samples will facilitate the design of tests to predict benefit from treatment with oncolytic viruses.

REFERENCES

1. Shen P et al. Factors predicting survival after intraperitoneal hyperthermic chemotherapy with mitomycin C after cytoreductive surgery for patients with peritoneal carcinomatosis. *Archives of Surgery.* 2003;138(1):26–33.

2. Culliford AT et al. Surgical debulking and intraperitoneal chemotherapy for established peritoneal metastases from colon and appendix cancer. *Annals of Surgical Oncology.* 2001;8(10):787–795.

3. Marcus EA et al. Prognostic factors affecting survival in patients with colorectal carcinomatosis. *Cancer Investigation.* 1999;17(4):249–252.

4. Glehen O et al. Surgery combined with peritonectomy procedures and intraperitoneal chemohyperthermia in abdominal cancers with peritoneal carcinomatosis: A phase II study. *Journal of Clinical Oncology.* 2003;21(5):799–806.

5. Levine EA et al. Intraperitoneal chemotherapy for peritoneal surface malignancy: Experience with 1,000 patients. *Journal of the American College of Surgeons.* 2014;218(4):573–585.

6. Yonemura Y et al. A new surgical approach (peritonectomy) for the treatment of peritoneal dissemination. *Hepatogastroenterology.* 1999;46(25):601–609.

7. Stephens AD et al. Morbidity and mortality analysis of 200 treatments with cytoreductive surgery and hyperthermic intraoperative intraperitoneal chemotherapy using the coliseum technique. *Annals of Surgical Oncology.* 1999;6(8):790–796.

8. Ahmad SA et al. Reduced morbidity following cytoreductive surgery and intraperitoneal hyperthermic chemoperfusion. *Annals of Surgical Oncology.* 2004;11(4):387–392.

9. Martuza RL et al. Experimental therapy of human glioma by means of a genetically engineered virus mutant. *Science.* 1991;252(5007):854–856.

10. Holman HA, MacLean AR. Neurovirulent factor ICP34.5 uniquely expressed in the herpes simplex virus type 1 Delta gamma 1 34.5 mutant 1716. *Journal of NeuroVirology.* 2008;14(1):28–40.

11. Rampling R et al. Toxicity evaluation of replication-competent herpes simplex virus (ICP 34.5 null mutant 1716) in patients with recurrent malignant glioma. *Gene Therapy.* 2000;7(10):859–866.

12. Goldstein DJ, Weller SK. Herpes simplex virus type 1-induced ribonucleotide reductase activity is dispensable for virus growth and DNA synthesis: Isolation and characterization of an ICP6 *lacZ* insertion mutant. *Journal of Virology.* 1988;62(1):196–205.

13. Mineta T, Rabkin SD, Martuza RL. Treatment of malignant gliomas using ganciclovir-hypersensitive, ribonucleotide reductase-deficient herpes simplex viral mutant. *Cancer Research.* 1994;54(15):3963–3966.

14. Aghi M et al. Oncolytic herpes virus with defective ICP6 specifically replicates in quiescent cells with homozygous genetic mutations in p16. *Oncogene.* 2008;27(30):4249–4254.

15. Mineta T et al. Attenuated multi-mutated herpes simplex virus-1 for the treatment of malignant gliomas. *Nature Medicine.* 1995;1(9):938–943.

16. Walker JR et al. Local and systemic therapy of human prostate adenocarcinoma with the conditionally replicating herpes simplex virus vector G207. *Human Gene Therapy.* 1999;10(13):2237–2243.

17. Loya SM, Zhang X. Enhancing the bystander killing effect of an oncolytic HSV by arming it with a secretable apoptosis activator. *Gene Therapy.* 2015;22:21–30.

18. Kaufman HL et al. Current status of granulocyte-macrophage colony-stimulating factor in the immunotherapy of melanoma. *Journal for Immunotherapy of Cancer.* 2014;2:11.

19. Pesonen S, Kangasniemi L, Hemminki A. Oncolytic adenoviruses for the treatment of human cancer: Focus on translational and clinical data. *Molecular Pharmaceutics.* 2011;8(1):12–28.

20. Van Dyke TA. Analysis of viral-host protein interactions and tumorigenesis in transgenic mice. *Seminars in Cancer Biology.* 1994;5(1):47–60.

21. Bett AJ, Prevec L, Graham FL. Packaging capacity and stability of human adenovirus type 5 vectors. *Journal of Virology.* 1993;67(10):5911–5921.

22. Bauzon M et al. Multigene expression from a replicating adenovirus using native viral promoters. *Molecular Therapy.* 2003;7(4):526 534.

23. Hawkins LK, Hermiston T. Gene delivery from the E3 region of replicating human adenovirus: Evaluation of the E3B region. *Gene Therapy.* 2001;8(15):1142–1148.

24. Toth K, Dhar D, Wold WS. Oncolytic (replication-competent) adenoviruses as anticancer agents. *Expert Opinion on Biological Therapy.* 2010;10(3):353–368.

25. Barzon L et al. Clinical trials of gene therapy, virotherapy, and immunotherapy for malignant gliomas. *Cancer Gene Therapy.* 2006;13(6):539–554.

26. Kirn D, Hermiston T, McCormick F. ONYX-015: Clinical data are encouraging. *Nature Medicine.* 1998;4(12):1341–1342.

27. Kirn D. Oncolytic virotherapy for cancer with the adenovirus dl1520 (Onyx-015): Results of phase I and II trials. *Expert Opinion on Biological Therapy.* 2001;1(3):525–538.

28. Bischoff JR et al. An adenovirus mutant that replicates selectively in p53-deficient human tumor cells. *Science.* 1996;274(5286):373–376.

29. Alemany R. Cancer selective adenoviruses. *Molecular Aspects of Medicine*. 2007;28(1):42–58.

30. Crompton AM, Kirn DH. From ONYX-015 to armed vaccinia viruses: The education and evolution of oncolytic virus development. *Current Cancer Drug Targets*. 2007;7(2):133–139.

31. Kirn DH, Thorne SH. Targeted and armed oncolytic poxviruses: A novel multi-mechanistic therapeutic class for cancer. *Nature Reviews Cancer*. 2009;9(1):64–71.

32. McCart JA et al. Systemic cancer therapy with a tumor-selective vaccinia virus mutant lacking thymidine kinase and vaccinia growth factor genes. *Cancer Research*. 2001;61(24):8751–8757.

33. Guo ZS et al. The enhanced tumor selectivity of an oncolytic vaccinia lacking the host range and anti-apoptosis genes SPI-1 and SPI-2. *Cancer Research*. 2005;65(21):9991–9998.

34. Kirn DH et al. Targeting of interferon-beta to produce a specific, multi-mechanistic oncolytic vaccinia virus. *PLoS Medicine*. 2007;4(12):e353.

35. Park BH et al. Use of a targeted oncolytic poxvirus, JX-594, in patients with refractory primary or metastatic liver cancer: A phase I trial. *The Lancet Oncology*. 2008;9(6):533–542.

36. Breitbach CJ et al. Intravenous delivery of a multi-mechanistic cancer-targeted oncolytic poxvirus in humans. *Nature*. 2011;477(7362):99–102.

37. Heo J et al. Randomized dose-finding clinical trial of oncolytic immunotherapeutic vaccinia JX-594 in liver cancer. *Nature Medicine*. 2013;19(3):329–336.

38. Kohanbash G et al. GM-CSF promotes the immunosuppressive activity of glioma-infiltrating myeloid cells through interleukin-4 receptor-alpha. *Cancer Research*. 2013;73(21):6413–6423.

39. Banaszynski LA et al. Chemical control of protein stability and function in living mice. *Nature Medicine*. 2008;14(10):1123–1127.

40. Wang LC et al. Treating tumors with a vaccinia virus expressing IFNbeta illustrates the complex relationships between oncolytic ability and immunogenicity. *Molecular Therapy*. 2012;20(4):736–748.

41. Chen H et al. Regulating cytokine function enhances safety and activity of genetic cancer therapies. *Molecular Therapy*. 2013;21(1):167–174.

42. Yu F et al. T-cell engager-armed oncolytic vaccinia virus significantly enhances antitumor therapy. *Molecular Therapy*. 2014;22(1):102–111.

43. Li J et al. Chemokine expression from oncolytic vaccinia virus enhances vaccine therapies of cancer. *Molecular Therapy*. 2011;19(4):650–657.

44. Blackham AU et al. Variation in susceptibility of human malignant melanomas to oncolytic vesicular stomatitis virus. *Surgery*. 2013;153(3):333–343.

45. Zhang Z et al. Intravenous administration of adenoviruses targeting transforming growth factor beta signaling inhibits established bone metastases in 4T1 mouse mammary tumor model in an immuno-competent syngeneic host. *Cancer Gene Therapy*. 2012;19(9):630–636.

46. Ahmed M, Cramer SD, Lyles DS. Sensitivity of prostate tumors to wild type and M protein mutant vesicular stomatitis viruses. *Virology*. 2004;330(1):34–49.

47. Chang G et al. Enhanced oncolytic activity of vesicular stomatitis virus encoding SV5-F protein against prostate cancer. *The Journal of Urology*. 2010;183(4):1611–1618.

48. Moussavi M et al. Oncolysis of prostate cancers induced by vesicular stomatitis virus in PTEN knockout mice. *Cancer Research*. 2010;70(4):1367–1376.

49. Galivo F et al. Interference of CD40L-mediated tumor immunotherapy by oncolytic vesicular stomatitis virus. *Human Gene Therapy*. 2010;21(4):439–450.

50. Wollmann G et al. Some attenuated variants of vesicular stomatitis virus show enhanced oncolytic activity against human glioblastoma cells relative to normal brain cells. *Journal of Virology*. 2010;84(3):1563–1573.

51. Blackham AU et al. Molecular determinants of susceptibility to oncolytic vesicular stomatitis virus in pancreatic adenocarcinoma. *Journal of Surgical Research*. 2014;187(2):412–426.

52. Randle RW et al. Oncolytic vesicular stomatitis virus as a treatment for neuroendocrine tumors. *Surgery*. 2013;154(6):1323–1329; discussion 1329–1330.

53. Stewart JH 4th et al. Vesicular stomatitis virus as a treatment for colorectal cancer. *Cancer Gene Therapy*. 2011;18(12):837–849.

54. Yuan H, Yoza BK, Lyles DS. Inhibition of host RNA polymerase II-dependent transcription by vesicular stomatitis virus results from inactivation of TFIID. *Virology*. 1998;251(2):383–392.

55. Yuan H, Puckett S, Lyles DS. Inhibition of host transcription by vesicular stomatitis virus involves a novel mechanism that is independent of phosphorylation of TATA-binding protein (TBP) or association of TBP with TBP-associated factor subunits. *Journal of Virology*. 2001;75(9):4453–4458.

56. Kopecky SA, Lyles DS. Contrasting effects of matrix protein on apoptosis in HeLa and BHK cells infected with vesicular stomatitis virus are due to inhibition of host gene expression. *Journal of Virology*. 2003;77(8):4658–4669.

57. Ahmed M, Lyles DS. Identification of a consensus mutation in M protein of vesicular stomatitis virus from persistently infected cells that affects inhibition of host-directed gene expression. *Virology*. 1997;237(2):378–388.

58. Ahmed M et al. Ability of the matrix protein of vesicular stomatitis virus to suppress beta interferon gene expression is genetically correlated with the inhibition of host RNA and protein synthesis. *Journal of Virology*. 2003;77(8):4646–4657.

59. Ziegler JL. Spontaneous remission in Burkitt's lymphoma. *Journal of the National Cancer Institute Monographs.* 1976;44:61–65.

60. Gross S. Measles and leukaemia. *Lancet.* 1971;1(7695):397–398.

61. Yanagi Y, Takeda M, Ohno S. Measles virus: Cellular receptors, tropism and pathogenesis. *Journal of General Virology.* 2006;87(Pt. 10):2767–2779.

62. Wild TF, Malvoisin E, Buckland R. Measles virus: Both the haemagglutinin and fusion glycoproteins are required for fusion. *Journal of General Virology.* 1991;72(Pt. 2):439–442.

63. Phuong LK et al. Use of a vaccine strain of measles virus genetically engineered to produce carcinoembryonic antigen as a novel therapeutic agent against glioblastoma multiforme. *Cancer Research.* 2003;63(10):2462–2469.

64. Peng KW et al. Systemic therapy of myeloma xenografts by an attenuated measles virus. *Blood.* 2001;98(7):2002–2007.

65. Lorence RM et al. Complete regression of human fibrosarcoma xenografts after local Newcastle disease virus therapy. *Cancer Research.* 1994;54(23):6017–6021.

66. Lorence RM et al. Complete regression of human neuroblastoma xenografts in athymic mice after local Newcastle disease virus therapy. *Journal of the National Cancer Institute.* 1994;86(16):1228–1233.

67. Lorence RM et al. Overview of phase I studies of intravenous administration of PV701, an oncolytic virus. *Current Opinion in Molecular Therapeutics.* 2003;5(6):618–624.

68. Yan Y et al. Effect of recombinant Newcastle disease virus transfection on lung adenocarcinoma A549 cells. *Oncology Letters.* 2014;8(6):2569–2576.

69. Yan Y et al. Apoptotic induction of lung adenocarcinoma A549 cells infected by recombinant RVG Newcastle disease virus (rL-RVG) in vitro. *Molecular Medicine Reports.* 2015;11(1):317–326.

70. Pecora AL et al. Phase I trial of intravenous administration of PV701, an oncolytic virus, in patients with advanced solid cancers. *Journal of Clinical Oncology.* 2002;20(9):2251–2266.

71. Hotte SJ et al. An optimized clinical regimen for the oncolytic virus PV701. *Clinical Cancer Research.* 2007;13(3):977–985.

72. Schulze T et al. Efficiency of adjuvant active specific immunization with Newcastle disease virus modified tumor cells in colorectal cancer patients following resection of liver metastases: Results of a prospective randomized trial. *Cancer Immunology, Immunotherapy.* 2009;58(1):61–69.

73. Bergmann M et al. A genetically engineered influenza A virus with ras-dependent oncolytic properties. *Cancer Research.* 2001;61(22):8188–8193.

74. Hatada E, Saito S, Fukuda R. Mutant influenza viruses with a defective NS1 protein cannot block the activation of PKR in infected cells. *Journal of Virology.* 1999;73(3):2425–2433.

75. Kasloff SB et al. Oncolytic activity of avian influenza virus in human pancreatic ductal adenocarcinoma cell lines. *Journal of Virology.* 2014;88(16):9321–9334.

76. Sturlan S et al. Endogenous expression of proteases in colon cancer cells facilitate influenza A viruses mediated oncolysis. *Cancer Biology & Therapy.* 2010;10(6):592–599.

77. Sabin AB. Reoviruses. A new group of respiratory and enteric viruses formerly classified as ECHO type 10 is described. *Science.* 1959;130(3386):1387–1389.

78. Van Den Wollenberg DJ et al. Modification of mammalian reoviruses for use as oncolytic agents. *Expert Opinion on Biological Therapy.* 2009;9(12):1509–1520.

79. Clarke P et al. Reovirus-induced apoptosis is mediated by TRAIL. *Journal of Virology.* 2000;74(17):8135–8139.

80. Twigger K et al. Enhanced in vitro and in vivo cytotoxicity of combined reovirus and radiotherapy. *Clinical Cancer Research.* 2008;14(3):912–923.

81. Errington F et al. Reovirus activates human dendritic cells to promote innate antitumor immunity. *Journal of Immunology.* 2008;180(9):6018–6026.

82. Maitra R, Ghalib MH, Goel S. Reovirus: A targeted therapeutic—Progress and potential. *Molecular Cancer Research.* 2012;10(12):1514–1525.

Pressurized intraperitoneal aerosol chemotherapy (PIPAC)

MARC A. REYMOND, W. SOLASS, AND C. TEMPFER

INTRODUCTION

To be most effective, anticancer drugs must penetrate tissue efficiently, reaching all the cancer cells that comprise the target population in a concentration sufficient to exert a therapeutic effect. Most research into the resistance of cancers to chemotherapy has concentrated on molecular mechanisms of resistance, whereas the role of limited drug distribution within tumors has been neglected [1].

The use of intraperitoneal drug delivery in the treatment of malignant disease confined to the peritoneal cavity is based on the theoretical potential for increased exposure of the tumor to antineoplastic agents leading to improved cytotoxicity. In patients with tumors confined to the peritoneal cavity, there is established pharmacokinetic and tumor biology–related evidence that intraperitoneal drug administration is advantageous. Clearly, intraperitoneal drug delivery is an important adjunct to surgery and systemic chemotherapy in selected patients [2].

However, there are practical and theoretical concerns about intraperitoneal chemotherapy including [3]

1. Adequacy of drug distribution throughout the entire peritoneal cavity
2. Limited direct penetration of drugs into tumor or normal tissue
3. Decrease in the delivery of drug to the tumor by capillary flow (through the systemic circulation) after regional delivery

4. Unique toxic effects associated with local delivery— e.g., abdominal pain, bowel perforation, infection, and obstruction
5. Added time, inconvenience, and cost associated with the specific requirements of regional delivery—e.g., catheter placement

These concerns explain why, despite the positive effect of initial intraperitoneal chemotherapy on progression-free and overall survival in selected patients with small volume peritoneal carcinomatosis, only few clinicians employ this management strategy other than in the trial setting.

The optimal form of drug delivery for intraperitoneal/intracavitary chemotherapy remains to be determined. The question now is how intraperitoneal chemotherapy should be distributed in order to be most effective, and least toxic. Ideally, this procedure should be of generic nature allowing customization for various indications and further developments in the future.

PRESSURIZED INTRAPERITONEAL AEROSOL CHEMOTHERAPY

A new way of intraperitoneal chemotherapy is the application of cytotoxics in form of a pressurized aerosol into the abdominal cavity. Pressurized intraperitoneal aerosol chemotherapy (PIPAC) was developed on the basis of the specification sheet defined in Table 35.1. PIPAC relies on logical physical principles: local administration into the

Table 35.1 Characteristics of an ideal technology for intraperitoneal drug delivery

Minimally invasive procedure
Procedure can be repeated
Homogeneous drug distribution within the body cavity
Effective/deep drug penetration into tumor nodes
Low systemic drug uptake, low systemic toxicity
Low dose of drug, low local toxicity
No need for previous cytoreductive surgery
Efficacy in the presence of diffuse small bowel invasion
Objective and early assessment of tumor response
Short-term/simultaneous administration with systemic chemotherapy possible
Administration of a large range of active substances (drugs, antibodies, genes, and nanomolecules)

body cavity to improve therapeutic ratio, gaseous form to achieve homogeneous drug distribution, pressure application to enhance convective drug uptake into tumor nodes, and minimally invasive approach to minimize operative trauma. PIPAC allows repeated therapy cycles and objective tumor response assessment.

PIPAC (Figure 35.1) is applied through a laparoscopic access using two balloon trocars in an operating room equipped with laminar airflow. In a first step, a normothermic capnoperitoneum is established with a pressure of 12 mmHg. A cytotoxic solution (about 10% of a normal systemic dose) is nebulized with a micropump into the abdominal cavity, and maintained for 30 minutes. The aerosol is then removed through a closed suction system. Applying an aerosol in the peritoneal cavity allows a homogeneous distribution of the chemotherapeutic agent within the abdomen. Furthermore, an artificial pressure gradient is generated that overcomes tumoral interstitial fluid pressure and results in higher local drug concentration compared to conventional intraperitoneal or intravenous chemotherapy [4]. At the same time, the plasma concentration of the chemotherapeutic agent remains low. Occupational health safety aspects are described elsewhere [5,6].

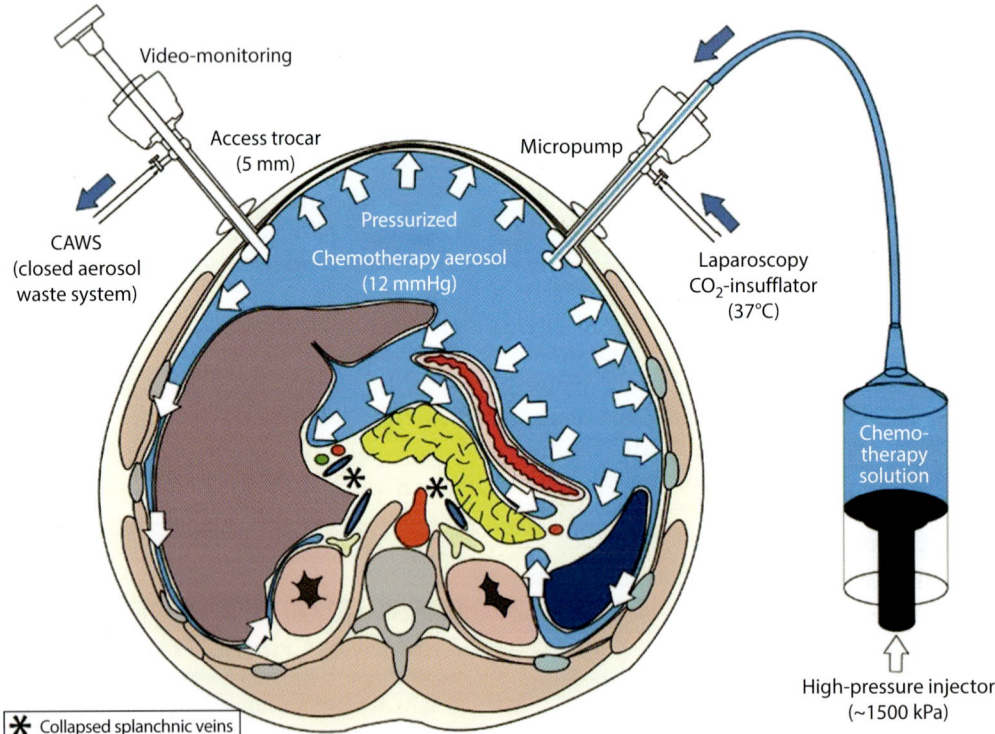

Figure 35.1 Technique of PIPAC. A capnoperitoneum of 12 mmHg is established as usual during laparoscopy. A chemotherapy aerosol is generated at the tip of a mechanical micropump introduced through a balloon trocar and maintained for 30 minutes at 37°C. Then, the toxic aerosol is exsufflated over a secured system (CAWS [closed aerosol waste system]) into the outside environment.

Adequacy of drug distribution throughout the entire peritoneal cavity

If anticancer drugs are unable to access all of the cells within a tumor that are capable of regenerating it (that is, clonogenic cells or tumor stem cells), then whatever their mode of action or potency, their effectiveness will be compromised. Perhaps more importantly, the effectiveness of new molecular medicines to treat cancer will be jeopardized if they cannot efficiently penetrate tumor tissue to reach all of the viable cells [7]. For a cancer treatment to be curative, it must have access to all such tumor cells, as the survival of one cell could form the focus of tumor recurrence (reviewed in [1]).

Various observations in experimental animals suggest limited exposure of the peritoneal surface under conditions of peritoneal dialysis. In general, definitive studies have not been conducted on the potential peritoneal surface area of human subjects. The likelihood exists that much of the residual tumor burden after surgery is untreated or undertreated by conventional intraperitoneal irrigation. If the peritoneal surfaces are not exposed to drug-containing solutions or if they are inadequately exposed, then the rationale for regional administration is compromised [8].

Experimental data obtained in the animal model suggest limited exposure of the peritoneal surface during conventional peritoneal lavage. When peritoneal dialysis was carried out in rodents with a solution containing methylene blue and bovine serum albumin, autopsy findings showed that large parts of the visceral and parietal peritoneum displayed no stain or very little stain [9]. In particular, the hidden aspects of the caecum and stomach as well as large portions of the small and large intestines and of the diaphragm remained unstained. Our experimental results in the large animal model confirm this finding, namely, that distribution of methylene blue within the peritoneal cavity of pigs is poor after peritoneal lavage [10].

During minimal-invasive surgery, pneumoperitoneum is applied in order to create a working space. This working space allows safe placement of access ports through the abdominal wall, outstanding visualization of organs, and completion of complex surgical procedures. Theoretical considerations suggest that the therapeutic capnoperitoneum should be capable of carrying microdroplets of active substances to all exposed peritoneal surfaces. These considerations were confirmed by several preclinical experiments, showing that the active principle is distributed relatively homogeneously throughout the abdomen (Figure 35.2), including hidden surfaces such caecum, stomach, inferior aspect of the liver, gallbladder, ligamentum falciforme, as well as large portions of the small and large intestines and of the diaphragm.

An aerosol is a suspension of particles (in our example of liquid droplets) in a gas (in our case carbon dioxide, CO_2). Hundreds of aerosol products are on the market, including therapeutic aerosols, in particular, in pulmonary medicine [11].

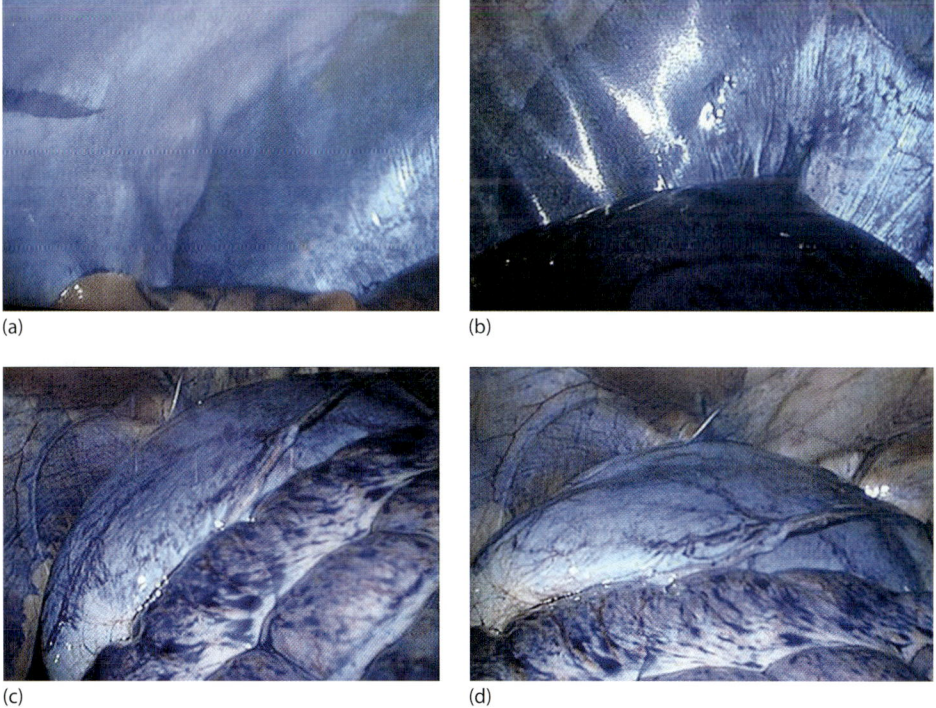

(a)

(b)

(c)

(d)

Figure 35.2 Real-time endoscopic monitoring of nebulization showed immediate staining of the complete abdominal cavity, including the anterior abdominal wall and diaphragmatic peritoneum (a, b), liver (b), and bowel loops and visceral peritoneum (c and d).

Usually, an inert gaseous compound under pressure serves as a propellant. The propellant serves several purposes:

- Pushing the product out of the can
- Vaporizing after leaving the container, producing a spray or foam
- Acting as a solvent for the product (in most cases)

PIPAC technology differs from usual aerosol can technology. No propellant gas is needed, but during PIPAC, a liquid solution is aerosolized into a gaseous (CO_2) environment using a specific nozzle. Energy is provided by applying an upstream mechanical force gradient over a period of time.

The size of the aerosol particles has a major influence on their behavioral properties, so the particle diameter is a key characteristic. During PIPAC, the micropump does not generate a monodisperse aerosol (i.e., all particles have the same size) but a polydisperse aerosol with a heterogeneous droplets diameter ranging from 3 to 15 μm after sedimentation (mean diameter = 11 μm).

Current PIPAC technology is derived from automobile industry, namely, from high-pressure injectors for diesel engines, whereas diesel is known to have a high viscosity, in particular, at lower temperature. Thus, the current micropump allows aerosolizing solutions with higher viscosity, including polymers, glucoses, and lipids. Moreover, it has been shown to work in environments highly saturated with humidity; in other words, it can generate fog in fog.

When applying therapeutic aerosols, it is useful to remember that they are subject to physical laws. These general laws, including size distribution, terminal velocity, aerodynamic diameter, dynamics and dynamics regime, partitioning, activation, and coagulation, are relatively complex [12]. Aerosols used in medicine produce particles that are usually less than 50 μm in size, which is also the case for PIPAC. This small size ensures that the dispersed droplets or particles will remain airborne for a prolonged period of time. A 1 second burst from a typical space spray will produce 120 million particles in which a substantial number will remain airborne for about an hour. Microdroplets produced during PIPAC measure around 11 μm in size and, as expected theoretically after a typical PIPAC application time (30 minutes), video endoscopy confirms that microdroplets are still in suspension in the gaseous environment at the end of the procedure.

Therapeutic aerosols have been best investigated in pulmonary medicine, and there is little knowledge about intraperitoneal aerosols. However, intra-abdominal or intrapleural administration appears much easier and more reproducible than pulmonary applications, for the following reasons [13]:

1. Physical laws governing aerosol deposition are concerned principally with inertial impaction and gravitational sedimentation. Inertial impaction occurs chiefly in pulmonary medicine with larger particles whenever the transporting airstream is fast, changing direction, or turbulent (for example, in the oropharynx or at bifurcation between successive airway). Inertial deposition is therefore influencing aerosol delivery by capturing a significant part of the therapeutic substance in the upper airways. This problem does not exist within the peritoneal cavity, where deposition mainly follows gravitational sedimentation.
2. One of the most critical maneuvers during pulmonary administration is to coordinate the actuation of the aerosol with the patient's inspiration. This problem does not exist during intraperitoneal administration.
3. Gas molecules travel in random paths and collide with one another and the organ walls. These collisions exert a pressure per unit area and also cause the gases to occupy a volume. Both the pressure and volume are affected by temperature. The interrelationships between these three variables were formulated by Boyle, Charles, and Gay-Lussac [14], and can be applied to pharmaceutical aerosols. PIPAC allows modification of the intra-abdominal or intrapleural temperature by applying cooled or heated CO_2, which is barely possible in pulmonary medicine.

Preclinical and clinical data support the superior distribution of a staining and/or therapeutic substance within the abdominal cavity after PIPAC. Results obtained in the large-animal model showed a more homogeneous and more intensive vital staining of the abdominal cavity after aerosolization than after lavage with methylene blue [10]. Ex vivo experiment on surgical specimen of human peritoneal carcinomatosis evidenced a homogeneous distribution of Dbait onto peritoneum, better than after conventional peritoneal lavage [15].

In the clinical setting, adhesions represent a significant limitation both for abdominal access and for intraperitoneal aerosol repartition. However, in our experience, this problem appears to be manageable. Since we are treating mostly patients with advanced, platin-resistant peritoneal carcinomatosis after exhaustion of guideline-recommended therapies, the vast majority of patients had previous surgery. As to date, it was not possible to create an adequate working space in 71 out of 658 procedures (11%), including primary and secondary nonaccess after at least 1 PIPAC procedure. In other words, PIPAC application was successful in 89% of patients. Systematic peritoneal biopsies in all four abdominal quadrants (upper and lower abdomen, left and right) showed homogeneous regressive changes after PIPAC therapy. However, in some patients in whom the lesser sac had not been opened during previous surgery, we observed isolated tumor progression in this closed anatomic space, as illustrated in Figure 35.3.

Limited direct penetration of drugs into tumor or normal tissue

Experimental and clinical data support the conclusion that the high concentrations of drugs observed after delivery directly into the peritoneal cavity will only be relevant for patients with microscopic disease or very small volume

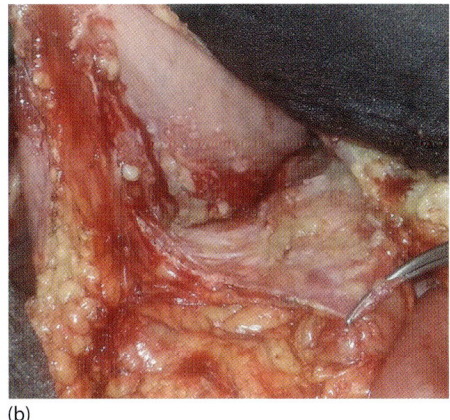

(a)   (b)

Figure 35.3 Repartition of the pressurized therapeutic aerosol under clinical conditions. Intraoperative finding during secondary cytoreductive surgery and HIPEC after repeated PIPAC. **(a)** Main abdominal cavity shows major regressive changes of the peritoneal surfaces and of the great omentum with complete regression of small bowel nodes and development of a fibrotic sheet around the omentum. **(b)** Same patient. Active tumor can still be observed in the lesser sac (bursa omentalis) that was obviously not reached effectively by the pressurized therapeutic aerosol.

macroscopic cancer (reviewed in [3]). This is in part explained by the high tumor interstitial fluid pressure. Interstitial fluid pressure is a barrier for efficient drug delivery (reviewed in [16]). It is well-established that the interstitial fluid pressure of most solid tumors is increased (reviewed in [17]). In the literature, values as high as 60 mmHg have been recorded, and our routine measurements of interstitial fluid pressure in diseased human peritoneal nodules showed interstitial fluid pressure up to 20 cm H_2O, depending on the size and degree of tumor regression (data on file).

Many drugs used for the systemic treatment of patients with cancer—high-molecular-weight compounds in particular—are transported from the circulatory system through the interstitial space by convection rather than by diffusion. Low-molecular-weight compounds, such as glucose or oxygen, are mainly transported by diffusion; that is, they move from an area of high concentration to an area of low concentration. Large molecules, such as soluble proteins, are mainly transported into the interstitium by convection; that is, they are carried by streaming of a flowing fluid [18]. Thus, increased interstitial fluid pressure leads to a decreased uptake of drugs or therapeutic antibodies into the tumor. Cancer cells are therefore exposed to a lower effective concentration of therapeutic agent than normal cells, lowering the therapeutic efficiency. Thus, elevated interstitial fluid pressure is an obstacle to cancer treatment [16]. Several studies indicate that high interstitial fluid pressure in the tumor is correlated with poor prognosis [19].

Measurement of local cisplatin (CDDP) concentrations using autogradiography in the kidney showed platinum penetration between 1 and 2 mm after intraperitoneal chemotherapy [20]. Experimental data support the potential benefit of increasing intraperitoneal hydrostatic pressure for increasing locoregional drug uptake. Esquis et al. demonstrated in a rat tumor model that increasing the intraperitoneal pressure resulted in a significantly higher cisplatin penetration in tumor tissue [4]. Similarly, Jacquet et al.

found a significant enhancement of doxorubicin uptake in the abdominal wall and diaphragm of rats when the intraperitoneal pressure was increased to 20–30 mmHg [21]. In a swine model, intra-abdominal high pressure enhanced diffusion of the drug in both the visceral and parietal peritoneum, using a liquid solution [22].

Increased intra-abdominal pressure is thought to generate a convective flux that forces the drug from the peritoneal cavity into the subperitoneal tissue. The clinical limit of usable intra-abdominal pressure enhancement is dictated by respiratory and hemodynamic tolerance. Clinical applications of hyperthermic intraperitoneal chemotherapy (HIPEC) with elevated intra-abdominal pressure had so far been limited to palliating debilitating malignant ascites with laparoscopic HIPEC at 10–15 mmHg [23].

Preclinical and clinical results obtained with PIPAC confirm the beneficial role of increasing intraperitoneal pressure for tissue drug uptake. Recently, oxaliplatin concentration, depth of penetration, and apoptosis induction after PIPAC were found to be superior to the effects obtained after HIPEC in a three-dimensional cell-line model in vitro (Marc Pocard, personal communication, August 2014). In the large animal model, direct penetration of stain into the peritoneum was enhanced by nebulization (with the application of a pressure of 12 mmHg) compared with the conventional lavage. Importantly, this difference was obtained despite the application of higher total methylene blue doses in the control animal. In the nebulization group, the stain reached the backside of the peritoneum, as demonstrated by the staining of isolated retroperitoneal capillary vessels [10]. Ex vivo with diseased human peritoneum, microscopic analysis revealed homogeneous peritoneal distribution of Dbait-Cy5 in the therapeutic capnoperitoneum sample, only minimal uptake in the lavage sample, and no staining in the control sample. Fluorescence was detected within the tumor up to 1 mm depth in the therapeutic capnoperitoneum sample but not in the lavage sample. Thus, aerosolization of the molecule allowed significantly better tumor access and better bioavailability of Dbait than conventional lavage. Biological results showed intranuclear phosphorylation of H2AX in the nebulized sample and almost no activity in the lavage sample. Detection of histone gamma-H2AX (phosphorylated H2AX) reveals the nuclear activation of DNA-dependent protein kinase (DNA-PK) by Dbait. Dbait was taken up by cancer cells, and a biological activity was detected up to 1 mm depth. Importantly, tumor nodules showed more activity at the tumor invasion front [15].

After the application of an artificial hydrostatic pressure of 10–12 mmHg in the human patient during PIPAC, doxorubicin was detected in significant concentrations in peritoneal carcinomatosis nodules, and nuclear staining was demonstrated throughout the peritoneum, up to deeply into the retroperitoneal fatty tissue. Although used in only 1/10 of the total dose, doxorubicin concentration in the aerosol (52 µM) is three times higher as in the intraperitoneal fluid usually used in HIPEC (18 µM)

without impairing tolerability, which was reported after applying higher concentrations of intraperitoneal chemotherapy [25].

In several patients, we have observed that PIPAC with low-dose cisplatin and doxorubicin is able to induce major or complete regression of tumor nodules with a diameter of several millimeters in the platin-resistant, salvage situation. This clinical observation might appear puzzling since the depth of doxorubicin penetration documented immediately after PIPAC is only less than 1 mm. A first possible explanation is that reported penetration of doxorubicin after HIPEC is only four to five cell layers [25], so that 0.5 mm appears to be a major progress. This hypothesis is confirmed by the high doxorubicin concentration measured in human peritoneal nodes after PIPAC application, up to 200× times the dose reported after HIPEC, with 10% of the dose applied [26].

A second possible explanation is that during PIPAC the drug penetrates deeply enough into the tumor node to induce cytostasis in the invasion front, which is located at the periphery of the nodule. Ex vivo experiments with Dbait in diseased human peritoneum showed a selective genotoxicity in the tumor invasion front (Figure 35.4 panel a).

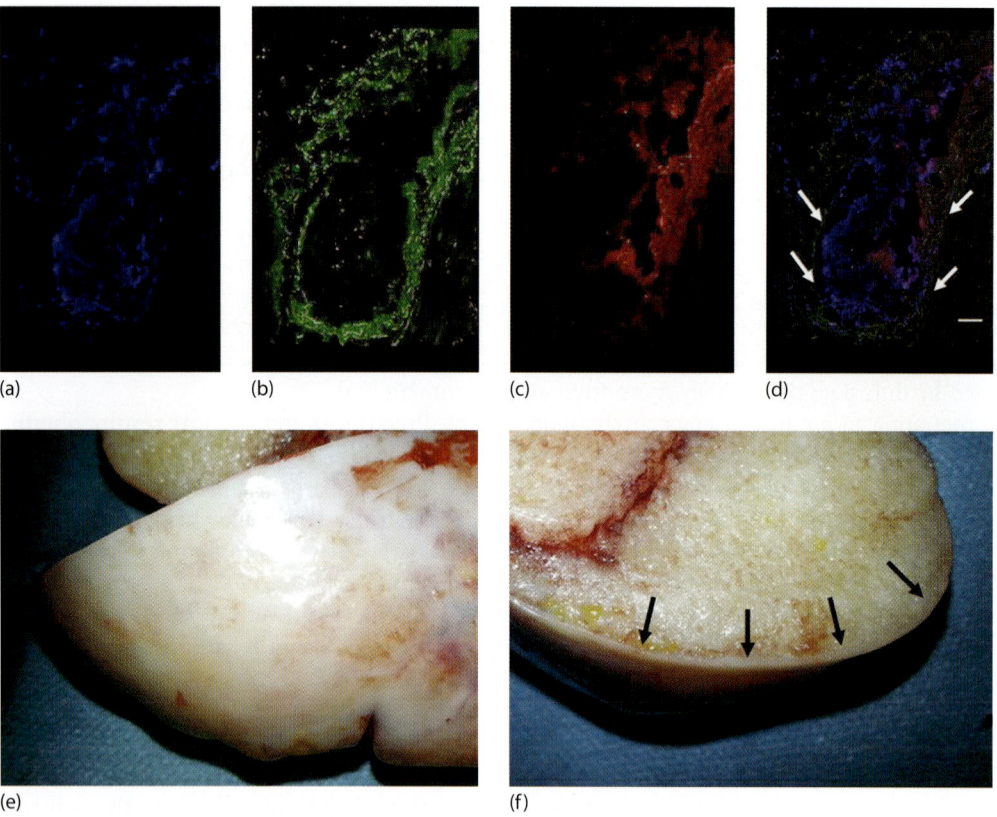

(a)   (b)   (c)   (d)

(e)   (f)

Figure 35.4 Influence of PIPAC on tumor invasion front. **(a–d)** Ex vivo experiment with diseased human peritoneum treated with PIPAC using small DNA fragments (Dbait). Detection of early Dbait activity marker: cryosection of human peritoneum; **(a)** blue: dapi staining (nucleus); **(b)** green: c-H2AX after nebulization of Dbait, **(c)** red: Dbait-Cy5 staining, **(d)** merged: genotoxicity (detected as H2AX activation) is maximal at the tumor invasion front (arrows). Scale bar: 100 µm. **(e and f)**: Macroscopy of the great omentum of a 64-year-old colorectal cancer patient after repeated PIPAC with oxaliplatin 92 mg/m² body surface. Complete secondary cytoreductive surgery (CC-0) and HIPEC was possible. A fibrotic capsule of 2–3 mm thickness (arrows) had developed in the periphery/at the outer invasion front of the tumor mass (8.4 × 7.4 × 4.6 cm). Patient is alive 11 months after salvage therapy with PIPAC with excellent quality of life.

In the clinical setting, pressurized aerosol chemotherapy induces a progressive nodular sclerosis, even in centimetric tumor nodes (Figure 35.4b). This can lead to the complete regression of tumor nodes of several mm diameters and might reduce the need for complete cytoreductive surgery, in particular, when these nodules are located on the serosal surface of the small intestine (Figure 35.5).

A further important feature is the repeated PIPAC application, in sharp contrast to HIPEC but analogous to systemic palliative chemotherapy, which is usually applied for several cycles. So far, we have only indicated PIPAC in advanced, therapy-resistant cases in palliative intent and we strongly believe that repeated application is needed to prolong time to progression. We are currently performing routinely three PIPAC cycles at 6-week intervals. In patients where complete or major tumor regression is documented in multiple biopsies and a piece of local peritonectomy, we then indicate PIPAC sessions in 3-month intervals.

Last but not least, peritoneal tumor nodes usually develop initially in the immediate vicinity of a mesenteric vessel, most commonly at the border between the mesenterium and the bowel itself. Although tumor cells can usually survive in an anaerobic environment, development of neovessels is necessary for the nodes to reach a significant volume. This neovascularization is fragile, is lying superficially, and might be sensitive to the high local chemotherapy concentrations induced by PIPAC application at the peritoneal surface.

Thus, PIPAC with low-dose cisplatin and doxorubicin (or oxaliplatin) can induce objective regression of peritoneal tumor nodes of several millimeters diameter.

Decrease in the delivery of drug to the tumor by capillary flow

Intra-abdominal pressure increases intratumoral drug concentration. At the same time, intra-abdominal pressure during PIPAC might counteract the hydraulic capillary pressure and slow the outflow of the drug to the body compartment, so that there is less or no decrease in the delivery of drug to the tumor by capillary flow. Such slow exit from the peritoneal cavity increases indeed the pharmacokinetic advantage associated with regional delivery.

Increasing the intra-abdominal pressure impairs not only the capillary flow, but also both portal and renal blood flow. As a consequence, renal function is decreased during capnoperitoneum, depending on the level of hydration, intra-abdominal pressure, patient positioning, and procedure duration [27].

Increased intra-abdominal pressure during laparoscopy also influences visceral flow [28]. An increase of the intra-abdominal pressure by 5 mmHg (from 10 to 15 mmHg)

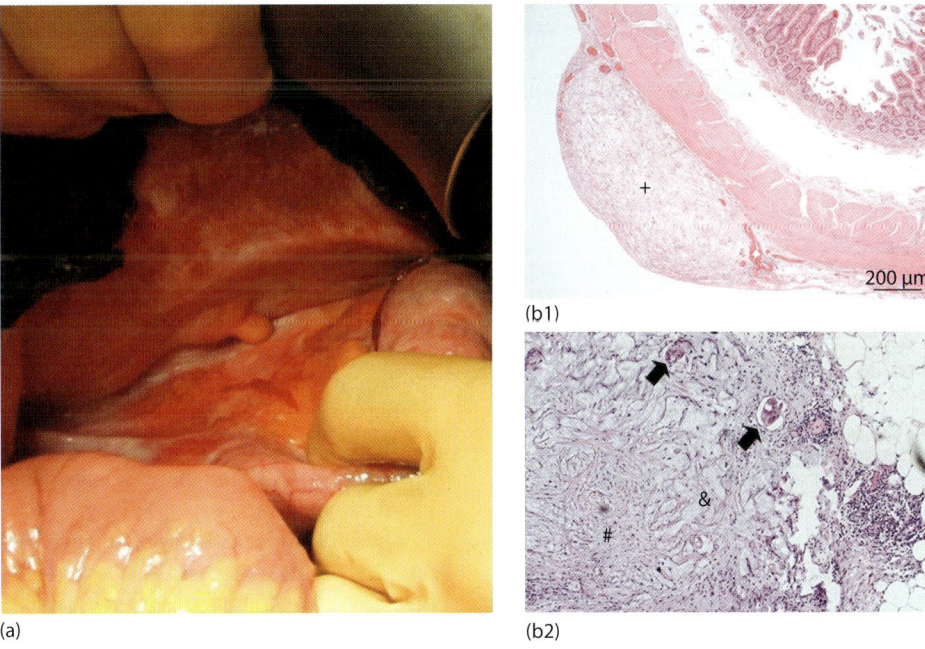

(a) (b1) (b2)

Figure 35.5 Fifty-eight-year-old patient with metachronous peritoneal carcinomatosis of colorectal cancer 27 months after diagnosis and after systemic chemotherapy (XELOX, then capecitabin alone due to side effects, and then FOLFIRI). The patient underwent secondary cytoreductive surgery (CC-0) and HIPEC with oxaliplatin 7 months after first PIPAC. **(a)** Macroscopy of the left upper abdomen showing limited peritoneal carcinomatosis (peritoneal carcinomatosis index = 3) with diffuse scarring. **(b1)** Four suspect millimetric nodes on the surface of the small bowel were resected, all of them were tumor-free (+). **(b2)** Vital tumor cells (arrows) were found in 3/9 peritoneal biopsies and in the omentum, together with extensive fibrosis (#) and large mucous areas (&) as a sign of tumor regression. Patient is alive 1 year after salvage therapy with PIPAC with excellent quality of life.

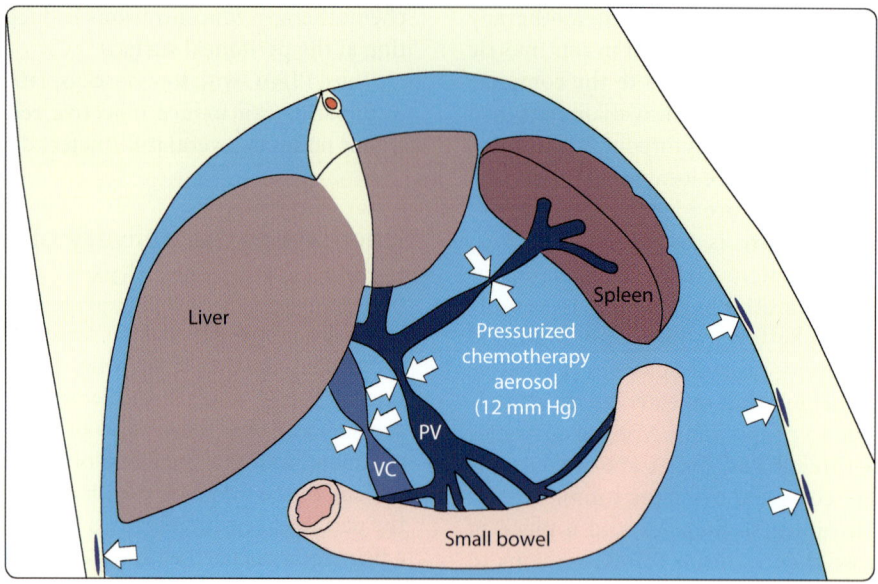

Figure 35.6 Artificial intra-abdominal hydrostatic pressure is impairing portal and cava venous flow and is slowing down the outflow of the drug from the abdominal cavity to other organs and body compartments. Moreover, it is assumed to counteract the hydraulic capillary pressure in the retroperitoneal tissue (arrows).

resulted in a blood flow decrease by 39% to the liver and by 60% to the peritoneum. In a pig model of living-donor nephrectomy, portal venous flow decreased almost by half during laparoscopy (974 vs. 547 mL/min; p = 0.001) [29]. Reduction of portal venous flow reduces the hepatic drug metabolism, which in turn reduces hepatic toxicity. This results in limited outflow from the splanchnic circulation to the systemic compartment, which leads to high tissue bioavailability and low systemic plasma concentration (Figure 35.6).

In the large animal model, direct penetration of the stain into the peritoneum was enhanced by PIPAC (with the application of a pressure of 12 mmHg) as compared to the conventional lavage. Importantly, the stain reached the backside of the peritoneum as demonstrated by the staining of isolated retroperitoneal capillary vessels [10]. The pharmacological data collected in our first patients confirm that the systemic AUC of doxorubicin after PIPAC is only about 1% of that of systemic administration and 5% of that of HIPEC administration [26]. This probably explains why we did not observe any significant renal toxicity and only minimal liver toxicity after PIPAC [30].

Specifically, only discrete signs of liver toxicity were observed after PIPAC with cisplatin 7.5 mg/m² body surface and doxorubicin 1.5 mg/m² body surface. First, we observed a doubling of serum gamma-GT levels with a peak on the fourth postoperative day (POD), followed by a decrease on POD 5 (one-way ANOVA, p = 0.22). Discrete liver cytolysis was detected, with maximal GPT (ALAT) serum level of 135 ± 177 U/L on POD 4 versus a preoperative value of 35 ± 31 U/L (p = 0.57). We also observed an increase of GOT (ASAT) serum levels, with a peak of 76 ± 33 U/L on POD 3 versus a preoperative value of 35 ± 8 U/L (p = 0.68). Liver synthesis was also discretely impaired after PIPAC application. Quick test dropped from 103% ± 8% (preoperatively) to 84% ± 2% on POD 4. However, the mean values remained within the normal range (70%–100%). Total bilirubin serum levels remained within the normal range, increasing slightly on POD 1 and then returning to the preoperative value within 4 days.

Renal function was not impaired: Serum creatinine levels remained within the normal range with a peak of 0.75 ± 0.19 mmol/L on POD 1 versus a preoperative mean value of 0.70 ± 0.17 mmol/L. No cumulative toxicity was observed after repeated PIPAC application at 4-week intervals. The preoperative mean serum creatinine level was not increased, as compared with the reference value before the first application, so that cumulative renal injury could be reasonably excluded. A similar pattern was observed for liver toxicity: serum GOT, GPT, and bilirubin as well as quick test did not increase significantly with repeated PIPAC application.

Thus, PIPAC can be applied several times without any relevant organ toxicities. This is indeed an important feature for developing effective locoregional chemotherapy regimen including several cycles and is a clear advantage over HIPEC, for which repeated application is exceptional. On the basis of data from the literature and our own observations, it appears reasonable to propose that PIPAC is advantageous over other delivery routes, because of limited blood inflow into the intra-abdominal organs during the uptake phase.

Unique toxic effects associated with local delivery

There has been concern that the added morbidity associated with regional drug delivery, e.g., abdominal pain, infection, and bowel obstruction cannot be justified [30]. There is some debate about the real incidence of such complications and a possible learning curve. Concern about the local toxic effects of regional delivery and the recognition that large tumor masses essentially never regressed, markedly reduced the enthusiasm for the management of peritoneal carcinomatosis with intraperitoneal chemotherapy, except to provide symptomatic relief in malignant ascites [31].

It remains uncertain whether the effect observed after intraperitoneal chemotherapy results from a direct cytotoxic effect, or might be due to an indirect effect caused by the sclerosing potential of cytotoxic drugs on the mesothelial cells lining the peritoneal cavity. Exposition of the peritoneal membrane to chemotherapeutic agents causes a chemical peritonitis. It is well known from peritoneal dialysis patients that repeated peritoneal exposition to bioincompatible solutions induces progressive fibrosis, angiogenesis, ultrafiltration failure, and, ultimately, peritoneal sclerosis. Peritoneal fibrosis (or sclerosis) is a term that comprises a wide spectrum of peritoneal structural alterations, ranging from mild inflammation to severe sclerosing peritonitis and its most complicated manifestation, encapsulating peritoneal sclerosis (reviewed in [32]). Simple sclerosis, an intermediate stage of peritoneal fibrosis, is the most common peritoneal lesion found in the patients after a few months on PD and could represent the initial phase of sclerosing peritonitis syndrome. The peritoneum has a normal thickness of 20 μm, but after a few months on peritoneal dialysis could reach up to 40 μm. The sclerosing peritonitis is a progressive sclerosis that is characterized by a dramatic thickening of the peritoneum (up to 4.000 μm) and is accompanied by inflammatory infiltrates, calcification, neovascularization, and dilatation of blood and lymphatic vessels, the thickening being the most commonly used pathological criterion for differential diagnosis.

Peritoneal sclerosis is a severe disease with no effective therapy that can lead to bowel obstruction [33,34] and, eventually, to death [35]. The development of peritoneal fibrosis is not recognized so far as a significant problem in peritoneal carcinomatosis patients, probably because this problem has a low relevance in patients with a short life expectation. Such an attitude might be acceptable in advanced, palliative situations but the problem will gain in importance when intraperitoneal chemotherapy might be applied earlier in the natural course of disease, for example, as a prophylaxis of peritoneal carcinomatosis in high-risk patients. By analogy, the intrapleural application of chemotherapy might induce a pleural fibrosis potentially inducing secondary restrictive lung disease. So far, there is a single report of interstitial pneumonia after hyperthermic intrathoracic chemotherapy (HITOC) [36].

Most patients referred to our tertiary center for PIPAC therapy had previous surgery. Adhesions are indeed a common problem after cancer surgery. However, access lesions during PIPAC were rare with 1.1%, a low figure considering the high incidence of previous surgical procedures. All but one access lesions were recognized intraoperatively and immediately repaired. The choice of blunt trocars for accessing the abdomen was certainly a decisive factor in keeping these iatrogenic injuries at a minimal level.

PIPAC with the drugs and the dose used was not responsible for any postoperative bowel perforation in our single-center cohort, so that procedure-related major local toxicity can be reasonably excluded.

In a handful of procedures, we observed a postoperative localized inflammation at a trocar insertion site. This complication developed after around 2 weeks and disappeared spontaneously or under symptomatic therapy about 1 week later. No patient required surgical intervention. This local problem is probably explained by undetected subcutaneous toxic emphysema during PIPAC procedure.

Patients with advanced peritoneal carcinomatosis usually report about gastrointestinal symptoms, including nausea, anorexia, and abdominal pain. As a rule, these symptoms are deteriorating until death. We performed a retrospective analysis of quality of life (QoL) data in 91 consecutive peritoneal carcinomatosis patients (M:F = 23:25, age 58 ± 10 years) with 158 PIPAC applications (at least 2 PIPAC q6w) in order to assess the effect of PIPAC. All patients had pretreated, platin-resistant, advanced peritoneal carcinomatosis (PCI = 15 ± 9). Quality of life was assessed with QLQ30 questionnaire of EORTC, filled out by the patient himself the day before PIPAC therapy. Global scores (QoL, physical, and health condition) were reduced at the beginning of treatment (65% ± 20%). After first PIPAC (during 6 weeks), the global scores further deteriorated slightly (63% ± 19%), but then improved after PIPAC # 2 (after 3 months, 70% ± 18%) and PIPAC # 3 (after 4.5 months, 70% ± 16%). Pain score deteriorated slightly after PIPAC # 1 (from 47% to 54%), but then improved again (48%). Gastrointestinal symptoms (nausea/vomiting, constipation, diarrhea, and anorexia) remained stable under PIPAC therapy. Thus, global quality of life improved slightly under PIPAC therapy in this group of patients with advanced, pretreated peritoneal carcinomatosis. Disease-related symptoms could be stabilized by means of PIPAC therapy during at least 4.5 months for the majority of patients. Except for a transient moderate increase in pain score, PIPAC hardly caused therapy-related symptoms, especially little gastrointestinal symptoms.

Added time, inconvenience, and cost associated with the specific requirements of regional delivery

Added time, inconvenience, and cost associated with the specific requirements of regional delivery are further practical and theoretical concerns about intraperitoneal chemotherapy. At the current early stage of development of PIPAC, it is too early to make any statements about the effectiveness of the procedure. In particular, it is not yet possible to balance the benefits of the procedure for the patient vs. the added costs for the healthcare system. However, PIPAC is a minimal-invasive procedure with short hospital stay and minimal general symptoms. Operating time is around 90 minutes, and no intensive care is necessary. The procedures were well tolerated and the surgical complication rate very low. Patient compliance for PIPAC was excellent. Of course, PIPAC cannot be directly compared to cytoreductive surgery and HIPEC, since the patients are not the same and the intention to treat is clearly different (palliative vs. curative). However, the impact of the procedure, the side effects, and the costs are clearly much higher after CRS and HIPEC than after PIPAC.

CLINICAL RESULTS

First in-human PIPAC application was performed on November 5, 2011, in three end-stage patients. In the meantime, we have performed 658 consecutive procedures in 286 patients. These procedures were first performed as compassionate use, then as off-label use, and, in the most common indications, within the framework of prospective clinical studies. For ethical reasons, we started treating patients with very limited life expectation. The current scientific evidence for PIPAC is summarized in Table 35.2. Of course, PIPAC is still in its infancy and it would be unfair to require prospective randomized trials at this stage of development. The best evidence has been collected in platin-resistant peritoneal carcinomatosis of ovarian cancer, since most patients (45%) treated with PIPAC in our institution are women diagnosed with this type of cancer. The results of the first regulatory Phase 2 study [37] have been presented in October 2014 at the Ninth International Congress on Peritoneal Surface Malignancies in Amsterdam. This study was completed within 1 year and results confirm superior efficacy of PIPAC with low-dose cisplatin and doxorubicin with a clinical benefit rate of 60% (per protocol, according to RECIST 1.1) in the third-line situation. Histological regression rate was 79% after 3 PIPAC. Safety data were excellent with favorable side effect profile: 12% adverse events CTCAE 3 (intention to treat) and no severe adverse events CTCAE 4 or death. A dose-escalation study has been started recently to optimize PIPAC dose in ovarian cancer [38]. Another Phase 2 trial is recruiting rapidly in patients with platin-resistant peritoneal carcinomatosis of gastric cancer in the second-line salvage situation [39].

CONCLUSION

Already at this early stage of development, it appears legitimate to claim that PIPAC has superior pharmacologic properties versus both intraperitoneal lavage and systemic chemotherapy for treating peritoneal carcinomatosis, since in vitro, animal model, ex vivo, and clinical data support this statement. In the meantime, these experimental and clinical results have been reproduced in part by other groups. It is legitimate to claim that PIPAC can induce regression of diffuse, platinum-resistant peritoneal carcinomatosis. Of course, it is much too early to claim PIPAC will allow a quantum leap in therapy of peritoneal or pleural surface malignances. However, carcinomatosis is indeed an unmet medical need and there is an urgent need for novel and better therapies—and PIPAC is a good candidate—in this fatal situation.

It is important to remember that PIPAC is a drug-delivering system taking advantages of physical laws to improve efficacy of locoregional drug delivery, and not a therapy by itself. Cytotoxic effect in the target organ is indeed determined by the drug applied, and not by the aerosol or by pressure itself. To start with this new therapeutic method, we applied approved drugs with proven efficacy in the cancer types concerned. However, PIPAC is a generic drug-delivery concept. The technology developed for generating pressurized therapeutic aerosols has potential applications in various pathologies, with various therapeutic principles, and in different anatomic locations (reviewed in [40]). Prevention and therapy of intraperitoneal cancer dissemination is certainly the most promising indication for PIPAC, followed by intrathoracic application (PITAC), which opens new research avenues in therapy of pleura mesothelioma. Since a therapeutic aerosol can also be distributed within organ cavities, potential applications such as Pressurized IntraVesical Aerosol Chemotherapy (PIVAC) in bladder cancer or intraluminal endoesophageal application in Barrett's dysplasia (PILAC) are under investigation in the animal model. Application of radiosensibilizers such as DT01 (Dbait) [41] might improve efficacy of radiochemotherapy [15], for example, for locally unresectable pancreatic cancer. Finally, administration of cytolytic viruses in the form of a pressurized aerosol might improve uptake into tumor tissues, a significant limitation in current protocols of intraperitoneal gene therapy [42].

It is realistic to expect that PIPAC and derived technologies will now be tested in numerous cancer types, in different anatomical locations, with many drugs and biologicals, in different indications, under various physicochemical conditions and in various combinations with other therapeutic modalities.

Table 35.2 Preclinical and clinical studies assessing the biological and clinical effects of PIPAC

	Author	Year	Oncological diagnosis	Study type	Number of patients	Drug	Adverse events	Outcome(s)
1	Solass et al.	2012	—	Experimental/ex vivo	—	DT01	—	Repartition; penetration; genotoxicity
2	Solass et al.	2012	—	Experimental/in vivo	Animal model (swine)	MB	—	Repartition; penetration
3	Solass et al.	2013	—	Observational	2	CIS	No toxicity	Occupational health safety (TRG402)
4	Oyais et al.	2014	—	Observational	1	CIS	No toxicity	Occupational health safety (TRG402)
5	Solass et al.	2014	GastricCa, appendicealCa, ovarianCa	Case series (first in human application)*	3	CIS+DOX	CTCAE grade < 3	Feasibility; pharmacology, penetration; histological regression; survival
6	Tempfer et al.	2014	OvarianCa	Retrospective*	18	CIS+DOX	CTCAE grade > 2: 28% Hospital mortality: n = 0	Radiological and histological regression; local and systemic toxicity, survival
7	Blanco et al.	2013	PC	Retrospective*	3	CIS+DOX	No measurable renal toxicity, low liver toxicity	Acute and cumulative renal and liver toxicity
8	Nadiradze et al.	2013 (abstract)	GastricCa	Retrospective*	24	CIS+DOX	CTCAE grade > 2: 37% Bowel perforation: n = 0 Hospital mortality: n = 2#	Radiological and histological regression; local and systemic toxicity, survival
9	Demtröder et al.	2014 (abstract)	ColonCa	Retrospective*	17	OX	CTCAE grade > 2: 23% Bowel perforation: n = 0 Hospital mortality: n = 0	Radiological and histological regression; local and systemic toxicity, survival
10	Solass et al.	2014 (abstract)	Peritoneal mesothelioma	Retrospective*	10	CIS+DOX	CTCAE grade > 2: 10% Bowel perforation: n = 0 Hospital mortality: n = 1#	Radiological and histological regression; local and systemic toxicity, survival
11	Giger–Pabst et al.	(submitted)	OvarianCa	Case report*	1	CIS+DOX	CTCAE grade 1–2	Radiological and histological regression; local and systemic toxicity, survival

(Continued)

Table 35.2 (Continued) Preclinical and clinical studies assessing the biological and clinical effects of PIPAC

	Author	Year	Oncological diagnosis	Study type	Number of patients	Drug	Adverse events	Outcome(s)
12	Tempfer et al.	(submitted)	PMP	Case report*	1	CIS+DOX	CTCAE grade 1–2	Radiological and histological regression; local and systemic toxicity, survival
13	EudraCT Nr. 2012-004397-26	2012	OvarianCa (third line situation)	AMG-study phase-II	45 (closed)	CIS+DOX	CTCAE grade 3: (12%, itt) No grade 4, no grade 5 toxicity	CBR pp: 60%, Histological regression 79% after 3 PIPAC
14	EudraCT Nr. 2013-002103-3	2013	GastricCa (second-line situation)	AMG-study phase-II	45 (open)	CIS+DOX	CTCAE	CBR according to RECIST 1.1
15	EudraCT Nr. 2014-001034-28	2014	OvarianCa	AMG-study phase-I	25 (open)	CIS+DOX	CTCAE	Dose-limiting toxicity
	Total	—	—	—	195	—	—	—

Note: CTCAE, common terminology criteria for adverse; PC, peritoneal carcinomatosis; PMP, pseudomyxoma peritonei; #, death due to disease progression; GastricCa, gastric cancer; OvarianCa, ovarian cancer; ColonCa, colorectal cancer. *, Off-label use application; AMG-study, regulatory study according to German Drug Act; pp, per protocol; itt, intention to treat. DT01, Dbait; MB, methylene blue; CIS + DOX, cisplatin 7.5 mg/m^2 and doxorubicin 1.5 mg/m^2 body surface; OX, oxaliplatin 92 mg/m^2 body surface.

REFERENCES

1. Minchinton AI, Tannock IF. Drug penetration in solid tumors. *Nature Reviews Cancer*. August 2006;6(8):583–592. Review.

2. Ceelen WP, Flessner MF. Intraperitoneal therapy for peritoneal tumors: Biophysics and clinical evidence. *Nature Reviews Clinical Oncology*. February 2010;7(2):108–115.

3. Markman M. Intraperitoneal antineoplastic drug delivery: Rationale and results. *Lancet Oncology*. May 2003;4(5):277–283. Review.

4. Esquis P, Consolo D, Magnin G, Pointaire P, Moretto P, Ynsa MD et al. High intra-abdominal pressure enhances the penetration and antitumor effect of intraperitoneal cisplatin on experimental peritoneal carcinomatosis. *Annals of Surgery*. July 2006;244(1):106–112.

5. Solass W, Giger-Pabst U, Zieren J, Reymond MA. Pressurized intraperitoneal aerosol chemotherapy (PIPAC): Occupational health and safety aspects. *Annals of Surgical Oncology*. October 2013;20(11):3504–3511.

6. Oyais A, Solass W, Zieren J, Reymond MA, Giger-Pabst U. Occupational health aspects of Pressurised Intraperitoneal Aerosol Chemotherapy (PIPAC): Confirmation of harmlessness. *Zentralblatt für Chirurgie*. February 4, 2014. [Epub ahead of print] German.

7. Jain RK. Barriers to drug delivery in solid tumors. *Scientific American*. 1994;271:59–65.

8. Dedrick RL, Flessner MF. Pharmacokinetic problems in peritoneal drug administration: Tissue penetration and surface exposure. *Journal of the National Cancer Institute*. 1997;89:480–487.

9. Flessner MF. Small-solute transport across specific peritoneal tissue surfaces in the rat. *Journal of the American Society of Nephrology*. 1996;7:225–233.

10. Solass W, Hetzel A, Nadiradze G, Sagynaliev E, Reymond MA. Description of a novel approach for intraperitoneal drug delivery and the related device. *Surgical Endoscopy*. July 2012;26(7):1849–1855.

11. Rubin BK, Williams RW. Emerging aerosol drug delivery strategies: from bench to clinic. *Advanced Drug Delivery Reviews*. August 2014;75:141–148.

12. Hinds WC (Ed.). *Aerosol Technology: Properties, Behavior, and Measurement of Airborne Particles*. 2nd edn., Hoboken, NJ: Wiley Interscience, 1999.

13. Labiris NR, Dolovich MB. Pulmonary drug delivery. Part I: Physiological factors affecting therapeutic effectiveness of aerosolized medications. *British Journal of Clinical Pharmacology*. December 2003;56(6):588–599. Review.

14. USC Eshelman School of Pharmacy, http://pharm-labs.unc.edu/labs/aerosols/physical_laws.htm, consulted on April 27, 2014.

15. Solass W, Herbette A, Schwarz T, Hetzel A, Sun JS, Dutreix M, Reymond MA. Therapeutic approach of human peritoneal carcinomatosis with Dbait in combination with capnoperitoneum: Proof of concept. *Surgical Endoscopy*. March 2012;26(3):847–852.

16. Heldin CH, Rubin K, Pietras K, Ostman A. High interstitial fluid pressure—An obstacle in cancer therapy. *Nature Reviews Cancer*. 2004;4(October (10)):806–813.

17. Jain RK. The next frontier of molecular medicine: Delivery of therapeutics. *Nature Medicine*. 1998;4:655–657.

18. Rippe B, Haraldsson B. Transport of macromolecules across microvascular walls: The two-pore theory. *Physiological Reviews*. 1994;74:163–219. Review.

19. Milosevic M, Fyles A, Hedley D, Pintilie M, Levin W, Manchul L, Hill R. Interstitial fluid pressure predicts survival in patients with cervix cancer independent of clinical prognostic factors and tumor oxygen measurements. *Cancer Research*. 2001;61:6400–6405.

20. Los G, Mutsaers PH, Lenglet WJ, Baldew GS, McVie JG. Platinum distribution in intraperitoneal tumors after intraperitoneal cisplatin treatment. *Cancer Chemotherapy and Pharmacology*. 1990;25:389–394.

21. Jacquet P, Stuart OA, Chang D, Sugarbaker PH. Effects of intra-abdominal pressure on pharmacokinetics and tissue distribution of doxorubicin after intraperitoneal administration. *Anticancer Drugs*. 1996;7:596–603.

22. Facy O, Al Samman S, Magnin G, Ghiringhelli F, Ladoire S, Chauffert B, Rat P, Ortega-Deballon P. High pressure enhances the effect of hyperthermia in intraperitoneal chemotherapy with oxaliplatin: An experimental study. *Annals of Surgery*. December 2012;256(6):1084–1088.

23. Garofalo A, Valle M, Garcia J, Sugarbaker PH. Laparoscopic hyperthermic chemotherapy for palliation of debilitating malignant ascites. *European Journal of Surgical Oncology*. 2006;32:682–685.

24. Ozols RF, Young RC, Speyer JL, Sugarbaker PH, Greene R, Jenkins J, Myers CE. Phase I and pharmacological studies of adriamycin administered intraperitoneally to patients with ovarian cancer. *Cancer Research*. 1982;42(10):4265–4269.

25. Ceelen WP, Påhlman L, Mahteme H. Pharmacodynamic aspects of intraperitoneal cytotoxic therapy. *Cancer Treatment and Research*. 2007;134:195–214. Review.

26. Solass W, Kerb R, Mürdter T, Giger-Pabst U, Strumberg D, Tempfer C, Zieren J, Schwab M, Reymond MA. Intraperitoneal chemotherapy of peritoneal carcinomatosis using pressurized aerosol as an alternative to liquid solution: First evidence for efficacy. *Annals of Surgical Oncology*. February 2014;21(2):553–559.

27. Demyttenaere S, Feldman LS, Fried GM. Effect of pneumoperitoneum on renal perfusion and function: A systematic review. *Surgical Endoscopy.* February 2007;21(2):152–160.

28. Schilling MK, Redaelli C, Krähenbühl L, Signer C, Büchler MW. Splanchnic microcirculatory changes during CO_2 laparoscopy. *Journal of the American College of Surgeons.* 1997;184:378–382.

29. Burgos FJ, Saenz J, Correa C, Linares A, Cuevas B, Pascual J, Villafruela J, Marcén R, Fernandez A, Galindo J, Asuero MS. Changes in visceral flow induced by aparoscopic and open living-donor nephrectomy: Experimental model. *Transplantation Proceedings.* July to August, 2009;41(6):2491–2492.

30. Blanco A, Giger-Pabst U, Solass W, Zieren J, Reymond MA. Renal and hepatic toxicities after pressurized intraperitoneal aerosol chemotherapy (PIPAC). *Annals of Surgical Oncology.* July 2013;20(7):2311–2316.

31. Ostrowski MJ. An assessment of the long-term results of controlling the reaccumulation of malignant effusions using intracavity bleomycin. *Cancer.* 1986;57:721–727.

32. Aguilera A, Loureiro J, Gónzalez-Mateo G, Selgas R, López-Cabrera M. The mesothelial to mesenchymal transition a pathogenic and therapeutic key for peritoneal membrane failure. In: Aguilera Peralta A, ed.,*The Latest in Peritoneal Dialysis*, InTech, 2013.

33. Chan WS, Bohmer R, McIntosh R, Blomfield P. Peritoneal fibrosis leading to small bowel obstruction two years after first-line intraperitoneal chemotherapy for optimally debulked ovarian cancer. *Australian and New Zealand Journal of Obstetrics and Gynaecology.* February 2011;51(1):91–92.

34. Vlasveld LT, Taal BG, Kroon BB, Gallee MP, Rodenhuis S. Intestinal obstruction due to diffuse peritoneal fibrosis at 2 years after the successful treatment malignant peritoneal mesothelioma with intraperitoneal mitoxantrone. *Cancer Chemotherapy and Pharmacology.* 1992;29(5):405–408. Erratum in: *Cancer Chemotherapy and Pharmacology.* 1992;30(3):249.

35. Minutolo V, Gagliano G, Angirillo G, Minutolo O, Morello A, Rinzivillo C. Intestinal obstruction due to idiopathic sclerosing encapsulating peritonitis. Clinical report and review of literature. *Giornale di Chirurgia* Apr 2008;29(4):173–176.

36. Zappa L, Savady R, Humphries GN, Sugarbaker PH. Interstitial pneumonitis following intrapleural chemotherapy. *World Journal of Surgical Oncology.* February 12, 2009;7:17.

37. Tempfer CB, Winnekendonk G, Solass W, Horvat R, Giger-Pabst U, Zieren J, Reznicek GA, Reymond MA. Pressurized intraperitoneal aerosol chemotherapy in women with recurrent ovarian cancer: A phase 2 study. *Gynecologic Oncology.* May 2015;137(2):223–228.

38. A phase I, single-arm (nonrandomized), open-label, three step dose escalation study with cisplatin and doxorubicin applied as pressurized intraperitoneal aerosol chemotherapy (PIPAC) in patients with recurrent ovarian cancer and peritoneal carcinomatosis. *EudraCT:* 2014-001034-28. https://eudract.ema.europa.eu/

39. Intraperitoneal Aerosol Chemotherapy in Gastric Cancer (PIPAC-GA01). NCT01854255. http://www.clinicaltrials.gov.

40. Khalili-Harbi N, Herath N, Solass W, Giger-Pabst U, Dutreix M, Reymond MA. Feasibility of Pressurized IntraLuminal Aerosol Chemotherapy (PILAC) in distal experiment. *Endoscopy,* in press.

41. Croset A, Cordelières FP, Berthault N, Buhler C, Sun JS, Quanz M, Dutreix M. Inhibition of DNA damage repair by artificial activation of PARP with siDNA. *Nucleic Acids Research.* August 2013;41(15):7344–7355.

42. Hartkopf AD, Bossow S, Lampe J, Zimmermann M, Taran FA, Wallwiener D, Fehm T, Bitzer M, Lauer UM. Enhanced killing of ovarian carcinoma using oncolytic measles vaccine virus armed with a yeast cytosine deaminase and uracil phosphoribosyltransferase. *Gynecologic Oncology.* August 2013;130(2):362–368.

Index